VOLUME ONE HUNDRED AND TWENTY EIGHT

ADVANCES IN CANCER RESEARCH

Immunotherapy of Cancer

VOLUME ONE HUNDRED AND TWENTY EIGHT

ADVANCES IN CANCER RESEARCH

Immunotherapy of Cancer

Edited by

XIANG-YANG WANG
Department of Human and Molecular Genetics, VCU Institute of Molecular Medicine, and VCU Massey Cancer Center, Virginia Commonwealth University School of Medicine, Richmond, Virginia, USA

PAUL B. FISHER
Department of Human and Molecular Genetics, VCU Institute of Molecular Medicine, and VCU Massey Cancer Center, Virginia Commonwealth University School of Medicine, Richmond, Virginia, USA

ELSEVIER

AMSTERDAM • BOSTON • HEIDELBERG • LONDON
NEW YORK • OXFORD • PARIS • SAN DIEGO
SAN FRANCISCO • SINGAPORE • SYDNEY • TOKYO
Academic Press is an imprint of Elsevier

Academic Press is an imprint of Elsevier
225 Wyman Street, Waltham, MA 02451, USA
525 B Street, Suite 1800, San Diego, CA 92101-4495, USA
125 London Wall, London, EC2Y 5AS, UK
The Boulevard, Langford Lane, Kidlington, Oxford OX5 1GB, UK

First edition 2015

ISBN: 978-0-12-802316-7
ISSN: 0065-230X

For information on all Academic Press publications
visit our website at store.elsevier.com

CONTENTS

CONTRIBUTORS

Daniel W. Beury
Department of Biological Sciences, University of Maryland Baltimore County, Baltimore, Maryland, USA

Eduardo Bonavita
IRCCS Istituto Clinico Humanitas, Rozzano, Italy

Sadna Budhu
Ludwig Collaborative and Swim Across America Laboratory, Memorial Sloan Kettering Cancer Center, New York, USA

Jose R. Conejo-Garcia
Tumor Microenvironment and Metastasis Program, The Wistar Institute, Philadelphia, Pennsylvania, USA

Olivier De Henau
Ludwig Collaborative and Swim Across America Laboratory, Memorial Sloan Kettering Cancer Center, New York, USA, and Department of Medical Oncology, Jules Bordet Institute, Universite Libre De Bruxelles, Brussels, Belgium

Victor H. Engelhard
Department of Microbiology, Immunology, and Cancer Biology, Carter Immunology Center, University of Virginia School of Medicine, Charlottesville, Virginia, USA

Paul B. Fisher
Department of Human and Molecular Genetics; VCU Institute of Molecular Medicine, and VCU Massey Cancer Center, Virginia Commonwealth University School of Medicine, Richmond, Virginia, USA

Maria Rosaria Galdiero
IRCCS Istituto Clinico Humanitas, Rozzano, and Division of Clinical Immunology and Allergy, University of Naples Federico II, Naples, Italy

Billel Gasmi
Ludwig Collaborative and Swim Across America Laboratory, Memorial Sloan Kettering Cancer Center, New York, USA

Chunqing Guo
Department of Human and Molecular Genetics; VCU Institute of Molecular Medicine, and VCU Massey Cancer Center, Virginia Commonwealth University School of Medicine, Richmond, Virginia, USA

Duane H. Hamilton
Laboratory of Tumor Immunology and Biology, Center for Cancer Research, National Cancer Institute, National Institutes of Health, Bethesda, Maryland, USA

Daniel Hirschhorn-Cymerman
Ludwig Collaborative and Swim Across America Laboratory, Memorial Sloan Kettering Cancer Center, New York, USA

Rikke B. Holmgaard
Ludwig Collaborative and Swim Across America Laboratory, Memorial Sloan Kettering Cancer Center, New York, USA

Sebastien Jaillon
IRCCS Istituto Clinico Humanitas, Rozzano, Italy

Michael Karin
Departments of Pharmacology and Pathology, Laboratory of Gene Regulation and Signal Transduction, School of Medicine, University of California, San Diego, California, USA

Danny N. Khalil
Ludwig Collaborative and Swim Across America Laboratory, and Department of Medicine, Memorial Sloan Kettering Cancer Center, New York, USA

Alberto Mantovani
IRCCS Istituto Clinico Humanitas, and Humanits University, Rozzano, Italy

Taha Merghoub
Ludwig Collaborative and Swim Across America Laboratory, and Department of Medicine, Memorial Sloan Kettering Cancer Center, New York, USA

Judith T. Murphy
Ludwig Collaborative and Swim Across America Laboratory, Memorial Sloan Kettering Cancer Center, New York, USA

Suzanne Ostrand-Rosenberg
Department of Biological Sciences, University of Maryland Baltimore County, Baltimore, Maryland, USA

Claudia Palena
Laboratory of Tumor Immunology and Biology, Center for Cancer Research, National Cancer Institute, National Institutes of Health, Bethesda, Maryland, USA

Katherine H. Parker
Department of Biological Sciences, University of Maryland Baltimore County, Baltimore, Maryland, USA

Alfredo Perales-Puchalt
Tumor Microenvironment and Metastasis Program, The Wistar Institute, Philadelphia, Pennsylvania, USA

J. David Peske
Department of Microbiology, Immunology, and Cancer Biology, Carter Immunology Center, University of Virginia School of Medicine, Charlottesville, Virginia, USA

Tamar Plitt
Ludwig Collaborative and Swim Across America Laboratory, Memorial Sloan Kettering Cancer Center, New York, USA

Melanie R. Rutkowski
Tumor Microenvironment and Metastasis Program, The Wistar Institute, Philadelphia, Pennsylvania, USA

Walter J. Storkus
Department of Immunology; Department of Dermatology, University of Pittsburgh School of Medicine, and University of Pittsburgh Cancer Institute, Pittsburgh, Pennsylvania, USA

John R. Subjeck
Department of Cellular Stress Biology, Roswell Park Cancer Institute, Buffalo, New York, USA

Nikolaos Svoronos
Tumor Microenvironment and Metastasis Program, The Wistar Institute, Philadelphia, Pennsylvania, USA

Kepeng Wang
Departments of Pharmacology and Pathology, Laboratory of Gene Regulation and Signal Transduction, School of Medicine, University of California, San Diego, California, USA

Xiang-Yang Wang
Department of Human and Molecular Genetics; VCU Institute of Molecular Medicine, and VCU Massey Cancer Center, Virginia Commonwealth University School of Medicine, Richmond, Virginia, USA

Aliyah M. Weinstein
Department of Immunology, University of Pittsburgh School of Medicine, Pittsburgh, Pennsylvania, USA

Jedd D. Wolchok
Ludwig Collaborative and Swim Across America Laboratory; Department of Medicine, Memorial Sloan Kettering Cancer Center, and Weill Cornell Medical College, New York, USA

Amber B. Woods
Department of Microbiology, Immunology, and Cancer Biology, Carter Immunology Center, University of Virginia School of Medicine, Charlottesville, Virginia, USA

Xiaofei Yu
Department of Human and Molecular Genetics; VCU Institute of Molecular Medicine, and VCU Massey Cancer Center, Virginia Commonwealth University School of Medicine, Richmond, Virginia, USA

Dmitriy Zamarin
Ludwig Collaborative and Swim Across America Laboratory; Department of Medicine, Memorial Sloan Kettering Cancer Center, and Weill Cornell Medical College, New York, USA

Roberta Zappasodi
Ludwig Collaborative and Swim Across America Laboratory, Memorial Sloan Kettering Cancer Center, New York, USA

PREFACE

The past two decades have witnessed a virtual explosion in our comprehension and practical applications of cancer immunotherapy. Recent clinical successes provide compelling evidence supporting the concept that therapeutic manipulation of the immune system can actually achieve meaningful antitumor effects in cancer patients. These accomplishments have stemmed from major advancements of basic and translational research expanding our understanding of the mechanism(s) underlying protective antitumor immunity. This thematic volume of ACR includes the contributions from internationally recognized experts in this evolving field of immunology and provides up-to-date reviews of the advances providing insights into the complexity of the immune system in cancer biology and the promise as well as successes/challenges of cancer immunotherapy.

The first three chapters describe current immunotherapeutic successes in clinical treatment of cancer, highlight novel vaccine strategies targeting adaptable cancer cells, and discuss the putative roles of tumor-mediated immunosuppressive mechanisms that impair or disable antitumor functions of immune effector cells. The authors review several promising immunotherapeutic approaches, including blockade of inhibitory signaling pathways to overcome immune checkpoints (CTLA-4 and PD-1/PD-L1), adoptive T cell therapy, as well as combination regimens that incorporate targeted therapies or standard chemotherapy and radiation therapy to provide a more efficacious and durable response. Considering a critical role of the epithelial–mesenchymal transition (EMT) in tumor progression, potential mechanisms of resistance to immune-mediated attack driven by EMT of cancer cells are summarized and creation of novel vaccines that target the process of tumor EMT to overcome cancer stemness and resistance to therapies is emphasized. Due to the potential role of myeloid-derived suppressor cells (MDSCs) in counteracting naturally and therapeutically induced antitumor immune response in cancer patients, the authors also provide insights into the immune suppressive mechanisms utilized by MDSCs, inflammation signaling that govern accumulation and suppressive activity of MDSCs, and recent therapeutics that target MDSCs to enhance antitumor immunity.

An intriguing and paradoxical role of immune or inflammatory components as well as inflammation in promoting neoplastic transformation or progression and limiting tumor responses to therapy is well recognized. Two chapters discuss the important role of cancer-related inflammation and tumor-elicited inflammation in promoting tumor growth and metastasis. The authors provide current views on tumor-associated macrophages and tumor-associated neutrophils that have long been overlooked and considered as a minor proinflammatory component, as well as their involvement in protecting cancer cells from cytotoxic therapies. Additionally, the functions and the mechanisms of induction of inflammatory cytokines during colorectal cancer development and novel anticancer therapies by modulating tumor-elicited inflammation are discussed in depth.

The tumor microenvironment (TME), which includes cellular and molecular components of the immune system, is critical in modulating tumor progression and responses to cancer treatment, including immunotherapies. Three chapters in this thematic volume provide new insights into how immune composition and characteristics of the TME regulate tumor invasion and antitumor immune responses. Inflammatory signaling pathways and formation of secondary lymphoid organs or "tertiary" lymphoid structures in the TME are discussed relative to their prognostic value in cancer patients as well as their therapeutic potential in the rational design of immunotherapies for improved clinical outcomes. Recent findings on the TME and systemic tumor macroenvironment, such as hormones, mucosal commensal microbiota, and myeloid cells, in coordinating malignant progression, invasion, and metastasis are also highlighted. Since the presence and frequency of cytotoxic $CD8^+$ T lymphocytes (CTLs) in tumors correlates with a positive prognosis in cancer patients, the authors also describe the factors as well as the tumor-associated vasculature as a gateway that determines tumor infiltration by CTLs, and discuss strategies to enhance infiltration of CTLs to overcome the established barrier of immunosuppression in the TME.

The final review in the thematic issue focuses on scavenger receptors, a major subset of innate pattern recognition receptors, which are emerging as important regulators of tumor behavior and host immune responses to cancer. The authors summarize recent investigations into diverse functions of scavenger receptors in cancer immunobiology and emphasize their potential use as diagnostic biomarkers and novel immune targets that can be exploited for enhanced therapeutic treatment of cancer.

The decades of research in tumor immunology is now providing tangible benefits and is culminating in the adoption of immunotherapies as standards of care in oncology. We believe that the reviews in this collective volume provide a comprehensive and timely summary of the advances in major areas of cancer immunology and immunotherapy, and offer new insights into future directions that will lead to the development of novel cancer immunotherapies for successful clinical translation.

Xiang-Yang Wang
Paul B. Fisher

CHAPTER ONE

The New Era of Cancer Immunotherapy: Manipulating T-Cell Activity to Overcome Malignancy

Danny N. Khalil*,†, Sadna Budhu*, Billel Gasmi*, Roberta Zappasodi*, Daniel Hirschhorn-Cymerman*, Tamar Plitt*, Olivier De Henau*,‡, Dmitriy Zamarin*,†,§, Rikke B. Holmgaard*, Judith T. Murphy*, Jedd D. Wolchok*,†,§, Taha Merghoub*,†,1

*Ludwig Collaborative and Swim Across America Laboratory, Memorial Sloan Kettering Cancer Center, New York, USA
†Department of Medicine, Memorial Sloan Kettering Cancer Center, New York, USA
‡Department of Medical Oncology, Jules Bordet Institute, Universite Libre De Bruxelles, Brussels, Belgium
§Weill Cornell Medical College, New York, USA
[1]Corresponding author: e-mail address: Merghout@mskcc.org

Contents

Advances in Cancer Research, Volume 128
ISSN 0065-230X
http://dx.doi.org/10.1016/bs.acr.2015.04.010

Abstract

Using the immune system to control cancer has been investigated for over a century. Yet it is only over the last several years that therapeutic agents acting directly on the immune system have demonstrated improved overall survival for cancer patients in phase III clinical trials. Furthermore, it appears that some patients treated with such agents have been cured of metastatic cancer. This has led to increased interest and acceleration in the rate of progress in cancer immunotherapy. Most of the current immunotherapeutic success in cancer treatment is based on the use of immune-modulating antibodies targeting critical checkpoints (CTLA-4 and PD-1/PD-L1). Several other immune-modulating molecules targeting inhibitory or stimulatory pathways are being developed. The combined use of these medicines is the subject of intense investigation and holds important promise. Combination regimens include those that incorporate targeted therapies that act on growth signaling pathways, as well as standard chemotherapy and radiation therapy. In fact, these standard therapies have intrinsic immune-modulating properties that can support antitumor immunity. In the years ahead, adoptive T-cell therapy will also be an important part of treatment for some cancer patients. Other areas which are regaining interest are the use of oncolytic viruses that immunize patients against their own tumors and the use of vaccines against tumor antigens. Immunotherapy has demonstrated unprecedented durability in controlling multiple types of cancer and we expect its use to continue expanding rapidly.

1. INTRODUCTION

Despite much recent attention to the field of cancer immunotherapy (Couzin-Frankel, 2013), the idea of recruiting the immune system against cancer predates our knowledge of the genetic basis of cancer and even modern genetics. The reason for the relative lack of attention to the field is debatable, but likely is in part due to important developments in other modes of cancer therapy such as surgery, radiation, cytotoxic chemotherapy, and most recently targeted therapy. While there are indications that ancient civilizations intentionally transferred microbes into tumors to control their growth, thereby unknowingly harnessing the immune system, modern cancer immunotherapy can be traced back to Dr. William Coley, a surgeon working in New York City who began treating cancer patients by injecting live *Streptococcus pyogenes* intratumorally after learning of a patient with prolonged remission of recurrent sarcoma after severe erysipelas (Coley, 1991).

In the century since the work of Coley, research in the field of cancer immunotherapy has continued mostly outside the spotlight of mainstream cancer research. While the first data from a phase III clinical trial demonstrating improved overall survival among patients with advanced cancer attributable to immunotherapy would not come until 2010 (Hodi et al., 2010), there were several instructive successes in the interim that have impacted standard of care. Cytokine therapy has been the most important such therapy for systemic disease. Interleukin-2 treatment has resulted in durable responses for patients with metastatic renal cell carcinoma and melanoma (Rosenberg, 2014; Rosenberg et al., 1994). Interferon-α has been developed for the treatment of melanoma, renal cell carcinoma, AIDS-related Kaposi sarcoma, follicular lymphoma, and hairy cell leukemia (Gajewski & Corrales, 2015; Jonasch & Haluska, 2001). The knowledge gained from the experience with these agents has been invaluable, and their role in controlling cancer remains an area of active research. They have demonstrated the extreme manifestations of attempting to engage the immune system in treating cancer, as patients have developed both severe toxicity as well as deep, durable disease control. In many ways, it was these results that motivated the strong interest in engaging the immune system with greater specificity. This resulted in a concerted effort to develop therapeutic cancer vaccines that dominated the field for more than a decade. The fact that this has yet to result in the approval of vaccination for the treatment of human cancer is instructive in itself, and while this remains an exciting field of translational cancer research, it suggests that educating the immune system to recognize disease-specific antigens, a highly effective method in preventing infectious disease, may not address the crucial barriers preventing a healthy immune system from eradicating tumors.

Although cancer immunotherapy has largely focused on the systemic control of cancer, it is important to recognize its historic contribution in the treatment of localized disease. Topical imiquimod, a TLR7 agonist, is indicated for the treatment of superficial basal cell carcinoma (Beutner et al., 1999); and the tuberculosis vaccine Bacillus Calmette-Guérin is used intravesically in the treatment of nonmuscle-invasive bladder cancer (Brandau & Suttmann, 2007).

Other standard treatments for cancer that are not always categorized as "immunotherapy" also rely, to a greater or lesser extent, on the immune system. The graft-versus-leukemia effect of allogeneic bone-marrow transplant is well known (Horowitz et al., 1990). Antigen presentation by dendritic cells (DCs) seems to be necessary for the potentially curative effect of extracorporeal photopheresis in cutaneous T-cell lymphoma (Edelson, 1999). The efficacy of antitumor monoclonal antibodies (mAbs) such as rituximab, trastuzumab) partially depends on immune-mediated destruction of targeted malignant cells even when the target is a growth factor receptor (Horlock et al., 2009; Tokuyama et al., 2008). Similarly, small molecules, including those developed to block cancer-cell signaling pathways (e.g., vemurafenib), also have profound effects on the antitumor immune response (Su et al., 2012). Along these lines, it is important to recognize that the immunologic impact of surgery, radiation therapy, and cytotoxic chemotherapy is also significant in some cases (Apetoh et al., 2007; Vittimberga, Foley, Meyers, & Callery, 1998).

The clinical success of immune checkpoint blockade and genetically engineered T cells has drawn tremendous interest. This has served not only to accelerate studies of how these tools can be implemented and improved, but it has also opened the door to investigation of new classes of immunotherapies, many of which are already in active clinical development. In this piece we provide an overview of the current state of therapeutic immune modulation in cancer, highlighting areas that we feel hold particular promise. We lay out the role of mAbs in blocking immune checkpoints and activating costimulatory molecules. This is followed by a description of adoptive T-cell therapy. We then describe a set of small-molecule inhibitors that are potentially potent immunomodulators. Finally, we review the place of radiotherapy and oncolytic virus therapy in mediating anticancer immune activity.

2. MODULATION OF T-CELL ACTIVITY WITH mAbs

After decades of research on educating the immune system to recognize specific antigens associated with cancers, primarily in the form of therapeutic anticancer vaccines, a very different approach in which inhibitory or activating immune cell receptors are targeted has recently gained interest

(Fig. 1). This method uses mAbs to block inhibitory receptors or to activate stimulatory receptors on T cells and other immune cells (Table 1). This approach has proved sufficient to mediate robust antitumor activity in the absence of an agent to direct the immune response to specific antigens.

2.1 CTLA-4

The finding that a mAb against the T-cell coinhibitory receptor CTLA-4 is sufficient to improve overall survival in patients with melanoma (Hodi et al., 2010) is considered one of the watershed moments in the history of cancer immunotherapy. After being used early in its development with anticancer vaccines (Phan et al., 2003), the anti-CTLA-4 mAb ipilimumab has subsequently been established as the first immune checkpoint inhibitor to demonstrate improved overall survival for any malignancy, and the first therapy to extend overall survival for patients with advanced melanoma in a phase III clinical trial. These dramatic results led to FDA approval of ipilimumab for advanced melanoma in 2011.

CTLA-4 (CD152) is important in modulating T-cell priming at the immunological synapse with antigen-presenting cells (APCs). T cells are classically primed to recognize novel or foreign antigens within secondary lymphoid organs such as lymph nodes. This is mediated by APCs, the most potent of which are the DCs (Steinman, Hawiger, & Nussenzweig, 2003). So-called signal one in T-cell priming occurs upon TCR engagement with its cognate peptide presented by the APC in the binding cleft of an MHC molecule. Importantly, signal one alone is insufficient to activate T cells. In fact, in the absence of a second signal, such an interaction will induce T-cell apoptosis or anergy in a process that is central to physiologic peripheral tolerance (Schwartz, 1990; Webb, Morris, & Sprent, 1990). One of the most established triggers for signal two is the stimulation of CD28 on T cells by CD80 or CD86 on APCs. As clinical studies with a CD28 agonist antibody suggest (Suntharalingam et al., 2006), this is an extremely potent means of T-cell stimulation and clonal expansion (Viola & Lanzavecchia, 1996). As such, an accessory mechanism for attenuation of this signal has evolved in the form of CTLA-4, the surface expression of which is induced upon CD28/TCR coligation. With peak expression at 24–48 h following TCR engagement (Perkins et al., 1996), CTLA-4 has a higher affinity for CD80/CD86 than CD28 and is able to outcompete CD28 for ligand (Krummel & Allison, 1995; Walunas

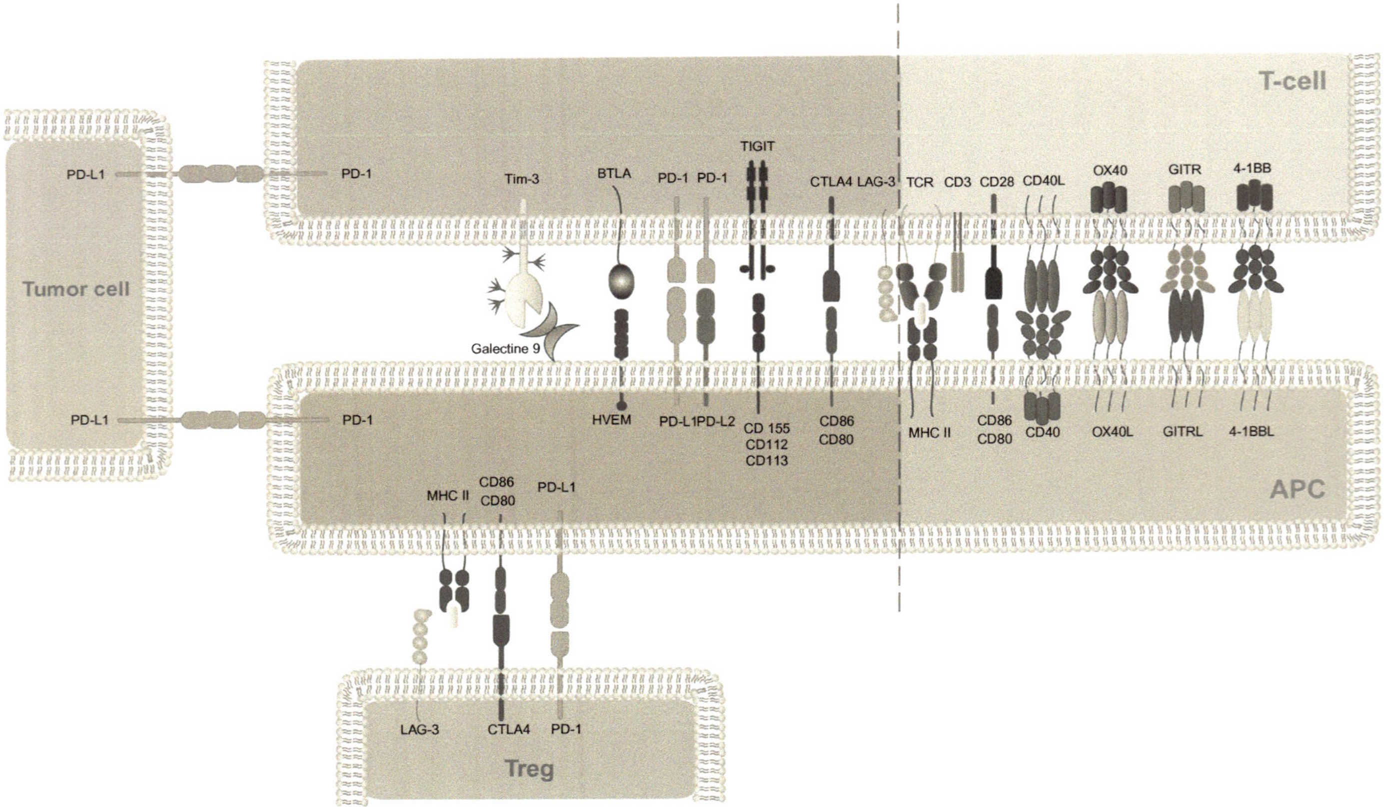

Figure 1 Overview of immunomodulatory cell-surface molecules on tumor cells, conventional T cells, regulatory T cells, and antigen-presenting cells: T-cell receptors to the left of the dashed line are inhibitory and those to the right are stimulatory. Agonist mAbs against stimulatory receptors and blocking mAbs against inhibitory receptors have demonstrated robust antitumor activity in clinical and preclinical studies. From PMID: 20307208, 22961161, 22261959, 25743219, 23334208, 16932752. (See the color plate.)

Table 1 Selection of Immunomodulatory Agents in Active Clinical Development

Target	Agent	Class	Current Clinical Status
Agonist mAbs			
OX40	MEDI6469 (9B12, Medimmune/AZ/AgonOX)	IgG1k mouse antihuman antibody	Multiple cancers (phase I, II)
OX40	Hu106–222 and Hu119–122 (UTMDACC)	IgG humanized monoclonal antibody	
GITR	TRX518 (GITR Inc.)	IgG1 fully humanized monoclonal antibody	Multiple solid cancers (phase I)
4-1BB	PF-05082566 (Pfizer)	IgG2 fully humanized monoclonal antibody	Multiple cancers (phase I)
4-1BB	Urelumab (BMS)		
CD40	CP-870,893 (Pfizer, VLST)	IgG2 fully human monoclonal antibody	Multiple solid cancers (phase I)
CD40	Dacetuzumab (Seattle Genetics)	IgG1 humanized monoclonal antibody	Multiple cancers (phase I, II)
CD40	Chi Lob 7/4 (University of Southampton)	IgG1 chimeric monoclonal antibody	Multiple cancers (phase I)
Antagonist mAbs			
CTLA-4	Tremelimumab (ticilimumab, CP-675,206, AZ)	IgG2 fully human monoclonal antibody	Multiple cancers (phase I, II)
PD-1	Nivolumab (MDX1106/BMS936558/BMS-ONO)	IgG4 fully human monoclonal antibody	Approved in unresectable or refractory metastatic melanoma; multiple cancers (phase I, II)
PD-1	Pembrolizumab (MK3475M, lambrolizumab, Merck)	IgG4 engineered humanized monoclonal antibody	Multiple cancers (phase I, II, III)

Continued

Table 1 Selection of Immunomodulatory Agents in Active Clinical Development—cont'd

Target	Agent	Class	Current Clinical Status
PD-1	Pidilizumab (CT-011, Cure Tech)	IgG1 humanized monoclonal antibody	Multiple cancers (phase I, II)
PD-1	AMP-224 (Amplimmune-GSK)	Fc-PD-L2 fusion protein	Multiple cancers (phase I)
PD-1	AMP-514 (MEDI0680, Amplimmune)	Monoclonal antibody	Multiple cancers (phase I)
PD-1	AUNP-12 (Pierre Fabre, Aurigene)	Branched 29-amino acid peptide	
PDL-1	BMS935559 (MDX-1105, BMS-ONO)	IgG4 fully human monoclonal antibody	Multiple cancers (phase I)
PDL-1	MPDL3280A (Genentech)	IgG1 engineered humanized monoclonal antibody	Multiple cancers (phase I, II)
PDL-1	MEDI4736 (MedImmune/AZ)	IgG1 engineered humanized monoclonal antibody	
PDL-1	MSB0010718C (Merck-Serono)	IgG1 monoclonal antibody	Multiple cancers (phase I)
PDL-2	rHIgM12B7 (Mayo Clinic)	IgM human monoclonal antibody	Melanoma (phase I)
LAG-3	BMS-986016 (BMS-ONO)	Monoclonal antibody	Multiple cancers (phase I)
LAG-3	GSK2831781 (GSK)	Humanized monoclonal afucosylated antibody	

Table 1 Selection of Immunomodulatory Agents in Active Clinical Development—cont'd

Target	Agent	Class	Current Clinical Status
LAG-3	IMP321 (Immuntep)	Soluble LAG-3	Multiple solid cancers (phase I, II)
BTLA	3B1 (Genentech)	Monoclonal antibody	
TIM-3	Anti-TIM3 antibody (Tesaro)	Fully human monoclonal antibody	

et al., 1994). In addition, upon ligation, CTLA-4 acts to inhibit intracellular signaling. Once stimulated, CTLA-4 recruits the tyrosine phosphatase SHP-2 via its cytoplasmic tail. SHP-2 in turn dephosphorylates TCRζ and p52SHC, thereby counteracting activation signals downstream of the TCR and CD28 (Lee et al., 1998; Marengère et al., 1996). CTLA-4 also appears to reduce T-cell activation by inhibiting AKT via its interaction with the serine/threonine phosphatase PP2A (Baroja et al., 2002; Chuang et al., 2000) and by stabilizing the ubiquitin ligase Cbl-b (Li et al., 2004). This results in the suppression of IL-2 secretion, curtailed T-cell expansion, and induction of T-cell anergy (Greenwald, Boussiotis, Lorsbach, Abbas, & Sharpe, 2001; Krummel & Allison, 1996; Walunas, Bakker, & Bluestone, 1996).

Phenotypic evidence of CTLA-4's capacity to dampen T-cell activation is well illustrated in CTLA-4 knockout mice. These animals develop marked T-cell expansion and infiltration into multiple tissue types, with mice succumbing to systemic autoimmune disease by 4 weeks of age (Tivol et al., 1995; Waterhouse et al., 1995). This lethal autoimmunity is dependent not only on TCR stimulation but also on signal two delivered via CD28 (Tai, Van Laethem, Sharpe, & Singer, 2007), suggesting that CTLA-4 is a potent negative regulator of T-cell costimulation by CD28. In mice, there is evidence that targeting both CD8 and CD4 T cells with anti-CTLA-4 is needed for maximal antitumor immunity. Other than its effect on conventional T cells, a portion of the antitumor activity of anti-CTLA-4 mAb treatment has been attributed to the antibody's effect on regulatory T cells (Tregs). Interestingly, Tregs constitutively express CTLA-4 at high levels (Takahashi et al., 2000) and appear to be dependent on CTLA-4 for some of their ability to suppress immune responses (Read, Malmström, & Powrie, 2000; Wing et al., 2008). Furthermore, anti-CTLA-4 mAb treatment can induce Fc-mediated Treg depletion (Selby et al., 2013; Simpson et al., 2013), raising the possibility that therapeutic antibodies against CTLA-4 induce antibody-dependent cell-mediated cytotoxicity (ADCC) or complement-dependent cytotoxicity of Tregs. Correlative evidence used to support this view includes the finding that the anti-CTLA-4 mAb therapy is associated with an increased effector-T:Treg and CD8:Treg ratio (Read et al., 2000; Takahashi et al., 2000).

Independent of the precise mechanism, the finding that Treg-specific CTLA-4 deletion results in a phenotype similar to that observed in mice with germline CTLA-4 deletion (Wing et al., 2008) implies that targeting CTLA-4 on Tregs is an important aspect of anti-CTLA-4 therapy. This conclusion should be tempered, however, by the fact that tremelimumab, an anti-CTLA-4 fully human IgG2 mAb in clinical development, maintains antimelanoma activity (Camacho et al., 2009) despite its relatively poor engagement of activating Fc receptors and thus its inability to mediate ADCC. Another argument against the centrality of Fc receptor-dependent depletion of Tregs by therapeutic anti-CTLA-4 mAbs is that Fc receptor FcγRIIIa or FcγRIIa polymorphisms to not seem to correlate with clinical response to ipilimumab (Korman et al., 2013).

Based on encouraging preclinical data (Leach, Krummel, & Allison, 1996; Peggs, Quezada, & Allison, 2008), in animal models of lymphoma, fibrosarcoma, prostate, colorectal, and renal cancer, anti-CTLA-4 has been investigated clinically in a broad range of malignancies. While CTLA-4 blockade has demonstrated activity in multiple malignancies, the most robust and consistent activity has been seen in melanoma (Hodi et al., 2010; Wolchok, Kluger et al., 2013). It is especially noteworthy that among advanced melanoma patients treated with single-agent ipilimumab, a fraction achieved durable responses not previously seen in this disease setting, with approximately 20% surviving beyond 4 years. Despite its antimelanoma activity mentioned above, tremelimumab (anti-CTLA-4 IgG2) did not demonstrate a survival advantage over standard chemotherapy in a phase III clinical trial (Ribas et al., 2013). The reason for this remains controversial, but possibilities include the unusual every-90-day dosing schedule, and the fact that patients enrolled in this trial were able to subsequently receive ipilimumab.

The experience with ipilimumab has rejuvenated interest in the field of cancer immunotherapy and in building on this success with combination therapies. At present, the most clinically promising approach to be used in combination with CTLA-4 blockade is PD-1 blockade (Wolchok, Kluger, et al., 2013). This treatment is based on the rationale that since CTLA-4 inhibition strengthens T-cell priming at the interface with the APC, it is rational to couple this with blockade of an inhibitory signal that T-cells can encounter at the interface with tumors (see next section). Other less traditional approaches have also gained interest. For example, combining localized radiation therapy with systemic CTLA-4 blockade is being actively studied based largely on encouraging data that radiation may potentiate a systemic (or "abscopal") antitumor response when combined with ipilimumab (Postow et al., 2012).

Besides generating interest in new strategies for treating cancer, this approach has also led to a revision of how the response to treatment is evaluated. Historically, cytotoxic chemotherapy has set the standard for judging a response to systemic cancer therapy. Given that immunotherapy enables the immune system to act on tumors, as opposed to cytotoxic chemotherapy which acts directly on cancer cells, there is no *a priori* reason to expect these two modalities to demonstrate comparable kinetics. In fact, immunotherapy can mediate delayed tumor regression prior to producing more sustained tumor control relative to traditional chemotherapy (Wolchok, Hodi, et al., 2013). There is even a remarkable case in the literature of a patient with metastatic pancreatic cancer treated with single-agent ipilimumab who went on to experience significant disease regression beginning approximately 6 weeks after starting treatment, after an initial period of marked on-treatment tumor growth (Royal et al., 2010). These observations have led to the development of immune-related response criteria (Wolchok et al., 2009) which are important for curtailing premature discontinuation of potentially active immunotherapies. It is important to note that delayed responses are not always observed with immunotherapy, and that continuing with treatment in the face of progression requires cautious clinical judgment. Standard response criteria such as RECIST do not fully capture the potential benefit of this class of therapy, and alternative methods for judging success in the setting of clinical trials, such as immune-related response criteria or the more traditional overall survival or landmark survival, are often more appropriate.

Not surprisingly, the novel mechanism of ipilimumab and tremelimumab goes hand in hand with a unique side effect profile. Patients treated with CTLA-4 blockade do not develop adverse events associated with cytotoxic chemotherapy or even targeted pathway inhibition. Instead, they are at risk for developing primarily on-target toxicity; that is, toxicity associated with T-cell disinhibition or so-called immune-related adverse events (Weber, 2007; Wolchok et al., 2010). Such toxicities include colitis, dermatitis, hypophysitis, hepatitis, and fatigue. Of note, a subset of such pathology may be related to factors other than nonspecific autoimmunity. For example, there are data showing that hypophysitis is attributable to CTLA-4 expression on cells of the pituitary gland (Iwama et al., 2014). Immune-related adverse events can potentially be severe; however, the collective clinical experience with anti-CTLA-4 therapy has led to marked improvement in the management of these side effects. In the setting of careful monitoring and early intervention, most immune-related adverse effects can be readily controlled with algorithm-based medical management.

There has been strong interest in identifying biomarkers to predict response to CTLA-4 blockade. The identification of such biomarkers would not only spare melanoma patients unlikely to respond from potentially toxic treatments but may also identify patients with other malignancies who may respond. Early findings suggested that C-reactive protein (Wilgenhof et al., 2013) levels and absolute lymphocyte count (>1000/μL) after the second dose of ipilimumab may predict for improved overall survival. Pretreatment circulating myeloid-derived suppressor cell (MDSC) levels were subsequently shown to predict for prolonged overall survival (Kitano et al., 2014). More recently, an elevated baseline level of soluble CD25 has been identified as a possible poor prognostic indicator for response to ipilimumab (Hannani et al., 2015). In a separate study analyzing tissue samples from melanoma patients using whole-exome sequencing, distinct novel tumor epitopes were found to be associated with long-term clinical benefit from ipilimumab (Snyder et al., 2014). This raises the exciting possibility that such epitopes can be used to screen patients for treatment with ipilimumab. Overall, CTLA-4 blockade has not only opened the door to a new class of anticancer treatment but also remains a promising approach for patients with malignancies other than melanoma. Such advances will likely be ushered into clinical practice by the continued development of increasingly precise biomarkers and increasingly potent combination strategies.

2.2 PD-1/PD-L1

Another critical immune checkpoint is the pathway between PD-1 (programmed cell death-1, CD279) and its ligand PD-L1 (B7-H1, CD274). PD-1 is a type I transmembrane cosignaling receptor of the CD28 immunoglobulin (Ig) superfamily. It is expressed on double-negative αβ and γδ T cells in the thymus and activated peripheral T and B cells (Okazaki & Honjo, 2007). Upon interaction with either of its two ligands, PD-L1 or PD-L2, PD-1 negatively regulates antigen receptor signaling by recruiting the protein tyrosine phosphatase SHP-2, which dephosphorylates downstream effector molecules, such as Syk and PI3K (phosphatidylinositol 3-kinase) in B cells and ZAP70 and CD3ζ in T cells (Okazaki, Maeda, Nishimura, Kurosaki, & Honjo, 2001; Parry et al., 2005). The involvement of PD-1 in immune tolerance has been demonstrated by the development of autoimmune diseases in PD-1-deficient mice across different strains (glomerulonephritis and arthritis in C57BL/6 (Nishimura, Nose, Hiai, Minato, & Honjo, 1999); autoimmune severe myocarditis in BALB/c (Nishimura et al., 2001); acceleration of type I diabetes in NOD mice (Wang et al., 2005)). Correspondingly, multiple groups have reported significant associations between single-nucleotide polymorphisms affecting PD-1 expression and autoimmunity in humans (Okazaki & Honjo, 2007). Overall, however, inhibition of this pathway is generally considered to have more limited side effects than CTLA-4 blockade (Okazaki & Honjo, 2006).

PD-L1 and PD-L2 are type I transmembrane glycoproteins with short cytoplasmic tails lacking any known motif for signal transduction, implying the potential inability of these ligands to back-signal upon interaction with PD-1 (Okazaki & Honjo, 2007). PD-L1 is expressed on resting B cells, T cells, macrophages, and DCs and is upregulated on these cells by various types of stimulation (Yamazaki et al., 2002). PD-L2 is rarely detected on either resting immune cells or activated B and T cells; however, it can be induced on macrophages and DCs upon activation. In contrast to PD-L2, PD-L1 can be expressed in nonhematopoietic cells, including microvascular endothelial cells, particularly at the site of immune privilege, such as heart and placenta, and also in lung, pancreas, and muscle (Okazaki & Honjo, 2007). Interestingly, PD-L1-null mice display virtually no phenotype unless exposed to pathogens or crossed onto an autoimmunity-prone background. Various tumors can upregulate both PD-L1 and/or PD-L2 as part of what is believed to be one of their immune-evasion mechanisms. In melanoma, for example, this seems to be the response to proinflammatory cytokines, such as interferon (IFN)-γ (Taube et al., 2012), released by tumor-infiltrating T cells. In other tumors, PD-L1 can be driven by intrinsic oncogenic events, such as loss of the tumor suppressor PTEN (Parsa et al., 2007). The finding that PD-1 is expressed by a large proportion of tumor-infiltrating lympho cytes (TILs) as a consequence of chronic self-antigen exposure

(Ahmadzadeh et al., 2009) and that PD-L1 in particular is upregulated in a number of cancers where its expression often correlates with unfavorable outcomes (Okazaki & Honjo, 2007) makes this pathway an attractive target for immunotherapeutic intervention. Accordingly, several animal studies have shown that blockade of PD-1 promotes therapeutic antitumor T-cell responses in models of melanoma (Blank et al., 2004), pancreatic (Okudaira et al., 2009), squamous cell (Strome et al., 2003), and colon carcinomas (Iwai, Terawaki, & Honjo, 2005). In addition, the combination of PD-L1-blockade with 4-1BB agonist antibodies demonstrated synergistic activity in a breast cancer model (Hirano et al., 2005). These promising preclinical results led to the generation of antihuman PD-1/PD-L1-blocking antibodies and their evaluation in the clinical setting. These studies demonstrated a striking 30–35% durable response rate in patients with advanced melanoma, leading to the FDA approval of the anti-PD1 antibodies pembrolizumab (humanized IgG4) (Robert et al., 2014; Topalian et al., 2012) and nivolumab (fully human IgG4) for melanoma in 2014 (Wolchok, Kluger, et al., 2013) and an extension of the FDA approval for nivolumab to squamous cell lung cancer in 2015. In view of these clinical successes, PD-1/L1-blocking antibodies are currently under investigation in patients with other malignancies, such as lung (Harvey, 2014), breast (Stagg & Allard, 2013), bladder (Powles et al., 2014), and renal cancer (Tykodi, 2014) as well as Hodgkin's lymphoma (Ansell et al., 2014). Whether PD-1 versus PD-L1 is a superior target has been a matter of ongoing debate. Both strategies have potential limitations. Inhibition of PD-1 leaves the interaction between PD-L1 and CD80 unaffected (Butte, Pena-Cruz, Kim, Freeman, & Sharpe, 2008), and PD-L1 blockade does not preclude PD-1 activation by PD-L2. This suggests that concurrent inhibition of PD-1 and PD-L1 may result in superior activity. Thus far, both anti-PD-1 and anti-PD-L1 antibodies have shown responses in multiple overlapping tumor types and no clear difference in adverse event profiles has been identified.

Similar to CTLA-4 blockade, one of the major challenges at the present time is identifying predictive biomarkers to guide selection of the patients likely to benefit from treatment with PD-1 or PD-L1 blockade. Despite initial evidence pointing to the association between tumor PD-L1 expression and clinical efficacy, responses have been observed in patients with PD-L1-negative tumors (Taube et al., 2014). Whether PD-L1 expression is accessory to PD-1 blockade or is simply a reflection of a favorable tumor microenvironment remains to be determined. It is also likely that this parameter needs to be integrated into a more complex model to improve prediction of clinical benefit. Systematic analysis of tumor immune infiltrates, proinflammatory cytokines, and TCR deep sequencing is now being pursued with the aim of defining the key variables determining patients' likelihood of responding to anti-PD-1/PD-L1 mAb therapy.

T-cell coinhibitory receptors other than CTLA-4 and PD-1 have been described. These inhibitory molecules are less developed in the clinic, yet have potential. They can act as molecules that set a threshold, as immune modulators, checkpoints, or feedback mechanisms that fine-tune the magnitude and quality of T-cell immune responses. We give a brief overview on Lag-3 (lymphocyte activation gene-3), Tim3, TIGIT, and BTLA (B and T lymphocyte attenuator) below.

2.3 LAG-3

LAG-3 (CD223) is an inhibitory receptor expressed on activated CD8 and CD4 T cells (including Tregs) (Huard, Gaulard, Faure, Hercend, & Triebel, 1994). It is also expressed on NK cells, B cells, and plasmacytoid DCs (Goldberg & Drake, 2011). LAG-3 is a member of the Ig superfamily containing four Ig loops, with structural similarity to the CD4 molecule. It has been shown to bind to MHC class II molecules at site distinct from CD4 but with higher affinity (Huard, Prigent, Tournier, Bruniquel, & Triebel, 1995). Unlike the CD4 molecule, LAG-3 contains an exposed extra loop region in the first Ig domain that appears to be important for its binding to MHC class II molecules (Baixeras et al., 1992). Studies in LAG-3 knockout mice demonstrated an inhibitory role for LAG-3 in controlling both CD4 and CD8 T-cell proliferation *in vitro* and *in vivo* (Grosso et al., 2007; Workman et al., 2004). This inhibitory function is dependent on a conserved KIEELE motif in the cytoplasmic tail of the protein (Workman, Dugger, & Vignali, 2002). Several preclinical studies in mice have documented a role for LAG-3 in T-cell exhaustion in chronic infections as well as cancers (Blackburn et al., 2009; Butler et al., 2012; Matsuzaki et al., 2010; Woo et al., 2012). In addition, LAG-3 expression on Tregs has been shown to be important for their suppressive function (Huang et al., 2004; Okamura et al., 2009). The coexpression of LAG-3 with the inhibitory receptor PD-1 on exhausted T cells or Tregs correlates with a greater state of effector T-cell exhaustion and the suppressive function of Tregs. Simultaneous blockade of both LAG-3 and PD-1 with mAbs in chronic viral infection and cancer models has shown more potent therapeutic efficacy than blockade of either receptor alone (Blackburn et al., 2009; Butler et al., 2012; Woo et al., 2012). A soluble form of LAG-3 has been identified in the sera of cancer patients, suggesting that cleavage of LAG-3 might have a functional role (Triebel, Hacene, & Pichon, 2006). Soluble LAG-3 has been associated with Th1 responses in cancer patients and such patients show higher overall survival and disease-free survival rates when detectable levels of soluble LAG-3 are present at diagnosis (Triebel et al., 2006). A soluble LAG-3-Ig fusion protein (Immutep IMP321) has been tested in patients with renal cell carcinoma (Brignone, Escudier, Grygar, Marcu, & Triebel, 2009). This drug was well tolerated, and while there were no objective responses, some patients displayed stable disease. In addition, this drug induced sustained CD8 T-cell activation and an increase in the fraction of long-lived effector memory CD8 T cells. When IMP321 was used in combination with chemotherapy (paclitaxel) in patients with metastatic breast cancer, the results were more promising (Brignone et al., 2010). Clinical benefit was observed in 90% of patients with an objective tumor response rate of 50% compared to 25% in historical controls. Clinical trials are currently underway to examine the effects of a LAG-3-blocking mAb (BMS-986016) in cancer patients as a single agent or in combination with PD-1 blockade (ClinicalTrials.gov: NCT02061761, NCT01968109).

2.4 TIM-3

T-cell immunoglobulin domain and mucin-domain-containing molecule-3 (TIM-3) is an inhibitory receptor expressed by several immune cell subsets (Anderson et al., 2007; Monney et al., 2002; Ndhlovu et al., 2012). There are four known ligands for TIM-3: galectin-9 (Zhu et al., 2005), HMGB1 (Chiba et al., 2012), phosphatidylserine (Nakayama et al., 2009), and CEACAM-1 (Huang et al., 2015) all of which are widely distributed on various tissues. TIM-3 appears to use different intracellular signaling pathways than other inhibitory receptors. The cytoplasmic tail of both mouse and human TIM-3 contains multiple tyrosine residues that correspond to putative phosphorylation sites (Ferris, Lu, & Kane, 2014). However, no inhibitory motifs (ITIM or ITSM) that are seen in other inhibitory molecules were found. TIM-3 interactions with a chaperone protein, Bat3, have been implicated in regulating T-cell responses (Rangachari et al., 2012). It is believed that Bat3 binding to the cytoplasmic tail of TIM-3 prevents the inhibitory downstream signaling of TIM-3. Once TIM-3 binds to its ligand (e.g., galectin-9), Bat3 is displaced allowing for inhibitory downstream signaling pathways to be engaged, ultimately leading to reduced T-cell proliferation and effector functions (Haining, 2012).

In mouse models of autoimmunity, TIM-3 binding to its ligand, galectin-9, on CD4 and CD8 T cells induces apoptosis and attenuates effector function of these cells, indicating that TIM-3 acts as a negative regulator of the adaptive immune response (Wang et al., 2007; Zhu et al., 2005). High TIM-3 expression has been reported on exhausted T cells (Jin et al., 2010; McMahan et al., 2010). In addition, coexpression of TIM-3 and PD-1 on CD8 T cells is associated with the most severely exhausted T-cell population in mouse models of chronic viral infections (Zhou et al., 2011) and cancer (Fourcade et al., 2010; Sakuishi et al., 2010). Blockade of TIM-3 with a mAb reversed T-cell exhaustion and elicited antitumor activity in several mouse tumor models (Ngiow et al., 2011; Sakuishi et al., 2010). Greater antitumor efficacy was achieved when anti-TIM-3 was administered in combination with PD-1 blockade. In addition, TIM-3 blockade of tumor antigen-specific CD8 T cells from melanoma patients restored proliferation and cytokine production *ex vivo* (Fourcade et al., 2010). TIM-3 expression on NK cells from melanoma patients increases as the tumor advances, with higher expression in patients with poor prognoses (da Silva et al., 2014). This high expression of TIM-3 correlates with NK cell exhaustion as measured by decreased cytotoxicity, IFNγ production, and proliferation. Moreover, blockade of TIM-3 *ex vivo* with mAbs reversed NK cell exhaustion. In addition to its expression on NK cells, TIM-3 is also expressed on innate cells such as monocytes, macrophages, and DCs. Initially, it was reported that TIM-3 ligation alone or in the presence of TLR stimulation on DCs led to enhanced TNFα production (Anderson et al., 2007). However, more recently, it was shown that TIM-3 acts as an inhibitory molecule on human monocytes (Zhang et al., 2012). TIM-3 has also been shown to bind and mediate the phagocytosis of apoptotic cells through recognition of phosphatidylserine, in a mechanism that may be important for cross-presentation of antigens from dying cells by DCs or macrophages within tumors or inflamed tissues (DeKruyff et al., 2010; Nakayama et al., 2009). The effects of TIM-3 blockade on multiple arms of the immune system make this approach an attractive candidate for clinical development.

2.5 TIGIT

T-cell immunoreceptor with Ig and ITIM domains (TIGIT) is one of the most recent immune checkpoints to be investigated as an immunotherapeutic target. TIGIT is a transmembrane glycoprotein receptor with an Ig-like V-type domain and an ITIM in its cytoplasmic domain. It is expressed on activated and memory T cells, NK cells, and Tregs. Binding to either of its two ligands on APCs, CD155 (PVR: poliovirus receptor) and CD112 (PVRL2, nectin-2), prevents their maturation and confers a tolerogenic phenotype (Yu et al., 2009). DNAX accessory molecule (DNAM-1, CD226) is an alternative low-affinity receptor for the same ligands, expressed by both naïve and effector T cells, which delivers costimulatory signals (Xu & Jin, 2010). This underscores a common immunoregulatory mechanism within the immunoglobulin superfamily receptors, whereby costimulatory and coinhibitory receptors compete for binding to the same ligands (CD28/CTLA4-CD80/86; BTLA/LIGHT-HVEM; TIGIT/CD226-CD155/CD112) to control T-cell functions.

Among CD4 T cells, TIGIT expression usually defines Foxp3$^+$ Tregs, whereas on CD8 T cells, it marks significantly dysfunctional cells that coexpress LAG-3, TIM-3, and PD-1 (Johnston et al., 2014; Lozano, Dominguez-Villar, Kuchroo, & Hafler, 2012; Stanietsky et al., 2009). The contribution of the TIGIT pathway to tumor immune evasion has been consistently verified in different preclinical settings. Despite the lack of spontaneous autoimmunity in TIGIT knockout mice, tumor growth is significantly reduced in these mice in a T and NK cell-dependent manner (Johnston et al., 2014; Kurtulus et al., 2014). Both human and murine tumor-infiltrating T cells express high levels of TIGIT, and TIGIT inhibition, by either genetic ablation or blocking mAbs, increases T-cell activation and proliferation in response to both polyclonal and antigen-specific stimulation (Johnston et al., 2014; Joller et al., 2011; Lozano et al., 2012). Importantly, TIGIT engagement has been shown to inhibit T cells not only indirectly via induction of tolerogenic DCs but also by impeding CD226 dimerization on T cells themselves, thus directly avoiding the delivery of costimulatory signals (Johnston et al., 2014). The latter effect has been found associated with the downregulation of the TCR activation pathway (Joller et al., 2011). To date, antagonist anti-TIGIT mAbs have not demonstrated dramatic antitumor activity as single agents. However, coblockade of TIGIT and either PD-L1 (Johnston et al., 2014) or TIM3 have proven synergistic against different solid tumors in mouse models (Kurtulus et al., 2014). It is therefore likely that TIGIT blockade will ultimately find application in combination with antagonist anti-PD1/PDL-1 or anti-Tim3 mAbs in the clinic.

2.6 BTLA

BTLA (CD272) is a type I transmembrane cosignaling receptor belonging to the CD28 Ig superfamily. It shares structural similarities with CTLA-4 and PD-1 and is mainly expressed on immune cells (Watanabe et al.,

2003). Naïve αβ T cells, NK cells, conventional DCs, and splenic macrophages express BTLA at low levels, whereas resting γδ T cells, activated αβ T cells, and resting B cells express BTLA at high levels (Sedy et al., 2005; Watanabe et al., 2003). In contrast to the general propensity toward binding structurally similar members of the immunoglobulin and TNF superfamilies, BTLA binds to the TNFR family member herpes virus entry mediator (HVEM) (Cai et al., 2008; Sedy et al., 2005; Steinberg, Cheung, & Ware, 2011). Upon interaction with HVEM, BTLA recruits the protein tyrosine phosphatases SHP-1 and SHP-2, thus inhibiting signaling cascades downstream of the TCR (Sedy et al., 2005) and BCR (Vendel et al., 2009). Interestingly, through a different domain, HVEM can bind its costimulatory ligand LIGHT (TNF superfamily member) and deliver costimulatory signals (Cai et al., 2008; Sedy et al., 2005). Accordingly, removal of the BTLA-binding domain from HVEM converts HVEM from a dominant coinhibitory receptor to an exclusively costimulatory receptor (Cai et al., 2008).

The immunosuppressive functions of BTLA have been demonstrated by the gradual development of autoantibodies and autoimmune hepatitis, and increased susceptibility to induced autoimmunity, in BTLA-deficient mice (Deppong et al., 2006; Oya et al., 2008; Watanabe et al., 2003). In addition, BTLA appears to contribute to Treg action on T effector (Teff) cells, as BTLA-deficient Teff cells are resistant to Treg suppression. Indeed, upon T-cell stimulation, HVEM increases on Tregs and BTLA on Teff cells, thus orienting inhibitory signals from Tregs to Teff (Tao, Wang, Murphy, Fraser, & Hancock, 2008).

In cancer patients, overexpression of BTLA has been detected in neoplastic cells from chronic lymphocytic leukemia, but not from other lymphomas (M'Hidi et al., 2009) and unexpectedly in melanoma (Haymaker et al., 2013). Furthermore, in melanoma patients, tumor antigen-specific effector CD8 T cells can express high levels of BTLA, which in association with PD-1 expression defines a particularly anergic T-cell phenotype (Baitsch et al., 2011; Derré et al., 2010). Interestingly, BTLA blockade has been shown to synergize with PD-1 and TIM-3 inhibition in enhancing *in vitro* proliferation and cytokine production of melanoma-specific CD8 T cells (Fourcade et al., 2012). Similarly, high expression of BTLA was found on tumor-reactive CD8 T cells from allogeneic transplant patients with hematologic malignancies and treatment with antagonist anti-BTLA antibody boosted expansion and cytokine production of antigen-specific CD8 T cells *in vitro* (Hobo et al., 2012). Blockade of BTLA may therefore be a novel approach to inhibit tumor growth and prevent negative signaling through BTLA in immune cells. Antagonist antihuman BTLA antibodies are currently in clinical development. However, before the potential of BTLA blockade can be fully realized, further insights into its biology, such as the potential compensatory effects of the other HVEM coinhibitory partner CD160, will need to be clarified.

While several molecules that target coinhibitory receptors have been developed, the outcome of the engagement of the T-cell receptor (TCR) is determined by both coinhibitory and costimulatory signals. Several agonist antibodies targeting costimulatory receptors have been developed preclinically and evaluation is underway in clinic. We will describe the most developed ones below (4-1BB, glucocorticoid-induced TNFR-related protein (GITR), OX40, and CD40).

2.7 4-1BB

4-1BB (CD137) is a costimulatory member of the tumor necrosis factor receptor superfamily that is upregulated on activated T cells, NK cells, NKT cells, and monocytes. 4-1BB is also expressed on Tregs and DCs. Its ligand 4-1BBL, a member of tumor necrosis factor superfamily, is expressed on activated APCs including DCs, macrophages, and B cells. The engagement of 4-1BB by either its natural ligand or an agonistic antibody enhanced T-cell proliferation and cytokine production, and protected T cells from activation-induced cell death via upregulation of antiapoptotic genes such as Bcl-xl, Bfl1, and C-flip (Cheuk, Mufti, & Guinn, 2004; Lee et al., 2002; Shuford et al., 1997; Stärck, Scholz, Dörken, & Daniel, 2005; Vinay & Kwon, 2014; Wilcox et al., 2002). 4-1BB ligation also induced proinflammatory cytokine production by DCs, macrophages, and neutrophils, and enhanced NK cell proliferation. *In vivo*, 4-1BB engagement enhanced the proliferation of B cells, NK cells, CD4 T cells, and particularly CD8 T cells. Numerous preclinical studies have shown that ligation of 4-1BB with an agonistic mAb induces an antitumor immune response in part by increasing cytotoxic lymphocyte (CTL) activity in some, but not all, of the studied murine models. Combination of 4-1BB with other therapies such as CTLA-4 blockade, CD40 agonism, cell-based vaccines, and radiation therapy (Shi & Siemann, 2006) demonstrated more potent antitumor effects than targeting 4-1BB alone (Curran, Kim, Montalvo, Al-Shamkhani, & Allison, 2011; Tirapu et al., 2004; Uno et al., 2006;

Xu et al., 2004). These combination therapies have a marked proliferative effect on both CD4 and CD8 T cells. CTLA-4 blockade combined with 4-1BB stimulation in the context of a B16 melanoma vaccine resulted in increased tumor rejection compared to either treatment alone in mice bearing B16 tumors (Curran et al., 2011). In addition, the combination of an anti-4-1BB mAb with adoptive T-cell therapy resulted in increased survival and resistance to rechallenge in the murine thymoma model E.G7 (Lin et al., 2010). Urelumab (BMS-663513), a human agonist mAb targeting 4-1BB, was investigated in patients with ovarian cancer, renal cell carcinoma, and melanoma (Sznol et al., 2008). In a phase I dose escalation study, three of four patients with melanoma had stable disease or better. However, a phase II study of urelumab was terminated due to a high incidence of hepatic toxicity, including two deaths. Other clinical trials are ongoing with urelumab as a single agent (NCT01471210) and in combination with rituximab (NCT01775631) in patients with B-cell non-Hodgkin's lymphoma. Combination therapies including urelumab with elotuzumab (anti-CS1, also known as CRACC, CD319 and SLAMF7) in patients with multiple myeloma (NCT02252263); with cetuximab (anti-EGFR) in patients with colorectal cancer or head and neck cancers (NCT02110082); and with nivolumab (anti-PD-1) in patients with advanced solid tumors and refractory B-cell non-Hodgkin's lymphoma (NCT01471210) are being investigated. These latter combinations with tumor targeting mAbs are designed based on encouraging preclinical data showing synergy of the combinations with anti-4-1BB, presumably due to upregulation of Fc receptors (Kohrt et al., 2012).

2.8 GITR

GITR (TNFRSF18, AITR, CD357) is a costimulatory receptor of the TNF superfamily, which is expressed at constitutively high levels on $Foxp3^{+}CD4$ Tregs and upregulated on activated T cells (Schaer, Cohen, & Wolchok, 2010). *In vitro* studies performed with murine cells have shown that GITR stimulation with agonist mAbs or the physiologic ligand (GITRL) promotes Teff proliferation, cytokine production (Kanamaru et al., 2004; Ronchetti et al., 2007), resistance to Treg suppression (Ko et al., 2005; Mitsui et al., 2010; Nishikawa et al., 2008; Shimizu, Yamazaki, Takahashi, Ishida, & Sakaguchi, 2002), and inhibition of Treg suppressive function (Valzasina et al., 2005). *In vivo*, the agonist anti-mouse GITR mAb (DTA-1) has shown antitumor activity, causing tumor eradication and the development of tumor-specific immunological memory in immunogenic tumor models such as MethA fibrosarcoma and CT26 colorectal carcinoma (Cohen et al., 2010; Ko et al., 2005; Turk, Guevara-Patiño, Rizzuto, Engelhorn, & Houghton, 2004). The therapeutic activity of DTA-1 is associated with reduction of intratumoral Treg accumulation and potentiation of antitumor CD8 Teff functions (Cohen et al., 2010; Ko et al., 2005; Mitsui et al., 2010; Sharma et al., 2008). Our group observed that the maximum antitumor effect of DTA-1 is achieved when both effector T cells (Teff) and Tregs express GITR in B16 melanoma-bearing mice (Cohen et al., 2010). Very recently, the activity of antibodies against costimulatory receptors, including GITR, has been reported to be dependent on engagement of activating Fc γ receptors and ADCC and antibody-dependent cellular phagocytosis of intratumoral Tregs in the CT26 colorectal cancer model (Bulliard et al., 2013, 2014). High GITR expression on intratumoral Tregs along with the accumulation of myeloid cells and NK cells in the tumor microenvironment is proposed to be the basis for the selective depletion of intratumor Tregs (Bulliard et al., 2013). In addition, we have shown that GITR ligation also affects the function of tumor-infiltrating Tregs by altering their lineage stability. Indeed, the remaining intratumoral Tregs after DTA-1 treatment in B16-bearing mice displayed reduced levels of Foxp3, Helios, and IL-10, features that are thought to be responsible for the suppressive activity of Tregs. Consequently, these Tregs also displayed increased T-bet, eomesodermin (Eomes), and IFNγ expression (Schaer et al., 2013), features associated with effector T-cell function suggesting a conversion to a Teff-like phenotype. Interestingly, loss of Foxp3 was tumor dependent, as adoptively transferred tumor-infiltrating, but not naïve, Tregs lose Foxp3 expression in DTA-1-treated hosts (Schaer et al., 2013). This is consistent with other studies showing that GITR stimulation does not affect Treg suppression in the periphery (spleen or tumor-draining lymph nodes) (Cohen et al., 2010; Mitsui et al., 2010). Taken as a whole, these findings indicate that anti-GITR therapy may specifically target "pathogenic" tumor-infiltrating Tregs, thus potentially limiting systemic autoimmunity. Based on the promising antitumor effects of GITR stimulation in preclinical models, and the underlying mechanisms associated with the therapy, a first-in-human phase 1 clinical trial has begun to evaluate the safety and immunologic activity of the agonist anti-human GITR mAb TRX518 (aglycosyl humanized IgG1) (Rosenzweig et al., 2010) in patients with advanced solid tumors (NCT01239134). Another anti-GITR mAB, MK-3474, is also in early clinical development.

2.9 CD40

CD40 (TNFRSF5) is a costimulatory type I membrane glycoprotein belonging to the tumor necrosis factor receptor superfamily. In contrast to 4-1BB, OX40, and GITR, which are primarily expressed on T cells, CD40 is mainly expressed on APCs including monocytes, macrophages, DCs, and B cells. CD40 is also expressed on several nonimmune cells and a variety of cancers such as Hodgkin and non-Hodgkin lymphomas, lymphocytic leukemias, acute myeloid leukemia, multiple myeloma, melanoma, lung, prostate, bladder, and ovarian cancers (Eliopoulos & Young, 2004; van Kooten & Banchereau, 2000). The CD40 primary ligand (CD40L, CD154) is a type II transmembrane protein predominantly expressed on activated T cells, and at low levels in some cancer cells such as non-Hodgkin lymphoma, Burkitt lymphoma, and chronic lymphocytic leukemia (Eliopoulos & Young, 2004).

The CD40–CD40L interaction is an important step in the initiation of an adaptive immune response. Ligation of CD40 on DCs increases the expression of MHC class II molecules and induces the secretion of proinflammatory cytokines leading to enhanced T-cell activation (van Kooten & Banchereau, 2000). In addition, CD40–CD40L ligation plays an important role in B-cell activation, proliferation, and differentiation as well as in macrophage activation (Fecteau & Néron, 2003). Inhibition of the CD40–CD40L interaction in humans as a result of a mutant CD40L causes the X-linked hyper IgM syndrome, a severe immunodeficiency characterized by the absence of serum IgG, IgA, and IgE (Callard, Armitage, Fanslow, & Spriggs, 1993) due to the inability of B cells to undergo class switching. CD40 signaling is mediated by adaptor proteins from the TNF receptor-associated factor (TRAF) family. The recruitment of these adaptor molecules triggers multiple signaling pathways including the transcription factor NF-κB (Tsukamoto, Kobayashi, Azuma, Yamamoto, & Inoue, 1999), PI3K, and the mitogen-activated protein kinase (MAPK) pathway (Davies, Mason, Wakelam, Young, & Eliopoulos, 2004). TRAF-independent signaling through the JAK–STAT pathway has also been described (Bishop, Moore, Xie, Stunz, & Kraus, 2007; Hanissian & Geha, 1997).

In contrast with the proliferative effect of CD40 engagement in normal B cells, preclinical experiments show that ligation of CD40 using agonist mAb in specific CD40-expressing B-cell malignancies had a direct antiproliferative effect (Burington et al., 2011). Engagement of CD40 protected

Table 2 Selected Anti-CD40 Therapeutic mAbs in Clinical Development

	Agonistic Anti-CD40 mAb			Antagonistic Anti-CD40 mAb
mAb	Dacetuzumab (SGN-40)	CP-870,893	Chi Lob 7/4	Lucatumumab
Developer	Seattle Genetics	Pfizer	University of Southampton	Novartis
Isotype	Humanized IgG1	Fully human IgG2	Chimeric IgG1	Humanized IgG1
Targeted malignancies	• Multiple myeloma • Non-Hodgkin's lymphoma • CLL • Others	• Melanoma • Breast cancer • NSCLC • Sarcoma • Pancreatic carcinoma • Others	Solid tumors—Diffuse large B-cell non-Hodgkin's lymphoma	Follicular lymphoma

not only against CD40-positive malignancies but also against cancers lacking CD40 expression. This antitumor effect is mediated by the ability of anti-CD40 to induce maturation of DCs leading to an enhanced activation of tumor-specific T cells. In addition, a T cell-independent antitumor effect involving macrophage activation with CD40 agonist mAb has been shown to have a potent antitumor effect perhaps through macrophage-mediated ADCC (Vonderheide et al., 2013). Table 2 shows therapeutic mAbs in clinical development.

2.10 OX40

Like 4-1BB, GITR, and CD40, OX40 (CD134) is a member of the TNFR superfamily of costimulatory molecules that is upregulated on lymphocyte activation (Al-Shamkhani et al., 1996; Bansal-Pakala, Halteman, Cheng, & Croft, 2004; Mallett, Fossum, & Barclay, 1990). While OX40 is primarily known to be expressed on activated CD4 and CD8 T cells, it has also been identified on other immune cells such as NK cells, NKT cells, and neutrophils (Baumann et al., 2004; Liu et al., 2008). Like other TNFR ligands, OX40 ligand (OX40L, CD252) is a trimer. It bears structural similarity and sequence homology to other molecules in the TNF superfamily (Baum et al., 1994). OX40L is primarily expressed on APCs such as activated

B cells (Stüber, Neurath, Calderhead, Fell, & Strober, 1995), mature DCs (Ohshima et al., 1997), plasmacytoid DCs (Ito et al., 2004; Liu et al., 2008), Langerhans cells (Sato et al., 2002), and macrophages (Weinberg, Wegmann, Funatake, & Whitham, 1999). Interestingly, OX40L has also been shown to be expressed other cell types such as NK cells (Zingoni et al., 2004), mast cells (Kashiwakura, Yokoi, Saito, & Okayama, 2004), endothelial cells (Imura et al., 1996), and activated T cells (Soroosh, Ine, Sugamura, & Ishii, 2006). Upon engaging its ligand, OX40 enhances T-cell expansion (Baum et al., 1994; Paterson et al., 1987), promotes long-term survival of CD4 T cells (Rogers, Song, Gramaglia, Killeen, & Croft, 2001), and induces both Th1 and Th2 cytokines (Arestides et al., 2002). Beyond augmenting the activity of effector T-cells, OX40 has also been shown to regulate the development, and reduce the suppressive function, of Tregs (Griseri, Asquith, Thompson, & Powrie, 2010; Piconese et al., 2010; Ruby et al., 2009; Takeda et al., 2004; Valzasina et al., 2005).

In light of its physiologic function, OX40 is seen as a promising target for antitumor immune activation (Schaer, Hirschhorn-Cymerman, & Wolchok, 2014). As monotherapy, OX40 agonism has been associated with antitumor activity in multiple animal models (Hirschhorn-Cymerman et al., 2009; Jensen et al., 2010; Weinberg et al., 2000). CD4 and CD8 cells were found to be necessary for the full antitumor activity of OX40 ligation, and immunological memory induced by OX40 activation can mediate resistance to tumor rechallenge (Pan, Zang, Weber, Meseck, & Chen, 2002).

Most importantly, OX40 activation has shown promising results in combination with a other immunomodulatory agents including IL-12 (Pan et al., 2002), IL-2 (Redmond, Triplett, Floyd, & Weinberg, 2012), 4-1BB agonism (Pan et al., 2002), CTLA-4 blockade (Watanabe et al., 2010), anti-CD25 (Watanabe et al., 2010) therapy, TLR-9 stimulation (Houot & Levy, 2009), TGF-beta inhibition (Garrison et al., 2012), and adoptive cell transfer (Watanabe et al., 2010). Interestingly, it has also been noted that the combination of OX40 and cyclophosphamide can mediate antitumor activity and robustly enhance the antitumor activity of adoptively transferred CD4 T cells (Hirschhorn-Cymerman et al., 2009). Anti-OX40 therapy has demonstrated safety and some evidence of antitumor activity in multiple tumor types in a single-agent phase I clinical trial (Curti et al., 2013). Given this, and the robust preclinical data, multiple combination treatments are now entering the clinic (e.g., NCT02205333, NCT01303705).

3. ADOPTIVE T-CELL TRANSFER

An important hurdle in mobilizing the immune system against cancers is that the precursor frequency of tumor-specific T cells is typically low or even nonexistent. This is because T cells that recognize antigens associated with tumors (generally self-antigens) undergo extensive negative selection by central and peripheral tolerance mechanisms. To circumvent the low precursor frequency of these cell, it is now possible to expand tumor-specific T cells *ex vivo* and adoptively transfer them to cancer patients (Chacon et al., 2014; Dudley & Rosenberg, 2003; Rosenberg, Restifo, Yang, Morgan, & Dudley, 2008; Fig. 2), so-called adoptive cell therapy (ACT).

3.1 TIL Therapy

One of the earliest approaches to ACT has been the therapeutic reinfusion of TILs from resected malignant tissues (Dudley et al., 2002; Rosenberg & Dudley, 2009). After resection, the tumor is dissociated, and a T-cell population with specificity for tumor antigens is expanded *ex vivo* using IL-2 and sometimes mitogenic agents such as anti-CD3 and anti-CD28 antibodies. The expanded T cells are subsequently infused back into the patient (Rosenberg, Spiess, & Lafreniere, 1986). *Ex vivo* expansion allows the T cells of interest to grow in an environment engineered to be free of immunosuppressive signals that are abundant within tumors. In a study by Hunder et al., patients with metastatic melanoma showed durable clinical responses when infused with *in vitro* expanded CD4 T cells specific for the tumor-associated antigen (TAA) NY-ESO-1 (Hunder et al., 2008). This class of antigen is termed cancer testis antigen (CT, described in greater details below). While there is an ongoing effort to extend this technique to treat a variety of cancers, the lack of precise antigen mapping of the expanded TILs can be problematic since a considerable number of T-cell clones will not recognize the tumor (Hinrichs & Rosenberg, 2014). Recently, TIL product has been shown to recognize mutational neoepitopes, indicating both the potential and complexity of this approach (Tran et al., 2014). The extraction of enough material for the expansion of sufficient effector T cells sometimes poses a technical burden (Svane & Verdegaal, 2014), as can the toxicities of lymphodepletion which is needed to allow for homeostatic expansion of the infused cells.

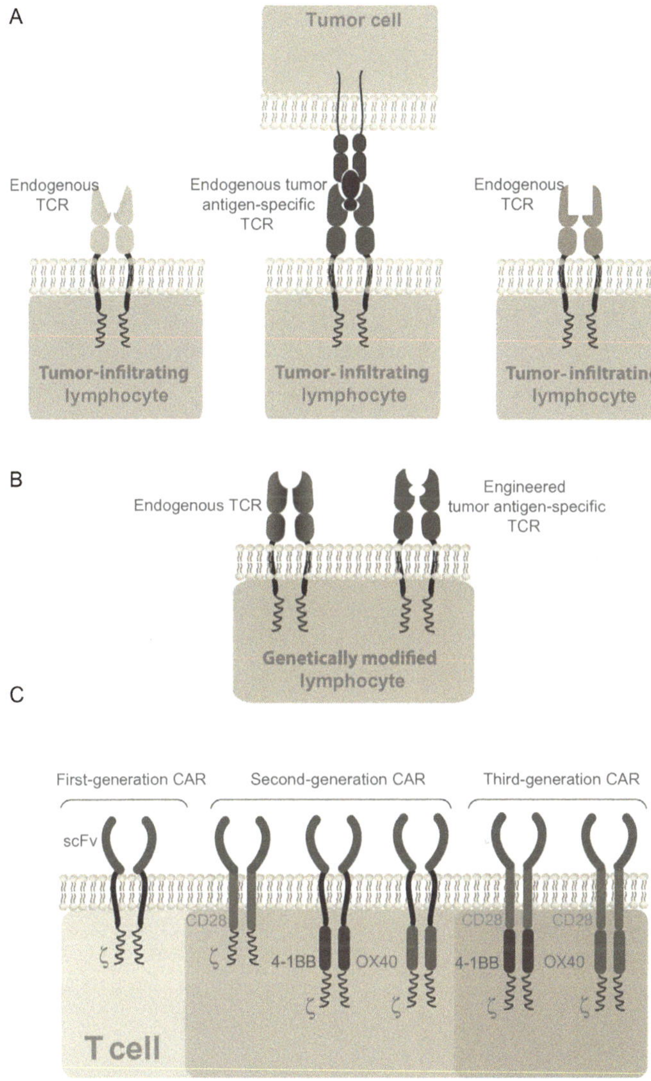

Figure 2 Evolution of cell-based immunotherapy: (A) TIL therapy in which patients are treated with T cells harvested and subsequently expanded from resected malignant tissue. In a more recent manifestation of this approach, tumor antigen-specific T cells are selectively enriched prior to infusion. (B) T cells genetically modified to express TCRs known to be antigen specific. (C) Three generations of CAR technology. Activation is stimulated by the binding of scFv on CAR T cells to their cognate antigen on the surface of antigen-expressing cells. First-generation CARs rely on a chimeric CD3 ζ chain to activate intracellular signaling. Subsequent generation CAR technology incorporates specific domains of 4-1BB, OX40, and CD28 chimeras either alone (second generation) or in combination (third generation) to augment signaling. From PMID: 23550147. (See the color plate.)

3.2 Transgenic TCRs

To overcome the possibility of expanding nonspecific T-cell clones, the ectopic expression of a known antitumor TCR has been explored (Hinrichs & Rosenberg, 2014). Using this approach, naive T cells purified from peripheral blood are expanded using anti-CD3 and anti-CD28 antibodies in the setting of specific growth factors. The proliferating lymphocytes are then transduced with a retrovirus or a lentivirus encoding α and β chains of a high-avidity TCR against a tumor antigen (Hughes et al., 2005; Morgan et al., 2006, 2003). The avidity of these TCRs can be further enhanced by *in vitro* mutagenesis techniques and further selection with phage display technology (Kershaw, Westwood, Slaney, & Darcy, 2014).

Both clinical and preclinical studies have demonstrated the efficacy of ACT-based immunotherapies. For example, it has been shown that long-term regression of metastatic melanoma lesions can be achieved in patients receiving autologous lymphocytes transduced with a retroviral vector expressing TCR for the melanoma antigen MART1 (Morgan et al., 2006). While ACT holds great promise, there are important caveats. It is possible that mismatched pairing of the transferred TCR α and β chains with the endogenous TCRs will occur in some cases, resulting in chimeric TCRs that are inert or that can cross-react with self-antigen (Kuball et al., 2007; Stanislawski et al., 2001; Voss et al., 2006). This can be partially overcome by using mouse TCR constant regions or by adding cysteine residues at specific sites to ensure precise pairing of the transferred TCRs (Kuball et al., 2007). A second potential challenge in this area is that the efficacy of transferred TCRs is dependent on antigen being processed and presented on MHC molecules within the tumor (Rosenberg et al., 2008; Sadelain, Rivière, & Brentjens, 2003).

3.3 CAR Therapy

MHC restriction can be circumvented with chimeric antigen receptor (CAR) T cells (Ho, Blattman, Dossett, Yee, & Greenberg, 2003; Sadelain et al., 2003). Pioneered by Zelig Eshhar and then further refined by the groups of June and Sadelain, CARs consist of a single-chain variable antibody fragment (scFv) that recognizes a tumor-specific antigen (TSA) and is genetically fused to the transmembrane region of the TCR signaling domain (CD3). This CAR construct is transduced into T cells purified from peripheral blood (Kershaw, Westwood, & Darcy, 2013). Once a CAR-modified T cell engages the antigen, the activated T cells will mediate tumor cell lysis. CAR technology has evolved significantly since its inception. Originally, CARs signaled through a lone CD3 signaling domain, which resulted in suboptimal activation and *in vivo* persistence (Kershaw et al., 2013). Second-generation CARs contain sequences from costimulatory molecules such as CD28, 4-1BB, or OX40 (Finney, Akbar, & Lawson, 2004; Hombach & Abken, 2011; Hombach et al., 2001). Third-generation CARs contain a combination of two or more signaling domains (typically CD28 and 4-1BB). Clinical protocols thus far have focused largely on targeting CD19, a protein expressed on B cells and B-cell malignancies (Brentjens et al., 2011; Kalos et al., 2011; Kochenderfer et al., 2012; Kochenderfer, Yu, Frasheri, Restifo, & Rosenberg, 2010). Patients infused with CD19 CAR T cells containing an intracellular 4-1BB signaling domain have achieved striking durable remissions (Kalos et al., 2011; Porter, Levine, Kalos, Bagg, & June, 2011). Comparable results have also been observed when the CD19-specific CARs contain a CD28 signaling domain (Brentjens et al., 2011; Kochenderfer et al., 2012, 2010; Patel, Dale, Vartabedian, Dey, & Selvaraj, 2014; Savoldo et al., 2011). The optimal intracellular signaling domain for use in this setting remains unclear.

An important consideration in adoptive T-cell transfer strategies is the state of the host at the time of cell transfer. It is necessary to precondition the host in order to allow T cells to achieve optimal antitumor properties (Gattinoni, Powell, Rosenberg, & Restifo, 2006; Gilham, 2011). Host preconditioning consists of whole-body irradiation and/or chemotherapy (Gattinoni et al., 2006). Given that the tumor microenvironment can be highly immunosuppressive, the potency of transferred T cells can be reduced as they approach the tumor. Preconditioning regimens can eliminate suppressive cellular components such as Tregs and MDSCs (Bronte & Zanovello, 2005; Gattinoni et al., 2006; North, 1982). In addition, lymphodepletion promotes homeostatic proliferation that can expand transferred T cells (Dudley et al., 2002, 2005; Gattinoni et al., 2006). Lastly, radiation and chemotherapy can directly lyse malignant cells releasing both tumor antigens and damage-associated molecular pattern molecules (DAMPs) which serve in turn to facilitate the priming of transferred T cells (Russo et al., 2000; Zhang, Louboutin, Zhu, Rivera, & Emerson, 2002).

The quality and quantity of the transferred cells themselves have a profound effect on antitumor activity. T cells with a central memory phenotype characterized by expression of CCR7, CD27, CD28, and CD62L appear more effective than terminally differentiated T cells that do not express these markers (Krummel & Allison, 1995). This may be due to the fact that memory T cells have greater pluripotency and replicative capacity than the more terminally differentiated CTL. In fact, dedifferentiated T cells exhibit greater engraftment, persistence, and antitumor activity as compared to more terminally differentiated T cells (Klebanoff, Gattinoni, & Restifo, 2012). There is thus great interest in increasing the number of tumor-reactive T cells with naive or even stem-like phenotypes. When tumor-reactive T cells are cultured in the presence of IL-21 instead of the more commonly used T-cell growth factor IL-2, the T cells retain a more naive phenotype with more robust antitumor properties (Hinrichs et al., 2008). With current technological advances in stem cell reprogramming, it is possible to redirect terminally differentiated T cells toward stem-like phenotypes. These T cells are capable of secreting the effector cytokine IFNγ when presented with cognate peptide; however, whether these cells can produce deep and durable responses remains an open question (Crompton, Sukumar, & Restifo, 2014). The T-cell dose is also a critical parameter in adoptive T-cell transfer. Intuitively, higher levels of T cells should provide superior antitumor efficacy. This has been the case in a mouse melanoma model where a direct correlation was found between the number of antigen-specific CD8 T cells transferred and the magnitude of tumor regression (Klebanoff et al., 2011). However, in a different model, larger numbers of transferred T cells actually impaired antitumor activity (Rizzuto et al., 2009). This observation is at least partially attributable to intraclonal competition among transferred T cells that prevents adequate T-cell priming (Rizzuto et al., 2009). Future studies are expected to clarify optimal precursor frequency in the setting of adoptive transfer protocols.

A key aspect in the design of adoptive transfer strategies is the selection of antigens to be targeted (Finn, 2008; Gilboa, 1999; Palucka & Banchereau, 2012; Parmiani, De Filippo, Novellino, & Castelli, 2007). Tumor antigens can be divided into two categories: TSAs and TAAs. TSAs are molecules that are expressed exclusively by tumor cells as a result of genomic mutations or viral infection (Finn, 2008; Novellino, Castelli, & Parmiani, 2005). TAAs are proteins expressed at higher levels in malignant cells than in benign cells. TAAs include tissue differentiation antigens and CT antigens. CT antigens frequently map to the X-chromosome and are primarily expressed in the male testis and occasionally in the ovary and trophoblast. Such sites are considered immune-privileged as they are not typically exposed to immune surveillance and thus are not subject to full immune tolerance. CT antigens, when aberrantly expressed in genetically unstable tumors, are thus attractive targets for immunologic intervention. Examples of CT antigens include

NY-ESO-1, MAGE-A, and SSX. In addition to targeting the tumor directly, targeting malignant stroma including tumor vasculature with transferred T cells may increase the therapeutic potential of ACT (Kakarla et al., 2013; Schuberth et al., 2013; Smith et al., 2013; Tran et al., 2013). While malignant cells can rapidly evolve owing to their genetic instability, and ability to downregulate antigens under selective pressure, nonmalignant tissues are thought to be more stable and thus susceptible to persistent immunologic attack. In fact, T cells redirected against stromal antigens have shown potent antitumor effects when transferred alone or in combination with T cells that target tumor antigens (Chinnasamy et al., 2012; Prewett et al., 1999; Shrimali et al., 2010; Tong et al., 2004).

It is important to keep in mind that transferred T cells are typically subject to the same immune suppressive mechanisms that allow the tumor to evade destruction by immune surveillance. Many tumors are highly infiltrated with suppressive cells such as regulatory T cells (Tregs), MDSCs, and so-called M2 suppressive macrophages. In addition, tumors cells and the associated stroma can express inhibitory molecules such as PD-L1, FAS, or TGF-β that can kill or inhibit transferred cells (Arina et al., 2014). One advantage of adoptive transfer protocols is that T cells can be manipulated *ex vivo* and strategies to overcome tumor-induced immune suppression can be directly engineered into them. IL-12-secreting CARs, for example, show increase resistance to suppression and retain a central memory-effector phenotype (Chmielewski, Hombach, & Abken, 2014; Pegram et al., 2012). Examples include the development of rapamycin-resistant effector T cells (T-Rapa) associated with increased effector function and antitumor activity (Easton & Houghton, 2006; Huye et al., 2011), and T cells engineered to express homing chemokine receptors such as CCR4 and/or CXCR2 exhibiting increased tumor infiltration (Di Stasi et al., 2009; Fisher et al., 2006; Griffith, Sokol, & Luster, 2014).

One major concern regarding ACT is the significant toxicities associated with this treatment. Such toxicities include the immune-related damage of off-target tissues and the marked systemic release of proinflammatory cytokines (Morgan et al., 2010; Tey, 2014), sometimes resulting in a clinical picture that resembles the graft-versus-host disease (Collins et al., 1997; Drobyski et al., 1993; Tey, 2014). In an effort to augment CAR specificity, T cells have been engineered to initiate TCR signaling only in the presence of two distinct antigens expressed on the target cell using so-called "AND logic" (Cordoba, Kong, & Pule, 2014). Another concern is that transferred cells themselves have malignant potential. Therefore, strategies that can limit the potency and longevity of transferred T cells are of interest. Modifying T cells to express a so-called suicide gene can increase their safety profile and facilitate their clinical development. Suicide genes such as herpes simplex thymidine kinase for use with ganciclovir are in clinical development (Bonini et al., 1997; Ciceri et al., 2009; Tiberghien et al., 2001, 1994). An important caveat, however, is that genes of this type are potentially immunogenic and thus may trigger an anti-T-cell immune response (Berger, Flowers, Warren, & Riddell, 2006). Strategies that induce the expression of endogenous apoptotic machinery such as FAS or caspase-9, however, may be a viable alternative (Di Stasi et al., 2011; Thomis et al., 2001). In one approach, the intracellular domain of caspase-9 is fused to chemical inducers of dimerization that can be triggered to eliminate engineered T cells (Clackson et al., 1998; Spencer, Wandless, Schreiber, & Crabtree, 1993). Transferred T cells have also been designed to express CD20 (Introna et al., 2000; Serafini, Bonamino, Golay, & Introna, 2004; Serafini et al., 2004), so that they can be eliminated with the therapeutic anti-CD20 mAb rituximab (Serafini, Bonamino, Golay, & Introna, 2004; Serafini, Manganini, et al., 2004), although in this case healthy B cells expressing CD20 would also be targeted (Rossig & Brenner, 2004).

The key distinguishing feature of ACT is that it relies on administering intact living cells to enhance the endogenous immune repertoire. This presents an enormous opportunity not only to directly and specifically kill cancer cells but also to control the tumor microenvironment with unprecedented flexibility. Transferred cells can be engineered to express a number of intracellular, membrane-bound, and secreted proteins. Such engineered cells can therefore, in principle, overcome elements in the microenvironment and on malignant cells that allow tumors to grow and persist.

4. SMALL MOLECULES FOR IMMUNE MODULATION

Aside from immunomodulation with mAbs and adoptive cell transfer, small-molecule inhibitors play a growing role mediating antitumor immune activity. Such small molecules target enzymes directly involved in immune regulation such as indoleamine 2,3-dioxygenase (IDO). Other small molecules that were initially designed to inhibit major oncogenic pathways such as the MAP kinase pathway are now recognized as playing an important role in immune modulation. The use of these inhibitors to modulate the immune response is currently under investigation in many cancer types as well as in inflammatory and autoimmune disease. In this section, we review some recent progress in the development of such "small-molecule immunomodulators" focusing on IDO, RAF, PI3K, and mTOR (mammalian target of rapamycin) inhibitors.

4.1 Indoleamine 2,3-Dioxygenase

In addition to the expression of ligands that directly inhibit T cells, some tumors exert immune suppression through depletion of essential metabolites, mediated by upregulation of enzymes such as IDO (Munn & Mellor, 2004). IDO inhibits immune responses through several mechanisms, including depletion of the essential amino acid tryptophan and the production of kynurenine, which binds the aryl hydrocarbon receptor and promotes Treg differentiation (Munn & Mellor, 2013). IDO is expressed by many cancer types, and abnormal levels of IDO have been correlated with poor prognosis (Munn, 2011). IDO expression in preclinical models prevents tumor rejection, and correspondingly, blockade of IDO activity can be immune-potentiating *in vivo* (Liu et al., 2010; Uyttenhove et al., 2003).

Inhibition of IDO is being pursued using various small-molecule inhibitors. Three potent small-molecule IDO inhibitors are in clinical development: indoximod (Soliman et al., 2012), NLG-919, and INCB024360 (Newton et al., 2012). Indoximod and INCB024360 have progressed through phase I clinical testing and biologically active doses that improve the tryptophan/kynurenine ratio have been established. Phase II single-agent studies have been initiated with both compounds. NLG-919 is currently in phase I trials (NCT02048709).

Preclinical combination studies with small-molecule inhibitors of IDO appear promising. It has previously been demonstrated that upregulation of IDO in the tumor microenvironment is a possible mechanism of resistance to anti-CTLA-4 immunotherapy (Holmgaard, Zamarin, Munn, Wolchok, & Allison, 2013; Spranger et al., 2014). Combination of IDO inhibitors with CTLA-4-blocking antibodies resulted in significant enhancement of therapeutic efficacy in different murine tumor models, an effect that was associated with significant increases in tumor-infiltrating CD8 T cells (Holmgaard et al., 2013; Spranger et al., 2014). Preliminary data from our laboratory have indicated that IDO inhibition combined with anti-PD-1/PD-L1 mAbs can also lead to potent immune-mediated tumor control *in vivo* (unpublished data). Evaluation of combinations of IDO inhibitors and CTLA-4 blockade is currently being pursued in clinical trials, with preliminary data showing activity of the combination in patients with metastatic melanoma (Gibney et al., 2014). Similar studies have demonstrated that IDO inhibitors display synergy with chemotherapeutic drugs, including cyclophosphamide, doxorubicin, paclitaxel, cisplatin, and gemcitabine (Hou et al., 2007; Muller, DuHadaway, Donover, Sutanto-Ward, & Prendergast, 2005). Phase I and II clinical trials with IDO inhibitors and either docetaxel or paclitaxel are currently ongoing (NCT01792050). Finally, preclinical studies have shown that responses to therapeutic vaccination could be significantly enhanced by concurrent administration of IDO inhibitors (Sharma et al., 2010, 2009). Thus, the fact that IDO inhibitors are synergistic with multiple therapeutic agents and in multiple different tumor types suggests that IDO plays a fundamental and broadly applicable biological role in helping suppress the host antitumor immune response following cancer therapy.

4.2 PI3 Kinase

PI3Ks are crucial coordinators of intracellular signaling in response to various extracellular stimuli. The many downstream pathways regulated by this lipid kinase family control diverse physiological functions and cellular processes including cell proliferation, growth, differentiation, survival, motility, and metabolism (Vanhaesebroeck, Guillermet-Guibert, Graupera, & Bilanges, 2010). These processes are critical not only for cancer development—PI3K is one of the most commonly mutated oncogenes in human cancer—but also for the function of normal cells including immune cells (Thorpe, Yuzugullu, & Zhao, 2015). In vertebrate genomes there are eight catalytic PI3K subunits divided into three classes based on sequence homology and domain structure. Each isoform has been implicated in different immune functions (Okkenhaug, 2013). Over the past decade, multiple studies leveraging pharmacologic inhibition or specific genetic deletion of signaling components in the PI3K pathway have contributed to a deep understanding of the individual functions of the PI3K catalytic and regulatory subunits as well as the selectivity of such isoform activity among different cell types. These findings have yielded the development of highly specific PI3K inhibitors (Fruman & Rommel, 2014).

Early development of nonselective, pan-PI3K inhibitors, in clinical trials was disappointing and highlighted the complexities of this pathway.

Nonselective inhibition of the PI3K pathway can either suppress or enhance immune responses depending on its effects on diverse subsets of innate and adaptive immune cells. The emergence of isoform-specific PI3K inhibitors has been met with great anticipation, driven by the recent therapeutic success of a p110δ-selective inhibitor, idelalisib (GS1101, CAL101) in relapsed chronic lymphocytic leukemia (Furman et al., 2014). Interestingly, in this setting the PI3K pathway is not mutationally activated but rather relays signals from the tumor microenvironment that are critical for tumor maintenance (Vanhaesebroeck & Khwaja, 2014).

Recent studies have evaluated the impact of isoform-specific inhibitors in the immune microenvironment of solid tumors. By studying the role of chemoattractant signals produced in tumor, Schmid et al. have shown that various inflammatory signals are transduced by a single PI3K γ isoform in myeloid cells, which control the expression of the α4β1 integrin promoting the recruitment of these cells in the tumor (Schmid Michael et al., 2011). Specific p110γ isoform inhibitors were able to suppress myeloid cell recruitment, angiogenesis, tumor inflammation, and progression without affecting the tumor cells directly. Similarly, by using genetic mouse models of p110γ−/− and pan-PI3K inhibitors, Joshi et al. demonstrate that a macrophage-dominant PI3K isoform (p110γ) also directs tumor growth, angiogenesis, metastasis, and the HIFa/VEGF axis in mice tumor models (Joshi, Singh, Zulcic, & Durden, 2014). Two other studies indicated that inhibition of the class I PI3K delta isoform (p110δ) impaired tumor growth by disrupting immune tolerance mediated by Tregs and MDSCs. In PI3K δ-deficient mice, it has been shown that the impairment of growth in a range of solid tumors is mediated by restoring the balance of Treg/CTLs in favor of cytotoxicity by blocking Treg immunosuppressive activity (Ali et al., 2014). In addition, prolonged survival in a spontaneous pancreatic tumor model was demonstrated by pharmacologically inhibiting PI3Kδ, which suppresses Treg activity and promotes CD8 T-cell accumulation in the pancreas. Abu-Eid et al. obtained similar results using PI3K-Akt inhibitors in various tumor models (Abu-Eid et al., 2014). Interestingly, the combination of the inhibitor with the E7 vaccine was able to enhance the vaccine induced immune control in a TC-1 tumor model, showing that the combined strategy of PI3K inhibition with other immunotherapeutic approaches may act synergistically. Along these lines, synergistic antitumor activity has been observed by combining a class I PI3K inhibitor and the TLR5 ligand flagellin (Marshall et al., 2012).

These findings emphasize the potential therapeutic effect of PI3K inhibitors as immunomodulatory agents. Among the wide range of drugs that target PI3K, the specific inhibitors for p110 δ and p110 γ seem to have the strongest immuotherapeutic effect as these PI3K isoforms are expressed selectively in myeloid and lymphoid cell subsets. Ultimately clinical trials will determine whether PI3K inhibition can augment antitumor immunotherapy, and we anticipate that such trials will be forthcoming in the future.

4.3 Mammalian Target of Rapamycin

mTOR is a protein kinase in the PI3K/Akt signaling pathway. Activation of mTOR in response to growth signals leads to an increase in protein synthesis and tumor development (Laplante & Sabatini, 2012). Consequently, mTOR inhibitors are currently extensively used for the treatment of various cancers (Chiarini, Evangelisti, McCubrey, & Martelli, 2014). Sirolimus derivatives (rapalogs) such as everolimus and temsirolimus are approved for the treatment of renal cell carcinoma (Chiarini et al., 2014). Temsirolimus is also approved for the treatment of mantle-cell lymphoma. More recently, everolimus combined with hormonal therapy was approved for the treatment of metastatic breast cancer (Chia et al., 2015). The mTOR protein complex is emerging as an important integrator of environmental cues critical for activation, differentiation, and function of immune cells (Powell, Pollizzi, Heikamp, & Horton, 2012). The reprogramming of T-cell metabolism is mediated by various environmental signals converging on mTOR complex 1 and 2 and fine-tuning of this pathway regulates T-cell differentiation (Pollizzi & Powell, 2015). Further studies have demonstrated the critical link between metabolic demands and cellular function in diverse immune cells, including neutrophils, mast cells, natural killer cells, γδ T cells, macrophages, DCs, and B cells (Thomson, Turnquist, & Raimondi, 2009; Weichhart & Säemann, 2009).

Interestingly, the mTOR inhibitors, which were previously developed as immunosuppressive drugs, could paradoxically promote some immune functions and antitumor immunity in mouse models. Treatment with rapamycin enhances CD8 T-cell memory and recall responses against virus and tumor after vaccination (Araki et al., 2009; Li et al., 2012; Pearce et al., 2009). The therapeutic potential of promoting memory responses with mTOR inhibitors was also demonstrated in murine studies using antigen-specific transgenic CD8 T-cells adoptively transferred into tumor-bearing mice, where the use of rapamycin enhanced the antitumor activity by inducing the proliferation of effector CD8 T cells (Rao, Li, Odunsi, & Shrikant, 2010). In another study, the combination of rapamycin with autologous DCs treated with TLR agonists resulted in improved generation of Ag-specific CD8 T cells *in vivo* and enhanced antitumor immunity (Amiel et al., 2012). These findings suggest that mTOR inhibitors could have context-dependent effects on T cells. Nonetheless, given the broad distribution of the target, the use of mTOR inhibitors to modulate the immune system could be complicated by undesirable immune (Marçais et al., 2014) and nonimmune adverse effects.

4.4 BRAF

BRAF inhibitors, such as vemurafenib and debrafenib, target tumors harboring the BRAF V600 mutations. These agents have shown significant clinical benefit in patients with advanced melanoma and other cancers. However, a significant drawback of such targeted therapy is that the durability of clinical responses remains limited. There is, however, emerging evidence that in addition to direct effects against cancer cells, BRAF inhibitors can affect the antitumor immune response raising hopes that in the future such therapy may be integrating into an immunomodulatory treatment regimen capable of imparting durable responses. One important feature of BRAF inhibitors is their ability to paradoxically stimulate wild-type BRAF (Callahan et al., 2014; Hall-Jackson et al., 1999; Hatzivassiliou et al., 2010; Hoeflich et al., 2009; Joseph et al., 2010; Poulikakos, Zhang, Bollag, Shokat, & Rosen, 2010) in other tissues. Clinically, this manifests as the progression of squamous cell skin cancer, and other MAPK-driven malignancies among patients receiving BRAF inhibitors (Robert, Arnault, & Mateus, 2011; Su et al., 2012). Crucially, the MAPK pathway is also important in transducing signals upon TCR ligation. Accordingly, it has been observed that BRAF inhibitors stimulate such signaling in healthy T cells which harbor wild-type BRAF (Poulikakos et al., 2010). This has led to studies focusing on the effects of BRAF inhibitors on the immune system. The immunomodulatory activity of a pan-RAF inhibitor BMS908662 was evaluated *in vitro* using Jurkat cells, a human CD4 T-cell line. Compared to cells treated with vehicle, cells treated with the drug significantly upregulated activation maker CD69 and proliferation marker Ki67 in a dose-dependent manner. Moreover, murine CD4 T cells specific for the CT antigen NY-ESO-1 displayed an increase of IFNγ production when activated in the presence of RAF inhibitor (Callahan et al., 2014).

Our group has found that systemic treatment with a BRAF inhibitor leads to a significant increase in antigen-specific T cells, particularly in combination with CTLA-4 blockade. Furthermore, splenocytes harvested from mice treated with the same drug were shown to be more sensitive to stimulation *ex vivo* as demonstrated by an increase in the levels of phosphorylated-ERK (Callahan et al., 2014).

In patients, treatment with BRAF inhibition led to a significant increase in intratumoral CD8 and CD4 T cells (Frederick et al., 2013; Wargo et al., 2011; Wilmott et al., 2012). Levels of T-cell cytotoxicity markers (e.g., perforin, granzyme B) were also increased, correlating with tumor regression (Frederick et al., 2013; Wilmott et al., 2012). Further characterization of TILs revealed an increase in expression of exhaustion markers such as PD-1 upon BRAF inhibition (Frederick et al., 2013). These findings suggest that there may be a place in the clinic for BRAF inhibition together with checkpoint blockade. Such studies will need to be undertaken with great caution as we have found that BRAF inhibition together with CTLA-4 blockade can be associated with significant hepatotoxicity (Ribas, Hodi, Callahan, Konto, & Wolchok, 2013).

5. OTHER APPROACHES

5.1 Radiotherapy and Immunomodulatory Effects of Radiation on Tumors

Radiation therapy is one of the most commonly used treatments for cancer. The abscopal effect, a phenomenon thought to be immune mediated in which local therapy is associated with the regression of distal cancer outside the site of treatment, has been observed with radiation therapy as a single modality; however, the frequency of this occurrence is exceedingly low (Siva, MacManus, Martin, & Martin, 2013). While radiation is generally thought to be immunosuppressive, there is evidence that radiation therapy can induce systemic changes in the immune system that are beneficial to cancer patients. Sublethal and lethal doses of radiation have been shown to induce immunogenic tumor cell death leading to a more robust immune response to tumor (Apetoh et al., 2007; Panaretakis et al., 2009). Radiation has been shown to upregulate the expression of calreticulin on the surface of dying tumor cells leading to better recognition and phagocytosis of dead tumor cells by DCs. These dying tumor cells can also release molecules such as HMGB1, which acts as a "danger" signal to enhance DC maturation (Gameiro et al., 2014). In addition to directly killing tumor cells, radiation has been shown to induce expression of proteins important for antigen presentation such as MHC class I and ICAM-1 which allow the surviving tumor cells to be more visible to the immune system, thereby leading to better elimination by cytotoxic CD8 T cells (Gameiro et al., 2014). Finally, radiation has been shown to induce the expression of CXCL16 by tumor cells, a chemokine that can recruit activated CD4 and CD8 effector T cells to sites of inflammation (Matsumura et al., 2008).

5.2 Combination of Radiation Therapy with Immunotherapy

There is accumulating clinical evidence to support the combination of local radiation therapy and immunotherapy for the treatment of cancer. Recently, three clinical reports of the abscopal effect in melanoma patients who received immunotherapy (anti-CTLA-4, IL-2) and local radiation therapy have renewed interest in the abscopal effect of local radiation (Okwan-Duodu, Pollack, Lawson, & Khan, 2015; Postow et al., 2012; Stamell, Wolchok, Gnjatic, Lee, & Brownell, 2013). In the case report by Postow et al., a patient on ipilimumab (anti-CTLA-4) exhibited an increase in antibody responses to the CT antigen NY-ESO-1, an increase in the activation state of CD4 T cells (as measured by an increase in ICOS expression), and a decrease in the fraction of MDSCs in the peripheral blood after local radiation therapy. In the report documented by Stamell et al., a patient on ipilimumab exhibited an increase in antibody responses to MAGE-A3 and PASD1. In addition to these findings, there are many preclinical reports of the abscopal effect in mouse studies. There is a wide range of radiation schedules and doses (single ablative doses vs. fractionated doses) as well as categories of immunotherapies that have been used in combination and showed benefit. In a B16 melanoma model (Lee et al., 2009), a single dose of 15 Gy local radiation was shown to increase T-cell priming in draining lymph nodes and lead to regression of the primary tumor and distant metastasis in a CD8 T-cell-dependent manner. This effect was not observed when the radiation was fractionated (5 Gy × 4), suggesting insufficient priming of the immune response. Another study using a two-flank mouse breast carcinoma model showed that fractionated and not single doses of local radiation with anti-CTLA-4 therapy induces the abscopal effect. This effect was associated with an increase in tumor-specific CD8 T-cell responses. It appears from these studies that local radiation can induce a systemic antitumor response that, depending on dose and schedule, may lead to regression of primary tumors and distant metastases.

5.3 Oncolytic Viruses

Oncolytic viruses represent a class of anticancer agents that have been in development since the 1950s (Kelly & Russell, 2007). The primary mechanism of action of oncolytic viruses was traditionally thought to be their inherent ability to replicate within, and ultimately lyse, cancer cells while sparing normal cells. The promising therapeutic efficacy of such viruses was demonstrated by their ability to lyse human cancer cells in culture and cause regression of human tumor xenografts (Russell, Peng, & Bell, 2012). With these findings, multiple oncolytic viruses have entered the clinical arena over the past 60 years, though the clinical results have not been as impressive. The major limitation of oncolytic viruses is the rapid development of neutralizing antibodies by the host, which limits the viral delivery to metastatic cancer sites and the therapeutic effect (Russell et al., 2012). Interestingly, with intravenous administration, in the few patients that did achieve response to oncolytic virotherapy, the observed clinical benefit was often durable even after completion of therapy, which suggested the involvement of an antitumor immune response (Lorence et al., 2007). With an evolving understanding of the interplay between oncolytic viruses and the immune system came the recognition that the virus-induced antitumor immune response, rather than direct tumor lysis, may be a dominant factor driving the efficacy of these therapies (Lichty, Breitbach, Stojdl, & Bell, 2014; Zamarin & Wolchok, 2014).

This immune phenomenon was recognized early on by some investigators, prompting evaluation of oncolytic viruses as immunotherapeutic rather than lytic agents. In the 1960s, Lindenmann and colleagues noted that infection of tumor cells with influenza virus increased immune responses directed toward tumor cell antigens (Lindenmann & Klein, 1967). Since then, multiple studies have demonstrated that in addition to tumor lysis, oncolytic viruses can potently activate innate immune responses in tumor cells and tumor-infiltrating APCs (Guo, Liu, & Bartlett, 2014). Activation of the antitumor immune response by oncolytic viruses proceeds through several mechanisms, all of which likely act in concert. First, direct infection of tumor cells activates innate immune signaling pathways, resulting in secretion of inflammatory mediators such as IFN-α, and upregulation of MHC, cell adhesion proteins, and costimulatory molecules

(Plitt & Zamarin, 2015). These inflammatory changes result in reversal of immune inhibition within the tumor microenvironment. *Ex vivo* studies demonstrated that TILs isolated from freshly resected melanomas do not proliferate when stimulated with autologous melanoma cells; however, proliferation can be restored when TILs are stimulated with autologous melanoma cells infected with the Newcastle disease virus (NDV) (Termeer, Schirrmacher, Bröcker, & Becker, 2000). Second, the mechanisms of tumor cell killing, which include immunogenic apoptosis, necrosis, and autophagy, have been described as associated with immunogenic cell death and result in the release of TAAs and DAMPs, which promote activation of tumor-infiltrating professional APCs (Guo et al., 2014). Finally, direct infection of tumor-infiltrating DCs and the inflammatory mediators secreted by the infected tumor cells promote DC activation and maturation (Melcher, Parato, Rooney, & Bell, 2011).

Taken together, the infection of tumor cells and the associated APCs produce a vaccination event, which creates conditions necessary for optimal T-cell priming in the setting of proinflammatory mediators. Several studies also demonstrate that infection with oncolytic viruses leads to inhibition of the suppressive cell populations in the tumors, such as Tregs and MDSCs (Fournier, Arnold, Wilden, & Schirrmacher, 2012; Kaufman et al., 2010; Ni, Galani, Cerwenka, Schirrmacher, & Fournier, 2011; Zamarin et al., 2014). Early recognition of such properties prompted evaluation of oncolytic viruses as vaccines. Perhaps the best-documented early examples of this are the studies with NDV in the 1970s, where autologous and allogeneic NDV-infected lysed melanoma cells were used to vaccinate patients with resected melanoma in the adjuvant setting. In these studies, an unprecedented 60% 10-year recurrence-free survival was reported (Batliwalla et al., 1998; Cassel & Murray, 1988, 1992). Similar studies, including those utilizing vaccinia oncolysates (Wallack et al., 1997), demonstrated evidence of clinical benefit in patients with melanoma, colorectal, breast, ovarian, and kidney cancer, as well as glioblastoma (Schirrmacher & Fournier, 2009; Zamarin & Palese, 2012).

With the advent of genetic engineering of oncolytic viruses, several studies explored whether modulation of the tumor microenvironment through expression of immunostimulatory ligands or cytokines could potentiate the antitumor efficacy of oncolytic viruses. For example, expression of the ligands of TNF receptor superfamily such as OX40L, 4-1BBL, and GITRL by has been demonstrated to enhance the efficacy of adenovirus and vaccinia vectors delivered intratumorally (Andarini et al., 2004; Calmels et al., 2005;

Kim, Kim-Schulze, Kim, & Kaufman, 2009). Most of the studies demonstrated that such viruses could induce stronger infiltration of immune cells into the virus-injected tumors; however, the question remained whether this was merely a reflection of an enhanced antiviral immune response and whether this would translate into a more effective systemic antitumor immunity. The latter is favored by the studies of talimogene laherparepvec (T-VEC), an oncolytic herpes simplex virus encoding GM-CSF. Intralesional administration of the virus to patients with advanced melanoma led to increase in TILs and therapeutic responses not only in the injected lesions but also at distant sites (Andtbacka et al., 2013; Kaufman et al., 2010, 2014). In a similar study, intratumoral injection of another oncolytic virus, coxsackievirus A21, in patients with melanoma similarly demonstrated responses in distant lesions (Andtbacka et al., 2014).

The data using intralesionally administered oncolytic viruses indicate that the limitations of systemic administration can perhaps be overcome by focusing on the immune-activating, rather than lytic properties of the viruses, as a significant part of therapeutic response is driven by the immune system (Andtbacka et al., 2014; Kaufman et al., 2014). These findings would argue that having an accessible tumor lesion for an "*in situ* vaccination" with an oncolytic virus should be sufficient to initiate an antitumor immune response, which could perhaps be further driven through the use of combinatorial strategies with other systemic immunotherapeutic agents such as immunomodulatory antibodies. To formally explore this possibility, oncolytic NDV was evaluated in animal models bearing bilateral flank tumors, with the virus administered intratumorally into a single site in combination with systemic CTLA-4 blockade (Zamarin et al., 2014). Such combination led to rejection of both virus-injected and contralateral tumors, with long-term survival in the majority of the animals, an effect that was dependent on NK cells, CD8 T cells, and type I and II IFNs. Importantly, the success of therapy was seen in several tumor models, independently of tumor cell line sensitivity to NDV-mediated lysis, highlighting the importance of the virus-induced antitumor immunity rather than direct oncolysis in the observed therapeutic efficacy (Zamarin et al., 2014). A similar study using systemic agonistic anti-GITR antibody together with intratumoral administration of adenovirus expressing IFNα also resulted in synergistic inhibition of the virus-injected and distant tumors (Aida et al., 2014). Taken together, these studies thus provide a strong rationale for further evaluation of oncolytic viruses as potentiators of immunotherapy with agents targeting immune costimulatory or coinhibitory receptors. These studies are currently underway both in animal models and in the clinic. Preliminary results evaluating the oncolytic T-VEC given intralesionally in combination with systemic anti-CTLA4 (ipilimumab) in 18 patients with advanced melanoma demonstrated promising activity with an objective response rate of 41% (Puzanov et al., 2014). While early, these results provide a clinical validation of the data seen in animal models.

These findings, while encouraging, generate multiple further questions. First, since most oncolytic viruses have not been compared head to head, it is difficult to make any conclusions regarding superiority of one virus over another, especially in clinical setting. In addition, it is unclear whether different viruses may be more suitable for different cancer types or different routes of delivery. The situation becomes even more complex with genetically engineered viruses expressing cytokines and other immunostimulatory proteins, as the immune responses to these ligands in the setting of tumor infection by the virus cannot be reliably predicted based on their known biology. Finally, it is also unclear whether certain viruses will demonstrate better synergy with systemic immunomodulatory antibodies and whether the combined therapies have a lesser or greater chances for toxicity. There is emerging evidence that such combination strategies may translate into therapeutic benefit where either therapy is ineffective alone; thus, understanding the interplay between the immune system and viral oncolysis will be crucial for rational engineering of oncolytic viruses and the development of appropriate combinatorial strategies.

6. CONCLUSION

The record of success for cancer immunotherapy has grown rapidly over the past several years as patients with a broad spectrum of malignancies have now benefited from such therapy. It is important to keep in mind, however, that the promise of cancer immunotherapy extends beyond what is immediately suggested by a review of the history up to this point. For example, recruiting the immune system to treat malignancies, as opposed to directly targeting cancer cells with drugs, carries with it the potential to stimulate immunological memory. Engaging a memory response that can develop with an evolving tumor may be the reason that durable responses occur in a significant fraction of patients. In fact, given that many of the most promising immunotherapy approaches have only entered clinical development recently, we have yet to obtain a full sense of how durable responses to most of these agents can be. Furthermore, unlike targeted cancer therapy, immunotherapy is not inherently disease specific. While certain cancers clearly respond better than others to current immunotherapy, and the proper place of biomarker screening to identify the ideal candidates for immunotherapy remains an open question, targeting healthy immune cells rather than malignant cells leaves open the possibility that such immunotherapy can be applied to an ever-expanding set of malignancies.

This raises a crucial point: the immunotherapy community is only at the first stage of testing rational drug combinations. Notwithstanding the robust activity found with dual immune checkpoint inhibition in melanoma (Wolchok, Kluger, et al., 2013), we still know relatively little about how broadly this therapy can be applied, and even less about other immunotherapy combinations. There are innumerable potential ways to combine the types of immunotherapy discussed in this review, including combinations of drug therapies and cellular therapies. Going forward, we may also discover that many previously studied approaches, including many types of therapeutic cancer vaccines that were previously deemed ineffective, may return to the forefront of active investigation in combination with contemporary approaches to immune modulation. Along these lines, we expect that in the future, immunotherapy will be combined with conventional cancer therapies in ways that cannot yet be completely anticipated. There are suggestions in the literature that immunotherapy can be effectively used with radiation therapy (Postow et al., 2012), surgery (Eggermont et al., 2014), cytotoxic chemotherapy (Hirschhorn-Cymerman et al., 2009), inhibitory small molecules (Puzanov et al., 2014), and tumor antigen-targeting mAbs (Westin et al., 2014).

As with any advance in science or medicine, progress in the field of immunotherapy brings with it a new set of challenges. For example, it has been suggested that some tumors may be able to exclude T-cell infiltration altogether (Kraman et al., 2010). Obviously, in such cases manipulating T-cell stimulation alone would not be expected to yield antitumor activity. Nevertheless, significant efforts to address this and related challenges are already underway and while it is impossible to predict precisely where the field will lead, we can be confident that future progress will be marked the same way that it has been in the past: with an ever-increasing number of cancer patients whose disease burden has been lessened and whose life has been extended.

ACKNOWLEDGMENTS

We are grateful for the support of Peter and Deborah Weinberg, the Frederick Adler Fund, the National Institutes of Health, Swim across America, the Ludwig Trust, the Melanoma Research Alliance, the Stand Up To Cancer–Cancer Research Institute Immunotherapy Dream Team, the Hazen Polsky Foundation, the STARR Cancer Consortium, and the Harry J. Lloyd Charitable Trust.

REFERENCES

Abu-Eid, R., Samara, R. N., Ozbun, L., Abdalla, M. Y., Berzofsky, J. A., Friedman, K. M., et al. (2014). Selective inhibition of regulatory T cells by targeting the PI3K–Akt pathway. *Cancer Immunology Research*, *2*(11), 1080–1089.

Ahmadzadeh, M., Johnson, L. A., Heemskerk, B., Wunderlich, J. R., Dudley, M. E., White, D. E., et al. (2009). Tumor antigen-specific CD8 T cells infiltrating the tumor express high levels of PD-1 and are functionally impaired. *Blood*, *114*(8), 1537–1544.

Aida, K., Miyakawa, R., Suzuki, K., Narumi, K., Udagawa, T., Yamamoto, Y., et al. (2014). Suppression of Tregs by anti-glucocorticoid induced TNF receptor antibody enhances the antitumor immunity of interferon-α gene therapy for pancreatic cancer. *Cancer Science*, *105*(2), 159–167.

Ali, K., Soond, D. R., Piñeiro, R., Hagemann, T., Pearce, W., Lim, E. L., et al. (2014). Inactivation of PI (3) K p110 [dgr] breaks regulatory T-cell-mediated immune tolerance to cancer. *Nature*, *510*(7505), 407–411.

Al-Shamkhani, A., Birkeland, M. L., Puklavec, M., Brown, M. H., James, W., & Barclay, A. N. (1996). OX40 is differentially expressed on activated rat and mouse T cells and is the sole receptor for the OX40 ligand. *European Journal of Immunology*, *26*(8), 1695–1699.

Amiel, E., Everts, B., Freitas, T. C., King, I. L., Curtis, J. D., Pearce, E. L., et al. (2012). Inhibition of mechanistic target of rapamycin promotes dendritic cell activation and enhances therapeutic autologous vaccination in mice. *The Journal of Immunology*, *189*(5), 2151–2158.

Andarini, S., Kikuchi, T., Nukiwa, M., Pradono, P., Suzuki, T., Ohkouchi, S., et al. (2004). Adenovirus vector-mediated in vivo gene transfer of OX40 ligand to tumor cells enhances antitumor immunity of tumor-bearing hosts. *Cancer Research*, *64*(9), 3281–3287.

Anderson, A. C., Anderson, D. E., Bregoli, L., Hastings, W. D., Kassam, N., Lei, C., et al. (2007). Promotion of tissue inflammation by the immune receptor Tim-3 expressed on innate immune cells. *Science*, *318*(5853), 1141–1143.

Andtbacka, R. H. I., Collichio, F. A., Amatruda, T., Senzer, N. N., Chesney, J., Delman, K. A., et al. (2013). OPTiM: A randomized phase III trial of talimogene laherparepvec (T-VEC) versus subcutaneous (SC) granulocyte-macrophage colony-stimulating factor (GM-CSF) for the treatment (tx) of unresected stage IIIB/C and IV melanoma. In *ASCO annual meeting proceedings 20 June 2013: LBA9008*.

Andtbacka, R., Curti, B., Kaufman, H., Daniels, G., Nemunaitis, J., Spitler, L., et al. (2014). CALM study: A phase II study of an intratumorally delivered oncolytic immunotherapeutic agent, coxsackievirus A21, in patients with stage IIIc and stage IV malignant melanoma. *Journal of Clinical Oncology*, *32*.

Ansell, S. M., Lesokhin, A. M., Borrello, I., Halwani, A., Scott, E. C., Gutierrez, M., et al. (2014). PD-1 blockade with nivolumab in relapsed or refractory Hodgkin's lymphoma. *New England Journal of Medicine*, *372*, 311–319.

Apetoh, L., Ghiringhelli, F., Tesniere, A., Obeid, M., Ortiz, C., Criollo, A., et al. (2007). Toll-like receptor 4-dependent contribution of the immune system to anticancer chemotherapy and radiotherapy. *Nature Medicine*, *13*(9), 1050–1059.
Araki, K., Turner, A. P., Shaffer, V. O., Gangappa, S., Keller, S. A., Bachmann, M. F., et al. (2009). mTOR regulates memory CD8 T-cell differentiation. *Nature*, *460*(7251), 108–112.
Arestides, R. S., He, H., Westlake, R. M., Chen, A. I., Sharpe, A. H., Perkins, D. L., et al. (2002). Costimulatory molecule OX40L is critical for both Th1 and Th2 responses in allergic inflammation. *European Journal of Immunology*, *32*(10), 2874–2880.
Arina, A., Schreiber, K., Binder, D. C., Karrison, T. G., Liu, R. B., & Schreiber, H. (2014). Adoptively transferred immune T cells eradicate established tumors despite cancer-induced immune suppression. *The Journal of Immunology*, *192*(3), 1286–1293.
Baitsch, L., Baumgaertner, P., Devêvre, E., Raghav, S. K., Legat, A., Barba, L., et al. (2011). Exhaustion of tumor-specific CD8+ T cells in metastases from melanoma patients. *The Journal of Clinical Investigation*, *121*(6), 2350.
Baixeras, E., Huard, B., Miossec, C., Jitsukawa, S., Martin, M., Hercend, T., et al. (1992). Characterization of the lymphocyte activation gene 3-encoded protein. A new ligand for human leukocyte antigen class II antigens. *The Journal of Experimental Medicine*, *176*(2), 327–337.
Bansal-Pakala, P., Halteman, B. S., Cheng, M. H., & Croft, M. (2004). Costimulation of CD8 T cell responses by OX40. *The Journal of Immunology*, *172*(8), 4821–4825.
Baroja, M. L., Vijayakrishnan, L., Bettelli, E., Darlington, P. J., Chau, T. A., Ling, V., et al. (2002). Inhibition of CTLA-4 function by the regulatory subunit of serine/threonine phosphatase 2A. *The Journal of Immunology*, *168*(10), 5070–5078.
Batliwalla, F. M., Bateman, B. A., Serrano, D., Murray, D., Macphail, S., Maino, V., et al. (1998). A 15-year follow-up of AJCC stage III malignant melanoma patients treated postsurgically with Newcastle disease virus (NDV) oncolysate and determination of alterations in the CD8 T cell repertoire. *Molecular Medicine*, *4*(12), 783.
Baum, P. R., Gayle, R., 3rd, Ramsdell, F., Srinivasan, S., Sorensen, R., Watson, M., et al. (1994). Molecular characterization of murine and human OX40/OX40 ligand systems: Identification of a human OX40 ligand as the HTLV-1-regulated protein gp34. *The EMBO Journal*, *13*(17), 3992.
Baumann, R., Yousefi, S., Simon, D., Russmann, S., Mueller, C., & Simon, H. (2004). Functional expression of CD134 by neutrophils. *European Journal of Immunology*, *34*(8), 2268–2275.
Berger, C., Flowers, M. E., Warren, E. H., & Riddell, S. R. (2006). Analysis of transgene-specific immune responses that limit the in vivo persistence of adoptively transferred HSV-TK-modified donor T cells after allogeneic hematopoietic cell transplantation. *Blood*, *107*(6), 2294–2302.
Beutner, K. R., Geisse, J. K., Helman, D., Fox, T. L., Ginkeld, A., & Owens, M. L. (1999). Therapeutic response of basal cell carcinoma to the immune response modifier imiquimod 5% cream. *Journal of the American Academy of Dermatology*, *41*(6), 1002–1007.
Bishop, G. A., Moore, C. R., Xie, P., Stunz, L. L., & Kraus, Z. J. (2007). TRAF proteins in CD40 signaling. *Advances in Experimental Medicine and Biology*, *597*, 131–151.
Blackburn, S. D., Shin, H., Haining, W. N., Zou, T., Workman, C. J., Polley, A., et al. (2009). Coregulation of CD8+ T cell exhaustion by multiple inhibitory receptors during chronic viral infection. *Nature Immunology*, *10*(1), 29–37.
Blank, C., Brown, I., Peterson, A. C., Spiotto, M., Iwai, Y., Honjo, T., et al. (2004). PD-L1/B7H-1 inhibits the effector phase of tumor rejection by T cell receptor (TCR) transgenic CD8+ T cells. *Cancer Research*, *64*(3), 1140–1145.
Bonini, C., Ferrari, G., Verzeletti, S., Servida, P., Zappone, E., Ruggieri, L., et al. (1997). HSV-TK gene transfer into donor lymphocytes for control of allogeneic graft-versus-leukemia. *Science*, *276*(5319), 1719–1724.

Brandau, S., & Suttmann, H. (2007). Thirty years of BCG immunotherapy for non-muscle invasive bladder cancer: A success story with room for improvement. *Biomedicine & Pharmacotherapy*, *61*(6), 299–305.
Brentjens, R. J., Rivière, I., Park, J. H., Davila, M. L., Wang, X., Stefanski, J., et al. (2011). Safety and persistence of adoptively transferred autologous CD19-targeted T cells in patients with relapsed or chemotherapy refractory B-cell leukemias. *Blood*, *118*(18), 4817–4828.
Brignone, C., Escudier, B., Grygar, C., Marcu, M., & Triebel, F. (2009). A phase I pharmacokinetic and biological correlative study of IMP321, a novel MHC class II agonist, in patients with advanced renal cell carcinoma. *Clinical Cancer Research*, *15*(19), 6225–6231.
Brignone, C., Gutierrez, M., Mefti, F., Brain, E., Jarcau, R., Cvitkovic, F., et al. (2010). First-line chemoimmunotherapy in metastatic breast carcinoma: Combination of paclitaxel and IMP321 (LAG-3Ig) enhances immune responses and antitumor activity. *Journal of Translational Medicine*, *8*(1), 71.
Bronte, V., & Zanovello, P. (2005). Regulation of immune responses by L-arginine metabolism. *Nature Reviews. Immunology*, *5*(8), 641–654.
Bulliard, Y., Jolicoeur, R., Windman, M., Rue, S. M., Ettenberg, S., Knee, D. A., et al. (2013). Activating Fc γ receptors contribute to the antitumor activities of immunoregulatory receptor-targeting antibodies. *The Journal of Experimental Medicine*, *210*(9), 1685–1693.
Bulliard, Y., Jolicoeur, R., Zhang, J., Dranoff, G., Wilson, N. S., & Brogdon, J. L. (2014). OX40 engagement depletes intratumoral Tregs via activating FcγRs, leading to antitumor efficacy. *Immunology and Cell Biology*, *92*(6), 475–480.
Burington, B., Yue, P., Shi, X., Advani, R., Lau, J. T., Tan, J., et al. (2011). CD40 pathway activation status predicts response to CD40 therapy in diffuse large B cell lymphoma. *Science Translational Medicine*, *3*(74), 74ra22.
Butler, N. S., Moebius, J., Pewe, L. L., Traore, B., Doumbo, O. K., Tygrett, L. T., et al. (2012). Therapeutic blockade of PD-L1 and LAG-3 rapidly clears established blood-stage Plasmodium infection. *Nature Immunology*, *13*(2), 188–195.
Butte, M. J., Pena-Cruz, V., Kim, M., Freeman, G. J., & Sharpe, A. H. (2008). Interaction of human PD-L1 and B7-1. *Molecular Immunology*, *45*(13), 3567–3572.
Cai, G., Anumanthan, A., Brown, J. A., Greenfield, E. A., Zhu, B., & Freeman, G. J. (2008). CD160 inhibits activation of human CD4+ T cells through interaction with herpesvirus entry mediator. *Nature Immunology*, *9*(2), 176–185.
Callahan, M. K., Masters, G., Pratilas, C. A., Ariyan, C., Katz, J., Kitano, S., et al. (2014). Paradoxical activation of T cells via augmented ERK signaling mediated by a RAF inhibitor. *Cancer Immunology Research*, *2*(1), 70–79.
Callard, R. E., Armitage, R. J., Fanslow, W. C., & Spriggs, M. K. (1993). CD40 ligand and its role in X-linked hyper-IgM syndrome. *Immunology Today*, *14*(11), 559–564.
Calmels, B., Paul, S., Futin, N., Ledoux, C., Stoeckel, F., & Acres, B. (2005). Bypassing tumor-associated immune suppression with recombinant adenovirus constructs expressing membrane bound or secreted GITR-L. *Cancer Gene Therapy*, *12*(2), 198–205.
Camacho, L. H., Antonia, S., Sosman, J., Kirkwood, J. M., Gajewski, T. F., Redman, B., et al. (2009). Phase I/II trial of tremelimumab in patients with metastatic melanoma. *Journal of Clinical Oncology*, *27*(7), 1075–1081.
Cassel, W. A., & Murray, D. R. (1988). Treatment of stage II malignant melanoma patients with a Newcastle disease virus oncolysate. *Natural Immunity and Cell Growth Regulation*, *7*(5-6), 351.
Cassel, W. A., & Murray, D. R. (1992). A ten-year follow-up on stage II malignant melanoma patients treated postsurgically with Newcastle disease virus oncolysate. *Medical Oncology and Tumor Pharmacotherapy*, *9*(4), 169–171.

Chacon, J., Sarnaik, A., Chen, J., Creasy, C., Kale, C., Robinson, J., et al. (2014). Manipulating the tumor microenvironment ex vivo for enhanced expansion of tumor-infiltrating lymphocytes for adoptive cell therapy. *Clinical Cancer Research, 21*(3), 611–621, 1934.2014.
Cheuk, A. T., Mufti, G. J., & Guinn, B. (2004). Role of 4-1BB: 4-1BB ligand in cancer immunotherapy. *Cancer Gene Therapy, 11*(3), 215–226.
Chia, S., Gandhi, S., Joy, A., Edwards, S., Gorr, M., Hopkins, S., et al. (2015). Novel agents and associated toxicities of inhibitors of the pi3k/Akt/mtor pathway for the treatment of breast cancer. *Current Oncology, 22*(1), 33.
Chiarini, F., Evangelisti, C., McCubrey, J. A., & Martelli, A. M. (2014). Current treatment strategies for inhibiting mTOR in cancer. *Trends in Pharmacological Sciences, 36*(2), 124–135.
Chiba, S., Baghdadi, M., Akiba, H., Yoshiyama, H., Kinoshita, I., Dosaka-Akita, H., et al. (2012). Tumor-infiltrating DCs suppress nucleic acid-mediated innate immune responses through interactions between the receptor TIM-3 and the alarmin HMGB1. *Nature Immunology, 13*(9), 832–842.
Chinnasamy, D., Yu, Z., Kerkar, S. P., Zhang, L., Morgan, R. A., Restifo, N. P., et al. (2012). Local delivery of lnterleukin-12 using T cells targeting VEGF receptor-2 eradicates multiple vascularized tumors in mice. *Clinical Cancer Research, 18*(6), 1672–1683.
Chmielewski, M., Hombach, A. A., & Abken, H. (2014). Of CARs and TRUCKs: Chimeric antigen receptor (CAR) T cells engineered with an inducible cytokine to modulate the tumor stroma. *Immunological Reviews, 257*(1), 83–90.
Chuang, E., Fisher, T. S., Morgan, R. W., Robbins, M. D., Duerr, J. M., Vander Heiden, M. G., et al. (2000). The CD28 and CTLA-4 receptors associate with the serine/threonine phosphatase PP2A. *Immunity, 13*(3), 313–322.
Ciceri, F., Bonini, C., Stanghellini, M. T. L., Bondanza, A., Traversari, C., Salomoni, M., et al. (2009). Infusion of suicide-gene-engineered donor lymphocytes after family haploidentical haemopoietic stem-cell transplantation for leukaemia (the TK007 trial): A non-randomised phase I–II study. *The Lancet Oncology, 10*(5), 489–500.
Clackson, T., Yang, W., Rozamus, L. W., Hatada, M., Amara, J. F., Rollins, C. T., et al. (1998). Redesigning an FKBP–ligand interface to generate chemical dimerizers with novel specificity. *Proceedings of the National Academy of Sciences of the United States of America, 95*(18), 10437–10442.
Cohen, A. D., Schaer, D. A., Liu, C., Li, Y., Hirschhorn-Cymmerman, D., Kim, S. C., et al. (2010). Agonist anti-GITR monoclonal antibody induces melanoma tumor immunity in mice by altering regulatory T cell stability and intra-tumor accumulation. *PLoS One, 5*(5), e10436.
Coley, W. B. (1991). The classic: The treatment of malignant tumors by repeated inoculations of erysipelas: with a report of ten original cases. *Clinical Orthopaedics and Related Research, 262*, 3–11.
Collins, R., Shpilberg, O., Drobyski, W. R., Porter, D. L., Giralt, S., Champlin, R., et al. (1997). Donor leukocyte infusions in 140 patients with relapsed malignancy after allogeneic bone marrow transplantation. *Journal of Clinical Oncology, 15*(2), 433–444.
Cordoba, S., Kong, K., & Pule, M. (2014). Chimeric antigen receptor logical AND gate based on CD45/CD148 phosphatases. *Molecular Therapy, 22*.
Couzin-Frankel, J. (2013). Cancer immunotherapy. *Science, 342*(6165), 1432–1433.
Crompton, J. G., Sukumar, M., & Restifo, N. P. (2014). Uncoupling T-cell expansion from effector differentiation in cell-based immunotherapy. *Immunological Reviews, 257*(1), 264–276.
Curran, M. A., Kim, M., Montalvo, W., Al-Shamkhani, A., & Allison, J. P. (2011). Combination CTLA-4 blockade and 4-1BB activation enhances tumor rejection by

increasing T-cell infiltration, proliferation, and cytokine production. *PLoS One*, *6*(4), e19499.
Curti, B. D., Kovacsovics-Bankowski, M., Morris, N., Walker, E., Chisholm, L., Floyd, K., et al. (2013). OX40 is a potent immune-stimulating target in late-stage cancer patients. *Cancer Research*, *73*(24), 7189–7198.
da Silva, I. P., Gallois, A., Baranda, S. J., Khan, S., Anderson, A. C., Kuchroo, V. K., et al. (2014). Reversal of NK cell exhaustion in advanced melanoma by Tim-3 blockade. *Cancer Immunology research*, *2*(5), 410–422, 0171.2013.
Davies, C. C., Mason, J., Wakelam, M. J., Young, L. S., & Eliopoulos, A. G. (2004). Inhibition of phosphatidylinositol 3-kinase-and ERK MAPK-regulated protein synthesis reveals the pro-apoptotic properties of CD40 ligation in carcinoma cells. *Journal of Biological Chemistry*, *279*(2), 1010–1019.
DeKruyff, R. H., Bu, X., Ballesteros, A., Santiago, C., Chim, Y. E., Lee, H., et al. (2010). T cell/transmembrane, Ig, and mucin-3 allelic variants differentially recognize phosphatidylserine and mediate phagocytosis of apoptotic cells. *The Journal of Immunology*, *184*(4), 1918–1930.
Deppong, C., Juehne, T. I., Hurchla, M., Friend, L. D., Shah, D. D., Rose, C. M., et al. (2006). Cutting edge: B and T lymphocyte attenuator and programmed death receptor-1 inhibitory receptors are required for termination of acute allergic airway inflammation. *The Journal of Immunology*, *176*(7), 3909–3913.
Derré, L., Rivals, J., Jandus, C., Pastor, S., Rimoldi, D., Romero, P., et al. (2010). BTLA mediates inhibition of human tumor-specific CD8+ T cells that can be partially reversed by vaccination. *The Journal of Clinical Investigation*, *120*(1), 157.
Di Stasi, A., De Angelis, B., Rooney, C. M., Zhang, L., Mahendravada, A., Foster, A. E., et al. (2009). T lymphocytes coexpressing CCR4 and a chimeric antigen receptor targeting CD30 have improved homing and antitumor activity in a Hodgkin tumor model. *Blood*, *113*(25), 6392–6402.
Di Stasi, A., Tey, S., Dotti, G., Fujita, Y., Kennedy-Nasser, A., Martinez, C., et al. (2011). Inducible apoptosis as a safety switch for adoptive cell therapy. *New England Journal of Medicine*, *365*(18), 1673–1683.
Drobyski, W. R., Keever, C. A., Roth, M. S., Koethe, S., Hanson, G., McFadden, P., et al. (1993). Salvage immunotherapy using donor leukocyte infusions as treatment for relapsed chronic myelogenous leukemia after allogeneic bone marrow transplantation: Efficacy and toxicity of a defined T-cell dose. *Blood*, *82*(8), 2310–2318.
Dudley, M. E., & Rosenberg, S. A. (2003). Adoptive-cell-transfer therapy for the treatment of patients with cancer. *Nature Reviews Cancer*, *3*(9), 666–675.
Dudley, M. E., Wunderlich, J. R., Robbins, P. F., Yang, J. C., Hwu, P., Schwartzentruber, D. J., et al. (2002). Cancer regression and autoimmunity in patients after clonal repopulation with antitumor lymphocytes. *Science*, *298*(5594), 850–854.
Dudley, M. E., Wunderlich, J. R., Yang, J. C., Sherry, R. M., Topalian, S. L., Restifo, N. P., et al. (2005). Adoptive cell transfer therapy following non-myeloablative but lymphodepleting chemotherapy for the treatment of patients with refractory metastatic melanoma. *Journal of Clinical Oncology*, *23*(10), 2346–2357.
Easton, J., & Houghton, P. (2006). mTOR and cancer therapy. *Oncogene*, *25*(48), 6436–6446.
Edelson, R. L. (1999). Sezary syndrome, cutaneous T-cell lymphoma, and extracorporeal photopheresis. *Archives of Dermatology*, *135*(5), 600–601.
Eggermont, A. M., Chiarion-Sileni, V., Grob, J. J., Dummer, R., Wolchok, J. D., Schmidt, H., et al. (2014). *Ipilimumab versus placebo after complete resection of stage III melanoma: Initial efficacy and safety results from the EORTC 18071 phase III trial.* ASCO Annual Meeting Proceedings.
Eliopoulos, A. G., & Young, L. S. (2004). The role of the CD40 pathway in the pathogenesis and treatment of cancer. *Current Opinion in Pharmacology*, *4*(4), 360–367.

Fecteau, J. F., & Néron, S. (2003). CD40 stimulation of human peripheral B lymphocytes: Distinct response from naive and memory cells. *The Journal of Immunology*, *171*(9), 4621–4629.

Ferris, R. L., Lu, B., & Kane, L. P. (2014). Too much of a good thing? Tim-3 and TCR signaling in T cell exhaustion. *The Journal of Immunology*, *193*(4), 1525–1530.

Finn, O. J. (2008). Cancer immunology. *New England Journal of Medicine*, *358*(25), 2704–2715.

Finney, H. M., Akbar, A. N., & Lawson, A. D. (2004). Activation of resting human primary T cells with chimeric receptors: Costimulation from CD28, inducible costimulator, CD134, and CD137 in series with signals from the TCRζ chain. *The Journal of Immunology*, *172*(1), 104–113.

Fisher, D. T., Chen, Q., Appenheimer, M. M., Skitzki, J., Wang, W., Odunsi, K., et al. (2006). Hurdles to lymphocyte trafficking in the tumor microenvironment: Implications for effective immunotherapy. *Immunological Investigations*, *35*(3-4), 251–277.

Fourcade, J., Sun, Z., Benallaoua, M., Guillaume, P., Luescher, I. F., Sander, C., et al. (2010). Upregulation of Tim-3 and PD-1 expression is associated with tumor antigen-specific CD8+ T cell dysfunction in melanoma patients. *The Journal of Experimental Medicine*, *207*(10), 2175–2186.

Fourcade, J., Sun, Z., Pagliano, O., Guillaume, P., Luescher, I. F., Sander, C., et al. (2012). CD8+ T cells specific for tumor antigens can be rendered dysfunctional by the tumor microenvironment through upregulation of the inhibitory receptors BTLA and PD-1. *Cancer Research*, *72*(4), 887–896.

Fournier, P., Arnold, A., Wilden, H., & Schirrmacher, V. (2012). Newcastle disease virus induces pro-inflammatory conditions and type I interferon for counter-acting Treg activity. *International Journal of Oncology*, *40*(3), 840–850.

Frederick, D. T., Piris, A., Cogdill, A. P., Cooper, Z. A., Lezcano, C., Ferrone, C. R., et al. (2013). BRAF inhibition is associated with enhanced melanoma antigen expression and a more favorable tumor microenvironment in patients with metastatic melanoma. *Clinical Cancer Research*, *19*(5), 1225–1231.

Fruman, D. A., & Rommel, C. (2014). PI3K and cancer: Lessons, challenges and opportunities. *Nature Reviews. Drug Discovery*, *13*(2), 140–156.

Furman, R. R., Sharman, J. P., Coutre, S. E., Cheson, B. D., Pagel, J. M., Hillmen, P., et al. (2014). Idelalisib and rituximab in relapsed chronic lymphocytic leukemia. *New England Journal of Medicine*, *370*(11), 997–1007.

Gajewski, T. F., & Corrales, L. (2015). New perspectives on type I IFNs in cancer. *Cytokine & Growth Factor Reviews*, *26*(2), 175–178.

Gameiro, S. R., Jammed, M. L., Wattenberg, M. M., Tsang, K. Y., Ferrone, S., & Hodge, J. W. (2014). Radiation-induced immunogenic modulation of tumor enhances antigen processing and calreticulin exposure, resulting in enhanced T-cell killing. *Oncotarget*, *5*(2), 403.

Garrison, K., Hahn, T., Lee, W., Ling, L. E., Weinberg, A. D., & Akporiaye, E. T. (2012). The small molecule TGF-β signaling inhibitor SM16 synergizes with agonistic OX40 antibody to suppress established mammary tumors and reduce spontaneous metastasis. *Cancer Immunology, Immunotherapy*, *61*(4), 511–521.

Gattinoni, L., Powell, D. J., Rosenberg, S. A., & Restifo, N. P. (2006). Adoptive immunotherapy for cancer: Building on success. *Nature Reviews. Immunology*, *6*(5), 383–393.

Gibney, G., Hamid, O., Gangadhar, T., Lutzky, J., Olszanski, A., Gajewski, T., et al. (2014). Preliminary results from a phase 1/2 study of INCB024360 combined with ipilimumab (ipi) in patients (pts) with melanoma. *Journal of Clinical Oncology*, *32*(Suppl. 15), 3010.

Gilboa, E. (1999). The makings of a tumor rejection antigen. *Immunity*, *11*(3), 263–270.

Gilham, D. E. (2011). Effective adoptive T-cell therapy for cancer in the absence of host lymphodepletion. *Immunotherapy*, *3*(2), 177–179.
Goldberg, M. V., & Drake, C. G. (2011). LAG-3 in cancer immunotherapy. *Current Topics in Microbiology and Immunology*, *344*, 269–278.
Greenwald, R. J., Boussiotis, V. A., Lorsbach, R. B., Abbas, A. K., & Sharpe, A. H. (2001). CTLA-4 regulates induction of anergy in vivo. *Immunity*, *14*(2), 145–155.
Griffith, J. W., Sokol, C. L., & Luster, A. D. (2014). Chemokines and chemokine receptors: Positioning cells for host defense and immunity. *Annual Review of Immunology*, *32*, 659–702.
Griseri, T., Asquith, M., Thompson, C., & Powrie, F. (2010). OX40 is required for regulatory T cell-mediated control of colitis. *The Journal of Experimental Medicine*, *207*(4), 699–709.
Grosso, J. F., Kelleher, C. C., Harris, T. J., Maris, C. H., Hipkiss, E. L., De Marzo, A., et al. (2007). LAG-3 regulates CD8 + T cell accumulation and effector function in murine self- and tumor-tolerance systems. *The Journal of Clinical Investigation*, *117*(11), 3383–3392.
Guo, Z. S., Liu, Z., & Bartlett, D. L. (2014). Oncolytic immunotherapy: Dying the right way is a key to eliciting potent antitumor immunity. *Frontiers in oncology*, *4*, 74.
Haining, W. N. (2012). Thinking inside the box: How T cell inhibitory receptors signal. *Nature Medicine*, *18*(9), 1338–1339.
Hall-Jackson, C. A., Eyers, P. A., Cohen, P., Goedert, M., Boyle, F. T., Hewitt, N., et al. (1999). Paradoxical activation of Raf by a novel Raf inhibitor. *Chemistry & Biology*, *6*(8), 559–568.
Hanissian, S. H., & Geha, R. S. (1997). Jak3 is associated with CD40 and is critical for CD40 induction of gene expression in B cells. *Immunity*, *6*(4), 379–387.
Hannani, D., Vétizou, M., Enot, D., Rusakiewicz, S., Chaput, N., Klatzmann, D., et al. (2015). Anticancer immunotherapy by CTLA-4 blockade: Obligatory contribution of IL-2 receptors and negative prognostic impact of soluble CD25. *Cell Research*, *25*(2), 208–224.
Harvey, R. D. (2014). Immunologic and clinical effects of targeting PD-1 in lung cancer. *Clinical Pharmacology & Therapeutics*, *96*(2), 214–223.
Hatzivassiliou, G., Song, K., Yen, I., Brandhuber, B. J., Anderson, D. J., Alvarado, R., et al. (2010). RAF inhibitors prime wild-type RAF to activate the MAPK pathway and enhance growth. *Nature*, *464*(7287), 431–435.
Haymaker, C., Chen, J. Q., Bernatchez, C., Kale, C., Torres-Cabala, C., & Radvanyi, L. (2013). Usurpation of a lymphocyte costimulatory molecule as a novel melanoma cell survival pathway (P2187). *The Journal of Immunology*, *190*(Meeting Abstracts 1), 170.50.
Hinrichs, C. S., & Rosenberg, S. A. (2014). Exploiting the curative potential of adoptive T-cell therapy for cancer. *Immunological Reviews*, *257*(1), 56–71.
Hinrichs, C. S., Spolski, R., Paulos, C. M., Gattinoni, L., Kerstann, K. W., Palmer, D. C., et al. (2008). IL-2 and IL-21 confer opposing differentiation programs to CD8 + T cells for adoptive immunotherapy. *Blood*, *111*(11), 5326–5333.
Hirano, F., Kaneko, K., Tamura, H., Dong, H., Wang, S., Ichikawa, M., et al. (2005). Blockade of B7-H1 and PD-1 by monoclonal antibodies potentiates cancer therapeutic immunity. *Cancer Research*, *65*(3), 1089–1096.
Hirschhorn-Cymerman, D., Rizzuto, G. A., Merghoub, T., Cohen, A. D., Avogadri, F., Lesokhin, A. M., et al. (2009). OX40 engagement and chemotherapy combination provides potent antitumor immunity with concomitant regulatory T cell apoptosis. *The Journal of Experimental Medicine*, *206*(5), 1103–1116.
Ho, W. Y., Blattman, J. N., Dossett, M. L., Yee, C., & Greenberg, P. D. (2003). Adoptive immunotherapy: Engineering T cell responses as biologic weapons for tumor mass destruction. *Cancer Cell*, *3*(5), 431–437.

Hobo, W., Norde, W. J., Schaap, N., Fredrix, H., Maas, F., Schellens, K., et al. (2012). B and T lymphocyte attenuator mediates inhibition of tumor-reactive CD8 + T cells in patients after allogeneic stem cell transplantation. *The Journal of Immunology, 189*(1), 39–49.

Hodi, F. S., O'Day, S. J., McDermott, D. F., Weber, R. W., Sosman, J. A., Haanen, J. B., et al. (2010). Improved survival with ipilimumab in patients with metastatic melanoma. *New England Journal of Medicine, 363*(8), 711–723.

Hoeflich, K. P., Herter, S., Tien, J., Wong, L., Berry, L., Chan, J., et al. (2009). Antitumor efficacy of the novel RAF inhibitor GDC-0879 is predicted by BRAFV600E mutational status and sustained extracellular signal-regulated kinase/mitogen-activated protein kinase pathway suppression. *Cancer Research, 69*(7), 3042–3051.

Holmgaard, R. B., Zamarin, D., Munn, D. H., Wolchok, J. D., & Allison, J. P. (2013). Indoleamine 2, 3-dioxygenase is a critical resistance mechanism in antitumor T cell immunotherapy targeting CTLA-4. *The Journal of Experimental Medicine, 210*(7), 1389–1402.

Hombach, A. A., & Abken, H. (2011). Costimulation by chimeric antigen receptors revisited the T cell antitumor response benefits from combined CD28-OX40 signalling. *International Journal of Cancer, 129*(12), 2935–2944.

Hombach, A., Sent, D., Schneider, C., Heuser, C., Koch, D., Pohl, C., et al. (2001). T-cell activation by recombinant receptors CD28 costimulation is required for interleukin 2 secretion and receptor-mediated T-cell proliferation but does not affect receptor-mediated target cell lysis. *Cancer Research, 61*(5), 1976–1982.

Horlock, C., Stott, B., Dyson, P., Morishita, M., Coombes, R., Savage, P., et al. (2009). The effects of trastuzumab on the CD4+ CD25+ FoxP3+ and CD4+ IL17A+ T-cell axis in patients with breast cancer. *British Journal of Cancer, 100*(7), 1061–1067.

Horowitz, M. M., Gale, R. P., Sondel, P. M., Goldman, J., Kersey, J., Kolb, H., et al. (1990). Graft-versus-leukemia reactions after bone marrow transplantation. *Blood, 75*(3), 555–562.

Hou, D., Muller, A. J., Sharma, M. D., DuHadaway, J., Banerjee, T., Johnson, M., et al. (2007). Inhibition of indoleamine 2, 3-dioxygenase in dendritic cells by stereoisomers of 1-methyl-tryptophan correlates with antitumor responses. *Cancer Research, 67*(2), 792–801.

Houot, R., & Levy, R. (2009). T-cell modulation combined with intratumoral CpG cures lymphoma in a mouse model without the need for chemotherapy. *Blood, 113*(15), 3546–3552.

Huang, C., Workman, C. J., Flies, D., Pan, X., Marson, A. L., Zhou, G., et al. (2004). Role of LAG-3 in regulatory T cells. *Immunity, 21*(4), 503–513.

Huang, Y., Zhu, C., Kondo, Y., Anderson, A. C., Gandhi, A., Russell, A., et al. (2015). CEACAM1 regulates TIM-3-mediated tolerance and exhaustion. *Nature, 517*(7534), 386–390.

Huard, B., Gaulard, P., Faure, F., Hercend, T., & Triebel, F. (1994). Cellular expression and tissue distribution of the human LAG-3-encoded protein, an MHC class II ligand. *Immunogenetics, 39*(3), 213–217.

Huard, B., Prigent, P., Tournier, M., Bruniquel, D., & Triebel, F. (1995). CD4/major histocompatibility complex class II interaction analyzed with CD4-and lymphocyte activation gene-3 (LAG-3)-Ig fusion proteins. *European Journal of Immunology, 25*(9), 2718–2721.

Hughes, M. S., Yu, Y. Y., Dudley, M. E., Zheng, Z., Robbins, P. F., Li, Y., et al. (2005). Transfer of a TCR gene derived from a patient with a marked antitumor response conveys highly active T-cell effector functions. *Human Gene Therapy, 16*(4), 457–472.

Hunder, N. N., Wallen, H., Cao, J., Hendricks, D. W., Reilly, J. Z., Rodmyre, R., et al. (2008). Treatment of metastatic melanoma with autologous CD4+ T cells against NY-ESO-1. *New England Journal of Medicine, 358*(25), 2698–2703.

Huye, L. E., Nakazawa, Y., Patel, M. P., Yvon, E., Sun, J., Savoldo, B., et al. (2011). Combining mTor inhibitors with rapamycin-resistant T cells: A two-pronged approach to tumor elimination. *Molecular Therapy*, *19*(12), 2239–2248.

Imura, A., Hori, T., Imada, K., Ishikawa, T., Tanaka, Y., Maeda, M., et al. (1996). The human OX40/gp34 system directly mediates adhesion of activated T cells to vascular endothelial cells. *The Journal of Experimental Medicine*, *183*(5), 2185–2195.

Introna, M., Barbui, A. M., Bambacioni, F., Casati, C., Gaipa, G., Borleri, G., et al. (2000). Genetic modification of human T cells with CD20: A strategy to purify and lyse transduced cells with anti-CD20 antibodies. *Human Gene Therapy*, *11*(4), 611–620.

Ito, T., Amakawa, R., Inaba, M., Hori, T., Ota, M., Nakamura, K., et al. (2004). Plasmacytoid dendritic cells regulate Th cell responses through OX40 ligand and type I IFNs. *The Journal of Immunology*, *172*(7), 4253–4259.

Iwai, Y., Terawaki, S., & Honjo, T. (2005). PD-1 blockade inhibits hematogenous spread of poorly immunogenic tumor cells by enhanced recruitment of effector T cells. *International Immunology*, *17*(2), 133–144.

Iwama, S., De Remigis, A., Callahan, M. K., Slovin, S. F., Wolchok, J. D., & Caturegli, P. (2014). Pituitary expression of CTLA-4 mediates hypophysitis secondary to administration of CTLA-4 blocking antibody. *Science Translational Medicine*, *6*(230), 230ra45.

Jensen, S. M., Maston, L. D., Gough, M. J., Ruby, C. E., Redmond, W. L., Crittenden, M., et al. (2010). Signaling through OX40 enhances antitumor immunity. *Seminars in Oncology*, *37*, 524–532, WB Saunders.

Jin, H., Anderson, A. C., Tan, W. G., West, E. E., Ha, S., Araki, K., et al. (2010). Cooperation of Tim-3 and PD-1 in CD8 T-cell exhaustion during chronic viral infection. *Proceedings of the National Academy of Sciences of the United States of America*, *107*(33), 14733–14738.

Johnston, R. J., Comps-Agrar, L., Hackney, J., Yu, X., Huseni, M., Yang, Y., et al. (2014). The immunoreceptor TIGIT regulates antitumor and antiviral CD8+ T cell effector function. *Cancer Cell*, *26*(6), 923–937.

Joller, N., Hafler, J. P., Brynedal, B., Kassam, N., Spoerl, S., Levin, S. D., et al. (2011). Cutting edge: TIGIT has T cell-intrinsic inhibitory functions. *The Journal of Immunology*, *186*(3), 1338–1342.

Jonasch, E., & Haluska, F. G. (2001). Interferon in oncological practice: Review of interferon biology, clinical applications, and toxicities. *The Oncologist*, *6*(1), 34–55.

Joseph, E. W., Pratilas, C. A., Poulikakos, P. I., Tadi, M., Wang, W., Taylor, B. S., et al. (2010). The RAF inhibitor PLX4032 inhibits ERK signaling and tumor cell proliferation in a V600E BRAF-selective manner. *Proceedings of the National Academy of Sciences of the United States of America*, *107*(33), 14903–14908.

Joshi, S., Singh, A. R., Zulcic, M., & Durden, D. L. (2014). A macrophage-dominant PI3K isoform controls hypoxia-induced HIF1α and HIF2α stability and tumor growth, angiogenesis, and metastasis. *Molecular Cancer Research*, *12*(10), 1520–1531.

Kakarla, S., Chow, K. K., Mata, M., Shaffer, D. R., Song, X., Wu, M., et al. (2013). Antitumor effects of chimeric receptor engineered human T cells directed to tumor stroma. *Molecular Therapy*, *21*(8), 1611–1620.

Kalos, M., Levine, B. L., Porter, D. L., Katz, S., Grupp, S. A., Bagg, A., et al. (2011). T cells with chimeric antigen receptors have potent antitumor effects and can establish memory in patients with advanced leukemia. *Science Translational Medicine*, *3*(95), 95ra73.

Kanamaru, F., Youngnak, P., Hashiguchi, M., Nishioka, T., Takahashi, T., Sakaguchi, S., et al. (2004). Costimulation via glucocorticoid-induced TNF receptor in both conventional and CD25+ regulatory CD4+ T cells. *The Journal of Immunology*, *172*(12), 7306–7314.

Kashiwakura, J., Yokoi, H., Saito, H., & Okayama, Y. (2004). T cell proliferation by direct cross-talk between OX40 ligand on human mast cells and OX40 on human T cells:

Comparison of gene expression profiles between human tonsillar and lung-cultured mast cells. *The Journal of Immunology*, *173*(8), 5247–5257.

Kaufman, H. L., Andtbacka, R. H. I., Collichio, F. A., Amatruda, T., Senzer, N. N., Chesney, J., et al. (2014). Primary overall survival (OS) from OPTiM, a randomized phase III trial of talimogene laherparepvec (T-VEC) versus subcutaneous (SC) granulocyte-macrophage colony-stimulating factor (GM-CSF) for the treatment (tx) of unresected stage IIIB/C and IV melanoma. In *ASCO annual meeting proceedings 20 May 2014: 9008a.*

Kaufman, H. L., Kim, D. W., DeRaffele, G., Mitcham, J., Coffin, R. S., & Kim-Schulze, S. (2010). Local and distant immunity induced by intralesional vaccination with an oncolytic herpes virus encoding GM-CSF in patients with stage IIIc and IV melanoma. *Annals of Surgical Oncology*, *17*(3), 718–730.

Kelly, E., & Russell, S. J. (2007). History of oncolytic viruses: Genesis to genetic engineering. *Molecular Therapy*, *15*(4), 651–659.

Kershaw, M. H., Westwood, J. A., & Darcy, P. K. (2013). Gene-engineered T cells for cancer therapy. *Nature Reviews Cancer*, *13*(8), 525–541.

Kershaw, M. H., Westwood, J. A., Slaney, C. Y., & Darcy, P. K. (2014). Clinical application of genetically modified T cells in cancer therapy. *Clinical & Translational Immunology*, *3*(5), e16.

Kim, H. S., Kim-Schulze, S., Kim, D. W., & Kaufman, H. L. (2009). Host lymphodepletion enhances the therapeutic activity of an oncolytic vaccinia virus expressing 4-1BB ligand. *Cancer Research*, *69*(21), 8516–8525.

Kitano, S., Postow, M. A., Ziegler, C. G., Kuk, D., Panageas, K., Cortez, C., et al. (2014). Computational algorithm driven evaluation of monocytic myeloid derived suppressor cell frequency for prediction of clinical outcomes. *Cancer Immunology Research*, *2*(8), 812–821, 0013.2014.

Klebanoff, C. A., Gattinoni, L., Palmer, D. C., Muranski, P., Ji, Y., Hinrichs, C. S., et al. (2011). Determinants of successful CD8+ T-cell adoptive immunotherapy for large established tumors in mice. *Clinical Cancer Research*, *17*(16), 5343–5352.

Klebanoff, C. A., Gattinoni, L., & Restifo, N. P. (2012). Sorting through subsets: Which T cell populations mediate highly effective adoptive immunotherapy? *Journal of Immunotherapy (Hagerstown, Md.: 1997)*, *35*(9), 651.

Ko, K., Yamazaki, S., Nakamura, K., Nishioka, T., Hirota, K., Yamaguchi, T., et al. (2005). Treatment of advanced tumors with agonistic anti-GITR mAb and its effects on tumor-infiltrating Foxp3+ CD25+ CD4+ regulatory T cells. *The Journal of Experimental Medicine*, *202*(7), 885–891.

Kochenderfer, J. N., Dudley, M. E., Feldman, S. A., Wilson, W. H., Spaner, D. E., Maric, I., et al. (2012). B-cell depletion and remissions of malignancy along with cytokine-associated toxicity in a clinical trial of anti-CD19 chimeric-antigen-receptor-transduced T cells. *Blood*, *119*(12), 2709–2720.

Kochenderfer, J. N., Yu, Z., Frasheri, D., Restifo, N. P., & Rosenberg, S. A. (2010). Adoptive transfer of syngeneic T cells transduced with a chimeric antigen receptor that recognizes murine CD19 can eradicate lymphoma and normal B cells. *Blood*, *116*(19), 3875–3886.

Kohrt, H. E., Houot, R., Weiskopf, K., Goldstein, M. J., Scheeren, F., Czerwinski, D., et al. (2012). Stimulation of natural killer cells with a CD137-specific antibody enhances trastuzumab efficacy in xenotransplant models of breast cancer. *The Journal of Clinical Investigation*, *122*(3), 1066.

Korman, A. J., Engelhardt, J., Shahabi, V., Yordanova, R., Henning, K., Chen, T., et al. (2013). Role of the immunoglobulin constant region in the antitumor activity of antibodies to cytotoxic T-lymphocyte antigen-4 (CTLA-4). *Journal of Clinical Oncology*, *31*, a9055.

Kraman, M., Bambrough, P. J., Arnold, J. N., Roberts, E. W., Magiera, L., Jones, J. O., et al. (2010). Suppression of antitumor immunity by stromal cells expressing fibroblast activation protein-α. *Science*, *330*(6005), 827–830.

Krummel, M. F., & Allison, J. P. (1995). CD28 and CTLA-4 have opposing effects on the response of T cells to stimulation. *The Journal of Experimental Medicine*, *182*(2), 459–465.

Krummel, M. F., & Allison, J. P. (1996). CTLA-4 engagement inhibits IL-2 accumulation and cell cycle progression upon activation of resting T cells. *The Journal of Experimental Medicine*, *183*(6), 2533–2540.

Kuball, J., Dossett, M. L., Wolfl, M., Ho, W. Y., Voss, R., Fowler, C., et al. (2007). Facilitating matched pairing and expression of TCR chains introduced into human T cells. *Blood*, *109*(6), 2331–2338.

Kurtulus, S., Sakuishi, K., Zhang, H., Joller, N., Tan, D., Smyth, M., et al. (2014). Mechanisms of TIGIT-driven immune suppression in cancer. *Journal for Immunotherapy of Cancer*, *2*(Suppl. 3), O13.

Laplante, M., & Sabatini, D. M. (2012). mTOR signaling in growth control and disease. *Cell*, *149*(2), 274–293.

Leach, D. R., Krummel, M. F., & Allison, J. P. (1996). Enhancement of antitumor immunity by CTLA-4 blockade. *Science*, *271*(5256), 1734–1736.

Lee, Y., Auh, S. L., Wang, Y., Burnette, B., Wang, Y., Meng, Y., et al. (2009). Therapeutic effects of ablative radiation on local tumor require CD8+ T cells: Changing strategies for cancer treatment. *Blood*, *114*(3), 589–595.

Lee, K., Chuang, E., Griffin, M., Khattri, R., Hong, D. K., Zhang, W., et al. (1998). Molecular basis of T cell inactivation by CTLA-4. *Science*, *282*(5397), 2263–2266.

Lee, H., Park, S., Choi, B. K., Kim, H. H., Nam, K., & Kwon, B. S. (2002). 4-1BB promotes the survival of CD8+ T lymphocytes by increasing expression of Bcl-xL and Bfl-1. *The Journal of Immunology*, *169*(9), 4882–4888.

Li, D., Gál, I., Vermes, C., Alegre, M., Chong, A. S., Chen, L., et al. (2004). Cutting edge: Cbl-b: One of the key molecules tuning CD28-and CTLA-4-mediated T cell costimulation. *The Journal of Immunology*, *173*(12), 7135–7139.

Li, Q., Rao, R., Vazzana, J., Goedegebuure, P., Odunsi, K., Gillanders, W., et al. (2012). Regulating mammalian target of rapamycin to tune vaccination-induced CD8+ T cell responses for tumor immunity. *The Journal of Immunology*, *188*(7), 3080–3087.

Lichty, B. D., Breitbach, C. J., Stojdl, D. F., & Bell, J. C. (2014). Going viral with cancer immunotherapy. *Nature Reviews Cancer*, *14*(8), 559–567.

Lin, G. H., Liu, Y., Ambagala, T., Kwon, B. S., Ohashi, P. S., & Watts, T. H. (2010). Evaluating the cellular targets of anti-4-1BB agonist antibody during immunotherapy of a pre-established tumor in mice. *PLoS One*, *5*(6), e11003.

Lindenmann, Jean, & Klein, Paul A. (1967). Viral oncolysis: Increased immunogenicity of host cell antigen associated with influenza virus. *The Journal of Experimental Medicine*, *126*(1), 93–108.

Liu, C., Lou, Y., Lizée, G., Qin, H., Liu, S., Rabinovich, B., et al. (2008). Plasmacytoid dendritic cells induce NK cell-dependent, tumor antigen-specific T cell cross-priming and tumor regression in mice. *The Journal of Clinical Investigation*, *118*(3), 1165.

Liu, X., Shin, N., Koblish, H. K., Yang, G., Wang, Q., Wang, K., et al. (2010). Selective inhibition of IDO1 effectively regulates mediators of antitumor immunity. *Blood*, *115*(17), 3520–3530.

Lorence, R. M., Scot Roberts, M., O'Neil, J. D., Groene, W. S., Miller, J. A., Mueller, S. N., et al. (2007). Phase 1 clinical experience using intravenous administration of PV701, an oncolytic Newcastle disease virus. *Current Cancer Drug Targets*, 7(2), 157–167.

Lozano, E., Dominguez-Villar, M., Kuchroo, V., & Hafler, D. A. (2012). The TIGIT/CD226 axis regulates human T cell function. *The Journal of Immunology, 188*(8), 3869–3875.

Mallett, S., Fossum, S., & Barclay, A. N. (1990). Characterization of the MRC OX40 antigen of activated CD4 positive T lymphocytes—A molecule related to nerve growth factor receptor. *The EMBO Journal, 9*(4), 1063.

Marçais, A., Cherfils-Vicini, J., Viant, C., Degouve, S., Viel, S., Fenis, A., et al. (2014). The metabolic checkpoint kinase mTOR is essential for IL-15 signaling during the development and activation of NK cells. *Nature Immunology, 15*(8), 749–757.

Marengère, L. E., Waterhouse, P., Duncan, G. S., Mittrücker, H., Feng, G., & Mak, T. W. (1996). Regulation of T cell receptor signaling by tyrosine phosphatase SYP association with CTLA-4. *Science, 272*(5265), 1170–1173.

Marshall, N. A., Galvin, K. C., Corcoran, A. B., Boon, L., Higgs, R., & Mills, K. H. (2012). Immunotherapy with PI3K inhibitor and Toll-like receptor agonist induces IFN-γ+ IL-17+ polyfunctional T cells that mediate rejection of murine tumors. *Cancer Research, 72*(3), 581–591.

Matsumura, S., Wang, B., Kawashima, N., Braunstein, S., Badura, M., Cameron, T. O., et al. (2008). Radiation-induced CXCL16 release by breast cancer cells attracts effector T cells. *The Journal of Immunology, 181*(5), 3099–3107.

Matsuzaki, J., Gnjatic, S., Mhawech-Fauceglia, P., Beck, A., Miller, A., Tsuji, T., et al. (2010). Tumor-infiltrating NY-ESO-1-specific CD8+ T cells are negatively regulated by LAG-3 and PD-1 in human ovarian cancer. *Proceedings of the National Academy of Sciences, 107*(17), 7875–7880.

McMahan, R. H., Golden-Mason, L., Nishimura, M. I., McMahon, B. J., Kemper, M., Allen, T. M., et al. (2010). Tim-3 expression on PD-1+ HCV-specific human CTLs is associated with viral persistence, and its blockade restores hepatocyte-directed in vitro cytotoxicity. *The Journal of Clinical Investigation, 120*(12), 4546.

Melcher, A., Parato, K., Rooney, C. M., & Bell, J. C. (2011). Thunder and lightning: Immunotherapy and oncolytic viruses collide. *Molecular Therapy, 19*(6), 1008–1016.

M'Hidi, H., Thibult, M., Chetaille, B., Rey, F., Bouadallah, R., Nicollas, R., et al. (2009). High expression of the inhibitory receptor BTLA in T-follicular helper cells and in B-cell small lymphocytic lymphoma/chronic lymphocytic leukemia. *American Journal of Clinical Pathology, 132*(4), 589–596.

Mitsui, J., Nishikawa, H., Muraoka, D., Wang, L., Noguchi, T., Sato, E., et al. (2010). Two distinct mechanisms of augmented antitumor activity by modulation of immunostimulatory/inhibitory signals. *Clinical Cancer Research, 16*(10), 2781–2791.

Monney, L., Sabatos, C. A., Gaglia, J. L., Ryu, A., Waldner, H., Chernova, T., et al. (2002). Th1-specific cell surface protein Tim-3 regulates macrophage activation and severity of an autoimmune disease. *Nature, 415*(6871), 536–541.

Morgan, R. A., Dudley, M. E., Wunderlich, J. R., Hughes, M. S., Yang, J. C., Sherry, R. M., et al. (2006). Cancer regression in patients after transfer of genetically engineered lymphocytes. *Science, 314*(5796), 126–129.

Morgan, R. A., Dudley, M. E., Yik, Y., Zheng, Z., Robbins, P. F., Theoret, M. R., et al. (2003). High efficiency TCR gene transfer into primary human lymphocytes affords avid recognition of melanoma tumor antigen glycoprotein 100 and does not alter the recognition of autologous melanoma antigens. *The Journal of Immunology, 171*(6), 3287–3295.

Morgan, R. A., Yang, J. C., Kitano, M., Dudley, M. E., Laurencot, C. M., & Rosenberg, S. A. (2010). Case report of a serious adverse event following the administration of T cells transduced with a chimeric antigen receptor recognizing ERBB2. *Molecular Therapy, 18*(4), 843–851.

Muller, A. J., DuHadaway, J. B., Donover, P. S., Sutanto-Ward, E., & Prendergast, G. C. (2005). Inhibition of indoleamine 2, 3-dioxygenase, an immunoregulatory target of the cancer suppression gene Bin1, potentiates cancer chemotherapy. *Nature Medicine*, *11*(3), 312–319.

Munn, D. (2011). Blocking IDO activity to enhance anti-tumor immunity. *Frontiers in Bioscience (Elite Edition)*, *4*, 734–745.

Munn, D. H., & Mellor, A. L. (2004). IDO and tolerance to tumors. *Trends in Molecular Medicine*, *10*(1), 15–18.

Munn, D. H., & Mellor, A. L. (2013). Indoleamine 2, 3 dioxygenase and metabolic control of immune responses. *Trends in Immunology*, *34*(3), 137–143.

Nakayama, M., Akiba, H., Takeda, K., Kojima, Y., Hashiguchi, M., Azuma, M., et al. (2009). Tim-3 mediates phagocytosis of apoptotic cells and cross-presentation. *Blood*, *113*(16), 3821–3830.

Ndhlovu, L. C., Lopez-Vergès, S., Barbour, J. D., Jones, R. B., Jha, A. R., Long, B. R., et al. (2012). Tim-3 marks human natural killer cell maturation and suppresses cell-mediated cytotoxicity. *Blood*, *119*(16), 3734–3743.

Newton, R. C., Scherle, P. A., Bowman, K., Liu, X., Beatty, G. L., O'Dwyer, P. J., et al. (2012). Pharmacodynamic assessment of INCB024360, an inhibitor of indoleamine 2, 3-dioxygenase 1 (IDO1), in advanced cancer patients. *Journal of Clinical Oncology*, *1*, 18.

Ngiow, S. F., von Scheidt, B., Akiba, H., Yagita, H., Teng, M. W., & Smyth, M. J. (2011). Anti-TIM3 antibody promotes T cell IFN-γ-mediated antitumor immunity and suppresses established tumors. *Cancer Research*, *71*(10), 3540–3551.

Ni, J., Galani, I. E., Cerwenka, A., Schirrmacher, V., & Fournier, P. (2011). Antitumor vaccination by Newcastle Disease Virus Hemagglutinin-Neuraminidase plasmid DNA application: Changes in tumor microenvironment and activation of innate anti-tumor immunity. *Vaccine*, *29*(6), 1185–1193.

Nishikawa, H., Kato, T., Hirayama, M., Orito, Y., Sato, E., Harada, N., et al. (2008). Regulatory T cell-resistant CD8+ T cells induced by glucocorticoid-induced tumor necrosis factor receptor signaling. *Cancer Research*, *68*(14), 5948–5954.

Nishimura, H., Nose, M., Hiai, H., Minato, N., & Honjo, T. (1999). Development of lupus-like autoimmune diseases by disruption of the PD-1 gene encoding an ITIM motif-carrying immunoreceptor. *Immunity*, *11*(2), 141–151.

Nishimura, H., Okazaki, T., Tanaka, Y., Nakatani, K., Hara, M., Matsumori, A., et al. (2001). Autoimmune dilated cardiomyopathy in PD-1 receptor-deficient mice. *Science*, *291*(5502), 319–322.

North, R. J. (1982). Cyclophosphamide-facilitated adoptive immunotherapy of an established tumor depends on elimination of tumor-induced suppressor T cells. *The Journal of Experimental Medicine*, *155*(4), 1063–1074.

Novellino, L., Castelli, C., & Parmiani, G. (2005). A listing of human tumor antigens recognized by T cells: March 2004 update. *Cancer Immunology, Immunotherapy*, *54*(3), 187–207.

Ohshima, Y., Tanaka, Y., Tozawa, H., Takahashi, Y., Maliszewski, C., & Delespesse, G. (1997). Expression and function of OX40 ligand on human dendritic cells. *The Journal of Immunology*, *159*(8), 3838–3848.

Okamura, T., Fujio, K., Shibuya, M., Sumitomo, S., Shoda, H., Sakaguchi, S., et al. (2009). CD4+ CD25–LAG3+ regulatory T cells controlled by the transcription factor Egr-2. *Proceedings of the National Academy of Sciences of the United States of America*, *106*(33), 13974–13979.

Okazaki, T., & Honjo, T. (2006). The PD-1–PD-L pathway in immunological tolerance. *Trends in Immunology*, *27*(4), 195–201.

Okazaki, T., & Honjo, T. (2007). PD-1 and PD-1 ligands: From discovery to clinical application. *International Immunology*, *19*(7), 813–824.

Okazaki, T., Maeda, A., Nishimura, H., Kurosaki, T., & Honjo, T. (2001). PD-1 immunoreceptor inhibits B cell receptor-mediated signaling by recruiting src homology 2-domain-containing tyrosine phosphatase 2 to phosphotyrosine. *Proceedings of the National Academy of Sciences of the United States of America*, *98*(24), 13866–13871.

Okkenhaug, K. (2013). Signaling by the phosphoinositide 3-kinase family in immune cells. *Annual Review of Immunology*, *31*, 675–704.

Okudaira, K., Hokari, R., Tsuzuki, Y., Okada, Y., Komoto, S., Watanabe, C., et al. (2009). Blockade of B7-H1 or B7-DC induces an anti-tumor effect in a mouse pancreatic cancer model. *International Journal of Oncology*, *35*(4), 741–749.

Okwan-Duodu, D., Pollack, B. P., Lawson, D., & Khan, M. K. (2015). Role of radiation therapy as immune activator in the era of modern immunotherapy for metastatic malignant melanoma. *American Journal of Clinical Oncology*, *38*(1), 119–125. http://dx.doi.org/10.1097/COC.0b013e3182940dc3.

Oya, Y., Watanabe, N., Owada, T., Oki, M., Hirose, K., Suto, A., et al. (2008). Development of autoimmune hepatitis-like disease and production of autoantibodies to nuclear antigens in mice lacking B and T lymphocyte attenuator. *Arthritis & Rheumatism*, *58*(8), 2498–2510.

Palucka, K., & Banchereau, J. (2012). Cancer immunotherapy via dendritic cells. *Nature Reviews Cancer*, *12*(4), 265–277.

Pan, P., Zang, Y., Weber, K., Meseck, M. L., & Chen, S. (2002). OX40 ligation enhances primary and memory cytotoxic T lymphocyte responses in an immunotherapy for hepatic colon metastases. *Molecular Therapy*, *6*(4), 528–536.

Panaretakis, T., Kepp, O., Brockmeier, U., Tesniere, A., Bjorklund, A., Chapman, D. C., et al. (2009). Mechanisms of pre-apoptotic calreticulin exposure in immunogenic cell death. *The EMBO Journal*, *28*(5), 578–590.

Parmiani, G., De Filippo, A., Novellino, L., & Castelli, C. (2007). Unique human tumor antigens: Immunobiology and use in clinical trials. *The Journal of Immunology*, *178*(4), 1975–1979.

Parry, R. V., Chemnitz, J. M., Frauwirth, K. A., Lanfranco, A. R., Braunstein, I., Kobayashi, S. V., et al. (2005). CTLA-4 and PD-1 receptors inhibit T-cell activation by distinct mechanisms. *Molecular and Cellular Biology*, *25*(21), 9543–9553.

Parsa, A. T., Waldron, J. S., Panner, A., Crane, C. A., Parney, I. F., Barry, J. J., et al. (2007). Loss of tumor suppressor PTEN function increases B7-H1 expression and immunoresistance in glioma. *Nature Medicine*, *13*(1), 84–88.

Patel, J. M., Dale, G. A., Vartabedian, V. F., Dey, P., & Selvaraj, P. (2014). Cancer CARtography: Charting out a new approach to cancer immunotherapy. *Immunotherapy*, *6*(6), 675–678.

Paterson, D., Jefferies, W., Green, J., Brandon, M., Corthesy, P., Puklavec, M., et al. (1987). Antigens of activated rat T lymphocytes including a molecule of 50,000 M r detected only on CD4 positive T blasts. *Molecular Immunology*, *24*(12), 1281–1290.

Pearce, E. L., Walsh, M. C., Cejas, P. J., Harms, G. M., Shen, H., Wang, L., et al. (2009). Enhancing CD8 T-cell memory by modulating fatty acid metabolism. *Nature*, *460*(7251), 103–107.

Peggs, K. S., Quezada, S. A., & Allison, J. P. (2008). Cell intrinsic mechanisms of T-cell inhibition and application to cancer therapy. *Immunological Reviews*, *224*(1), 141–165.

Pegram, H. J., Lee, J. C., Hayman, E. G., Imperato, G. H., Tedder, T. F., Sadelain, M., et al. (2012). Tumor-targeted T cells modified to secrete IL-12 eradicate systemic tumors without need for prior conditioning. *Blood*, *119*(18), 4133–4141.

Perkins, D., Wang, Z., Donovan, C., He, H., Mark, D., Guan, G., et al. (1996). Regulation of CTLA-4 expression during T cell activation. *The Journal of Immunology*, *156*(11), 4154–4159.

Phan, G. Q., Yang, J. C., Sherry, R. M., Hwu, P., Topalian, S. L., Schwartzentruber, D. J., et al. (2003). Cancer regression and autoimmunity induced by cytotoxic T lymphocyte-associated antigen 4 blockade in patients with metastatic melanoma. *Proceedings of the National Academy of Sciences of the United States of America, 100*(14), 8372–8377.

Piconese, S., Pittoni, P., Burocchi, A., Gorzanelli, A., Carè, A., Tripodo, C., et al. (2010). A non-redundant role for OX40 in the competitive fitness of Treg in response to IL-2. *European Journal of Immunology, 40*(10), 2902–2913.

Plitt, T., & Zamarin, D. (2015). Cancer therapy with Newcastle disease virus: Rationale for new immunotherapeutic combinations. *Clinical Investigation, 5*(1), 75–87.

Pollizzi, K. N., & Powell, J. D. (2015). Regulation of T cells by mTOR: The known knowns and the known unknowns. *Trends in Immunology, 36*(1), 13–20.

Porter, D. L., Levine, B. L., Kalos, M., Bagg, A., & June, C. H. (2011). Chimeric antigen receptor-modified T cells in chronic lymphoid leukemia. *New England Journal of Medicine, 365*(8), 725–733.

Postow, M. A., Callahan, M. K., Barker, C. A., Yamada, Y., Yuan, J., Kitano, S., et al. (2012). Immunologic correlates of the abscopal effect in a patient with melanoma. *New England Journal of Medicine, 366*(10), 925–931.

Poulikakos, P. I., Zhang, C., Bollag, G., Shokat, K. M., & Rosen, N. (2010). RAF inhibitors transactivate RAF dimers and ERK signalling in cells with wild-type BRAF. *Nature, 464*(7287), 427–430.

Powell, J. D., Pollizzi, K. N., Heikamp, E. B., & Horton, M. R. (2012). Regulation of immune responses by mTOR. *Annual Review of Immunology, 30*, 39.

Powles, T., Eder, J. P., Fine, G. D., Braiteh, F. S., Loriot, Y., Cruz, C., et al. (2014). MPDL3280A (anti-PD-L1) treatment leads to clinical activity in metastatic bladder cancer. *Nature, 515*(7528), 558–562.

Prewett, M., Huber, J., Li, Y., Santiago, A., O'Connor, W., King, K., et al. (1999). Anti-vascular endothelial growth factor receptor (fetal liver kinase 1) monoclonal antibody inhibits tumor angiogenesis and growth of several mouse and human tumors. *Cancer Research, 59*(20), 5209–5218.

Puzanov, I., Callahan, M. K., Linette, G. P., Patel, S. P., Luke, J. J., Sosman, J. A., et al. (2014). *Phase 1 study of the BRAF inhibitor dabrafenib (D) with or without the MEK inhibitor trametinib (T) in combination with ipilimumab (Ipi) for V600E/K mutation-positive unresectable or metastatic melanoma (MM)*. ASCO annual meeting proceedings.

Puzanov, I., Milhem, M. M., Andtbacka, R. H. I., Minor, D. R., Hamid, O., Li, A., et al. (2014). Primary analysis of a phase 1b multicenter trial to evaluate safety and efficacy of talimogene laherparepvec (T-VEC) and ipilimumab (ipi) in previously untreated, unresected stage IIIB-IV melanoma. In *ASCO annual meeting proceedings 20 May 2014: 9029*.

Rangachari, M., Zhu, C., Sakuishi, K., Xiao, S., Karman, J., Chen, A., et al. (2012). Bat3 promotes T cell responses and autoimmunity by repressing Tim-3-mediated cell death and exhaustion. *Nature Medicine, 18*(9), 1394–1400.

Rao, R. R., Li, Q., Odunsi, K., & Shrikant, P. A. (2010). The mTOR kinase determines effector versus memory CD8+ T cell fate by regulating the expression of transcription factors T-bet and Eomesodermin. *Immunity, 32*(1), 67–78.

Read, S., Malmström, V., & Powrie, F. (2000). Cytotoxic T lymphocyte-associated antigen 4 plays an essential role in the function of CD25+ CD4+ regulatory cells that control intestinal inflammation. *The Journal of Experimental Medicine, 192*(2), 295–302.

Redmond, W. L., Triplett, T., Floyd, K., & Weinberg, A. D. (2012). Dual anti-OX40/IL-2 therapy augments tumor immunotherapy via IL-2R-mediated regulation of OX40 expression. *PLoS One, 7*(4), e34467.

Ribas, A., Hodi, F. S., Callahan, M., Konto, C., & Wolchok, J. (2013). Hepatotoxicity with combination of vemurafenib and ipilimumab. *New England Journal of Medicine, 368*(14), 1365–1366.

Ribas, A., Kefford, R., Marshall, M. A., Punt, C. J., Haanen, J. B., Marmol, M., et al. (2013). Phase III randomized clinical trial comparing tremelimumab with standard-of-care chemotherapy in patients with advanced melanoma. *Journal of Clinical Oncology, 31*(5), 616–622.

Rizzuto, G. A., Merghoub, T., Hirschhorn-Cymerman, D., Liu, C., Lesokhin, A. M., Sahawneh, D., et al. (2009). Self-antigen-specific CD8+ T cell precursor frequency determines the quality of the antitumor immune response. *The Journal of Experimental Medicine, 206*(4), 849–866.

Robert, C., Arnault, J., & Mateus, C. (2011). RAF inhibition and induction of cutaneous squamous cell carcinoma. *Current Opinion in Oncology, 23*(2), 177–182.

Robert, C., Ribas, A., Wolchok, J. D., Hodi, F. S., Hamid, O., Kefford, R., et al. (2014). Anti-programmed-death-receptor-1 treatment with pembrolizumab in ipilimumab-refractory advanced melanoma: A randomised dose-comparison cohort of a phase 1 trial. *The Lancet, 384*(9948), 1109–1117.

Rogers, P. R., Song, J., Gramaglia, I., Killeen, N., & Croft, M. (2001). OX40 promotes Bcl-xL and Bcl-2 expression and is essential for long-term survival of CD4 T cells. *Immunity, 15*(3), 445–455.

Ronchetti, S., Nocentini, G., Bianchini, R., Krausz, L. T., Migliorati, G., & Riccardi, C. (2007). Glucocorticoid-induced TNFR-related protein lowers the threshold of CD28 costimulation in CD8+ T cells. *The Journal of Immunology, 179*(9), 5916–5926.

Rosenberg, S. A. (2014). IL-2: The first effective immunotherapy for human cancer. *The Journal of Immunology, 192*(12), 5451–5458.

Rosenberg, S. A., & Dudley, M. E. (2009). Adoptive cell therapy for the treatment of patients with metastatic melanoma. *Current Opinion in Immunology, 21*(2), 233–240.

Rosenberg, S. A., Restifo, N. P., Yang, J. C., Morgan, R. A., & Dudley, M. E. (2008). Adoptive cell transfer: A clinical path to effective cancer immunotherapy. *Nature Reviews Cancer, 8*(4), 299–308.

Rosenberg, S. A., Spiess, P., & Lafreniere, R. (1986). A new approach to the adoptive immunotherapy of cancer with tumor-infiltrating lymphocytes. *Science, 233*(4770), 1318–1321.

Rosenberg, S. A., Yang, J. C., Topalian, S. L., Schwartzentruber, D. J., Weber, J. S., Parkinson, D. R., et al. (1994). Treatment of 283 consecutive patients with metastatic melanoma or renal cell cancer using high-dose bolus interleukin 2. *Journal of American Medical Association, 271*(12), 907–913.

Rosenzweig, M., Ponte, J., Apostolou, I., Doty, D., Guild, J., Slavonic, M., et al. (2010). Development of TRX518, an aglycosyl humanized monoclonal antibody (Mab) agonist of huGITR. In *ASCO annual meeting proceedings*.

Rossig, C., & Brenner, M. K. (2004). Genetic modification of T lymphocytes for adoptive immunotherapy. *Molecular Therapy, 10*(1), 5–18.

Royal, R. E., Levy, C., Turner, K., Mathur, A., Hughes, M., Kammula, U. S., et al. (2010). Phase 2 trial of single agent Ipilimumab (anti-CTLA-4) for locally advanced or metastatic pancreatic adenocarcinoma. *Journal of Immunotherapy, 33*(8), 828–833.

Ruby, C. E., Yates, M. A., Hirschhorn-Cymerman, D., Chlebeck, P., Wolchok, J. D., Houghton, A. N., et al. (2009). Cutting Edge: OX40 agonists can drive regulatory T cell expansion if the cytokine milieu is right. *The Journal of Immunology, 183*(8), 4853–4857.

Russell, S. J., Peng, K. W., & Bell, J. C. (2012). Oncolytic virotherapy. *Nature Biotechnology, 30*(7), 658–670.

Russo, V., Tanzarella, S., Dalerba, P., Rigatti, D., Rovere, P., Villa, A., et al. (2000). Dendritic cells acquire the MAGE-3 human tumor antigen from apoptotic cells and induce a class I-restricted T cell response. *Proceedings of the National Academy of Sciences of the United States of America, 97*(5), 2185–2190.

Sadelain, M., Rivière, I., & Brentjens, R. (2003). Targeting tumours with genetically enhanced T lymphocytes. *Nature Reviews Cancer, 3*(1), 35–45.

Sakuishi, K., Apetoh, L., Sullivan, J. M., Blazar, B. R., Kuchroo, V. K., & Anderson, A. C. (2010). Targeting Tim-3 and PD-1 pathways to reverse T cell exhaustion and restore anti-tumor immunity. *The Journal of Experimental Medicine*, *207*(10), 2187–2194.

Sato, T., Ishii, N., Murata, K., Kikuchi, K., Nakagawa, S., Ndhlovu, L. C., et al. (2002). Consequences of OX40-OX40 ligand interactions in Langerhans cell function: Enhanced contact hypersensitivity responses in OX40L-transgenic mice. *European Journal of Immunology*, *32*(11), 3326–3335.

Savoldo, B., Ramos, C. A., Liu, E., Mims, M. P., Keating, M. J., Carrum, G., et al. (2011). CD28 costimulation improves expansion and persistence of chimeric antigen receptor-modified T cells in lymphoma patients. *The Journal of Clinical Investigation*, *121*(5), 1822.

Schaer, D. A., Budhu, S., Liu, C., Bryson, C., Malandro, N., Cohen, A., et al. (2013). GITR pathway activation abrogates tumor immune suppression through loss of regulatory T-cell lineage stability. *Cancer Immunology Research*, *1*(5), 320–331.

Schaer, D. A., Cohen, A. D., & Wolchok, J. D. (2010). Anti-GITR antibodies—Potential clinical applications for tumor immunotherapy. *Current Opinion in Investigational Drugs (London, England: 2000)*, *11*(12), 1378–1386.

Schaer, D. A., Hirschhorn-Cymerman, D., & Wolchok, J. D. (2014). Targeting tumor-necrosis factor receptor pathways for tumor immunotherapy. *Journal of Immunotherapy Cancer*, *2*(7), 7.

Schirrmacher, V., & Fournier, P. (2009). Newcastle disease virus: A promising vector for viral therapy, immune therapy, and gene therapy of cancer. *Gene Therapy of Cancer*, *542*, 565–605.

Schmid Michael, C., Avraamides Christie, J., Dippold Holly, C., Franco, I., Foubert, P., & Ellies Lesley, G. (2011). Receptor tyrosine kinases and TLR/IL1Rs unexpectedly activate myeloid cell PI3Kg, a single convergent point promoting tumor inflammation and progression. *Cancer Cell*, *19*, 715–727.

Schuberth, P. C., Hagedorn, C., Jensen, S. M., Gulati, P., van den Broek, M., Mischo, A., et al. (2013). Treatment of malignant pleural mesothelioma by fibroblast activation protein-specific re-directed T cells. *Journal of Translational Medicine*, *11*, 187.

Schwartz, R. H. (1990). A cell culture model for T lymphocyte clonal anergy. *Science*, *248*(4961), 1349–1356.

Sedy, J. R., Gavrieli, M., Potter, K. G., Hurchla, M. A., Lindsley, R. C., Hildner, K., et al. (2005). B and T lymphocyte attenuator regulates T cell activation through interaction with herpesvirus entry mediator. *Nature Immunology*, *6*(1), 90–98.

Selby, M., Engelhardt, J., Quigley, M., Henning, K., Chen, T., & Srinivasan, M. (2013). Anti-CTLA-4 antibodies of IgG2a isotype enhance antitumor activity through reduction of intratumoral regulatory T cells. *Cancer Immunology Research*, *1*, 32–42, CIR-13-0013.

Serafini, M., Bonamino, M., Golay, J., & Introna, M. (2004). Elongation factor 1 (EF1alpha) promoter in a lentiviral backbone improves expression of the CD20 suicide gene in primary T lymphocytes allowing efficient rituximab-mediated lysis. *Haematologica*, *89*(1), 86–95.

Serafini, M., Manganini, M., Borleri, G., Bonamino, M., Imberti, L., Biondi, A., et al. (2004). Characterization of CD20-transduced T lymphocytes as an alternative suicide gene therapy approach for the treatment of graft-versus-host disease. *Human Gene Therapy*, *15*(1), 63–76.

Sharma, S., Dominguez, A. L., Manrique, S. Z., Cavallo, F., Sakaguchi, S., & Lustgarten, J. (2008). Systemic targeting of CpG-ODN to the tumor microenvironment with anti-neu-CpG hybrid molecule and t regulatory cell depletion induces memory responses in BALB-neuT tolerant mice. *Cancer Research*, *68*(18), 7530–7540.

Sharma, M. D., Hou, D., Baban, B., Koni, P. A., He, Y., Chandler, P. R., et al. (2010). Reprogrammed Foxp^{3+} regulatory T cells provide essential help to support cross-presentation and CD8^{+} T cell priming in naive mice. *Immunity*, *33*(6), 942–954.

Sharma, M. D., Hou, D., Liu, Y., Koni, P. A., Metz, R., Chandler, P., et al. (2009). Indoleamine 2, 3-dioxygenase controls conversion of Foxp3+ Tregs to TH17-like cells in tumor-draining lymph nodes. *Blood*, *113*(24), 6102–6111.

Shi, W., & Siemann, D. W. (2006). Augmented antitumor effects of radiation therapy by 4-1BB antibody (BMS-469492) treatment. *Anticancer Research*, *26*(5A), 3445–3453.

Shimizu, J., Yamazaki, S., Takahashi, T., Ishida, Y., & Sakaguchi, S. (2002). Stimulation of CD25+ CD4+ regulatory T cells through GITR breaks immunological self-tolerance. *Nature Immunology*, *3*(2), 135–142.

Shrimali, R. K., Yu, Z., Theoret, M. R., Chinnasamy, D., Restifo, N. P., & Rosenberg, S. A. (2010). Antiangiogenic agents can increase lymphocyte infiltration into tumor and enhance the effectiveness of adoptive immunotherapy of cancer. *Cancer Research*, *70*(15), 6171–6180.

Shuford, W. W., Klussman, K., Tritchler, D. D., Loo, D. T., Chalupny, J., Siadak, A. W., et al. (1997). 4-1BB costimulatory signals preferentially induce CD8+ T cell proliferation and lead to the amplification in vivo of cytotoxic T cell responses. *The Journal of Experimental Medicine*, *186*(1), 47–55.

Simpson, T. R., Li, F., Montalvo-Ortiz, W., Sepulveda, M. A., Bergerhoff, K., Arce, F., et al. (2013). Fc-dependent depletion of tumor-infiltrating regulatory T cells co-defines the efficacy of anti-CTLA-4 therapy against melanoma. *The Journal of Experimental Medicine*, *210*(9), 1695–1710.

Siva, S., MacManus, M. P., Martin, R. F., & Martin, O. A. (2013). Abscopal effects of radiation therapy: A clinical review for the radiobiologist. *Cancer Letters*, *356*(1), 82–90.

Smith, N. R., Baker, D., Farren, M., Pommier, A., Swann, R., Wang, X., et al. (2013). Tumor stromal architecture can define the intrinsic tumor response to VEGF-targeted therapy. *Clinical Cancer Research*, *19*(24), 6943–6956.

Snyder, A., Makarov, V., Merghoub, T., Yuan, J., Zaretsky, J. M., Desrichard, A., et al. (2014). Genetic basis for clinical response to CTLA-4 blockade in melanoma. *New England Journal of Medicine*, *371*(23), 2189–2199.

Soliman, H. H., Neuger, A., Noyes, D., Vahanian, N. N., Link, C. J., Munn, D., et al. (2012). A phase I study of 1-methyl-D-tryptophan in patients with advanced malignancies. *Journal of Clinical Oncology*, *30*, abstr 2501.

Soroosh, P., Ine, S., Sugamura, K., & Ishii, N. (2006). OX40-OX40 ligand interaction through T cell-T cell contact contributes to CD4 T cell longevity. *The Journal of Immunology*, *176*(10), 5975–5987.

Spencer, D. M., Wandless, T. J., Schreiber, S. L., & Crabtree, G. R. (1993). Controlling signal transduction with synthetic ligands. *Science*, *262*(5136), 1019–1024.

Spranger, S., Koblish, H. K., Horton, B., Scherle, P. A., Newton, R., & Gajewski, T. F. (2014). Mechanism of tumor rejection with doublets of CTLA-4, PD-1/PD-L1, or IDO blockade involves restored IL-2 production and proliferation of CD8+ T cells directly within the tumor microenvironment. *Journal for immunotherapy of cancer*, *2*(1), 3.

Stagg, J., & Allard, B. (2013). Immunotherapeutic approaches in triple-negative breast cancer: Latest research and clinical prospects. *Therapeutic Advances in Medical Oncology*, *5*(3), 169–181.

Stamell, E. F., Wolchok, J. D., Gnjatic, S., Lee, N. Y., & Brownell, I. (2013). The abscopal effect associated with a systemic anti-melanoma immune response. *International Journal of Radiation Oncology, Biology, Physics*, *85*(2), 293–295.

Stanietsky, N., Simic, H., Arapovic, J., Toporik, A., Levy, O., Novik, A., et al. (2009). The interaction of TIGIT with PVR and PVRL2 inhibits human NK cell cytotoxicity.

Proceedings of the National Academy of Sciences of the United States of America, 106(42), 17858–17863.

Stanislawski, T., Voss, R., Lotz, C., Sadovnikova, E., Willemsen, R. A., Kuball, J., et al. (2001). Circumventing tolerance to a human MDM2-derived tumor antigen by TCR gene transfer. *Nature Immunology, 2*(10), 962–970.

Stärck, L., Scholz, C., Dörken, B., & Daniel, P. T. (2005). Costimulation by CD137/4-1BB inhibits T cell apoptosis and induces Bcl-xL and c-FLIPshort via phosphatidylinositol 3-kinase and AKT/protein kinase B. *European Journal of Immunology, 35*(4), 1257–1266.

Steinberg, M. W., Cheung, T. C., & Ware, C. F. (2011). The signaling networks of the herpesvirus entry mediator (TNFRSF14) in immune regulation. *Immunological Reviews, 244*(1), 169–187.

Steinman, R. M., Hawiger, D., & Nussenzweig, M. C. (2003). Tolerogenic dendritic cells. *Annual Review of Immunology, 21*(1), 685–711.

Strome, S. E., Dong, H., Tamura, H., Voss, S. G., Flies, D. B., Tamada, K., et al. (2003). B7-H1 blockade augments adoptive T-cell immunotherapy for squamous cell carcinoma. *Cancer Research, 63*(19), 6501–6505.

Stüber, E., Neurath, M., Calderhead, D., Fell, H. P., & Strober, W. (1995). Cross-linking of OX40 ligand, a member of the TNF/NGF cytokine family, induces proliferation and differentiation in murine splenic B cells. *Immunity, 2*(5), 507–521.

Su, F., Viros, A., Milagre, C., Trunzer, K., Bollag, G., Spleiss, O., et al. (2012). RAS mutations in cutaneous squamous-cell carcinomas in patients treated with BRAF inhibitors. *New England Journal of Medicine, 366*(3), 207–215.

Suntharalingam, G., Perry, M. R., Ward, S., Brett, S. J., Castello-Cortes, A., Brunner, M. D., et al. (2006). Cytokine storm in a phase 1 trial of the anti-CD28 monoclonal antibody TGN1412. *New England Journal of Medicine, 355*(10), 1018–1028.

Svane, I. M., & Verdegaal, E. M. (2014). Achievements and challenges of adoptive T cell therapy with tumor-infiltrating or blood-derived lymphocytes for metastatic melanoma: What is needed to achieve standard of care? *Cancer Immunology, Immunotherapy, 63*(10), 1081–1091.

Sznol, M., Hodi, F., Margolin, K., McDermott, D., Ernstoff, M., Kirkwood, J., et al. (2008). Phase I study of BMS-663513, a fully human anti-CD137 agonist monoclonal antibody, in patients (pts) with advanced cancer (CA). In *ASCO annual meeting proceedings*.

Tai, X., Van Laethem, F., Sharpe, A. H., & Singer, A. (2007). Induction of autoimmune disease in CTLA-4 −/− mice depends on a specific CD28 motif that is required for in vivo costimulation. *Proceedings of the National Academy of Sciences of the United States of America, 104*(34), 13756–13761.

Takahashi, T., Tagami, T., Yamazaki, S., Uede, T., Shimizu, J., Sakaguchi, N., et al. (2000). Immunologic self-tolerance maintained by CD25+ CD4+ regulatory T cells constitutively expressing cytotoxic T lymphocyte-associated antigen 4. *The Journal of Experimental Medicine, 192*(2), 303–310.

Takeda, I., Ine, S., Killeen, N., Ndhlovu, L. C., Murata, K., Satomi, S., et al. (2004). Distinct roles for the OX40-OX40 ligand interaction in regulatory and nonregulatory T cells. *The Journal of Immunology, 172*(6), 3580–3589.

Tao, R., Wang, L., Murphy, K. M., Fraser, C. C., & Hancock, W. W. (2008). Regulatory T cell expression of herpesvirus entry mediator suppresses the function of B and T lymphocyte attenuator-positive effector T cells. *The Journal of Immunology, 180*(10), 6649–6655.

Taube, J. M., Anders, R. A., Young, G. D., Xu, H., Sharma, R., McMiller, T. L., et al. (2012). Colocalization of inflammatory response with B7-h1 expression in human melanocytic lesions supports an adaptive resistance mechanism of immune escape. *Science Translational Medicine, 4*(127), 127ra37.

Taube, J. M., Klein, A., Brahmer, J. R., Xu, H., Pan, X., Kim, J. H., et al. (2014). Association of PD-1, PD-1 ligands, and other features of the tumor immune microenvironment with response to anti-PD-1 therapy. *Clinical Cancer Research*, *20*(19), 5064–5074.

Termeer, C. C., Schirrmacher, V., Bröcker, E., & Becker, J. C. (2000). Newcastle disease virus infection induces B7-1/B7-2-independent T-cell costimulatory activity in human melanoma cells. *Cancer Gene Therapy*, *7*(2), 316–323.

Tey, S. (2014). Adoptive T-cell therapy: Adverse events and safety switches. *Clinical & Translational Immunology*, *3*(6), e17.

Thomis, D. C., Marktel, S., Bonini, C., Traversari, C., Gilman, M., Bordignon, C., et al. (2001). A Fas-based suicide switch in human T cells for the treatment of graft-versus-host disease. *Blood*, *97*(5), 1249–1257.

Thomson, A. W., Turnquist, H. R., & Raimondi, G. (2009). Immunoregulatory functions of mTOR inhibition. *Nature Reviews. Immunology*, *9*(5), 324–337.

Thorpe, L. M., Yuzugullu, H., & Zhao, J. J. (2015). PI3K in cancer: Divergent roles of isoforms, modes of activation and therapeutic targeting. *Nature Reviews Cancer*, *15*(1), 7–24.

Tiberghien, P., Ferrand, C., Lioure, B., Milpied, N., Angonin, R., Deconinck, E., et al. (2001). Administration of herpes simplex-thymidine kinase-expressing donor T cells with a T-cell-depleted allogeneic marrow graft. *Blood*, *97*(1), 63–72.

Tiberghien, P., Reynolds, C. W., Keller, J., Spence, S., Deschaseaux, M., Certoux, J., et al. (1994). Ganciclovir treatment of herpes simplex thymidine kinase-transduced primary T lymphocytes: An approach for specific in vivo donor T-cell depletion after bone marrow transplantation? *Blood*, *84*(4), 1333–1341.

Tirapu, I., Arina, A., Mazzolini, G., Duarte, M., Alfaro, C., Feijoo, E., et al. (2004). Improving efficacy of interleukin-12-transfected dendritic cells injected into murine colon cancer with anti-CD137 monoclonal antibodies and alloantigens. *International Journal of Cancer*, *110*(1), 51–60.

Tivol, E. A., Borriello, F., Schweitzer, A. N., Lynch, W. P., Bluestone, J. A., & Sharpe, A. H. (1995). Loss of CTLA-4 leads to massive lymphoproliferation and fatal multiorgan tissue destruction, revealing a critical negative regulatory role of CTLA-4. *Immunity*, *3*(5), 541–547.

Tokuyama, H., Hagi, T., Mattarollo, S. R., Morley, J., Wang, Q., Fai-So, H., et al. (2008). Vγ9Vδ2 T cell cytotoxicity against tumor cells is enhanced by monoclonal antibody drugs—Rituximab and trastuzumab. *International Journal of Cancer*, *122*(11), 2526–2534.

Tong, R. T., Boucher, Y., Kozin, S. V., Winkler, F., Hicklin, D. J., & Jain, R. K. (2004). Vascular normalization by vascular endothelial growth factor receptor 2 blockade induces a pressure gradient across the vasculature and improves drug penetration in tumors. *Cancer Research*, *64*(11), 3731–3736.

Topalian, S. L., Hodi, F. S., Brahmer, J. R., Gettinger, S. N., Smith, D. C., McDermott, D. F., et al. (2012). Safety, activity, and immune correlates of anti-PD-1 antibody in cancer. *New England Journal of Medicine*, *366*(26), 2443–2454.

Tran, E., Chinnasamy, D., Yu, Z., Morgan, R. A., Lee, C. R., Restifo, N. P., et al. (2013). Immune targeting of fibroblast activation protein triggers recognition of multipotent bone marrow stromal cells and cachexia. *The Journal of Experimental Medicine*, *210*(6), 1125–1135.

Tran, E., Turcotte, S., Gros, A., Robbins, P. F., Lu, Y., Dudley, M. E., et al. (2014). Cancer immunotherapy based on mutation-specific CD4+ T cells in a patient with epithelial cancer. *Science*, *344*(6184), 641–645.

Triebel, F., Hacene, K., & Pichon, M. (2006). A soluble lymphocyte activation gene-3 (sLAG-3) protein as a prognostic factor in human breast cancer expressing estrogen or progesterone receptors. *Cancer Letters*, *235*(1), 147–153.

Tsukamoto, N., Kobayashi, N., Azuma, S., Yamamoto, T., & Inoue, J. (1999). Two differently regulated nuclear factor κB activation pathways triggered by the cytoplasmic tail of CD40. *Proceedings of the National Academy of Sciences of the United States of America*, *96*(4), 1234–1239.

Turk, M. J., Guevara-Patiño, J. A., Rizzuto, G. A., Engelhorn, M. E., & Houghton, A. N. (2004). Concomitant tumor immunity to a poorly immunogenic melanoma is prevented by regulatory T cells. *The Journal of Experimental Medicine*, *200*(6), 771–782.

Tykodi, S. S. (2014). PD-1 as an emerging therapeutic target in renal cell carcinoma: Current evidence. *OncoTargets and Therapy*, *7*, 1349.

Uno, T., Takeda, K., Kojima, Y., Yoshizawa, H., Akiba, H., Mittler, R. S., et al. (2006). Eradication of established tumors in mice by a combination antibody-based therapy. *Nature Medicine*, *12*(6), 693–698.

Uyttenhove, C., Pilotte, L., Théate, I., Stroobant, V., Colau, D., Parmentier, N., et al. (2003). Evidence for a tumoral immune resistance mechanism based on tryptophan degradation by indoleamine 2,3-dioxygenase. *Nature Medicine*, *9*(10), 1269–1274.

Valzasina, B., Guiducci, C., Dislich, H., Killeen, N., Weinberg, A. D., & Colombo, M. P. (2005). Triggering of OX40 (CD134) on CD4+ CD25+ T cells blocks their inhibitory activity: A novel regulatory role for OX40 and its comparison with GITR. *Blood*, *105*(7), 2845–2851.

Vanhaesebroeck, B., Guillermet-Guibert, J., Graupera, M., & Bilanges, B. (2010). The emerging mechanisms of isoform-specific PI3K signalling. *Nature Reviews. Molecular Cell Biology*, *11*(5), 329–341.

Vanhaesebroeck, B., & Khwaja, A. (2014). PI3Kδ inhibition hits a sensitive spot in B cell malignancies. *Cancer Cell*, *25*(3), 269–271.

van Kooten, C., & Banchereau, J. (2000). CD40-CD40 ligand. *Journal of Leukocyte Biology*, *67*(1), 2–17.

Vendel, A. C., Calemine-Fenaux, J., Izrael-Tomasevic, A., Chauhan, V., Arnott, D., & Eaton, D. L. (2009). B and T lymphocyte attenuator regulates B cell receptor signaling by targeting Syk and BLNK. *The Journal of Immunology*, *182*(3), 1509–1517.

Vinay, D. S., & Kwon, B. S. (2014). 4-1BB (CD137), an inducible costimulatory receptor, as a specific target for cancer therapy. *BMB Reports*, *47*(3), 122.

Viola, A., & Lanzavecchia, A. (1996). T cell activation determined by T cell receptor number and tunable thresholds. *Science*, *273*(5271), 104–106.

Vittimberga, F. J., Jr., Foley, D. P., Meyers, W. C., & Callery, M. P. (1998). Laparoscopic surgery and the systemic immune response. *Annals of Surgery*, *227*(3), 326.

Vonderheide, R. H., Bajor, D. L., Winograd, R., Evans, R. A., Bayne, L. J., & Beatty, G. L. (2013). CD40 immunotherapy for pancreatic cancer. *Cancer Immunology, Immunotherapy*, *62*(5), 949–954.

Voss, R., Kuball, J., Engel, R., Guillaume, P., Romero, P., Huber, C., et al. (2006). Redirection of T cells by delivering a transgenic mouse-derived MDM2 tumor antigen-specific TCR and its humanized derivative is governed by the CD8 coreceptor and affects natural human TCR expression. *Immunologic Research*, *34*(1), 67–87.

Wallack, M. K., Sivanandham, M., Ditaranto, K., Shaw, P., Balch, C. M., Urist, M. M., et al. (1997). Increased survival of patients treated with a vaccinia melanoma oncolysate vaccine: Second interim analysis of data from a phase III, multi-institutional trial. *Annals of Surgery*, *226*(2), 198.

Walunas, T. L., Bakker, C., & Bluestone, J. A. (1996). CTLA-4 ligation blocks CD28-dependent T cell activation. *The Journal of Experimental Medicine*, *183*(6), 2541–2550.

Walunas, T. L., Lenschow, D. J., Bakker, C. Y., Linsley, P. S., Freeman, G. J., Green, J. M., et al. (1994). CTLA-4 can function as a negative regulator of T cell activation. *Immunity*, *1*(5), 405–413.

Wang, F., He, W., Zhou, H., Yuan, J., Wu, K., Xu, L., et al. (2007). The Tim-3 ligand galectin-9 negatively regulates CD8+ alloreactive T cell and prolongs survival of skin graft. *Cellular Immunology*, *250*(1), 68–74.

Wang, J., Yoshida, T., Nakaki, F., Hiai, H., Okazaki, T., & Honjo, T. (2005). Establishment of NOD-Pdcd1-/- mice as an efficient animal model of type I diabetes. *Proceedings of the National Academy of Sciences of the United States of America*, *102*(33), 11823–11828.

Wargo, J. A., Cogdill, A., Dang, P., Gupta, R., Piris, A., Boni, A., et al. (2011). Treatment with a selective inhibitor of BRAFV600E increases melanocyte antigen expression and CD8 T cell infiltrate in tumors of patients with metastatic melanoma. *Cancer Research*, *71*(8 Suppl.), 958.

Watanabe, N., Gavrieli, M., Sedy, J. R., Yang, J., Fallarino, F., Loftin, S. K., et al. (2003). BTLA is a lymphocyte inhibitory receptor with similarities to CTLA-4 and PD-1. *Nature Immunology*, *4*(7), 670–679.

Watanabe, A., Hara, M., Chosa, E., Nakamura, K., Sekiya, R., Shimizu, T., et al. (2010). Combination of adoptive cell transfer and antibody injection can eradicate established tumors in mice—An in vivo study using anti-OX40mAb, anti-CD25mAb and anti-CTLA4mAb. *Immunopharmacology and Immunotoxicology*, *32*(2), 238–245.

Waterhouse, P., Penninger, J. M., Timms, E., Wakeham, A., Shahinian, A., Lee, K. P., et al. (1995). Lymphoproliferative disorders with early lethality in mice deficient in Ctla-4. *Science*, *270*(5238), 985–988.

Webb, S., Morris, C., & Sprent, J. (1990). Extrathymic tolerance of mature T cells: Clonal elimination as a consequence of immunity. *Cell*, *63*(6), 1249–1256.

Weber, J. (2007). Review: Anti-CTLA-4 antibody ipilimumab: Case studies of clinical response and immune-related adverse events. *The Oncologist*, *12*(7), 864–872.

Weichhart, T., & Säemann, M. D. (2009). The multiple facets of mTOR in immunity. *Trends in Immunology*, *30*(5), 218–226.

Weinberg, A. D., Rivera, M., Prell, R., Morris, A., Ramstad, T., Vetto, J. T., et al. (2000). Engagement of the OX-40 receptor in vivo enhances antitumor immunity. *The Journal of Immunology*, *164*(4), 2160–2169.

Weinberg, A. D., Wegmann, K. W., Funatake, C., & Whitham, R. H. (1999). Blocking OX-40/OX-40 ligand interaction in vitro and in vivo leads to decreased T cell function and amelioration of experimental allergic encephalomyelitis. *The Journal of Immunology*, *162*(3), 1818–1826.

Westin, J. R., Chu, F., Zhang, M., Fayad, L. E., Kwak, L. W., Fowler, N., et al. (2014). Safety and activity of PD1 blockade by pidilizumab in combination with rituximab in patients with relapsed follicular lymphoma: A single group, open-label, phase 2 trial. *The Lancet Oncology*, *15*(1), 69–77.

Wilcox, R. A., Chapoval, A. I., Gorski, K. S., Otsuji, M., Shin, T., Flies, D. B., et al. (2002). Cutting edge: Expression of functional CD137 receptor by dendritic cells. *The Journal of Immunology*, *168*(9), 4262–4267.

Wilgenhof, S., Du Four, S., Vandenbroucke, F., Everaert, H., Salmon, I., Liénard, D., et al. (2013). Single-center experience with ipilimumab in an expanded access program for patients with pretreated advanced melanoma. *Journal of Immunotherapy*, *36*(3), 215–222.

Wilmott, J. S., Long, G. V., Howle, J. R., Haydu, L. E., Sharma, R. N., Thompson, J. F., et al. (2012). Selective BRAF inhibitors induce marked T-cell infiltration into human metastatic melanoma. *Clinical Cancer Research*, *18*(5), 1386–1394.

Wing, K., Onishi, Y., Prieto-Martin, P., Yamaguchi, T., Miyara, M., Fehervari, Z., et al. (2008). CTLA-4 control over Foxp3+ regulatory T cell function. *Science*, *322*(5899), 271–275.

Wolchok, J. D., Hodi, F. S., Weber, J. S., Allison, J. P., Urba, W. J., Robert, C., et al. (2013). Development of ipilimumab: A novel immunotherapeutic approach for the treatment of advanced melanoma. *Annals of the New York Academy of Sciences*, *1291*(1), 1–13.

Wolchok, J. D., Hoos, A., O'Day, S., Weber, J. S., Hamid, O., Lebbé, C., et al. (2009). Guidelines for the evaluation of immune therapy activity in solid tumors: Immune-related response criteria. *Clinical Cancer Research, 15*(23), 7412–7420.

Wolchok, J. D., Kluger, H., Callahan, M. K., Postow, M. A., Rizvi, N. A., Lesokhin, A. M., et al. (2013). Nivolumab plus ipilimumab in advanced melanoma. *New England Journal of Medicine, 369*(2), 122–133.

Wolchok, J. D., Neyns, B., Linette, G., Negrier, S., Lutzky, J., Thomas, L., et al. (2010). Ipilimumab monotherapy in patients with pretreated advanced melanoma: A randomised, double-blind, multicentre, phase 2, dose-ranging study. *The Lancet Oncology, 11*(2), 155–164.

Woo, S., Turnis, M. E., Goldberg, M. V., Bankoti, J., Selby, M., Nirschl, C. J., et al. (2012). Immune inhibitory molecules LAG-3 and PD-1 synergistically regulate T-cell function to promote tumoral immune escape. *Cancer Research, 72*(4), 917–927.

Workman, C. J., Cauley, L. S., Kim, I., Blackman, M. A., Woodland, D. L., & Vignali, D. A. (2004). Lymphocyte activation gene-3 (CD223) regulates the size of the expanding T cell population following antigen activation in vivo. *The Journal of Immunology, 172*(9), 5450–5455.

Workman, C. J., Dugger, K. J., & Vignali, D. A. (2002). Cutting edge: Molecular analysis of the negative regulatory function of lymphocyte activation gene-3. *The Journal of Immunology, 169*(10), 5392–5395.

Xu, D., Gu, P., Pan, P., Li, Q., Sato, A. I., & Chen, S. (2004). NK and CD8+ T cell-mediated eradication of poorly immunogenic B16-F10 melanoma by the combined action of IL-12 gene therapy and 4-1BB costimulation. *International Journal of Cancer, 109*(4), 499–506.

Xu, Z., & Jin, B. (2010). A novel interface consisting of homologous immunoglobulin superfamily members with multiple functions. *Cellular & Molecular Immunology*, 7(1), 11–19.

Yamazaki, T., Akiba, H., Iwai, H., Matsuda, H., Aoki, M., Tanno, Y., et al. (2002). Expression of programmed death 1 ligands by murine T cells and APC. *The Journal of Immunology, 169*(10), 5538–5545.

Yu, X., Harden, K., Gonzalez, L. C., Francesco, M., Chiang, E., Irving, B., et al. (2009). The surface protein TIGIT suppresses T cell activation by promoting the generation of mature immunoregulatory dendritic cells. *Nature Immunology, 10*(1), 48–57.

Zamarin, D., Holmgaard, R. B., Subudhi, S. K., Park, J. S., Mansour, M., Palese, P., et al. (2014). Localized oncolytic virotherapy overcomes systemic tumor resistance to immune checkpoint blockade immunotherapy. *Science Translational Medicine*, *6*(226), 226ra32.

Zamarin, D., & Palese, P. (2012). Oncolytic Newcastle disease virus for cancer therapy: Old challenges and new directions. *Future Microbiology*, 7(3), 347–367.

Zamarin, D., & Wolchok, J. D. (2014). Potentiation of immunomodulatory antibody therapy with oncolytic viruses for treatment of cancer. *Molecular Therapy—Oncolytics, 1*, 14004.

Zhang, Y., Louboutin, J., Zhu, J., Rivera, A. J., & Emerson, S. G. (2002). Preterminal host dendritic cells in irradiated mice prime CD8+ T cell-mediated acute graft-versus-host disease. *The Journal of Clinical Investigation, 109*(10), 1335–1344.

Zhang, Y., Ma, C. J., Wang, J. M., Ji, X. J., Wu, X. Y., Moorman, J. P., et al. (2012). Tim-3 regulates pro-and anti-inflammatory cytokine expression in human CD14+ monocytes. *Journal of Leukocyte Biology, 91*(2), 189–196.

Zhou, Q., Munger, M. E., Veenstra, R. G., Weigel, B. J., Hirashima, M., Munn, D. H., et al. (2011). Coexpression of Tim-3 and PD-1 identifies a CD8+ T-cell exhaustion phenotype in mice with disseminated acute myelogenous leukemia. *Blood, 117*(17), 4501–4510.

Zhu, C., Anderson, A. C., Schubart, A., Xiong, H., Imitola, J., Khoury, S. J., et al. (2005). The Tim-3 ligand galectin-9 negatively regulates T helper type 1 immunity. *Nature Immunology*, *6*(12), 1245–1252.

Zingoni, A., Sornasse, T., Cocks, B. G., Tanaka, Y., Santoni, A., & Lanier, L. L. (2004). Cross-talk between activated human NK cells and CD4+ T cells via OX40-OX40 ligand interactions. *The Journal of Immunology*, *173*(6), 3716–3724.

CHAPTER TWO

Immune Targeting of Tumor Epithelial–Mesenchymal Transition via Brachyury-Based Vaccines

Claudia Palena[1], Duane H. Hamilton[1]
Laboratory of Tumor Immunology and Biology, Center for Cancer Research, National Cancer Institute, National Institutes of Health, Bethesda, Maryland, USA
[1]Corresponding authors: e-mail address: palenac@mail.nih.gov; hamiltondh@mail.nih.gov

Contents

Abstract

As a manifestation of their inherent plasticity, carcinoma cells undergo profound phenotypic changes during progression toward metastasis. One such phenotypic modulation is the epithelial–mesenchymal transition (EMT), an embryonically relevant process that can be reinstated by tumor cells, resulting in the acquisition of metastatic propensity, stem-like cell properties, and resistance to a variety of anticancer therapies, including chemotherapy, radiation, and some small-molecule targeted therapies. Targeting of the EMT is emerging as a novel intervention against tumor progression. This review focuses on the potential use of cancer vaccine strategies targeting tumor cells that exhibit mesenchymal-like features, with an emphasis on the current status of

Advances in Cancer Research, Volume 128
ISSN 0065-230X
http://dx.doi.org/10.1016/bs.acr.2015.04.001

development of vaccine platforms directed against the T-box transcription factor brachyury, a novel cancer target involved in tumor EMT, stemness, and resistance to therapies. Also presented is a summary of potential mechanisms of resistance to immune-mediated attack driven by EMT and the development of novel combinatorial strategies based on the use of agents that alleviate tumor EMT for an optimized targeting of plastic tumor cells that are responsible for tumor recurrence and the establishment of therapeutic refractoriness.

1. INTRODUCTION

Metastatic disease, the main cause of cancer-related deaths, is driven by the ability of malignant tumors to disseminate and to colonize sites that are distant from the location of the primary mass (Hanahan & Weinberg, 2000). Frequently, tumor dissemination is also associated with refractoriness to a range of conventional anticancer therapies, including chemotherapy and radiation (Braun et al., 2000), and several molecular-targeted therapies (Thomson et al., 2005; Thomson, Petti, Sujka-Kwok, Epstein, & Haley, 2008). In light of the recent advances in the field of cancer immunotherapy, an attractive therapeutic alternative to address the problem of metastatic disease is the generation of a sustained immune response directed against essential molecular drivers of tumor progression. This chapter focuses on the current status of development of immune-mediated anticancer interventions aimed at preventing and/or treating metastatic disease. Among the topics discussed here are (a) the role of the epithelial–mesenchymal transition (EMT) in tumor dissemination and metastasis, (b) the association of EMT with tumor stemness and resistance to multiple anticancer therapies, (c) how therapeutic cancer vaccines can be used to target regulators of EMT, and (d) the potential for mitigation of metastatic disease by the use of combinatorial therapies of cancer vaccines and other agents that alleviate tumor EMT. While this chapter does not discuss in detail the numerous factors involved in the design and development of therapeutic cancer vaccines, comprehensive reviews on this topic can be found in the literature (Palena & Schlom, 2010; Schlom, 2012; Schlom et al., 2014).

2. TUMOR EMT

2.1 EMT and Tumor Invasiveness

In order to metastasize, cancer cells undergo a series of events known collectively as the metastatic cascade, a process that involves their detachment from the primary tumor mass and invasion into the surrounding tissues, entrance into the circulation, homing in on distant organs, and survival and proliferation at secondary sites (Nguyen, Bos, & Massague, 2009; Nguyen & Massague, 2007). Multiple studies have now demonstrated that carcinoma cells undergo profound phenotypic changes during progression toward metastasis. These phenotypic fluctuations allow tumor cells to reversibly or irreversibly shift from (a) a relatively stationary state into an invasive one, (b) a proliferative state into a comparatively quiescent one, and (c) from being responsive to antitumor therapies into a refractory, non-responsive state. Altogether, these phenotypic modulations can be considered as manifestations of the inherent plasticity of cancer cells, which allows the tumor to dynamically adapt and to effectively progress toward metastatic disease (Nieto, 2013).

EMT has recently gained much attention within the field of cancer research due to its potentially critical role during carcinoma progression (Kalluri & Weinberg, 2009; Thiery, 2002). While EMT is normally involved in the morphogenetic events of embryogenesis, it is now understood that epithelial neoplasms can also aberrantly undergo a similar phenotypic switch in favor of acquiring an invasive, metastatic phenotype (Thiery, 2003; Thiery, Acloque, Huang, & Nieto, 2009). During passage through EMT, epithelial cells lose their stationary behavior, cell polarity, intercellular junctions, and epithelial markers (E-cadherin and cytokeratines) and upregulate the expression of proteins normally expressed by mesenchymal cells (Fibronectin, Vimentin, and N-cadherin), while acquiring motility and invasiveness, two properties that are fundamental for the initial steps of the metastatic cascade (Yang & Weinberg, 2008; Fig. 1). Like the embryogenesis-related EMT, tumor-related EMT is thought to be a reversible process, where the reacquisition of epithelial features by tumor cells may take place at the site of metastasis through a process designated as mesenchymal–epithelial transition (MET) (Fig. 1; Iwatsuki et al., 2010).

There are several reports that document the involvement of EMT in human carcinomas *in vivo*; however, the number of such studies is trivial compared to the extensive amount of data describing the occurrence and consequences of EMT in preclinical models *in vitro*. A recent report, for example, has shown that in breast cancer patients undergoing adjuvant therapy, recurring tumors after treatment with standard chemotherapy had an increased proportion of cells expressing EMT-associated genes, highlighting the importance of EMT in therapeutic resistance and breast cancer

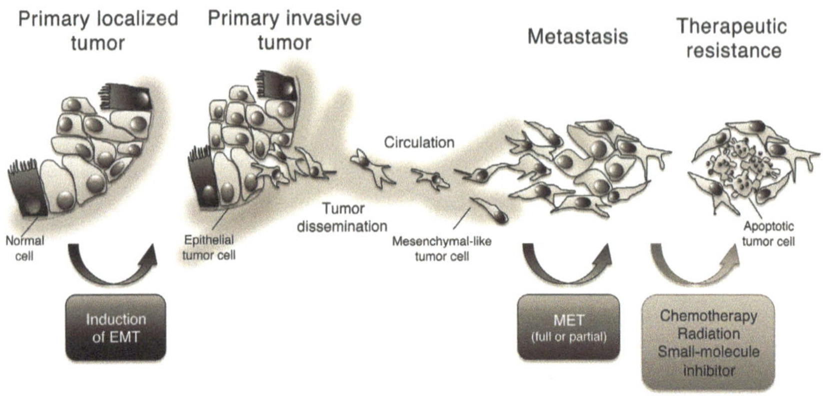

Figure 1 Role of the EMT–MET phenomena in tumor metastasis and acquisition of therapeutic resistance. *Adapted from Palena, Fernando, and Hamilton (2014).* (See the color plate.)

recurrence (Creighton et al., 2009). Another relevant report has demonstrated that circulating tumor cells (CTCs) from breast cancer patients express both mesenchymal and epithelial markers, with mesenchymal CTCs being associated with disease progression (Yu et al., 2013), thus supporting the idea that EMT may play a role in the blood-borne dissemination of breast cancer. Interestingly, the same report demonstrated that reversible shifts between the epithelial and mesenchymal phenotype of CTCs take place along cycles of treatment and disease progression, a manifestation of the plastic character of cancer cells. In line with the idea that EMT is a plastic, reversible modulation of tumor phenotype, it has been observed, for example, that epithelial E-cadherin can be reexpressed in metastatic lesions of breast cancer patients, even when the primary tumor demonstrates low levels of E-cadherin (Bukholm, Nesland, & Borresen-Dale, 2000).

2.2 EMT and Tumor Stemness

The existence of a subpopulation of tumor cells with self-renewal and tumor-initiating properties within an individual tumor mass, designated as cancer stem cells (CSCs), has been a matter of intensive investigation in the past few years. The original understanding of the hierarchical phenomenon of stem cell division recognized in normal tissues and hematological malignancies (Chao, Seita, & Weissman, 2008; Reya, Morrison, Clarke, & Weissman, 2001) has now been broadened to include the idea that, in solid tumors, differentiated cancer cells could adopt stem-like properties themselves, via plastic phenotypic modulations (Scheel & Weinberg,

2011, 2012). This idea has been fueled by the detection of a link between tumor EMT and the acquisition of features normally attributable to stem cells (i.e., tumor stemness), which includes the ability to initiate tumor formation, quiescence, resistance to apoptosis, and metastatic propensity (Polyak & Weinberg, 2009). To cite a few examples of the association between EMT and stemness, induction of EMT in human mammary epithelial cells has been shown to increase the proportion of cells bearing markers associated with stem-like cells (CD44 high/CD24 low) (Mani et al., 2008). In the clinical setting, the EMT–stemness association has been seen where residual breast tumor cell populations surviving post-conventional treatments were enriched in CD44+/CD24−/low cells that also exhibited mesenchymal features (Creighton et al., 2009).

It has now been demonstrated by many groups that EMT is not a twofold process, but instead a dynamic modulation of phenotype that generates tumor cells with shared epithelial and mesenchymal features (Tan et al., 2014). Interestingly, some recent studies have demonstrated that these intermediate cells harbor more characteristics of stem-like cells, including resistance to cell death and ability to form spheroids, than purely epithelial or mesenchymal cells (Huang, Wong, et al., 2013; Jordan, Johnson, & Abell, 2011).

Another example of the association between tumor EMT and the establishment of a stem cell-like state comes from studies on the role of inflammatory chemokine IL-8 in tumor biology (Palena, Hamilton, & Fernando, 2012). In breast cancer, for example, expression of the IL-8 receptor A (IL-8RA) has been shown to be predominant among populations of breast CSCs, and the addition of IL-8 to breast cancer cell lines enhanced the number, motility, and invasiveness of CSCs (Charafe-Jauffret et al., 2009; Ginestier et al., 2010). In parallel studies, it has been shown that induction of EMT in breast carcinoma cells results in a marked induction of the IL-8/IL-8R axis which, in an autocrine fashion, was able to maintain the EMT phenotype of the tumor cells (Fernando, Castillo, Litzinger, Hamilton, & Palena, 2011). Thus, the phenomena of EMT and CSCs in breast carcinomas appear to be linked by the activation of the IL-8/IL-8R axis.

2.3 EMT and Tumor Resistance

A major consequence of the transition from an epithelial to a mesenchymal-like phenotype by tumor cells is the acquisition of tumor resistance to a variety of cell death-inducing signals. For example, induction of oxaliplatin resistance in colorectal cancer cells (Yang et al., 2006), paclitaxel- or radioresistance in ovarian cancer cells (Kajiyama et al., 2007; Kurrey et al., 2009), and gemcitabine resistance in pancreatic carcinoma cells (Shah et al., 2007) has been associated with a switch from an epithelial to a mesenchymal-like phenotype. Intriguingly, one point of intersection connecting the concepts of EMT, stem-like state, and therapy resistance is that of proliferative restraint. In multiple experimental model systems, the induction of tumor EMT has been demonstrated to trigger a significant inhibition of cell cycle due to the modulation of cell cycle-associated proteins, including p21 and Cyclin D1, among others (Huang, Cohen, et al., 2013; Larocca et al., 2013; Mejlvang et al., 2007; Vega et al., 2004). As conventional cancer therapies, such as chemotherapy and radiation, require cell cycle processes to trigger apoptosis and target rapidly proliferating cells, it seems likely that inhibition of cell cycle during the EMT could allow tumor cells to initiate repair mechanisms, potentially preventing cytotoxicity (Fig. 1).

In addition to inducing resistance to conventional therapeutics, acquisition of mesenchymal features by carcinoma cells has been also associated with resistance to a range of molecularly targeted therapies, including resistance to epidermal growth factor receptor (EGFR) kinase inhibitors (Byers et al., 2013; Thomson et al., 2005, 2008) and acquired resistance to HER-2-directed therapy (Kim et al., 2014).

3. TARGETING OF EMT

Due to its critical role in cancer progression, targeting of EMT as a means of preventing metastasis, and possibly, of eliminating cancer cells that would otherwise resist most currently available therapies, is being considered as an attractive therapeutic alternative to the problem of metastatic disease (Palena et al., 2011). Some of the possible approaches that are being explored to inhibit the EMT involve the use of small-molecule agents that block the signaling pathways initiated by multiple cytokines, growth factors, or extracellular compartment components that are responsible for the initiation and/or maintenance of EMT. These agents include, but are not limited to, specific inhibitors of the EGFR, Axl, and Wnt-signaling pathways (Nantajit, Lin, & Li, 2014; Wilson et al., 2014; Zhang et al., 2009). Similarly, various TGF-β receptor I inhibitors have been used to revert the TGF-β-induced EMT in murine or human cancer cells *in vitro* (Halder, Beauchamp, & Datta, 2005;

Peng et al., 2005). One caveat of these approaches, however, is that the signaling pathways that control EMT are typically redundant, and the blockade of one such pathway might not be efficient when other alternative signaling pathways that mediate EMT are turned on.

3.1 EMT Transcription Factors

A different alternative being explored to lessen the occurrence of tumor EMT is the direct targeting of the transcriptional drivers of EMT, commonly designated as "EMT transcription factors" (EMT-TFs) (Palena, Fernando, et al., 2014). In general, the EMT-TFs are expressed in the early embryo, where they participate in the control of developmental EMT, and are subsequently overexpressed in tumor cells undergoing a plastic transition of phenotype. Perhaps, the most studied among the EMT-TFs are those that directly repress the E-cadherin gene, including the zinc finger proteins Snail and Slug, as the event of E-cadherin loss is considered a hallmark of EMT. Both proteins have been shown to trigger EMT in multiple model systems (Bolos et al., 2003; Cano et al., 2000), and their expression has been correlated with progression in human tumors of breast and cervical origin (Blanco et al., 2002; Lee, Chou, Tang, & Shen, 2008). Another regulator of EMT that participates directly or indirectly in the repression of E-cadherin is Twist (Yang et al., 2004), which is also increased in various types of human cancer, including breast, prostate, and cervical cancer. Twist has been correlated with poor disease outcome or more advanced disease status in various types of carcinomas (Kwok et al., 2005; Shibata et al., 2008).

A more recently described EMT-TF is the T-box transcription factor brachyury (also known as T), which is critically involved in embryonic development by promoting the formation of the posterior mesoderm via an EMT (Cunliffe & Smith, 1992; Kispert, Koschorz, & Herrmann, 1995; Muller & Herrmann, 1997). High levels of brachyury have been demonstrated in several human tumors, including chordomas (Tirabosco et al., 2008; Vujovic et al., 2006; Yang et al., 2009), hemangioblastomas (Barresi et al., 2012), and a range of human carcinomas such as lung (Hamilton, Fernando, Schlom, & Palena, 2014; Haro et al., 2013; Roselli et al., 2012), breast (Palena, Roselli, et al., 2014), colon (Kilic et al., 2011), and prostate, among others (Pinto et al., 2014), while brachyury is absent in the majority of normal tissues evaluated, with a few exceptions (Hamilton, Litzinger, Fernando, Huang, & Palena, 2012; Palena et al., 2007; Roselli et al., 2012). It has now been demonstrated in multiple preclinical experimental systems that brachyury promotes carcinoma cells to undergo an EMT *in vitro* (Fernando et al., 2011, 2010; Larocca et al., 2013), characterized by loss of epithelial markers (including E-cadherin), overexpression of mesenchymal-associated proteins, and gain of motility and invasiveness, while facilitating the metastatic dissemination of human tumor xenografts *in vivo*. In addition to its role in tumor EMT, the levels of brachyury have now been shown to positively correlate with the resistance of malignant cells to various chemotherapies and radiation (Huang, Cohen, et al., 2013; Larocca et al., 2013), and several studies have demonstrated the association between robust brachyury expression and poor clinical outcome in patients with various types of carcinomas. For example, the expression of brachyury has been reported to positively correlate with tumor progression in lung (Haro et al., 2013) and breast (Palena, Roselli, et al., 2014), and brachyury has been recently proposed to play a predominant role in triple-negative versus nontriple-negative breast tumors (Ben-Hamo, Gidoni, & Efroni, 2014). In line with these observations, experiments conducted with human breast cancer cell lines showed that overexpression of brachyury drives tumor invasiveness and, at the same time, upregulates the expression of markers of stemness, including the pluripotency regulators sex determining region Y box 2 (SOX2), NANOG, and octamer-binding transcription factor 4 (OCT-4), and enhances the tumor's ability to form mammospheres *in vitro*, a feature associated with stem cells. Brachyury-high breast tumor cells also manifested lower cell proliferation rates *in vitro* and were more resistant to the cytotoxic effects of docetaxel (Palena, Roselli, et al., 2014). These results are in agreement with the observation that high expression of brachyury in primary tumors of breast cancer patients treated with tamoxifen adjuvant therapy for 5 years is associated with poor prognosis, further supporting the involvement of brachyury in resistance to drug therapy.

3.2 Advantage of an Immune Approach Against EMT

The therapeutic alternative of targeting EMT-TFs as a means of alleviating EMT implies the targeting of intracellular molecules, a fact that precludes the use of monoclonal antibodies. In addition, conventional pharmacological approaches have been so far unsuccessful for the targeting of transcription factors due to their lack of a specific groove for tight binding of an inhibitor. In this context, T-cell-mediated immunotherapy offers a distinct possibility. Because T cells recognize a target in the form of short peptides presented in the context of the major histocompatibility complex (MHC) on the surface of target cells, T-cell-mediated immunotherapy can be used to target molecules irrespective of their cellular localization. By immunizing the patient against one of the relevant EMT-TFs, an effective T-cell immune response could be elicited that, in turn, could selectively eradicate tumor cells expressing the EMT driver of choice.

3.3 Immunotherapeutic Approaches Against Cancer

The aim of an immunotherapeutic approach against cancer is to elicit or to enhance a tumor-specific immune response in the host that, in turn, could mediate tumor control in the long range. There are several approaches currently under investigation to achieve this objective, including (i) vaccination of the patient against a tumor-specific antigen(s), (ii) adoptive transfer of tumor-specific T cells, and (iii) the blockade of immune inhibitory pathways (immune checkpoints) that mediate tumor evasion by restricting T-cell activation or effector function.

3.3.1 Cancer Vaccines

Therapeutic cancer vaccines are designed to stimulate a tumor-specific immune response by immunizing the patient against one or several tumor antigens, and may utilize one of four basic platforms: recombinant vectors, dendritic cell (DC)-based vaccines, whole tumor cell vaccines, and peptide/protein vaccines (Palena & Schlom, 2010). Unlike standard cancer treatments, therapeutic cancer vaccines have shown no associated toxicities and their immunotherapeutic effect could be long lasting. Vector-based vaccines are perhaps one of the most flexible vaccine delivery systems; among the vectors being evaluated are poxviruses, alphaviruses, bacterial (Salmonella, Listeria), and yeast vectors. In general, the "off-the-shelf" nature of vector vaccines renders them suitable for large, multicenter randomized trials. For example, a poxviral-based vaccine (PROSTVAC) encoding for prostate-specific antigen (PSA) and a triad of costimulatory molecules (B7.1, ICAM-1, LFA-3, designated TRICOM) is currently being evaluated in an international, Phase III randomized clinical trial in metastatic castration-resistant prostate cancer patients (Madan, Bilusic, Heery, Schlom, & Gulley, 2012; Singh & Gulley, 2014). The pros and cons of each vaccine platform as well as their current status of clinical development have been extensively reviewed elsewhere (Disis, 2014; Larocca & Schlom, 2011; Schlom et al., 2014).

3.3.2 Immune Checkpoint Inhibition

In addition to tumor cells being poorly immunogenic, the tumor microenvironment is known to further decrease the effectiveness of antitumor immune responses by potentiating different immunosuppressive mechanisms (Drake, Jaffee, & Pardoll, 2006; Igney & Krammer, 2002; Rabinovich, Gabrilovich, & Sotomayor, 2007). These inhibitory pathways, normally required for maintaining homeostasis within the immune system, can be functional in tumors where they could limit antitumor T-cell activation and effector functions. The molecules perhaps most studied in this respect are the cytotoxic T lymphocyte antigen-4 (CTLA-4) and programmed cell death-1 (PD-1) and its ligands, PDL-1 and PDL-2 (Shin & Ribas, 2015). CTLA-4 is expressed on the surface of activated T cells and delivers a negative signal upon ligation of B7-1 and B7-2; its blockade with the antibody ipilimumab has shown durable responses in patients with advance melanoma (Hodi et al., 2010). PD-1 is also expressed by activated T cells and binds PDL-1 and PDL-2 that are expressed in malignant cells; blockade of the PD-1/PD-L1 pathway has shown remarkable clinical responses in patients with advanced melanoma and some types of carcinomas, including lung cancer (Hamid et al., 2013; Hodi et al., 2010; Topalian, Drake, & Pardoll, 2012; Topalian, Hodi, et al., 2012). The use of immune checkpoint inhibitors is being extended to many different cancer types, and it is likely that the combination of these agents with therapeutic cancer vaccines will represent an exciting step forward in cancer treatments.

3.4 The Choice of Tumor Antigen

One fundamental aspect in the development of cancer vaccine approaches is the selection of the tumor antigen to be delivered to the host's immune system. In general, tumor antigens can be classified into one of two major categories. The first category corresponds to "tumor-specific antigens," which are molecules expressed *de novo* by the tumor cells, such as mutated proteins or virally derived products in tumors driven by infectious agents (Palena & Schlom, 2010). Most antigens so far studied, however, fall within a second category of "tumor-associated antigens," which are proteins overexpressed in tumors that could be also expressed at low levels in normal adult tissues or were expressed in early embryonic development. EMT-TFs belong to the second category, as they are molecules normally expressed during embryo development but minimally expressed in adult tissues, and reexpressed in neoplastic cells. An additional attractive feature of EMT-TFs as targets for immunotherapy relates to their functional relevance. In general, cancer cells are able to acquire multiple mechanisms that allow them to evade immune recognition and rejection, including the loss of a targeted antigen and the establishment of antigen-negative tumor clones (DuPage, Mazumdar, Schmidt, Cheung, & Jacks, 2012). Because of their critical role in the establishment of a metastatic phenotype, targeting of an EMT-TF could potentially minimize the effects of antigenic loss as tumor cells that downregulate the expression of the targeted EMT-TF will not be able to metastasize.

3.5 Brachyury as a Tumor Antigen

Brachyury fulfills two major requisites for a molecule to be used as a cancer vaccine target: (a) tumor specificity, as its expression is almost exclusively confined to neoplastic tissues in the adult and (b) immunogenicity. This last feature was first revealed when experiments conducted *in vitro* demonstrated that brachyury-specific cytotoxic $CD8^+$ T cells could be expanded from the blood of cancer patients by repeated stimulation with a nonameric brachyury-derived peptide (Palena et al., 2007). The peptide, an HLA-A0201-restricted epitope (WLLPGTSTL), was identified via a binding prediction algorithm and utilized *in vitro* for pulsing of DCs and subsequent stimulation of autologous T cells from the blood of colorectal and ovarian cancer patients. These brachyury-specific T cells were then shown to be able to lyse carcinoma cells that present endogenously processed epitopes of brachyury in the context of MHC class I molecules, including lung, colorectal, and breast carcinoma cells (Palena et al., 2007; Palena, Roselli, et al., 2014; Roselli et al., 2012). The epitope was subsequently modified by substitution of an amino acid involved in MHC binding and the resulting agonist epitope of brachyury (WLLPGTSTV) was shown to be more efficient than the native counterpart at expanding brachyury-specific T cells from the blood of cancer patients and at lysing cancer cells expressing the native brachyury protein. The immunogenicity of this peptide was also demonstrated *in vivo* by vaccination of A2.1/Kb transgenic mice using peptide in adjuvant (Tucker et al., 2014).

Another demonstration of the immunogenicity of brachyury arose from observations that some patients receiving cancer vaccines directed against PSA or carcinoembryonic antigen (CEA) also developed spontaneous CD8+ T-cell responses to brachyury, as measured directly from peripheral blood via the ELISPOT assay (Madan, Mohebtash, et al., 2012). As the patients received a vaccine targeting proteins other than brachyury, it is presumed that the expansion of brachyury-specific CD8+ T cells is a manifestation of the phenomenon of antigen spreading, i.e., the generation of an immune response against tumor antigens cross-presented to the immune system following tumor destruction in response to the vaccine. These studies together demonstrated that brachyury is an immunogenic protein with the potential to serve as a target for anticancer vaccination.

Potentially, EMT-TFs other than brachyury that are known to control human tumor progression could be explored as novel tumor antigens for the targeting of metastatic disease, provided that they also meet the criteria of tumor specificity and immunogenicity.

3.6 Therapeutic Vaccines Against Brachyury

3.6.1 Yeast-Based Brachyury Vaccine

One type of vector-based vaccine platform is a heat-killed recombinant strain of *Saccharomyces cerevisiae*, a nonpathogenic yeast species that efficiently activates DCs via Toll-like receptors and induces the production of high levels of type I cytokines, including IL-2, TNF-α, and IFN-γ (Bernstein et al., 2008; Remondo et al., 2009). Yeast vectors can be readily engineered to express one or more tumor antigens and have been well characterized in various preclinical and clinical studies. For example, a recombinant yeast-CEA vaccine has been used *in vitro* to expand murine and human T cells directed against the CEA protein, as well as *in vivo* for vaccination of mice bearing CEA-expressing tumors, resulting in antitumor activity (Bernstein et al., 2008; Boehm, Higgins, Franzusoff, Schlom, & Hodge, 2010; Cereda et al., 2011; Remondo et al., 2009; Wansley et al., 2008). In clinical studies, heat-killed yeast vaccines have been used in multicenter trials in patients with Hepatitis C, lung, and pancreatic carcinomas, and in patients with metastatic CEA-expressing carcinomas (Bilusic et al., 2014; Chaft et al., 2014; Hartley, Bade, Prins, Ampie, & Marshall, 2014). All of these studies demonstrated that yeast-based vaccines (a) can be injected repeatedly without inducing neutralizing responses, (b) possess excellent safety and tolerability profiles, and (c) are able to induce measurable tumor-specific immune responses.

A heat-killed recombinant yeast has been developed (designated as GI-6301) that expresses the full-length human brachyury protein. This vaccine has been initially used in preclinical studies to activate and promote the maturation of human DCs *in vitro* as well as to expand human brachyury-specific CD8+ and CD4+ T cells from the peripheral blood of healthy donors and cancer patients (Hamilton et al., 2013). The vaccine was also evaluated *in vivo*, where the administration of heat-killed brachyury-expressing yeast to mice was able to elicit brachyury-specific CD4+ and CD8+ T-cell responses that were capable of reducing tumor burden in an experimental model of brachyury-driven metastasis, in the absence of toxicity (Hamilton et al., 2013; Palena, Fernando, et al., 2014). Based on these studies, a Phase I clinical trial has been initiated with the yeast–brachyury vaccine GI-6301 to treat patients with advanced carcinomas as well as chordomas (www.clinicaltrials.gov, 2013). The initial results of this Phase I trial have been reported (Heery et al., 2014; Singh et al., 2014); the yeast–brachyury vaccine was well tolerated and brachyury-specific CD8+ and/or CD4+ T-cell responses were present in the blood of some patients post- versus pre-vaccination. These results demonstrated, for the first time in humans, that an EMT-TF could be targeted immunologically via vaccination.

3.6.2 Poxvirus-Based Brachyury Vaccine

Members of the poxvirus family, including vaccinia, modified vaccinia strain Ankara (MVA), and the avipox virus fowlpox, are being explored as cancer vaccine delivery systems in a variety of clinical studies. Poxviruses offer several advantages as vaccine delivery systems, including (a) the ability to accept large inserts of foreign DNA, allowing for the inclusion of multiple transgenes, (b) viral replication and transcription of the poxvirus genome takes place in the cytosol of the infected cell, thereby minimizing the risk of random insertion into the host's DNA, and (c) the encoded transgenes can be processed and presented by both MHC class I and II pathways, leading to activation of CD8+ and CD4+ T-cell responses. One particular recombinant poxvirus platform that has been extensively characterized both preclinically and clinically consists of a recombinant vaccinia or fowlpox virus that encodes for transgenes for one or more tumor-associated antigens (PSA, CEA, MUC-1) and the TRICOM triad of costimulatory molecules including B7.1, ICAM-1, and LFA-3. For a comprehensive review of the clinical development of poxviral-based cancer vaccines, see Madan, Bilusic, et al. (2012).

MVA is a highly attenuated strain of vaccinia virus that does not replicate productively in human cells, which has been administered to a large number of individuals in the final stages of the smallpox eradication campaign in Germany and Turkey (Blanchard, Alcami, Andrea, & Smith, 1998; Im & Hanke, 2004; Mayr & Danner, 1978). The absence of undesired effects among vaccinated individuals, including those with immune deficiencies, makes MVA a safe, ideal poxviral vector to use in immunotherapeutic approaches against cancer (Cosma et al., 2003; Im & Hanke, 2004). Recently, an MVA-poxviral vaccine encoding human brachyury and the TRICOM molecules has been developed and its testing in a Phase I clinical trial in patients with advanced carcinomas is currently ongoing (www.clinicaltrials.gov, 2014).

To our knowledge, yeast–brachyury and MVA–brachyury–TRICOM are the first vaccines targeting a driver of EMT that have successfully entered clinical development. Although it is still early to understand the mechanism of action of brachyury-based vaccine approaches, we speculate that the immune targeting of tumor cells undergoing brachyury-mediated EMT could have different outcomes when used at various stages of disease. If employed at an early stage of disease, the elimination of tumor cells that upregulate the expression of brachyury could prevent the establishment of metastatic lesions by eradicating tumor cells with migratory and invasive properties. At later stages of disease, however, once metastases have been established, it is also possible that a brachyury vaccine could potentially limit the acquisition of chemo- or radioresistance by eliminating therapy-resistant, stem-like cancer cells.

Because of the variety of tumor types showing some level of brachyury expression, brachyury-based vaccines could potentially be applied towards the treatment of several types of common carcinomas. As the phenomenon of EMT, which brachyury regulates, is considered to be transient, it is important to point out that, unlike with the targeting of proteins that are constitutively expressed in cancer cells, expression of brachyury in tumors should be thought of as a dynamic and reversible event. Thus, brachyury might be restricted to a minority of tumor cells or be detectable only at a given time along tumor progression. This fact should be taken into consideration when evaluating its expression in a biopsy specimen, which would measure the level of brachyury in a specific site and at that one moment in time. In agreement with these postulates, expression of brachyury, for example, has been observed in a minority of cells in the primary tumor, while a higher proportion of brachyury-positive tumor cells and higher levels of expression have been observed in metastatic lymph nodes or distal metastases derived from the same patient (Palena, Roselli, et al., 2014).

4. OVERCOMING POTENTIAL TUMOR IMMUNE RESISTANCE

While the associations of tumor EMT with tumor escape from conventional antineoplastic interventions or certain small-molecule targeted therapies, such as EGFR inhibitors, have been extensively documented, few reports have investigated whether tumor plasticity mediated by EMT could also mediate resistance to immune-mediated attack, potentially contributing to tumor escape from host immune surveillance and failure of immune-mediated rejection.

Some of the most studied mechanisms of immune evasion involve defects in any of the multiple components of the antigen-processing and/or presentation machinery, including the loss or reduction of MHC expression and the loss of antigen. However, recent reports have also started to implicate the phenomenon of EMT in the resistance of tumor cells to immune-mediated lysis. For example, it has been recently shown that the acquisition of EMT properties by tumor cells triggers the mechanism of autophagy that, in turn, protects tumor cells from cytotoxic T-cell-mediated lysis (Akalay, Janji, Hasmim, Noman, Andre, et al., 2013; Akalay, Janji, Hasmim, Noman, Thiery, et al., 2013). Another example of the potential negative impact of tumor EMT in immune-mediated lysis is the case of tumor cells that express very high levels of the transcription factor brachyury. The analysis of the cytotoxic response of human carcinoma cell lines with a range of brachyury expression demonstrated that the cytotoxic lysis of tumor cells with very high levels of brachyury is significantly reduced compared to that of brachyury-intermediate/low cells in response to brachyury-specific CD8 + T cells (Hamilton, Huang, Fernando, Tsang, & Palena, 2014). Interestingly, the impairment of immune effector-mediated lysis of tumor cells with very high levels of brachyury was also extended to antigen-independent lysis mediated by innate natural killer or lymphokine-activated killer cells, as well as to lysis mediated by other antigen-specific T cells, even in the presence of normal levels of the corresponding target antigen(s). This paradoxical observation that tumor lysis diminished in the presence of very high levels of the target antigen led to the hypothesis that very high levels of brachyury, as it is observed in some tumor tissues (oval, Fig. 2), could impart resistance to immune-mediated antitumor interventions. As seen in this proposed model, the majority of human carcinomas exhibit intermediate or low levels of brachyury and would be optimally lysed by brachyury-specific

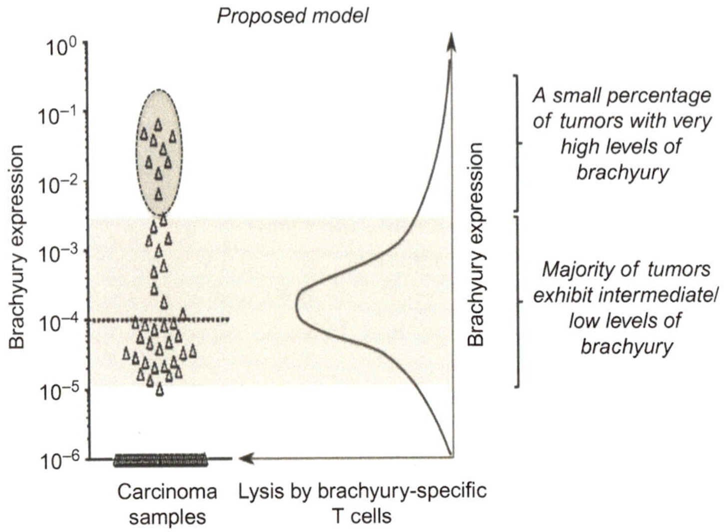

Figure 2 Expression of brachyury in lung cancer tissues (triangles); shaded area indicates the range of brachyury expression (low/intermediate) corresponding to optimal lysis by brachyury-specific T cells, according to the bell-shaped model shown at right. Tumors with very high levels of brachyury (oval) could escape immune-mediated lysis by brachyury-specific T cells. *Adapted from Roselli et al. (2012).* (See the color plate.)

T cells; however, a small percentage of tumors with very high levels of brachyury (red oval, Fig. 2) could escape immune-mediated lysis and contribute to tumor resistance to immune attack.

Mechanistic studies to understand the resistance of tumor cells with very high levels of brachyury showed that the defective lysis of those cells is due to inefficient caspase-dependent apoptotic death, a defect that takes place even in the presence of normal levels of fully activated effector caspases. The major apoptotic defect identified in those cells, however, was the absence of degradation of nuclear lamins due to a profound reduction on the levels of the cell cycle-associated kinase CDK1 (Fig. 3). The nuclear lamin, a component of the nuclear envelope, is a fibrillar mesh formed by the filament lamins A–C, which must be phosphorylated to undergo degradation by caspases during the last steps of apoptosis (McKeon, Kirschner, & Caput, 1986; Rao, Perez, & White, 1996). In tumor cells with very high brachyury levels, the levels of CDK1 protein are reduced and, as a consequence, lamins are not properly phosphorylated, thus precluding the degradation of the nuclear lamina during apoptosis.

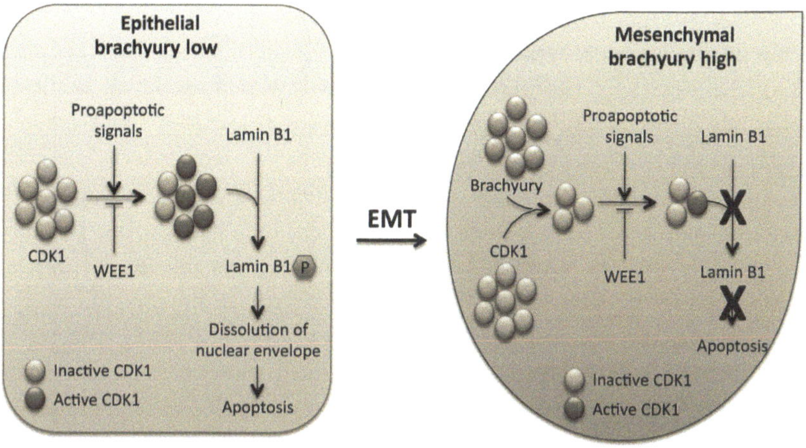

Figure 3 Schematic representation of the mechanisms of caspase-dependent lysis of brachyury-low versus -high cells indicating that loss of CDK1 kinase in the presence of high brachyury levels results in reduced phosphorylation of nuclear lamins and reduced apoptosis. *Adapted from Hamilton, Huang, et al. (2014).* (See the color plate.)

As the defective apoptosis of tumor cells with very high levels of brachyury is due to the enhanced degradation of the CDK1 protein, it has been proposed that restoration of threshold levels of CDK1 activity could allow nuclear apoptosis to proceed in those cells. This has been achieved by inhibiting the activity of the cell cycle kinase WEE1, which normally inactivates CDK1 by phosphorylating Tyr15 (Ottaviano & Gerace, 1985). A specific small-molecule inhibitor of WEE1, designated as AZD1775 (previously MK1775), is currently being tested in Phase I and II clinical trials for the treatment of multiple solid tumor types in combination with chemotherapies or radiation. It has been shown in preclinical studies with human carcinoma cells that WEE1 blockade by AZD1775 is able to fully revert the resistance of brachyury-high tumor cells to caspase-dependent cell death induced by immune effector mechanisms (Hamilton, Huang, et al., 2014). This was presumably achieved by restoration of threshold levels of CDK1 activity in brachyury-high cells, which would allow the proper phosphorylation of lamins and their subsequent degradation by caspases.

It is important to point out that, as of this writing, there is no clear understanding of what mechanisms are preferred by immune effector cells (caspase-dependent vs. caspase-independent) to lyse tumor cells *in vivo*. It has been shown, for example, with renal cell carcinoma cells in murine preclinical studies that the lytic pathway employed by antigen-specific T cells during tumor lysis is determined by the level of MHC class I/peptide, where the FAS lytic pathway is preferred at low peptide level, while the preference is lost at high peptide levels (Shanker et al., 2009). In particular, it has been shown that the efficient lysis of brachyury-high tumor cells could still take place if the effector cell mechanisms involved the perforin/granzyme pathway. This is consistent with the idea that during perforin/granzyme-dependent apoptosis, granzymes directly cleave the nuclear lamins, thus being able to overcome the defective lamin phosphorylation that is needed for the caspase-dependent lysis (Hamilton, Huang, et al., 2014). These results also indicated that immunotherapeutic approaches able to maximize the activation of effector cells for high production of granzymes should be able to effectively eliminate tumor cells with epithelial or mesenchymal features, the latter otherwise resistant to most antitumor interventions.

5. CONCLUDING REMARKS

Progress in elucidating the molecular mechanisms that govern the process of metastasis, including a full understanding of the role of tumor EMT and its association with tumor stemness and resistance to therapies, will help in designing therapies better fitted at preventing and/or treating metastatic disease. Cancer vaccines able to specifically target metastatic tumor cells constitute a very attractive methodology. Unlike other modalities, vaccines may be able to generate a long-lasting antitumor response; until now, they have demonstrated no associated toxicities, making them ideal for combination therapies, including the use of agents that alleviate tumor EMT for an optimized targeting of plastic tumor cells that are responsible for tumor recurrence and the establishment of therapeutic refractoriness.

ACKNOWLEDGMENTS

The authors thank Debra Weingarten for editorial assistance in preparation of this chapter.

REFERENCES

Akalay, I., Janji, B., Hasmim, M., Noman, M. Z., Andre, F., De Cremoux, P., et al. (2013). Epithelial-to-mesenchymal transition and autophagy induction in breast carcinoma promote escape from T-cell-mediated lysis. *Cancer Research*, *73*, 2418–2427.

Akalay, I., Janji, B., Hasmim, M., Noman, M. Z., Thiery, J. P., Mami-Chouaib, F., et al. (2013). EMT impairs breast carcinoma cell susceptibility to CTL-mediated lysis through autophagy induction. *Autophagy*, *9*, 1104–1106.

Barresi, V., Vitarelli, E., Branca, G., Antonelli, M., Giangaspero, F., & Barresi, G. (2012). Expression of brachyury in hemangioblastoma: Potential use in differential diagnosis. *The American Journal of Surgical Pathology*, *36*, 1052–1057.

Ben-Hamo, R., Gidoni, M., & Efroni, S. (2014). PhenoNet: Identification of key networks associated with disease phenotype. *Bioinformatics*, *30*, 2399–2405.

Bernstein, M. B., Chakraborty, M., Wansley, E. K., Guo, Z., Franzusoff, A., Mostbock, S., et al. (2008). Recombinant Saccharomyces cerevisiae (yeast-CEA) as a potent activator of murine dendritic cells. *Vaccine*, *26*, 509–521.

Bilusic, M., Heery, C. R., Arlen, P. M., Rauckhorst, M., Apelian, D., Tsang, K. Y., et al. (2014). Phase I trial of a recombinant yeast-CEA vaccine (GI-6207) in adults with metastatic CEA-expressing carcinoma. *Cancer Immunology, Immunotherapy*, *63*, 225–234.

Blanchard, T. J., Alcami, A., Andrea, P., & Smith, G. L. (1998). Modified vaccinia virus Ankara undergoes limited replication in human cells and lacks several immunomodulatory proteins: Implications for use as a human vaccine. *The Journal of General Virology*, *79*(Pt 5), 1159–1167.

Blanco, M. J., Moreno-Bueno, G., Sarrio, D., Locascio, A., Cano, A., Palacios, J., et al. (2002). Correlation of Snail expression with histological grade and lymph node status in breast carcinomas. *Oncogene*, *21*, 3241–3246.

Boehm, A. L., Higgins, J., Franzusoff, A., Schlom, J., & Hodge, J. W. (2010). Concurrent vaccination with two distinct vaccine platforms targeting the same antigen generates phenotypically and functionally distinct T-cell populations. *Cancer Immunology, Immunotherapy*, *59*, 397–408.

Bolos, V., Peinado, H., Perez-Moreno, M. A., Fraga, M. F., Esteller, M., & Cano, A. (2003). The transcription factor Slug represses E-cadherin expression and induces epithelial to mesenchymal transitions: A comparison with Snail and E47 repressors. *Journal of Cell Science*, *116*, 499–511.

Braun, S., Kentenich, C., Janni, W., Hepp, F., de Waal, J., Willgeroth, F., et al. (2000). Lack of effect of adjuvant chemotherapy on the elimination of single dormant tumor cells in bone marrow of high-risk breast cancer patients. *Journal of Clinical Oncology*, *18*, 80–86.

Bukholm, I. K., Nesland, J. M., & Borresen-Dale, A. L. (2000). Re-expression of E-cadherin, alpha-catenin and beta-catenin, but not of gamma-catenin, in metastatic tissue from breast cancer patients. *The Journal of Pathology*, *190*, 15–19.

Byers, L. A., Diao, L., Wang, J., Saintigny, P., Girard, L., Peyton, M., et al. (2013). An epithelial-mesenchymal transition gene signature predicts resistance to EGFR and PI3K inhibitors and identifies Axl as a therapeutic target for overcoming EGFR inhibitor resistance. *Clinical Cancer Research*, *19*, 279–290.

Cano, A., Perez-Moreno, M. A., Rodrigo, I., Locascio, A., Blanco, M. J., del Barrio, M. G., et al. (2000). The transcription factor snail controls epithelial-mesenchymal transitions by repressing E-cadherin expression. *Nature Cell Biology*, *2*, 76–83.

Cereda, V., Vergati, M., Huen, N. Y., di Bari, M. G., Jochems, C., Intrivici, C., et al. (2011). Maturation of human dendritic cells with Saccharomyces cerevisiae (yeast) reduces the number and function of regulatory T cells and enhances the ratio of antigen-specific effectors to regulatory T cells. *Vaccine*, *29*, 4992–4999.

Chaft, J. E., Litvak, A., Arcila, M. E., Patel, P., D'Angelo, S. P., Krug, L. M., et al. (2014). Phase II study of the GI-4000 KRAS vaccine after curative therapy in patients with stage I-III lung adenocarcinoma harboring a KRAS G12C, G12D, or G12V mutation. *Clinical Lung Cancer*, *15*, 405–410.

Chao, M. P., Seita, J., & Weissman, I. L. (2008). Establishment of a normal hematopoietic and leukemia stem cell hierarchy. *Cold Spring Harbor Symposia on Quantitative Biology*, *73*, 439–449.

Charafe-Jauffret, E., Ginestier, C., Iovino, F., Wicinski, J., Cervera, N., Finetti, P., et al. (2009). Breast cancer cell lines contain functional cancer stem cells with metastatic capacity and a distinct molecular signature. *Cancer Research*, *69*, 1302–1313.

Cosma, A., Nagaraj, R., Buhler, S., Hinkula, J., Busch, D. H., Sutter, G., et al. (2003). Therapeutic vaccination with MVA-HIV-1 nef elicits Nef-specific T-helper cell responses in chronically HIV-1 infected individuals. *Vaccine*, *22*, 21–29.

Creighton, C. J., Li, X., Landis, M., Dixon, J. M., Neumeister, V. M., Sjolund, A., et al. (2009). Residual breast cancers after conventional therapy display mesenchymal as well as tumor-initiating features. *Proceedings of the National Academy of Sciences of the United States of America*, *106*, 13820–13825.

Cunliffe, V., & Smith, J. C. (1992). Ectopic mesoderm formation in Xenopus embryos caused by widespread expression of a Brachyury homologue. *Nature*, *358*, 427–430.

Disis, M. L. (2014). Mechanism of action of immunotherapy. *Seminars in Oncology*, *41*(Suppl. 5), S3–S13.

Drake, C. G., Jaffee, E., & Pardoll, D. M. (2006). Mechanisms of immune evasion by tumors. *Advances in Immunology*, *90*, 51–81.

DuPage, M., Mazumdar, C., Schmidt, L. M., Cheung, A. F., & Jacks, T. (2012). Expression of tumour-specific antigens underlies cancer immunoediting. *Nature*, *482*, 405–409.

Fernando, R. I., Castillo, M. D., Litzinger, M., Hamilton, D. H., & Palena, C. (2011). IL-8 signaling plays a critical role in the epithelial-mesenchymal transition of human carcinoma cells. *Cancer Research*, *71*, 5296–5306.

Fernando, R. I., Litzinger, M., Trono, P., Hamilton, D. H., Schlom, J., & Palena, C. (2010). The T-box transcription factor Brachyury promotes epithelial-mesenchymal transition in human tumor cells. *The Journal of Clinical Investigation*, *120*, 533–544.

Ginestier, C., Liu, S., Diebel, M. E., Korkaya, H., Luo, M., Brown, M., et al. (2010). CXCR1 blockade selectively targets human breast cancer stem cells in vitro and in xenografts. *The Journal of Clinical Investigation*, *120*, 485–497.

Halder, S. K., Beauchamp, R. D., & Datta, P. K. (2005). A specific inhibitor of TGF-beta receptor kinase, SB-431542, as a potent antitumor agent for human cancers. *Neoplasia*, *7*, 509–521.

Hamid, O., Robert, C., Daud, A., Hodi, F. S., Hwu, W. J., Kefford, R., et al. (2013). Safety and tumor responses with lambrolizumab (anti-PD-1) in melanoma. *The New England Journal of Medicine*, *369*, 134–144.

Hamilton, D. H., Fernando, R. I., Schlom, J., & Palena, C. (2014). Aberrant expression of the embryonic transcription factor brachyury in human tumors detected with a novel rabbit monoclonal antibody. *Oncotarget*, *6*(7), 4853–4862, [Epub online], December 26.

Hamilton, D. H., Huang, B., Fernando, R. I., Tsang, K. Y., & Palena, C. (2014). WEE1 inhibition alleviates resistance to immune attack of tumor cells undergoing epithelial-mesenchymal transition. *Cancer Research*, *74*, 2510–2519.

Hamilton, D. H., Litzinger, M. T., Fernando, R. I., Huang, B., & Palena, C. (2012). Cancer vaccines targeting the epithelial-mesenchymal transition: Tissue distribution of brachyury and other drivers of the mesenchymal-like phenotype of carcinomas. *Seminars in Oncology*, *39*, 358–366.

Hamilton, D. H., Litzinger, M. T., Jales, A., Huang, B., Fernando, R. I., Hodge, J. W., et al. (2013). Immunological targeting of tumor cells undergoing an epithelial-mesenchymal transition via a recombinant brachyury-yeast vaccine. *Oncotarget*, *4*, 1777–1790.

Hanahan, D., & Weinberg, R. A. (2000). The hallmarks of cancer. *Cell*, *100*, 57–70.

Haro, A., Yano, T., Kohno, M., Yoshida, T., Koga, T., Okamoto, T., et al. (2013). Expression of Brachyury gene is a significant prognostic factor for primary lung carcinoma. *Annals of Surgical Oncology*, *20*(Suppl. 3), S509–S516.

Hartley, M. L., Bade, N. A., Prins, P. A., Ampie, L., & Marshall, J. L. (2014). Pancreatic cancer, treatment options, and GI-4000. *Human Vaccines & Immunotherapeutics*, *10*, 3347–3353.

Heery, C. R., Singh, H., Marte, J. L., Madan, R. A., O'Sullivan Coyne, G. H., Farsaci, B., et al. (2014). NCI experience using yeast–brachyury vaccine (GI-6301) in patients with advanced chordoma. *Journal of Clinical Oncology, 32*, 5s, Suppl. abstr 3081.

Hodi, F. S., O'Day, S. J., McDermott, D. F., Weber, R. W., Sosman, J. A., Haanen, J. B., et al. (2010). Improved survival with ipilimumab in patients with metastatic melanoma. *The New England Journal of Medicine, 363*, 711–723.

Huang, B., Cohen, J. R., Fernando, R. I., Hamilton, D. H., Litzinger, M. T., Hodge, J. W., et al. (2013). The embryonic transcription factor Brachyury blocks cell cycle progression and mediates tumor resistance to conventional antitumor therapies. *Cell Death & Disease, 4*, e682.

Huang, R. Y., Wong, M. K., Tan, T. Z., Kuay, K. T., Ng, A. H., Chung, V. Y., et al. (2013). An EMT spectrum defines an anoikis-resistant and spheroidogenic intermediate mesenchymal state that is sensitive to e-cadherin restoration by a src-kinase inhibitor, saracatinib (AZD0530). *Cell Death & Disease, 4*, e915.

Igney, F. H., & Krammer, P. H. (2002). Immune escape of tumors: Apoptosis resistance and tumor counterattack. *Journal of Leukocyte Biology, 71*, 907–920.

Im, E. J., & Hanke, T. (2004). MVA as a vector for vaccines against HIV-1. *Expert Review of Vaccines, 3*, S89–S97.

Iwatsuki, M., Mimori, K., Yokobori, T., Ishi, H., Beppu, T., Nakamori, S., et al. (2010). Epithelial-mesenchymal transition in cancer development and its clinical significance. *Cancer Science, 101*, 293–299.

Jordan, N. V., Johnson, G. L., & Abell, A. N. (2011). Tracking the intermediate stages of epithelial-mesenchymal transition in epithelial stem cells and cancer. *Cell Cycle, 10*, 2865–2873.

Kajiyama, H., Shibata, K., Terauchi, M., Yamashita, M., Ino, K., Nawa, A., et al. (2007). Chemoresistance to paclitaxel induces epithelial-mesenchymal transition and enhances metastatic potential for epithelial ovarian carcinoma cells. *International Journal of Oncology, 31*, 277–283.

Kalluri, R., & Weinberg, R. A. (2009). The basics of epithelial-mesenchymal transition. *The Journal of Clinical Investigation, 119*, 1420–1428.

Kilic, N., Feldhaus, S., Kilic, E., Tennstedt, P., Wicklein, D., Wasielewski, R., et al. (2011). Brachyury expression predicts poor prognosis at early stages of colorectal cancer. *European Journal of Cancer, 47*, 1080–1085.

Kim, H. P., Han, S. W., Song, S. H., Jeong, E. G., Lee, M. Y., Hwang, D., et al. (2014). Testican-1-mediated epithelial-mesenchymal transition signaling confers acquired resistance to lapatinib in HER2-positive gastric cancer. *Oncogene, 33*, 3334–3341.

Kispert, A., Koschorz, B., & Herrmann, B. G. (1995). The T protein encoded by Brachyury is a tissue-specific transcription factor. *The EMBO Journal, 14*, 4763–4772.

Kurrey, N. K., Jalgaonkar, S. P., Joglekar, A. V., Ghanate, A. D., Chaskar, P. D., Doiphode, R. Y., et al. (2009). Snail and slug mediate radioresistance and chemoresistance by antagonizing p53-mediated apoptosis and acquiring a stem-like phenotype in ovarian cancer cells. *Stem Cells, 27*, 2059–2068.

Kwok, W. K., Ling, M. T., Lee, T. W., Lau, T. C., Zhou, C., Zhang, X., et al. (2005). Up-regulation of TWIST in prostate cancer and its implication as a therapeutic target. *Cancer Research, 65*, 5153–5162.

Larocca, C., Cohen, J. R., Fernando, R. I., Huang, B., Hamilton, D. H., & Palena, C. (2013). An autocrine loop between TGF-beta1 and the transcription factor brachyury controls the transition of human carcinoma cells into a mesenchymal phenotype. *Molecular Cancer Therapeutics, 12*, 1805–1815.

Larocca, C., & Schlom, J. (2011). Viral vector-based therapeutic cancer vaccines. *Cancer Journal, 17*, 359–371.

Lee, M. Y., Chou, C. Y., Tang, M. J., & Shen, M. R. (2008). Epithelial-mesenchymal transition in cervical cancer: Correlation with tumor progression, epidermal growth factor receptor overexpression, and snail up-regulation. *Clinical Cancer Research*, *14*, 4743–4750.

Madan, R. A., Bilusic, M., Heery, C., Schlom, J., & Gulley, J. L. (2012). Clinical evaluation of TRICOM vector therapeutic cancer vaccines. *Seminars in Oncology*, *39*, 296–304.

Madan, R. A., Mohebtash, M., Arlen, P. M., Vergati, M., Rauckhorst, M., Steinberg, S. M., et al. (2012). Ipilimumab and a poxviral vaccine targeting prostate-specific antigen in metastatic castration-resistant prostate cancer: A phase 1 dose-escalation trial. *The Lancet Oncology*, *13*, 501–508.

Mani, S. A., Guo, W., Liao, M. J., Eaton, E. N., Ayyanan, A., Zhou, A. Y., et al. (2008). The epithelial-mesenchymal transition generates cells with properties of stem cells. *Cell*, *133*, 704–715.

Mayr, A., & Danner, K. (1978). Vaccination against pox diseases under immunosuppressive conditions. *Developments in Biological Standardization*, *41*, 225–234.

McKeon, F. D., Kirschner, M. W., & Caput, D. (1986). Homologies in both primary and secondary structure between nuclear envelope and intermediate filament proteins. *Nature*, *319*, 463–468.

Mejlvang, J., Kriajevska, M., Vandewalle, C., Chernova, T., Sayan, A. E., Berx, G., et al. (2007). Direct repression of cyclin D1 by SIP1 attenuates cell cycle progression in cells undergoing an epithelial mesenchymal transition. *Molecular Biology of the Cell*, *18*, 4615–4624.

Muller, C. W., & Herrmann, B. G. (1997). Crystallographic structure of the T domain-DNA complex of the Brachyury transcription factor. *Nature*, *389*, 884–888.

Nantajit, D., Lin, D., & Li, J. J. (2014). The network of epithelial-mesenchymal transition: Potential new targets for tumor resistance. *Journal of Cancer Research and Clinical Oncology*. http://dx.doi.org/10.1007/s00432-014-1840y, [Epub ahead of print], October 1.

Nguyen, D. X., Bos, P. D., & Massague, J. (2009). Metastasis: From dissemination to organ-specific colonization. *Nature Reviews. Cancer*, *9*, 274–284.

Nguyen, D. X., & Massague, J. (2007). Genetic determinants of cancer metastasis. *Nature Reviews. Genetics*, *8*, 341–352.

Nieto, M. A. (2013). Epithelial plasticity: A common theme in embryonic and cancer cells. *Science*, *342*, 1234850.

Ottaviano, Y., & Gerace, L. (1985). Phosphorylation of the nuclear lamins during interphase and mitosis. *The Journal of Biological Chemistry*, *260*, 624–632.

Palena, C., Fernando, R. I., & Hamilton, D. H. (2014). An immunotherapeutic intervention against tumor progression: Targeting a driver of the epithelial-to-mesenchymal transition. *Oncoimmunology*, *3*, e27220.

Palena, C., Fernando, R. I., Litzinger, M. T., Hamilton, D. H., Huang, B., & Schlom, J. (2011). Strategies to target molecules that control the acquisition of a mesenchymal-like phenotype by carcinoma cells. *Experimental Biology and Medicine (Maywood, N.J.)*, *236*, 537–545.

Palena, C., Hamilton, D. H., & Fernando, R. I. (2012). Influence of IL-8 on the epithelial-mesenchymal transition and the tumor microenvironment. *Future Oncology*, *8*, 713–722.

Palena, C., Polev, D. E., Tsang, K. Y., Fernando, R. I., Litzinger, M., Krukovskaya, L. L., et al. (2007). The human T-box mesodermal transcription factor Brachyury is a candidate target for T-cell-mediated cancer immunotherapy. *Clinical Cancer Research*, *13*, 2471–2478.

Palena, C., Roselli, M., Litzinger, M. T., Ferroni, P., Costarelli, L., Spila, A., et al. (2014). Overexpression of the EMT driver brachyury in breast carcinomas: Association with poor prognosis. *Journal of the National Cancer Institute*, *106*, pii: dju054.

Palena, C., & Schlom, J. (2010). Vaccines against human carcinomas: Strategies to improve antitumor immune responses. *Journal of Biomedicine & Biotechnology*, *2010*, 380697, [Epub 2010] March 16.

Peng, S. B., Yan, L., Xia, X., Watkins, S. A., Brooks, H. B., Beight, D., et al. (2005). Kinetic characterization of novel pyrazole TGF-beta receptor I kinase inhibitors and their blockade of the epithelial-mesenchymal transition. *Biochemistry, 44*, 2293–2304.

Pinto, F., Pertega-Gomes, N., Pereira, M. S., Vizcaino, J. R., Monteiro, P., Henrique, R. M., et al. (2014). T-box transcription factor Brachyury is associated with prostate cancer progression and aggressiveness. *Clinical Cancer Research, 20*, 4949–4961.

Polyak, K., & Weinberg, R. A. (2009). Transitions between epithelial and mesenchymal states: Acquisition of malignant and stem cell traits. *Nature Reviews. Cancer, 9*, 265–273.

Rabinovich, G. A., Gabrilovich, D., & Sotomayor, E. M. (2007). Immunosuppressive strategies that are mediated by tumor cells. *Annual Review of Immunology, 25*, 267–296.

Rao, L., Perez, D., & White, E. (1996). Lamin proteolysis facilitates nuclear events during apoptosis. *The Journal of Cell Biology, 135*, 1441–1455.

Remondo, C., Cereda, V., Mostbock, S., Sabzevari, H., Franzusoff, A., Schlom, J., et al. (2009). Human dendritic cell maturation and activation by a heat-killed recombinant yeast (Saccharomyces cerevisiae) vector encoding carcinoembryonic antigen. *Vaccine, 27*, 987–994.

Reya, T., Morrison, S. J., Clarke, M. F., & Weissman, I. L. (2001). Stem cells, cancer, and cancer stem cells. *Nature, 414*, 105–111.

Roselli, M., Fernando, R. I., Guadagni, F., Spila, A., Alessandroni, J., Palmirotta, R., et al. (2012). Brachyury, a driver of the epithelial-mesenchymal transition, is overexpressed in human lung tumors: An opportunity for novel interventions against lung cancer. *Clinical Cancer Research, 18*, 3868–3879.

Scheel, C., & Weinberg, R. A. (2011). Phenotypic plasticity and epithelial-mesenchymal transitions in cancer and normal stem cells? *International Journal of Cancer, 129*, 2310–2314.

Scheel, C., & Weinberg, R. A. (2012). Cancer stem cells and epithelial-mesenchymal transition: Concepts and molecular links. *Seminars in Cancer Biology, 22*, 396–403.

Schlom, J. (2012). Therapeutic cancer vaccines: Current status and moving forward. *Journal of the National Cancer Institute, 104*, 599–613.

Schlom, J., Hodge, J. W., Palena, C., Tsang, K. Y., Jochems, C., Greiner, J. W., et al. (2014). Therapeutic cancer vaccines. *Advances in Cancer Research, 121*, 67–124.

Shah, A. N., Summy, J. M., Zhang, J., Park, S. I., Parikh, N. U., & Gallick, G. E. (2007). Development and characterization of gemcitabine-resistant pancreatic tumor cells. *Annals of Surgical Oncology, 14*, 3629–3637.

Shanker, A., Brooks, A. D., Jacobsen, K. M., Wine, J. W., Wiltrout, R. H., Yagita, H., et al. (2009). Antigen presented by tumors in vivo determines the nature of CD8+ T-cell cytotoxicity. *Cancer Research, 69*, 6615–6623.

Shibata, K., Kajiyama, H., Ino, K., Terauchi, M., Yamamoto, E., Nawa, A., et al. (2008). Twist expression in patients with cervical cancer is associated with poor disease outcome. *Annals of Oncology, 19*, 81–85.

Shin, D. S., & Ribas, A. (2015). The evolution of checkpoint blockade as a cancer therapy: What's here, what's next? *Current Opinion in Immunology, 33C*, 23–35.

Singh, B. H., & Gulley, J. L. (2014). Therapeutic vaccines as a promising treatment modality against prostate cancer: Rationale and recent advances. *Therapeutic Advances in Vaccines, 2*, 137–148.

Singh, H., Heery, C. R., Marte, J. L., Farsaci, B., Madan, R. A., O'Sullivan Coyne, G. H., et al. (2014). A phase I study of a yeast-based therapeutic cancer vaccine, GI-6301, targeting brachyury in patients with metastatic carcinoma. *Journal of Clinical Oncology, 32*(Suppl.; abstr e14026).

Tan, T. Z., Miow, Q. H., Miki, Y., Noda, T., Mori, S., Huang, R. Y., et al. (2014). Epithelial-mesenchymal transition spectrum quantification and its efficacy in deciphering survival and drug responses of cancer patients. *EMBO Molecular Medicine, 6*, 1279–1293.

Thiery, J. P. (2002). Epithelial-mesenchymal transitions in tumour progression. *Nature Reviews. Cancer, 2*, 442–454.

Thiery, J. P. (2003). Epithelial-mesenchymal transitions in development and pathologies. *Current Opinion in Cell Biology, 15*, 740–746.

Thiery, J. P., Acloque, H., Huang, R. Y., & Nieto, M. A. (2009). Epithelial-mesenchymal transitions in development and disease. *Cell, 139*, 871–890.

Thomson, S., Buck, E., Petti, F., Griffin, G., Brown, E., Ramnarine, N., et al. (2005). Epithelial to mesenchymal transition is a determinant of sensitivity of non-small-cell lung carcinoma cell lines and xenografts to epidermal growth factor receptor inhibition. *Cancer Research, 65*, 9455–9462.

Thomson, S., Petti, F., Sujka-Kwok, I., Epstein, D., & Haley, J. D. (2008). Kinase switching in mesenchymal-like non-small cell lung cancer lines contributes to EGFR inhibitor resistance through pathway redundancy. *Clinical & Experimental Metastasis, 25*, 843–854.

Tirabosco, R., Mangham, D. C., Rosenberg, A. E., Vujovic, S., Bousdras, K., Pizzolitto, S., et al. (2008). Brachyury expression in extra-axial skeletal and soft tissue chordomas: A marker that distinguishes chordoma from mixed tumor/myoepithelioma/parachordoma in soft tissue. *The American Journal of Surgical Pathology, 32*, 572–580.

Topalian, S. L., Drake, C. G., & Pardoll, D. M. (2012). Targeting the PD-1/B7-H1(PD-L1) pathway to activate anti-tumor immunity. *Current Opinion in Immunology, 24*, 207–212.

Topalian, S. L., Hodi, F. S., Brahmer, J. R., Gettinger, S. N., Smith, D. C., McDermott, D. F., et al. (2012). Safety, activity, and immune correlates of anti-PD-1 antibody in cancer. *The New England Journal of Medicine, 366*, 2443–2454.

Tucker, J. A., Jochems, C., Boyerinas, B., Fallon, J., Greiner, J. W., Palena, C., et al. (2014). Identification and characterization of a cytotoxic T-lymphocyte agonist epitope of brachyury, a transcription factor involved in epithelial to mesenchymal transition and metastasis. *Cancer Immunology, Immunotherapy, 63*, 1307–1317.

Vega, S., Morales, A. V., Ocana, O. H., Valdes, F., Fabregat, I., & Nieto, M. A. (2004). Snail blocks the cell cycle and confers resistance to cell death. *Genes & Development, 18*, 1131–1143.

Vujovic, S., Henderson, S., Presneau, N., Odell, E., Jacques, T. S., Tirabosco, R., et al. (2006). Brachyury, a crucial regulator of notochordal development, is a novel biomarker for chordomas. *The Journal of Pathology, 209*, 157–165.

Wansley, E. K., Chakraborty, M., Hance, K. W., Bernstein, M. B., Boehm, A. L., Guo, Z., et al. (2008). Vaccination with a recombinant Saccharomyces cerevisiae expressing a tumor antigen breaks immune tolerance and elicits therapeutic antitumor responses. *Clinical Cancer Research, 14*, 4316–4325.

Wilson, C., Ye, X., Pham, T., Lin, E., Chan, S., McNamara, E., et al. (2014). AXL inhibition sensitizes mesenchymal cancer cells to antimitotic drugs. *Cancer Research, 74*, 5878–5890.

http://www.clinicaltrials.gov. (2013). Open label study to evaluate the safety and tolerability of GI-6301 a vaccine consisting of whole heat-killed recombinant yeast genetically modified to express brachyury protein in adults with solid tumors. Retrieved February 5, 2013.

http://www.clinicaltrials.gov. (2014). Safety and tolerability of a modified vaccinia Ankara (MVA)-based vaccine modified to express brachyury and T-cell costimulatory molecules (MVA-Brachyury-TRICOM). Retrieved September 3, 2014.

Yang, A. D., Fan, F., Camp, E. R., van Buren, G., Liu, W., Somcio, R., et al. (2006). Chronic oxaliplatin resistance induces epithelial-to-mesenchymal transition in colorectal cancer cell lines. *Clinical Cancer Research, 12*, 4147–4153.

Yang, J., Mani, S. A., Donaher, J. L., Ramaswamy, S., Itzykson, R. A., Come, C., et al. (2004). Twist, a master regulator of morphogenesis, plays an essential role in tumor metastasis. *Cell, 117*, 927–939.

Yang, X. R., Ng, D., Alcorta, D. A., Liebsch, N. J., Sheridan, E., Li, S., et al. (2009). T (brachyury) gene duplication confers major susceptibility to familial chordoma. *Nature Genetics*, *41*, 1176–1178.

Yang, J., & Weinberg, R. A. (2008). Epithelial-mesenchymal transition: At the crossroads of development and tumor metastasis. *Developmental Cell*, *14*, 818–829.

Yu, M., Bardia, A., Wittner, B. S., Stott, S. L., Smas, M. E., Ting, D. T., et al. (2013). Circulating breast tumor cells exhibit dynamic changes in epithelial and mesenchymal composition. *Science*, *339*, 580–584.

Zhang, D., LaFortune, T. A., Krishnamurthy, S., Esteva, F. J., Cristofanilli, M., Liu, P., et al. (2009). Epidermal growth factor receptor tyrosine kinase inhibitor reverses mesenchymal to epithelial phenotype and inhibits metastasis in inflammatory breast cancer. *Clinical Cancer Research*, *15*, 6639–6648.

CHAPTER THREE

Myeloid-Derived Suppressor Cells: Critical Cells Driving Immune Suppression in the Tumor Microenvironment

Katherine H. Parker[1], Daniel W. Beury[1], Suzanne Ostrand-Rosenberg[2]
Department of Biological Sciences, University of Maryland Baltimore County, Baltimore, Maryland, USA
[2]Corresponding author: e-mail address: srosenbe@umbc.edu

Contents

[1] K.H.P. and D.W.B. are dual-first authors.

Advances in Cancer Research, Volume 128
ISSN 0065-230X
http://dx.doi.org/10.1016/bs.acr.2015.04.002

Abstract

Myeloid-derived suppressor cells (MDSCs) are a heterogeneous population of immature myeloid cells that suppress innate and adaptive immunity. MDSCs are present in many disease settings; however, in cancer, they are a major obstacle for both natural antitumor immunity and immunotherapy. Tumor and host cells in the tumor microenvironment (TME) produce a myriad of pro-inflammatory mediators that activate MDSCs and drive their accumulation and suppressive activity. MDSCs utilize a variety of mechanisms to suppress T cell activation, induce other immune-suppressive cell populations, regulate inflammation in the TME, and promote the switching of the immune system to one that tolerates and enhances tumor growth. Because MDSCs are present in most cancer patients and are potent immune-suppressive cells, MDSCs have been the focus of intense research in recent years. This review describes the history and identification of MDSCs, the role of inflammation and intracellular signaling events governing MDSC accumulation and suppressive activity, immune-suppressive mechanisms utilized by MDSCs, and recent therapeutics that target MDSCs to enhance antitumor immunity.

1. MYELOID-DERIVED SUPPRESSOR CELL HISTORY

Abnormal myelopoiesis and neutrophilia were observed in cancer patients for many years; however, the role of these pathologies was not appreciated until relatively recently, when myeloid-derived suppressor cells (MDSCs) were identified and associated with immune suppression. Studies from the early and middle 1980s in tumor-free mice identified a population of so-called natural suppressor cells that inhibited T cell proliferation and the generation of cytotoxic T lymphocytes in an antigen and MHC-independent manner (Strober, 1984). In the 1990s, studies of patients with head and neck cancer described $CD34^{+}$-suppressive myeloid cells that had the capacity to differentiate into dendritic cells (DCs) (Garrity et al., 1997). Soon after their identification in head and neck cancer patients, similar cells were discovered in patients with various other forms of cancer. These cells prevented the *in vivo* and *in vitro* activation of T cells and were chemoattracted to the tumor microenvironment (TME) by tumor-produced vascular endothelial growth factor (VEGF) (Almand et al., 2001; Young et al., 2001). Mice with transplanted or spontaneous tumors also produced suppressive myeloid cells (Gabrilovich, Velders, Sotomayor, & Kast, 2001; Melani, Chiodoni, Forni, & Colombo, 2003), which expressed the granulocyte and macrophage markers Gr1 and CD11b/Mac1, respectively. Their accumulation correlated with tumor-produced granulocyte/monocyte-colony-stimulating factor (GM-CSF) (Bronte et al., 1999), and they inhibited antigen-specific $CD8^+$ T cell activation in a contact-dependent manner (Gabrilovich et al., 2001). Early studies used a variety of terms to identify the cells, including "immature myeloid cells (IMCs)," "immature macrophages (iMacs)," or "myeloid suppressor cells (MSCs)." In 2007, the terminology "myeloid-derived suppressor cells" (MDSCs) was adopted to reflect that the cells are the product of abnormal myelopoiesis (Gabrilovich et al., 2007).

MDSCs differentiate from a common myeloid progenitor cell that also gives rise to normal DCs, monocytes, macrophages, and granulocytes (Fig. 1). Unlike other fully differentiated myeloid cells that are relatively homogeneous, MDSCs are a heterogeneous population of cells since they represent varied stages in myelopoiesis. This heterogeneity is tumor dependent and is most likely spawned from the unique inflammatory milieu released by different tumors. These tumor-released factors, in turn, modulate the recruitment and suppressive potency of tumor-infiltrating MDSCs. The phenotype and functions of MDSCs may also vary with cancer progression since tumor cells evolve and change through immunoediting (Dunn, Bruce, Ikeda, Old, & Schreiber, 2002). Within this wide array of variation, human and mouse MDSCs have been separated into two major categories: monocytic (MO-MDSC) and granulocytic (PMN-MDSC).

1.1 Mouse MDSCs

MDSCs have been identified in the bone marrow, liver, blood, spleen, and tumor of tumor-bearing mice based on their expression of surface markers and their ability to prevent T cell activation. All murine MDSCs express the plasma membrane markers Gr1 and CD11b. The granulocyte marker Gr1

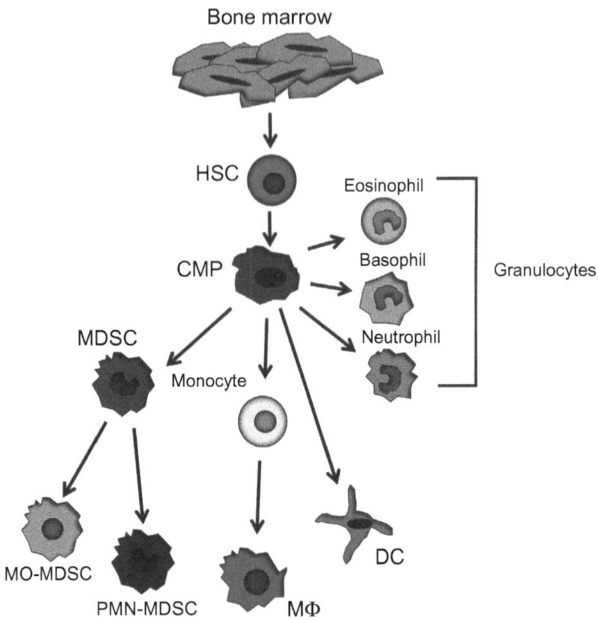

Figure 1 Myeloid cell differentiation under normal and tumor-induced conditions. Myeloid cells originate from bone marrow-derived hematopoietic stem cells (HSCs) that differentiate into common myeloid progenitors (CMPs). During normal myelopoiesis, CMPs differentiate into granulocytes including eosinophils, basophils, and neutrophils, as well as monocytes, macrophages, and dendritic cells. MDSCs also differentiate from CMPs and are categorized as MO-MDSCs or PMN-MDSCs. HSC, hematopoietic stem cell; CMP, common myeloid progenitor; DC, dendritic cell; MΦ, macrophage; MO-MDSCs, monocytic myeloid-derived suppressor cells; PMN-MDSCs, polymorphonuclear myeloid-derived suppressor cells. (See the color plate.)

includes the isoforms Ly6C and Ly6G. The differential expression of these molecules distinguishes MO-MDSCs from PMN-MDSCs. MO-MDSCs are $CD11b^{+}Ly6C^{+}Ly6G^{low/-}$; PMN-MDSCs are $CD11b^{+}Ly6C^{-}Ly6G^{+}$. MO-MDSCs are mononuclear and side $scatter^{low}$, while PMN-MDSCs are polymorphonuclear and side $scatter^{hi}$. The two subsets use different modes of suppression. PMN-MDSCs utilize reactive oxygen species (ROS) and the enzyme arginase 1 (ARG1), while MO-MDSCs use nitric oxide synthase 2 (NOS2) and ROS. These phenotypes apply to tumor-infiltrating MDSCs, as well as MDSCs residing in the spleen and blood of tumor-bearing mice. Tumor-infiltrating MDSCs are more suppressive than blood or splenic MDSCs on a per cell basis. Tumor-free mice contain cells with the same phenotype ($Gr1^{+}CD11b^{+}$) in the blood, spleen, and bone marrow; however, they are present at much lower levels compared to tumor-bearing mice (Sinha et al., 2008, 2011).

The markers Gr1 and CD11b as well as the polymorphonuclear morphology of PMN-MDSCs are also characteristics of neutrophils, raising the question of whether MDSCs are different from neutrophils. MDSCs are not neutrophils; however, MDSCs can differentiate into neutrophils. Tumor-associated neutrophils have been categorized as N1, antitumorigenic, and as N2, protumorigenic, with their induction dependent on the presence of IFNβ or TGFβ, respectively (Fridlender et al., 2009; Jablonska, Leschner, Westphal, Lienenklaus, & Weiss, 2010). N1 neutrophils are characterized as $TNF\alpha^{hi}$, $CCL3^{hi}$, $ICAM\text{-}1^{hi}$, and $ARG1^{low}$, while N2 neutrophils are high in CCL2, 3, 4, 8, 12, and 17 as well as in CXCL1, 2, 6, and 16 (Sionov, Fridlender, & Granot, 2014). In contrast to MDSCs, neutrophils do not express CD244 (M-CSF receptor), are more phagocytic than MDSCs, produce lower levels of ROS, have enhanced chemokine secretion, express higher levels of TNFα, and most importantly cannot suppress T cell activation (Youn, Collazo, Shalova, Biswas, & Gabrilovich, 2012).

1.2 Human MDSCs

Human MDSCs have been isolated from patients with solid tumors who display elevated MDSC levels that directly correlate with clinical cancer stage and metastatic burden. MDSCs have been found in patients with breast cancer (Alizadeh et al., 2014; Diaz-Montero et al., 2009), head and neck squamous cell carcinoma (Brandau et al., 2011), nonsmall cell lung cancer (Huang et al., 2013; Srivastava et al., 2008), colon and colorectal cancer (OuYang et al., 2015), renal cell carcinoma (Rodriguez et al., 2009), bladder cancer (Eruslanov et al., 2012), gastrointestinal cancer (Wang et al., 2013), pancreatic adenocarcinoma (Porembka et al., 2012), esophageal cancer (Gabitass, Annels, Stocken, Pandha, & Middleton, 2011), prostate cancer (Vuk-Pavlović et al., 2010), urothelial tract cancer (Brandau et al., 2011), sarcoma, carcinoid, gall bladder, adrenocortical, thyroid, and hepatocellular carcinoma (Shen, Wang, He, Wang, & Zheng, 2014). Patients with multiple myeloma and non-Hodgkin's lymphoma also exhibit elevated levels of MDSCs in their blood (Brimnes et al., 2010; Lin et al., 2011).

Since humans lack an analog to Gr1, human MDSCs are characterized by the monocyte/macrophage marker CD11b, the monocyte differentiation antigen CD14, the mature monocyte marker CD15, the myeloid lineage markers CD33, and the absence of HLA-DR, which is commonly expressed on myeloid cells (Dumitru, Moses, Trellakis, Lang, & Brandau, 2012). Similar to murine MDSCs, human MDSCs lack lineage markers characteristic of other hematopoietic-derived cells. Human PMN-MDSCs are $CD11b^{+}CD14^{-}CD15^{+}HLA\text{-}DR^{low/-}CD33^{+}$; MO-MDSCs are $CD11b^{+}CD14^{+}CD15^{-}IL4R\alpha^{+}HLA\text{-}DR^{low}CD33^{+}$ (Montero, Diaz-Montero, Kyriakopoulos, Bronte, & Mandruzzato, 2012). Since none of the individual markers are unique to MDSCs, definitive identification of MDSCs requires demonstration of immune-suppressive function.

2. MDSC DEVELOPMENT AND SUPPRESSIVE FUNCTIONS ARE INDUCED BY INFLAMMATION

Studies evaluating patients on long-term use of nonsteroidal anti-inflammatory drugs, epidemiological analyses, and trials involving blockade of inflammatory molecules have demonstrated that inflammation contributes to the onset of cancer (Balkwill & Mantovani, 2001). Four main sources of inflammation promote carcinogenesis: environmental inflammation, therapy-induced inflammation, tumor-associated inflammation, and chronic inflammation or infection.

Particulates from tobacco smoke are an example of an environmental source of inflammation. They cause chronic obstructive pulmonary disease which is associated with increased lung cancer (Punturieri, Szabo, Croxton, Shapiro, & Dubinett, 2009). Therapy-induced inflammation occurs following radiation and chemotherapy. It causes necrotic death of cancer cells and tumor stromal cells and initiates an inflammatory response similar to wound-healing (Zong & Thompson, 2006). Therapy-induced inflammation may enhance presentation of tumor antigens; however, it may also create tumor-promoting inflammation (Zitvogel, Apetoh, Ghiringhelli, & Kroemer, 2008). Many tumors are inherently inflammatory due to their production of inflammatory mediators such as IL-6 and prostaglandins. The resulting inflammation recruits immunosuppressive cells that also release cytokines and feed the inflammatory environment. As solid tumors outpace their blood supply and become deprived of nutrients and oxygen, necrosis sets in causing the chronic release of pro-inflammatory mediators such as IL-1 and high-mobility group box 1 (HMGB1), which in turn promote neoangiogenesis (Vakkila & Lotze, 2004). Long-term infection may also cause chronic inflammation and increased cancer risk. Examples include hepatocellular carcinoma in patients infected with hepatitis B or C viruses

(Karin, 2006), and bladder and colon cancer in individuals infected with Schistosoma or Bacteroides, respectively (Mostafa, Sheweita, & O'Connor, 1999; Wu et al., 2009).

Chronic inflammation promotes tumor development through various mechanisms including the production of proangiogenic factors, matrix metalloproteinases (MMPs), and damage-associated molecular pattern molecules (DAMPs), all of which drive MDSC accumulation and MDSC suppressive functions. Proangiogenic factors such as VEGF stimulate tumor neovascularization, while MMPs facilitate invasion and metastasis (Shacter & Weitzman, 2002). DAMPs such as S100A8/A9 chemoattract leukocytes and promote the expansion of MDSCs leading to an influx of inflammatory molecules within the TME (Cheng et al., 2008; Sinha et al., 2008).

The TME is a complex network that includes both tumor cells and host cells. MDSCs in this environment are therefore subjected to diverse pro-inflammatory factors. Since the TME varies between tumor types and individuals with cancer, as well as with stage of tumor progression, it is not surprising that MDSCs are a heterogeneous population that may vary from individual to individual.

Almost a decade ago, the connection between MDSCs and inflammation was established with the findings that the pro-inflammatory cytokines IL-1β, IL-6, and PGE_2 promote MDSC accumulation and suppressive function (Bunt, Sinha, Clements, Leips, & Ostrand-Rosenberg, 2006; Bunt et al., 2007; Ezernitchi et al., 2006; Sinha, Clements, Fulton, & Ostrand-Rosenberg, 2007; Song et al., 2005). Other studies demonstrated that additional cytokines, transcription factors, and DAMPs, including, but not limited to, C5a, PGE_2, COX_2, VEGF, GM-CSF, G-CSF, IL-17, IDO, HMGB1, and S100A8/A9, C/EBPβ, and chop, also drive MDSCs. The effects of these factors are discussed in the following section and are illustrated in Fig. 2.

2.1 Vascular Endothelial Growth Factor

VEGF is a pro-inflammatory growth factor that stimulates angiogenesis, and tumors producing high levels of VEGF have a poor prognosis. VEGF inhibits nuclear factor kappa-light-chain-enhancer (NF-κB) activation which blocks DC development while simultaneously driving MDSC accumulation (Gabrilovich et al., 1998). MDSCs express the VEGF receptor enabling VEGF to function as a chemoattractant for MDSCs. ROS

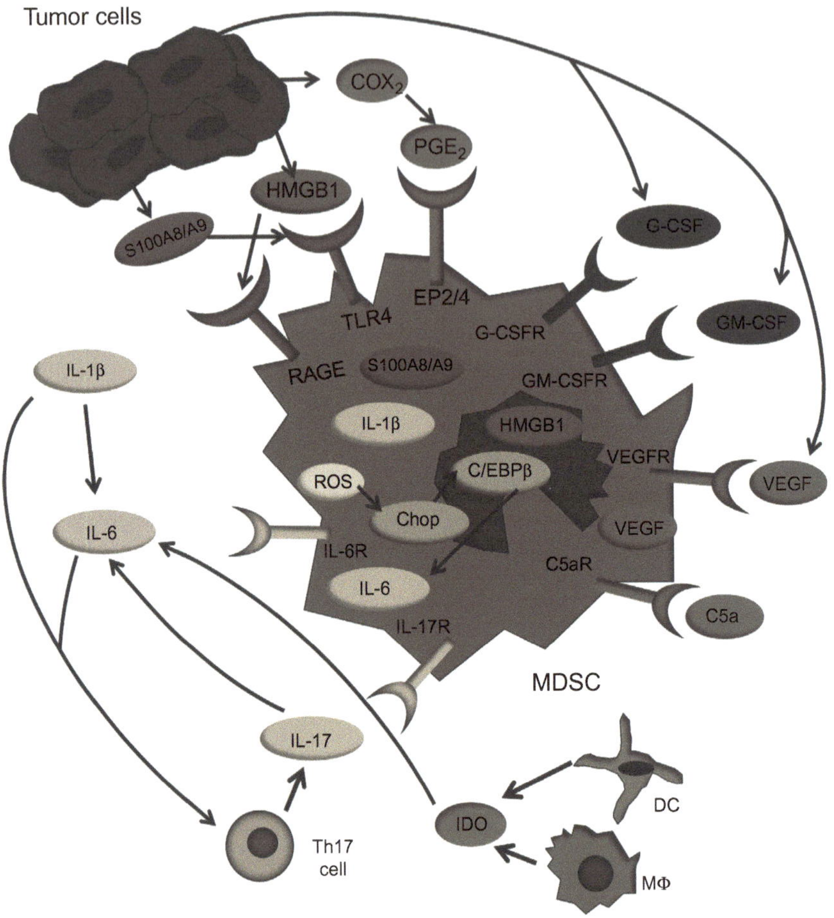

Figure 2 Inflammation drives MDSC development and function. Chronic inflammation induces the production of HMGB1, S100A8/A9, IL-1β, IL-6, C5a, and IL-17, all of which induce the accumulation of MDSC. Induction of MDSCs by IL-1β is mediated through IL-17 and IL-6. IL-1β induces Th17 cells to produce IL-17 which induces the production of IL-6. IL-6 production is also upregulated by IDO produced by DCs and macrophages (MΦ). C/EBPβ, which is activated by chop following MDSC production of ROS, also induces IL-6. MDSCs also produce VEGF, IL-6, IL-1β, HMGB1, and S100A8/A9, thereby perpetuating their accumulation. Tumor cells may produce COX_2, PGE_2, VEGF, IL-6, G-CSF, GM-CSF, S100A8/A9, and HMGB1 all of which induce the accumulation of MDSCs and may increase the suppressive potency of MDSCs. (See the color plate.)

production by MDSCs increases oxidative stress which upregulates MDSC expression of the VEGF receptor (Kusmartsev et al., 2008). Since other factors in solid tumors also contribute to oxidative stress, the TME is a critical factor in determining the responsiveness of MDSCs to VEGF.

In addition to tumor cells, MDSCs themselves produce VEGF, thereby creating an autocrine feedback loop that sustains MDSC accumulation (Kujawski et al., 2008). VEGF has been shown to be released from the extracellular matrix by MMP9, a matrix degrading enzyme (Bergers et al., 2000). Soluble MMP9 is produced by tumor cells and promotes MDSC accumulation and tumor angiogenesis (Melani, Sangaletti, Barazzetta, Werb, & Colombo, 2007). Therefore, MDSCs have multiple modes of generating VEGF.

2.2 Granulocyte-Macrophage Colony-Stimulating Factor and Granulocyte Colony-Stimulating Factor

GM-CSF is a growth factor for leukocytes. It is required for DC differentiation and is used to expand DC *ex vivo*. However, high levels of GM-CSF induce MDSC accumulation *in vivo* and *in vitro*, while *in vivo* knockdown of GM-CSF reduces MDSC expansion (Morales, Kmieciak, Knutson, Bear, & Manjili, 2010; Serafini et al., 2004). Inclusion of GM-CSF in cultures of bone marrow progenitor cells drives the differentiation of MDSCs, demonstrating that GM-CSF is a growth factor for MDSCs (Nefedova et al., 2004).

MDSC differentiation is also positively regulated by the growth factor granulocyte colony-stimulating factor (G-CSF). G-CSF plays a critical role in mobilizing bone marrow stem cells and is essential for differentiation of granulocytic lineages (Lieschke et al., 1994). Administration of G-CSF to tumor-bearing mice drives tumor growth and angiogenesis, while blockade of G-CSF reduces MDSC levels (Okazaki et al., 2006). G-CSF also preconditions metastatic sites by mobilizing MDSCs (Kowanetz et al., 2010). When G-CSF and VEGF are both inhibited, tumor growth is reduced (Okazaki et al., 2006). While the role of G-CSF in MDSC development is clear, the impact of G-CSF on MDSC function is more complicated. In mice bearing MCA203 sarcomas, G-CSF induced $Gr1^{hi}CD11b^{+}$ cells that were less suppressive than $Gr1^{int}CD11b^{+}$ cells, while in MMTV-PyMT transgenic mice with mammary carcinoma, G-CSF caused $CD11b^{+}Ly6G^{+}Ly6C^{+}$ cells to secret Bv8. Bv8 is an endocrine analog of VEGF and functions as a proangiogenic protein that promotes hematopoiesis (Dolcetti et al., 2010; Kowanetz et al., 2010). Therefore, G-CSF differentially affects MDSC function depending on the type of tumor.

2.3 Prostaglandin E2 and Cyclooxygenase 2

Prostaglandin E2 (PGE_2) is a potent inflammatory mediator that is generated by cyclooxygenase 2 (COX_2) conversion of arachidonic acid. PGE_2 supports tumor growth by promoting angiogenesis, stimulating tumor-cell proliferation, and protecting tumor cells from apoptosis. Many human and mouse tumors as well as tumor-infiltrating cells produce COX_2 and PGE_2. PGE_2 promotes MDSC differentiation at the expense of DC, while inhibition of COX_2 or PGE_2 in tumor-bearing mice blocks MDSC differentiation and delays tumor progression (Eruslanov, Daurkin, Ortiz, Vieweg, & Kusmartsev, 2010; Sinha, Clements, Fulton, et al., 2007). In the TME, PGE_2 mediates its effects through four integral membrane G-protein-coupled prostanoid receptors: EP1, EP2, EP3, and EP4. Mice deficient in EP2 display delayed tumor progression and reduced MDSC levels (Sinha, Clements, Fulton, et al., 2007). Blockade of PGE_2 or EP4 in tumor-bearing mice reduces MDSC production of ARG1 (Rodriguez et al., 2005). PGE_2 promotes the differentiation of progenitor cells in human blood to MDSCs ($CD11b^{+}CD33^{+}$ cells) from human blood progenitor cells that have elevated levels of NOS2, ARG1, IL-10, and IL-4Rα (Obermajer, Muthuswamy, Lesnock, Edwards, & Kalinski, 2011). Therefore, for mouse and human MDSCs, PGE_2 not only regulates the differentiation of MDSCs, but several suppressive mechanisms as well.

2.4 CCAAT/Enhancer Binding Protein β and C/EBP Homologous Protein

C/EBP proteins are a family of leucine zipper transcription factors that regulate inflammation and myeloid cell differentiation. While there are various isoforms of C/EBP proteins, CCAAT/enhancer binding protein β (C/EBPβ) acts during stress/inflammation-induced myelopoiesis. C/EBPβ has three isoforms: LAP* and LAP (liver-enriched activator proteins), and LIP (liver-enriched inhibitory protein). LAP* and LIP are transcriptional activators that drive inflammatory myelopoiesis by inducing IL-6 and ARG1. In contrast, LIP inhibits LAP signaling promoting an anti-inflammatory response. In inflammatory settings such as the TME, LAP* and LAP are active and drive inflammation-induced myelopoiesis. C/EBPβ is also required for the *ex vivo* generation of immunosuppressive MDSCs from bone marrow progenitor cells, via IL-6 and GM-CSF (Marigo et al., 2010).

2.5 Complement Component C5a

C5a (also known as anaphylatoxin) is a pro-inflammatory member of the complement and lectin pathway. When the complement pathway is activated, C5a in the blood becomes fixed in tissues. C5a triggers degranulation of mast cells (MCs), aids in vascular permeability, and stimulates smooth muscle contraction. In a tumor setting, C5a increases MDSC-mediated immune suppression by chemoattracting C5a receptor^{+} MDSCs to tumor vasculature and by increasing MDSC production of ROS and ARG1 (Markiewski et al., 2008).

2.6 S100A8/A9

S100A8/A9 proteins are pro-inflammatory danger signals. They are calcium binding proteins that are localized in the cytoplasm or nucleus of myeloid cells, and are released in response to cell damage, infection, or inflammation. Mice deficient in S100A9 reject transplanted tumors, while elevated expression of S100A8/A9 in solid tumors perpetuates inflammation by chemoattracting leukocytes that produce additional inflammatory molecules (Cheng et al., 2008; Sinha et al., 2008). MDSCs are one of the leukocyte populations that are chemoattracted by S100A8/A9, and chemoattraction is dependent on signaling through receptor for advanced glycation end-products (RAGE) (Sinha et al., 2008). Heterodimeric S100A8/A9 mediates it's pro-inflammatory effects by binding to the plasma membrane receptors TLR4, carboxylated N-glycans, RAGE, or heparin sulfate (Bresnick, Weber, & Zimmer, 2015). MDSCs amplify their own accumulation by secreting S100A8/A9, thus creating a self-sustained feedback loop (Sinha et al., 2008).

2.7 High-Mobility Group Box 1

HMGB1 is the second most abundant protein within a cell and is released from myeloid cells as a danger response to sepsis, infection, or arthritis. HMGB1 can signal through a number of receptors including thrombospondin, CD24, TLR2, 4, 7, and 9, as well as RAGE. HMGB1 consists of two functional domains, the A and B boxes, and an acidic tail. The A box is a RAGE antagonist and prevents HMGB1-mediated release of IL-1β and TNFα. The B box and part of the linker before the acidic tail is a RAGE agonist with pro-inflammatory properties (Bianchi & Manfredi, 2007). The B box signals via TLR4 on macrophages which initiate the release of

IL-1β, IL-6, TNFα, MIP-2, and IL-10. The A box is anti-inflammatory as it prevents HMGB1-mediated release of IL-1β and TNFα. Whether HMGB1 functions in a pro-inflammatory or anti-inflammatory manner is determined by its redox state. In the normal extracellular environment, the disulfide bridge between residues Cys_{23} and Cys_{45} maintains the A box in a dysfunctional conformation, so the B box is exclusively active. With inflammation, the microenvironment becomes oxidatively stressed and ROS is produced. ROS terminally oxidizes Cys_{23} and Cys_{45}, thereby breaking the disulfide bridge and allowing A box to resolve the inflammation (Venereau et al., 2012).

Elevated levels of HMGB1 are associated with numerous cancers and are known to directly promote tumor growth. However, HMGB1 also drives tumor progression by modulating MDSCs. Inhibition of HMGB1 prevents the expansion of MDSCs from bone marrow progenitor cells *in vitro*, demonstrating that HMGB1 is required for the differentiation of MDSCs. *In vivo* inhibition of HMGB1 in tumor-bearing mice reduces MDSC levels in the tumor, spleen, and blood, confirming HMGB1 as a driver of MDSCs. MDSC-mediated downregulation of T cell L-selectin (CD62L) is also HMGB1 dependent, since HMGB1 increases MDSC extracellular expression of A disintegrin and metalloproteinase 17 (ADAM17), a protease that cleaves L-selectin. Secretion of the protumor cytokines IL-10 and IL-1β by MDSCs is also increased by HMGB1 (Parker, Sinha, Horn, Clements, & Ostrand-Rosenberg, 2014), and HMGB1-driven MDSC accumulation facilitates metastasis (Li et al., 2013). Preliminary studies indicate that HMGB1 mediates its effects on MDSCs through RAGE and/or TLR4 (K.H. Parker & S. Ostrand-Rosenberg, unpublished). HMGB1 also binds to other receptors, but it is unknown if MDSCs are activated through additional receptors.

2.8 IL-1β, IL-6, and Indoleamine 2,3-Dioxygenase

The causative relationship between inflammation, cancer, and immune suppression was first proposed following the finding that IL-1β was a potent inducer of MDSC accumulation and suppressive activity (Ostrand-Rosenberg & Sinha, 2009). Mice bearing 4T1 tumor cells that were transfected to constitutively express high levels of IL-1β exhibit increased MDSC accumulation and more suppressive MDSCs compared to mice bearing parental 4T1 tumors. 4T1 tumor-bearing mice that lack the IL-1 receptor antagonist, an inhibitor for IL-1β, also develop elevated levels of MDSCs that are more suppressive. Similarly, mice deficient for the IL-1R display slower tumor growth and their MDSCs are less suppressive (Bunt et al., 2006, 2007; Elkabets et al., 2010; Song et al., 2005). Since IL-1β induces the production of other mediators, including VEGF, IL-6, PGE_2, and GM-CSF, some of the effects of IL-1β on MDSCs may be indirect. 4T1 tumor cells transfected to constitutively express IL-6 induce elevated levels of MDSCs and restore MDSC levels in tumor-bearing IL-1 receptor knockout mice, indicating that IL-6 effects on MDSCs are either downstream of IL-1β, or have an overlapping mechanism of action with IL-1β (Bunt et al., 2007). Since MDSCs produce IL-6 and IL-1β, these studies also raise the question of whether MDSC production of IL-6 is regulated by IL-1β, and if MDSC production of IL-1β enhances MDSC production of IL-6. Indole amine 2,3 dioxygenase (IDO), which is utilized by MDSCs as an immune-suppressive mechanism, also regulates IL-6, and tumor-bearing IDO1-deficient mice have less suppressive MDSCs, reduced levels of IL-6, and delayed primary tumor growth and metastatic disease (Smith et al., 2012). Provision of IL-6 to tumor-bearing indoleamine 2,3-dioxygenase (IDO) knockout mice restores MDSC levels and suppressive potency (Smith et al., 2012).

2.9 IL-17

IL-17 is a pro-inflammatory cytokine secreted by CD4 Th17 and CD8 Tc17 cells. Tumor growth is suppressed and MDSC levels are decreased in IL-17-deficient mice, while administration of IL-17 raises MDSC levels (He et al., 2010; Wang et al., 2009). Patients with gastrointestinal cancers show a strong positive correlation between serum IL-17 and MDSC levels, further supporting a role for IL-17 as an inducer of MDSCs (Yazawa et al., 2013). The effects of IL-17 may be either direct or indirect. Most cells have IL-17 receptors so MDSCs may be directly impacted. However, IL-17 triggers the production of IL-6 which in turn activates STAT3, so many effects on MDSCs may be directly mediated by IL-6 and indirectly by IL-17 (Chatterjee et al., 2013; Wang et al., 2009).

3. MDSC ARE REGULATED BY MULTIPLE MOLECULAR MECHANISMS

Multiple signal transduction pathways, transcription factors, and microRNAs (miRNAs) regulate MDSC accumulation and function (Fig. 3).

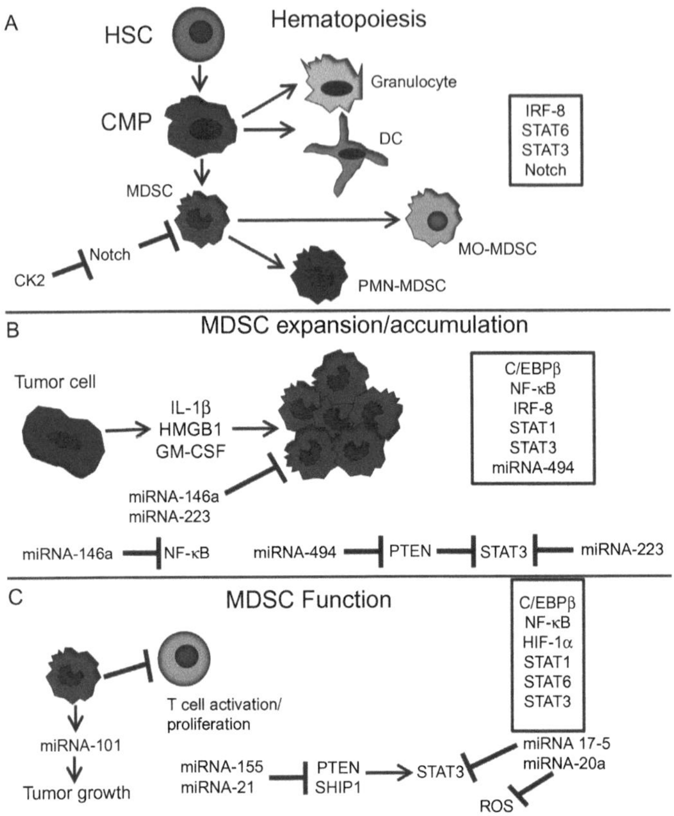

Figure 3 Multiple signal transduction pathways, transcription factors, and microRNAs regulate MDSC accumulation and function. (A) The differentiation of MDSCs from HSC and CMP is regulated by the transcription factors IRF-8, Notch, STAT6, and STAT3. IRF-8 and STAT6 regulate normal myelopoiesis and the differentiation of CMP to mature granulocytes and DCs. During abnormal myelopoiesis, which occurs in individuals with cancer, immature myeloid cells fail to terminally differentiate giving rise to elevated levels of MDSCs. Notch inhibits the differentiation of MDSCs, while CK2 blocks Notch and thereby increases MDSCs. STAT3 promotes MDSC development and suppressive potency. (B) Tumor and host cells produce multiple inflammatory molecules that perturb myelopoiesis and induce the expansion of MDSCs by activating or inactivating transcription factors. Pro-inflammatory mediators in the tumor microenvironment, such as IL-1β, HMGB1, and GM-CSF, drive the expansion of MDSCs by activating C/EBPβ, NF-κB, STAT1, STAT3, and miRNA-494 and downregulating IRF-8. Induction of miRNAs 146a and 223 prevents the expansion of MDSC. miRNA-494 promotes the expression of MMPs and inhibits PTEN function resulting in STAT3 induction. miRNA-146a inhibits NF-κB signaling, while miRNA-223 blocks C/EBPβ from binding to the c-myc promoter which downregulates STAT3 expression. (C) MDSC function is positively regulated by C/EBPβ, NF-κB, HIF-1α, STAT1, STAT6, and STAT3. The miRNAs 155 and 21 inhibit PTEN and SHIP1, negative regulators of STAT3, resulting in the activation of STAT3 and increased MDSC function. miRNAs 17-5 and 20a have the opposite effect by blocking STAT3 and ROS which negatively regulates MDSC function. MDSCs themselves also promote tumor growth by activating miRNA-101 in cancer cells. (See the color plate.)

3.1 Signal Transducer and Activator of Transcription 1

MDSC function is positively regulated by STAT1. STAT1 is activated by IFNγ or IL-1β and regulates the induction of NOS2 and ARG1 (Kusmartsev & Gabrilovich, 2005). MDSC accumulation is also dependent on STAT1 as tumor-bearing mice deficient in STAT1 exhibit reduced MDSC levels (Hix et al., 2013). Whether IFNγ is the ligand that activates MO-MDSCs is unclear. Early studies indicated that IFNγ was essential for the development of MO-MDSCs (Movahedi et al., 2008); however, subsequent experiments demonstrated that MDSC function, accumulation, and phenotype are independent of IFNγ as tumor-bearing $IFN\gamma^{+/+}$, $IFN\gamma^{-/-}$, $IFN\gamma R^{+/+}$, and $IFN\gamma R^{-/-}$ mice with equal-sized tumors contained equal numbers of equivalently suppressive MDSCs (Sinha, Parker, Horn, & Ostrand-Rosenberg, 2012).

3.2 Signal Transducer and Activator of Transcription 3 and 6

MDSC accumulation and function are enhanced by activation of both STAT3 and STAT6. Activation of STAT6 occurs from the binding of IL-4 or IL-13 to IL-4Rα resulting in the upregulation of ARG1 and TGFβ (Bronte et al., 2003; Sinha, Clements, & Ostrand-Rosenberg, 2005a; Terabe et al., 2003). In STAT6-deficient mice, signaling through IL-4Rα does not occur, MDSCs are less suppressive and accumulate more slowly, and spontaneous metastatic disease is delayed (Sinha, Clements, & Ostrand-Rosenberg, 2005b). STAT3 activation increases the half-life and proliferation of both human and mouse MDSCs by driving the expression of the antiapoptotic genes Bcl-xL, c-myc, and the proliferation gene cyclin D1 (Nefedova et al., 2005; Xin et al., 2009). STAT3 also increases the differentiation of MDSCs by inducing the pro-inflammatory mediators S100A8/A9 (Cheng et al., 2008) and by downregulating the transcription factor PKCβ II in hematopoietic progenitor cells (Farren, Carlson, & Lee, 2010). Since MDSCs and DCs are derived from a common progenitor cell, the increase in MDSC differentiation is accompanied by a decrease in DC expansion. In addition to regulating MDSC expansion, STAT3 also enhances MDSC suppressive activity (Kujawski et al., 2008). Tumor-derived exosomes containing heat-shock protein 72 on their membranes induce MDSC production of IL-6 which subsequently activates STAT3 and increases MDSC-mediated T cell suppression (Chalmin et al., 2010).

C/EBPβ is another transcription factor activated by STAT3. Activated C/EBPβ binds to the c-myc promoter and induces c-myc expression which stimulates cell proliferation. C/EBPβ is a key molecule for induction of MDSCs since multiple factors (GM-CSF, G-CSF, and IL-6) activate MDSCs via C/EBPβ, (Marigo et al., 2010). C/EBPβ regulation of MDSCs is associated with chop. ROS produced by tumors upregulates MDSC expression of chop (Thevenot et al., 2014). Chop expression in MDSCs activates C/EBPβ and induces STAT3 signaling. MDSCs from chop-deficient mice have decreased ability to inhibit T cell proliferation and accumulate to lower levels. This reduced accumulation and decreased potency of MDSCs is attributed to lower levels of IL-6 and reduced phosphorylation of STAT3. Overexpression of IL-6 in chop-deficient mice rescues MDSC suppressive activity (Thevenot et al., 2014).

MDSC production of ROS is also regulated by STAT3. ROS are generated intracellularly by the NAD(P)H oxidase enzyme complex (NOX), which consists of membrane-bound gp91 and p22, and cytosolic p40, p47, and p67. This complex catalyzes the production of superoxide through the reduction of oxygen, with NAD(P)H serving as the one electron donor. Activation of STAT3 increases ROS levels through upregulation of p47 and gp91 (Corzo et al., 2009); however, it is not known which of the several activators of STAT3 upregulate p47 and gp91. Solid tumors contain oxidatively stressed hypoxic regions, and cells within these regions contain activated hypoxia-inducible factor-1 alpha (HIF-1α). Activated HIF-1α induces STAT3 signaling. Therefore, STAT3 induction of ROS may be regulated by HIF-1α.

3.3 Nuclear Factor Kappa-Light-Chain-Enhancer

Activation of NF-κB also promotes MDSC accumulation and function and occurs following ligation of MyD88-dependent TLRs. Exposure to a variety of pro-inflammatory mediators including S100A8/A9, HMGB1, and IL-1β activates the NF-κB pathway in MDSCs (Parker et al., 2014; Sinha et al., 2008; Tu et al., 2008).

3.4 Interferon Regulatory Factor-8

Interferon regulatory factor 8 (IRF-8) is a transcription factor that is essential for the normal development of granulocyte/monocyte lineage cells. IRF-8-deficient mice have myeloproliferative disorders and accumulate high levels of MDSCs. Expression of IRF-8 is downregulated by G-CSF and GM-CSF, so treating mice with these cytokines blocks IRF-8 activation and drives the accumulation of MDSCs (Stewart, Liewehr, Steinberg, Greeneltch, &

Abrams, 2009; Waight et al., 2013). IRF-8 may also negatively regulate MDSC survival as IRF-8 downregulates antiapoptotic genes Bcl-2 and Bcl-xL and upregulates the proapoptotic gene caspase-3 (Burchert et al., 2004; Gabriele et al., 1999). Inhibition of Bcl-2 and Bcl-xL enhances MDSC susceptibility to Fas-mediated apoptosis (Hu et al., 2013).

3.5 Notch

Another transcription factor implicated in the development of MDSCs from hematopoietic progenitor cells is Notch. Notch signaling permits the differentiation of MDSCs into DCs. Inhibition of notch signaling by casein kinase 2 (CK2) drives abnormal myeloid cell differentiation (Cheng et al., 2014).

3.6 Hypoxia-Inducible Factor-1 Alpha

The HIF complex consists of the subunits HIF-1α and HIF-1β, both of which are constitutively expressed. Hypoxia stabilizes HIF-1α and allows it to translocate from the cytoplasm into the nucleus where it dimerizes with HIF-1β. The HIF complex upregulates multiple target genes (e.g., VEGF, NOS2, and MMPs) by associating with their hypoxia response elements. HIF-1α is overexpressed in various cancers, where it increases MDSC expression of ARG1 and NOS2, rendering MDSCs more immune suppressive and facilitating their conversion to tumor-associated macrophages (TAMs) (Corzo et al., 2010). The capacity of HIF-1α to modulate the function of MDSCs highlights the plasticity of MDSCs and further demonstrates that MDSC function is governed by their environment.

3.7 MicroRNAs

miRNAs are noncoding single-stranded RNAs approximately 22 nucleotides long that regulate gene expression. miRNAs in the RNA-induced silencing complex bind to complementary target mRNAs causing target mRNA degradation. The generation of miRNAs is regulated by cell- and tissue-specific transcription factors as well as proteins involved in the processing of miRNA, both of which can be influenced by chronic inflammation (El Gazzar & McCall, 2012).

miRNAs enhance and inhibit MDSC accumulation and suppressive potency. For example, miRNAs 146a and 223 prevent MDSC accumulation (Boldin et al., 2011; Liu et al., 2011). miRNA-146a blocks inflammation, while miRNA-223 is needed for the development of granulocytes. In contrast, miRNAs 494, 155, and 21 facilitate the accumulation of MDSCs.

miRNA-494 induces MMPs 2, 13, and 14 which drive MDSC growth and survival signals, and by inhibiting phosphatase and tensin homolog (PTEN) which promotes STAT3 activation (Liu et al., 2012). miRNAs 155 and 21 promote MDSC accumulation by activating STAT3, which, as previously discussed, drives both MDSC accumulation and suppressive potency (Li et al., 2014). miRNAs also negatively regulate MDSC suppressive function. These include miRNAs 17-5 and 20a which silence STAT3, thereby reducing MDSC production of ROS and hydrogen peroxide (H_2O_2) (Zhang et al., 2011).

MDSCs also use miRNAs to modulate cancer cell growth. An example is the MDSC-mediated activation of miRNA-101 in ovarian cancer cells (Cui et al., 2013). miRNA-101 increases cancer cell stemness as well as metastatic and tumorigenic potential (Cui et al., 2013).

3.8 MDSC Turnover

MDSC turnover *in vitro* and *in vivo* varies with tumor type, with half-life ranging for only a few days. T cells may contribute to this rapid turnover since when activated, T cells express FasL and cause apoptosis of Fas^+ MDSCs. Inflammation counteracts the T cell effect by increasing MDSC resistance to Fas-mediated lysis (Chornoguz et al., 2011; Sinha et al., 2011).

4. MDSCs UTILIZE A NETWORK OF EFFECTOR AND SIGNALING MOLECULES TO MODULATE THE INFLAMMATORY MILIEU AND DECREASE IMMUNE SURVEILLANCE

MDSCs utilize multiple suppressive mechanisms to induce a tolerogenic, tumor-promoting environment. MDSCs directly suppress T cells by starving them of amino acids, inducing apoptosis, reducing homing to lymph nodes, or inhibiting their intracellular signaling pathways required for activation. MDSCs also indirectly suppress T cells by altering the ability of antigen-presenting cells (APCs) to activate T cells and by inducing immunosuppressive T regulatory cells (Tregs). In addition, MDSCs impact other cells involved in an antitumor response because they alter the inflammatory milieu in the TME by cross talk with macrophages, tumor cells, and MCs. These mechanisms are described below and are illustrated in Fig. 4.

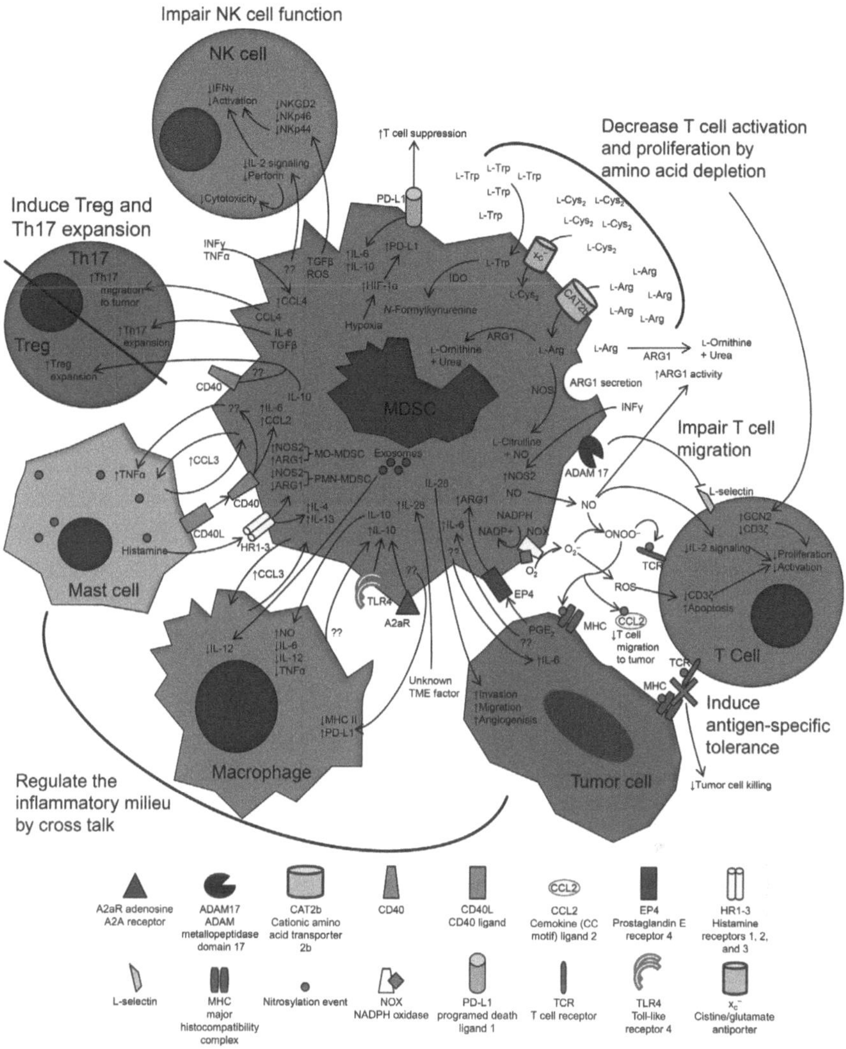

Figure 4 MDSCs suppress T cells and regulate the inflammatory milieu by multiple mechanisms. MDSCs regulate antitumor immunity by (i) secretion of IL-10, which induces Tregs; (ii) secretion of IL-6 and TGFβ, which induces Th17 cells; (iii) production of ROS and TGFβ, which inhibits NK cell function; (iv) degradation of amino acids essential for T cell activation and proliferation; (v) production of NO and O_2^-, which induces apoptosis and inhibits the activation and proliferation of T cells, and generates PNT that nitrates/nitrosylates MHC and TCR; and (vi) participation in cross talk with macrophages, tumor cells, and mast cells to generate a protumor environment. Question marks denote an unknown mechanism or signaling molecule. (See the color plate.)

4.1 MDSC Depletion of Amino Acids

Following initial contact with antigen, T cells undergo metabolic changes that are essential for their activation and clonal expansion. MDSCs limit several amino acids necessary for these processes and thereby inhibit T cell activation. An early event of amino-acid starvation is the accumulation of empty aminoacyl tRNAs, which activate serine–threonine kinase GCN2. GCN2 phosphorylates eIF2α, which binds eIF2B and suppresses the translation initiation complex from binding charged aminoacyl tRNA, thereby causing a global decrease in protein translation. Simultaneously, GCN2 enhances the translation of GCN4, which results in the transcription of genes required for the synthesis of amino acids (Wang & Green, 2012). MDSCs deplete the local environment of L-arginine (L-Arg), L-tryptophan (L-Trp), and L-cysteine (L-Cys) through different mechanisms.

One of the first suppressive mechanisms attributed to MDSCs was the inhibition of T cell activation and proliferation by the depletion of L-Arg. L-Arg is a nonessential amino acid and is a substrate for several enzymes: (i) NOS 1, 2, and 3 which metabolize L-Arg into L-citrulline and nitric oxide (NO); (ii) ARG 1 and 2 which convert L-Arg to L-ornithine and urea; (iii) arginine:glycine amidinotransferase which transfers the amidino group from L-Arg to L-glycine, yielding L-ornithine and glycocyamine; and (iv) arginine decarboxylase, which catalyzes the reaction of L-Arg to agmatine and CO_2 (Bronte & Zanovello, 2005).

In the absence of L-Arg, T cells decrease their expression of CD3ζ, which is required for signal transduction through the antigen-specific T cell receptor (TCR) (Rodriguez et al., 2002; Zea et al., 2004). L-Arg-depleted T cells are arrested in G_0–G_1 due to the failure to upregulate cyclin D3 and cyclin-dependent kinase 4 (cdk4). Cyclin D3 and cdk4 are not upregulated due to decreased mRNA stability and lower translation rates (Rodriguez et al., 2010). Despite their inability to proliferate, L-Arg-starved T cells express early activation markers and secrete IL-2, indicating that the early events of T cell activation are not L-Arg dependent (Fletcher et al., 2015). *In vivo* studies confirmed the critical role of MDSCs in L-Arg depletion since renal cell carcinoma patients and mice with chronic inflammation have elevated levels of MDSCs and low levels of serum L-Arg, which is correlated with decreased T cell activation (Ezernitchi et al., 2006; Zea et al., 2005). Depletion of L-Arg is mediated by ARG1, and MDSC synthesis of ARG1 is regulated by PGE_2 (Rodriguez et al., 2005). Tumor-derived MDSCs deplete their local environment of L-Arg by internalizing L-Arg through the cationic amino-acid transporter 2B (Rodriguez et al., 2004) and by secreting ARG1 (Rodriguez et al., 2009).

L-Trp metabolism by MDSCs also facilitates T cell suppression. MDSCs express IDO, which degrades the essential amino-acid L-Trp into *N*-formylkynurenine. IDO causes T cell suppression by enhancing GCN2 kinase in a similar manner as L-Arg starvation (Munn et al., 2005). Expression of IDO in MDSCs is regulated by STAT3 (Yu et al., 2013). However, not all MDSCs express IDO (Smith et al., 2012), indicating that IDO is not a universal mechanism utilized by MDSCs to suppress T cell activation.

MDSCs also prevent T cell activation by sequestering L-Cys. In the extracellular oxidizing environment, L-Cys exists as the dipeptide cystine (L-Cys_2). Naïve T cells must acquire L-Cys from APCs because they lack the cystine transporter x_c^- and therefore cannot import L-Cys_2, and cannot *de novo* synthesize L-Cys because they lack cystathionase, the enzyme that converts methionine to L-Cys. MDSCs also lack cystathionase and therefore must scavenge L-Cys_2. Since MDSCs do not export L-Cys due to their lack of the neutral amino-acid alanine-serine-cysteine transporter 1 (ASC), high levels of MDSCs quickly deplete their local environment of L-Cys_2, thereby limiting the ability of APCs to provide T cells with L-Cys. The role of MDSCs and their biological relevance in L-Cys depletion is supported by the correlation between high levels of MDSCs and reduced serum L-Cys_2 in tumor-bearing mice (Srivastava, Sinha, Clements, Rodriguez, & Ostrand-Rosenberg, 2010). Since activated T cells express x_c^-, theoretically they should be resistant to this suppressive mechanism (Levring et al., 2012). However, since ARG1 production by MDSCs suppresses T cell activation, it is unclear if T cell upregulation of x_c^- is functionally relevant.

4.2 MDSC Production of NO

NOS also catabolizes L-Arg and contributes to MDSC-mediated immune suppression (Bronte & Zanovello, 2005; Raber et al., 2014). MDSCs produce NO by the action of NOS2 and NOS3. PMN-MDSCs are $NOS2^{low}NOS3^{hi}$, while MO-MDSCs are $NOS2^{hi}NOS3^{low}$ (Raber et al., 2014). NOS2 generates more NO than NOS3 and is induced by pro-inflammatory cytokines, endotoxin, hypoxia, and oxidative stress, while NOS3 is constitutively expressed (Fukumura, Kashiwagi, & Jain, 2006).

NO is labile and reacts with multiple compounds to produce many toxic and regulatory factors. For example, NO reacts with (i) cysteine thiol groups on proteins and peptides, which form S-nitrosothiols, thereby altering a protein's tertiary structure; (ii) superoxide anions (O_2^-), which form peroxynitrite (PNT, $ONOO^-$), a molecule that alters protein structure; (iii) divalent cations (e.g., Fe^{2+} and Zn^{2+}), which regulate the function of various transcription factors and enzymes; (iv) nucleic acids, which cause mutagenesis; and (v) unsaturated lipids, which lead to the formation of nitrolipids that can have pro- or anti-inflammatory activity (Bogdan, 2015). Since NO influences many biological processes, it is not surprising that NO is capable of pro- and antitumor activity. NO can induce tumor-cell apoptosis and inhibit metastasis, or enhance tumor-cell invasion, proliferation, and angiogenesis (Fukumura et al., 2006). However, MDSC-produced NO negatively impacts T cells. NO inhibits JAK3, STAT5, ERK, and AKT, which prevents IL-2 signaling, thereby impairing the generation of effector and memory T cells (Mazzoni et al., 2002). NO directly inhibits these signaling proteins by S-nitrosothiolation, or indirectly by activating guanylate cyclase and cyclic-GMP-dependent kinases (Serafini, 2013). S-nitrosothiolation of ARG1 enhances ARG1 affinity for L-Arg which subsequently increases ARG1 activity, thereby establishing a synergistic relationship between ARG1- and NO-mediated immune suppression (Santhanam et al., 2007).

4.3 MDSC Production of ROS

NOX is a membrane-bound enzyme complex that is utilized by MDSCs to suppress T cell activation. MDSCs from tumor-bearing mice have enhanced expression of the NOX subunits gp91, p22, and p47 and produce more ROS than MDSCs from tumor-free mice (Corzo et al., 2009). NOX generates superoxide which spontaneously reacts with many molecules to produce a variety of ROS including H_2O_2, hydroxyl radical, and hypochlorous acid. These ROS damage proteins, lipids, and nucleic acids, thereby enhancing inflammation and promoting apoptosis. For example, H_2O_2 production in cancer patients reduces T cell production of cytokines and expression of CD3ζ (Schmielau & Finn, 2001). Superoxide also reacts with NO to form PNT, which is produced by PMN-MDSCs through the action of gp91 and NOS3 (Raber et al., 2014). PNT nitrates/nitrosylates the TCR and MHC (Lu & Gabrilovich, 2012), thereby disrupting TCR-MHC I/peptide binding and rendering tumor cells resistant to CTL-mediated apoptosis (Lu et al., 2011). Due to the short half-life of PNT, these reactions are limited to short distances and require close cell-to-cell contact. PNT also reacts with the chemoattractant CCL2, thereby inhibiting T cell infiltration into tumors (Molon et al., 2011).

4.4 MDSCs Inhibit T Cell Migration by Downregulating L- and E-Selectins

Activation of tumor-reactive T cells requires entry of naïve T cells into tumor-draining lymph nodes or migration to the TME. L-selectin mediates the first step in extravasation by facilitating T cell adhesion to high endothelial venules (HEVs). Naïve T cells with low expression of L-selectin do not adhere efficiently to HEVs and fail to enter lymph nodes (J. Mihich, S. Evans, S. Abrams, & S. Ostrand-Rosenberg, unpublished data). In tumor-bearing mice, MDSCs prevent T cell entry into lymph nodes by downregulating L-selection through their extracellular expression of ADAM17, the enzyme that cleaves L-selectin on naïve T cells (Hanson, Clements, Sinha, Ilkovitch, & Ostrand-Rosenberg, 2009; Parker et al., 2014).

In squamous cell carcinoma patients, MDSCs also prevent the homing of T cells to tumor sites by downregulating E-selectin on tumor vessels. In order for T cells to adhere to tumor vessels and subsequently enter the tumor mass, they must first bind to E-selectin. However, NO produced by MDSCs decreases E-selectin levels, thereby limiting T cell access to tumor (Gehad et al., 2012).

4.5 MDSCs Express Programmed Death-Ligand 1

Tumor cells escape antitumor immunity through their expression of programmed death-ligand 1 (PD-L1). When PD-L1 binds to its receptor PD-1 on T cells, it induces T cell exhaustion/apoptosis. MDSCs from some tumor-bearing mice and patients express PD-L1 (Youn, Nagaraj, Collazo, & Gabrilovich, 2008; Zhang, Wang, et al., 2013). Some tumor-infiltrating MDSCs have elevated expression of PD-L1 due to hypoxia-induced upregulation of HIF-1α (Noman et al., 2014). However, MDSCs do not universally express PD-L1, and PD-L1 blockade does not always decrease MDSC suppressive activity (Youn et al., 2008).

4.6 MDSCs Induce Tregs and Th17 Cells

Tregs play an important role in the control of immune reactivity against self- and non-self-antigens, and in some animal models, they protect tumors from antitumor immunity. Tregs are characterized as $CD4^+FoxP3^+$ cells. MDSCs induce/expand Tregs *in vitro* and *in vivo* in multiple tumor models (Adeegbe et al., 2011; Huang et al., 2006; MacDonald et al., 2005; Zoso et al., 2014). MDSCs induce Tregs by secreting IL-10 and TGFβ (Hoechst et al., 2008; Huang et al., 2006) and activate Tregs by presenting tumor-specific antigens in an ARG-dependent and TGFβ-independent manner (Serafini, Mgebroff, Noonan, & Borrello, 2008). MDSC expression of CD40 is required for MDSC-mediated Treg induction, since CD40-deficient MDSCs do not drive Treg expansion (Pan et al., 2010). Given the link between MDSCs and Tregs, therapies targeting MDSCs may also reduce Treg populations.

Th17 cells are a pro-inflammatory $CD4^+$ T cell subset ($CD4^+ROR\gamma t^+IL\text{-}17^+$). Since they have both pro- and antitumor effects, their role in antitumor immunity is controversial (Ye, Livergood, & Peng, 2013). MDSCs induce Th17 cells by producing IL-6 and TGFβ (Chatterjee et al., 2013). IFNγ- or TNFα-activated MDSCs also recruit Th17 cells through their production of CCL4, which is a Th17 chemoattractant (Ortiz et al., 2015). As previously mentioned, IL-17 drives the accumulation of MDSCs. Therefore, MDSCs and Th17 cells may induce each other.

4.7 MDSCs Impair NK Cell-Mediated Cytotoxicity

MDSCs impair NK function via contact-dependent mechanisms. MDSCs produce TGFβ and H_2O_2 which decrease NK cell expression of the activating receptors NKG2D, NKp46, and NKp44, thereby making NK cells more difficult to activate (Elkabets et al., 2010; Mao et al., 2014). MDSCs also decrease the ability of NK cells to induce apoptosis by downregulating NK cell production of perforin which is essential for NK-mediated target cell lysis. In addition, MDSCs suppress NK cells by limiting their response to IL-2, a growth factor that enhances NK cell proliferation and cytolytic activity (Liu et al., 2007).

4.8 Cross Talk Between MDSCs, Macrophages, Tumor Cells, and MCs Enhances Inflammation and Promotes MDSC Suppressive Activity

Solid tumors are a complex and frequently inflamed microenvironment. Both tumor and host (macrophages, DCs, MCs, MDSCs, and fibroblasts) cells within solid tumors participate in cross talk that regulates the release of pro- and anti-inflammatory cytokines and drive the accumulation and suppressive function of immune-suppressive cells such as Tregs, TAMs, and MDSCs.

Macrophages can be either tumoricidal (M1-like) or tumor-promoting (M2-like) (Sica & Mantovani, 2012). MDSCs subvert macrophages toward an M2 phenotype through their production of IL-10 which downregulates macrophage production of IL-12 and TNFα, while simultaneously enhancing macrophage production of NO (Beury et al., 2014; Sinha, Clements, Bunt, Albelda, & Ostrand-Rosenberg, 2007). IL-12 downregulation is mediated by both intact MDSCs and MDSC-derived exosomes (Burke, Choksawangkarn, Edwards, Ostrand-Rosenberg, & Fenselau, 2014). MDSC production of IL-10 involves TLR4 signaling and is increased by inflammation and direct cell-to-cell contact with macrophages (Bunt, Clements, Hanson, Sinha, & Ostrand-Rosenberg, 2009; Sinha, Clements, Bunt, et al., 2007), and via the adenosine A2A receptor (Cekic, Day, Sag, & Linden, 2014). MDSCs also decrease macrophage expression of MHC II through both IL-10-dependent and -independent mechanisms (P. Sinha, D. Beury, V. Clements, & S. Ostrand-Rosenberg, unpublished) and upregulate PD-L1 on macrophages in the liver (Ilkovitch & Lopez, 2009).

MDSCs and tumor cells also participate in cross talk. Tumor cells increase MDSC production of IL-6, and in turn, MDSCs enhance tumor-cell production of IL-6. IL-6 also increases MDSC suppressive activity, but inhibits MDSC production of IL-10 (Beury et al., 2014). In addition, tumor cells enhance MDSC production of IL-28, which facilitates tumor-cell invasion, migration, and angiogenesis (Mucha, Majchrzak, Taciak, Hellmen, & Krol, 2014).

MCs and MDSCs also interact. MDSC and MC cross talk drives inflammation by increasing production of TNFα, CCL3, IL-4, IL-13, IL-6, and CCL2 (Danelli et al., 2015; Martin et al., 2014; Saleem et al., 2012). The latter two molecules are regulated by ligation of MC CD40L to CD40 on MDSCs. Activated MCs release histamine which signals through histamine receptors 1, 2, and 3 on MDSCs and enhances MDSC expression of IL-4 and IL-13. Histamine upregulates ARG1 and NOS2 in MO-MDSCs and decreases ARG1 and NOS2 in PMN-MDSCs (Martin et al., 2014). Since histamine increases MO-MDSC production of NO and downregulates immune-suppressive mediators of PMN-MDSC, the net effect of histamine is to increase MO-MDSC suppressive activity (Danelli et al., 2015).

5. MDSCs IN NONCANCER SETTINGS

MDSCs are also elevated in noncancer settings, where they can be either detrimental or beneficial. For example, elevated levels of MDSC decrease immune responsiveness in patients with toxoplasmosis (Voisin, Buzoni-Gatel, Bout, & Velge-Roussel, 2004) and trypanosomiasis (Goñi, Alcaide, & Fresno, 2002). MDSCs are also elevated in mice with antigen-induced autoimmune enterocolitis, where adoptive transfer of additional MDSCs reduces disease symptoms, suggesting a protective role for MDSCs (Haile et al., 2008). Likewise, mice with experimental autoimmune encephalomyelitis have elevated levels of immune-suppressive MDSCs in their spleens and blood, which are likely to be beneficial in limiting autoreactivity (Zhu et al., 2007). Elevated levels of MDSCs are also found in the serum of patients with sepsis where they polarize immunity toward an antibody-promoting Type 2 response (Delano et al., 2007). Whether the MDSCs are beneficial or detrimental in sepsis is unclear.

Both stress and aging are also associated with increased MDSC levels. For example, postsurgery traumatic stress in mice is accompanied by increased levels of splenic MDSCs that suppress T cell proliferation by an ARG1-dependent mechanism (Makarenkova, Bansal, Matta, Perez, & Ochoa, 2006). Psychological stress in breast cancer patients further elevates circulating MDSCs (Mundy-Bosse, Thornton, Yang, Andersen, & Carson, 2011). MDSCs also increase with aging as shown in a study of adults ages 19–59, 61–76 (seniors), and 67–99 (elderly). The elderly cohort had the highest levels of MDSCs as well as increased serum levels of IL-6 and IL-1β (Verschoor et al., 2013). Studies in aging mice similarly show increases in MDSCs (Grizzle et al., 2007; Hanson et al., 2009).

MDSCs have also been implicated in driving asthma, an allergy caused by a hyper Th2 response that disrupts the normal Th1/Th2 balance. Children with asthma have elevated serum levels of MDSCs and IL-10, and reduced levels of IL-12 (Zhang, Luan, et al., 2013). Since MDSCs produce IL-10 which decreases macrophage production of IL-12 (Sinha, Clements, Bunt, et al., 2007), MDSCs are likely increasing the severity of disease by exacerbating polarization toward a type 2 response. In contrast, in a mouse asthma model, MDSCs appear to reduce disease because injection of tumor-derived MDSCs restored the Th1/Th2 balance by reducing the type 2 cytokine IL-4 and increasing the type 1 cytokine IFN-γ (Song et al., 2014).

MDSCs may play a beneficial role in obesity, which is considered a chronic low-grade inflammatory disease. Obese individuals have elevated levels of MDSCs in their peripheral tissues. These MDSCs counterbalance some of the detrimental effects of obesity by promoting insulin sensitivity and reducing inflammation. This latter effect occurs because MDSCs in adipose tissue skew macrophages toward an anti-inflammatory M2 phenotype (Xia et al., 2011), possibly by their production of IL-10. However, MDSCs may be detrimental in obese individuals undergoing vaccination, since mice with diet-induced obesity and elevated levels of MDSC displayed decreased antigen-specific T cell responses following vaccination (Chen et al., 2015).

Because of their immunosuppressive potency, MDSCs have been tested as therapeutic agents for autoimmune diseases or when tolerance is required. For example, adoptive transfer of bone marrow-generated MDSCs has been used to combat graft-versus-host disease (Highfill et al., 2010), ameliorate experimental autoimmune encephalomyelitis (Ioannou et al., 2012), aid in the retention of allogeneic islet grafts (Chou et al., 2012), and induce Tregs to protect against type1 diabetes (Yin et al., 2010). MDSCs may also be needed in mice to maintain maternal–fetal tolerance during the development of allogeneic fetuses (P. Sinha & S. Ostrand-Rosenberg, unpublished). The presence of elevated levels of immune-suppressive MDSCs in both mice and women pregnant with allogeneic embryos further supports the concept that MDSCs contribute to maternal–fetal tolerance and suggests that reduced levels of MDSCs in pregnant women could lead to miscarriage (Köstlin et al., 2014).

6. THERAPEUTIC TARGETING OF MDSCs

Because of their central role in immune suppression, many investigators have focused on neutralizing MDSCs in individuals with cancer. Strategies include targeting MDSC suppressive mechanisms, inducing MDSCs to differentiate into nonsuppressive mature APCs, blocking development of MDSCs, and killing of MDSCs. Table 1 lists recent approaches. Older therapies are reviewed in Wesolowski, Markowitz, and Carson (2013). It should be noted that none of these approaches universally neutralize MDSCs.

Table 1 Recently Reported Experimental Therapies Targeting MDSC Development, Viability, or Function

Therapy	Mechanism	Model	Effect
[a]2aG4 (phosphatidyl-serine antibody)	Reverses immunosuppressive effects by phosphatidyl-serine	LNCaP and PC3 prostate cancers (SCID mice)	Induces MDSC differentiation into M1 macrophages and DC; reduces MDSC numbers in tumor
[b]5-AZA (5-azacytidine)	Inhibits DNA methyltransferase	TRAMP-C2 prostate adenoma and TC-1/A9 pancreatic adenoma (C57BL/6 mice)	Reduces MDSC ARG1 expression, VEGF production, and suppressive activity; reduces MDSC accumulation.
[c]5-AZA + ENT (entinostat)	ENT is a class I HDAC inhibitor	CT26 colon carcinoma and 4T1 mammary carcinoma (BALB/c mice)	ENT causes apoptosis of PMN-MSDC *in vitro*, while 5-AZA has no effect on MDSCs; causes rejection of tumor when 5-AZA + ENT is used in combination with αPD-1 + αCTLA-4 immunotherapy
[d]ABT-737	Inhibitor of Bcl-2, Bcl-xL, and Bcl-w	CT26 colon carcinoma and 4T1 mammary carcinoma (BALB/c mice)	Increases MDSC susceptibility to FASL-mediated apoptosis; increases apoptosis of MDSC *in vivo*, not *in vitro*; decreases MDSC accumulation
[e]Antaxinib	VEGFR antagonist	RENCA renal cell carcinoma (BALB/c mice)	Inhibits STAT3 in MDSC; decreases MDSC ROS and ARG1; increases MDSC apoptosis
[f]ATRA (all-*trans* retinoic acid)	Agonist for retinoic acid receptor	SCLC patients	Causes apoptosis of PMN-MDSCs; differentiates MO-MDSCs to macrophages and DCs; reduces MDSCs in SCLC patients; enhanced the number of responders to p53 vaccine

[g]CD16XCD33 BiKE	Targets NK cells to $CD33^+$ cells	Myelodysplastic syndrome (MDS) patients	Induces NK cell-mediated killing of MDSCs
[h]Corosolic acid (Triterpenoid from apple pomace)	Blocks activation of STAT3 and NF-κB; inhibits polarization of macrophages to M2 phenotype	LM85 osteosarcoma (C3H mice)	Reduces MDSC suppressive activity
[i]Dopamine	Signals through D1-like DA receptors which inhibited MO-MDSC decreasing NO	LLC and B16 melanoma (C57BL/6 mice)	Reduces MDSC suppressive activity
[j]Gemcitabine + Capecitabine	Gemcitabine is a nucleoside analog. Capecitabine is a prodrug that is enzymatically converted to fluorouracil	Pancreatic cancer patients	No direct effect on MDSCs alone, but reduces MDSCs in patients receiving GM-CSF as an adjuvant for GV1001 (GV1001 is a telomerase vaccine)
[k]Gemcitabine + Rosiglitazone	Rosiglitazone activates PPARγ, thereby acting as an anti-inflammatory agent	Panc02 pancreatic carcinoma (C57BL/6 mice)	Rosiglitazone reduces early MDSC accumulation; combination therapy reduces late-stage MDSC accumulation
[c]J32	PI3K inhibitor	4T1 mammary carcinoma (BALB/c mice)	Causes PMN-MDSC apoptosis; no effect on tumor growth alone; causes tumor rejection in mice when used in combination with αPD-1 + αCTLA-4 immunotherapy
[l]Lenalidomide (thalidomide derivative)	Inhibits NF-κB, COX-2 activity, and angiogenesis; has immunomodulatory effects	A20 lymphoma (BALB/c mice)	Reduces MDSCs *in vivo*, but does not alter MDSC levels in naïve mice

Continued

Table 1 Recently Reported Experimental Therapies Targeting MDSC Development, Viability, or Function—cont'd

Therapy	Mechanism	Model	Effect
[m]MI-319	HDM2 inhibitor	Human renal cell carcinoma (nude mice)	Reverses sunitinib-induced MDSC infiltration into tumor (sunitinib is a RTK inhibitor and reduces angiogenesis)
[n]Polyphenon E (green tea extract)	Unknown mechanism	Neuroblastoma mouse models: TH-MYCN transgenic mice, human SHSY5Y (NOD/SCID mice), Neuro 2A (A/J mice)	Differentiates MO-MDSCs into PMN-MDSCs; reduces suppressive activity of MO-MDSCs; decreases ARG1 in MDSCs
[o]SAR131675	Inhibits VEGFR-3 tyrosine kinase	4T1 mammary carcinoma (BALB/c mice)	Reduces the number of MDSCs in tumor; promotes M1 macrophages
[p]Silibinin	Anti-inflammatory flavonoid	4T1 mammary carcinoma (BALB/c mice)	Reduces tumor volume, increases survival of tumor-bearing mice; decreases total number of MDSCs
[q]Tadalafil	PDE5 inhibitor	Human HNSCC patients	Lowers MDSCs and Treg numbers; increases tumor-specific $CD8^+$ T cells in a dose-dependent manner
[r]TCBA (tetrabromocinnamic acid)	Restores Notch signaling	EL4 lymphoma (C57BL/6 mice), CT26 colon carcinoma and MethA sarcoma (BALB/c mice)	Induces differentiation of MDSCs to DCs
[s]Vemurafenib	Inhibitor of $B\text{-}RAF^{V600E}$, a mutation leading to constitutive activation of MAP kinase pathway	Cutaneous melanoma patients	Inhibits the release of soluble factors from melanoma cells involved in the generation of MO-MDSC *in vitro*; decreases MO-MDSC *in vivo*

[t]Withaferin A (extract from ashwagandha plant)	Antioxidant with antitumor effects; inhibits Notch signaling and NF-κB activation	4T1 mammary carcinoma (BALB/c mice)	Decreases MDSC production of ROS and IL-10; decreases MDSC suppressive activity; reduces MDSC accumulation

[a]Yin, Huang, Lynn, and Thorpe (2013).
[b]Mikyskova et al. (2014).
[c]Kim et al. (2014).
[d]Hu et al. (2013).
[e]Yuan et al. (2014).
[f]Iclozan, Antonia, Chiappori, Chen, and Gabrilovich (2013).
[g]Gleason et al. (2014).
[h]Horlad et al. (2013).
[i]Wu et al. (2015).
[j]Annels et al. (2014).
[k]Bunt, Mohr, Bailey, Grandgenett, and Hollingsworth (2013).
[l]Sakamaki et al. (2014).
[m]Panka, Liu, Geissler, and Mier (2013).
[n]Santilli et al. (2013).
[o]Espagnolle et al. (2014).
[p]Forghani, Khorramizadeh, and Waller (2014).
[q]Weed et al. (2015).
[r]Cheng et al. (2014).
[s]Schilling et al. (2013).
[t]Sinha and Ostrand-Rosenberg (2013).

7. CONCLUSIONS

MDSCs encompass a range of immature immune-suppressive myeloid cells. Their suppressive activity and accumulation are induced by many inflammatory mediators with unique and redundant signaling pathways. MDSCs inhibit antitumor immunity through several mechanisms including (i) depletion of the local environment of the amino acids L-Arg, L-Trp, and L-Cys, which inhibits T cell activation and/or proliferation; (ii) secretion of NO, PNT, and ROS, which causes T cell apoptosis, inhibits peptide recognition by T cells, and inhibits T cell activation; (iii) induction of immunosuppressive Tregs; and (iv) impairment of T cell trafficking to lymph nodes. MDSCs also alter the inflammatory milieu by inducing inflammatory Th17 cells, participating in cross talk with macrophages, tumor cells, and MCs which promotes a protumor environment that enhances tumor-cell growth, invasion, and metastasis. Therefore, neutralizing MDSCs is an obvious strategy to enhance natural antitumor immunity and boost the efficacy of immunotherapies.

The concept of activating a patient's immune system to destroy their endogenous cancer cells has been a goal of immunotherapy for many years. Unfortunately, many cancer immunotherapy clinical trials have failed to show therapeutic efficacy. MDSCs may be responsible for at least some of these failures since they are present in many cancer patients, and have the ability to prevent T cell activation. Analysis of blood samples from non-responder patients indicated a correlation between lack of response and MDSC levels (Kimura et al., 2013). Regardless of the outcome of such studies, it is likely that cancer immunotherapies involving *in vivo* activation or proliferation of tumor-reactive T cells will require adjunctive treatment that neutralizes MDSCs.

Accumulation and suppressive potency of MDSCs are regulated by a complex milieu of inflammatory mediators. Environmental conditions such as hypoxia and inflammation act through similar signaling networks. These networks converge on common transcription factors such as STAT3 and NF-κB and regulate additional transcription factors, miRNAs, and proteins that mediate MDSC accumulation and suppression. Since multiple ligands initiate signaling through these pathways, MDSC regulation is highly redundant. This redundancy allows for the development of MDSCs under a broad range of conditions and may explain why MDSCs are so widespread in cancer patients. The redundancy also complicates therapeutic approaches for neutralizing MDSCs, since different inducers compensate for each other.

The past decade has seen remarkable progress in recognizing MDSCs as key players that inhibit antitumor immunity and facilitate tumor progression. Advances in understanding the mechanisms that drive MDSC accumulation and function have also been extensive. Hopefully, these studies will lead to the development of therapeutic strategies that are universally effective in neutralizing or eliminating MDSCs in cancer patients.

REFERENCES

Adeegbe, D., Serafini, P., Bronte, V., Zoso, A., Ricordi, C., & Inverardi, L. (2011). In vivo induction of myeloid suppressor cells and CD4(+)Foxp3(+) T regulatory cells prolongs skin allograft survival in mice. *Cell Transplantation*, *20*, 941–954.

Alizadeh, D., Trad, M., Hanke, N. T., Larmonier, C. B., Janikashvili, N., Bonnotte, B., et al. (2014). Doxorubicin eliminates myeloid-derived suppressor cells and enhances the efficacy of adoptive T-cell transfer in breast cancer. *Cancer Research*, *74*, 104–118.

Almand, B., Clark, J. I., Nikitina, E., van Beynen, J., English, N. R., Knight, S. C., et al. (2001). Increased production of immature myeloid cells in cancer patients: A mechanism of immunosuppression in cancer. *Journal of Immunology*, *166*, 678–689.

Annels, N. E., Shaw, V. E., Gabitass, R. F., Billingham, L., Corrie, P., Eatock, M., et al. (2014). The effects of gemcitabine and capecitabine combination chemotherapy and of low-dose adjuvant GM-CSF on the levels of myeloid-derived suppressor cells in patients with advanced pancreatic cancer. *Cancer Immunology, Immunotherapy*, *63*, 175–183.

Balkwill, F., & Mantovani, A. (2001). Inflammation and cancer: Back to Virchow? *Lancet*, *357*, 539–545.

Bergers, G., Brekken, R., McMahon, G., Vu, T. H., Itoh, T., Tamaki, K., et al. (2000). Matrix metalloproteinase-9 triggers the angiogenic switch during carcinogenesis. *Nature Cell Biology*, *2*, 737–744.

Beury, D. W., Parker, K. H., Nyandjo, M., Sinha, P., Carter, K. A., & Ostrand-Rosenberg, S. (2014). Cross-talk among myeloid-derived suppressor cells, macrophages, and tumor cells impacts the inflammatory milieu of solid tumors. *Journal of Leukocyte Biology*, *96*, 1109–1118.

Bianchi, M. E., & Manfredi, A. A. (2007). High-mobility group box 1 (HMGB1) protein at the crossroads between innate and adaptive immunity. *Immunological Reviews*, *220*, 35–46.

Bogdan, C. (2015). Nitric oxide synthase in innate and adaptive immunity: An update. *Trends in Immunology*, *36*, 161–178.

Boldin, M. P., Taganov, K. D., Rao, D. S., Yang, L., Zhao, J. L., Kalwani, M., et al. (2011). miR-146a is a significant brake on autoimmunity, myeloproliferation, and cancer in mice. *The Journal of Experimental Medicine*, *208*, 1189–1201.

Brandau, S., Trellakis, S., Bruderek, K., Schmaltz, D., Steller, G., Elian, M., et al. (2011). Myeloid-derived suppressor cells in the peripheral blood of cancer patients contain a subset of immature neutrophils with impaired migratory properties. *Journal of Leukocyte Biology*, *89*, 311–317.

Bresnick, A. R., Weber, D. J., & Zimmer, D. B. (2015). S100 proteins in cancer. *Nature Reviews. Cancer*, *15*, 96–109.

Brimnes, M. K., Vangsted, A. J., Knudsen, L. M., Gimsing, P., Gang, A. O., Johnsen, H. E., et al. (2010). Increased level of both CD4+FOXP3+ regulatory T cells and CD14+HLA-DR^{-}/low myeloid-derived suppressor cells and decreased level of dendritic cells in patients with multiple myeloma. *Scandinavian Journal of Immunology*, *72*, 540–547.

Bronte, V., Chappell, D. B., Apolloni, E., Cabrelle, A., Wang, M., Hwu, P., et al. (1999). Unopposed production of granulocyte-macrophage colony-stimulating factor by tumors inhibits CD8+ T cell responses by dysregulating antigen-presenting cell maturation. *Journal of Immunology, 162*, 5728–5737.

Bronte, V., Serafini, P., De Santo, C., Marigo, I., Tosello, V., Mazzoni, A., et al. (2003). IL-4-induced arginase 1 suppresses alloreactive T cells in tumor-bearing mice. *Journal of Immunology, 170*, 270–278.

Bronte, V., & Zanovello, P. (2005). Regulation of immune responses by L-arginine metabolism. *Nature Reviews. Immunology, 5*, 641–654.

Bunt, S. K., Clements, V. K., Hanson, E. M., Sinha, P., & Ostrand-Rosenberg, S. (2009). Inflammation enhances myeloid-derived suppressor cell cross-talk by signaling through Toll-like receptor 4. *Journal of Leukocyte Biology, 85*, 996–1004.

Bunt, S. K., Mohr, A. M., Bailey, J. M., Grandgenett, P. M., & Hollingsworth, M. A. (2013). Rosiglitazone and Gemcitabine in combination reduces immune suppression and modulates T cell populations in pancreatic cancer. *Cancer Immunology, Immunotherapy, 62*, 225–236.

Bunt, S. K., Sinha, P., Clements, V. K., Leips, J., & Ostrand-Rosenberg, S. (2006). Inflammation induces myeloid-derived suppressor cells that facilitate tumor progression. *Journal of Immunology, 176*, 284–290.

Bunt, S. K., Yang, L., Sinha, P., Clements, V. K., Leips, J., & Ostrand-Rosenberg, S. (2007). Reduced inflammation in the tumor microenvironment delays the accumulation of myeloid-derived suppressor cells and limits tumor progression. *Cancer Research, 67*, 10019–10026.

Burchert, A., Cai, D., Hofbauer, L. C., Samuelsson, M. K., Slater, E. P., Duyster, J., et al. (2004). Interferon consensus sequence binding protein (ICSBP; IRF-8) antagonizes BCR/ABL and down-regulates bcl-2. *Blood, 103*, 3480–3489.

Burke, M., Choksawangkarn, W., Edwards, N., Ostrand-Rosenberg, S., & Fenselau, C. (2014). Exosomes from myeloid-derived suppressor cells carry biologically active proteins. *Journal of Proteome Research, 13*, 836–843.

Cekic, C., Day, Y. J., Sag, D., & Linden, J. (2014). Myeloid expression of adenosine A2A receptor suppresses T and NK cell responses in the solid tumor microenvironment. *Cancer Research, 74*, 7250–7259.

Chalmin, F., Ladoire, S., Mignot, G., Vincent, J., Bruchard, M., Remy-Martin, J. P., et al. (2010). Membrane-associated Hsp72 from tumor-derived exosomes mediates STAT3-dependent immunosuppressive function of mouse and human myeloid-derived suppressor cells. *The Journal of Clinical Investigation, 120*, 457–471.

Chatterjee, S., Das, S., Chakraborty, P., Manna, A., Chatterjee, M., & Choudhuri, S. K. (2013). Myeloid derived suppressor cells (MDSCs) can induce the generation of Th17 response from naive CD4+ T cells. *Immunobiology, 218*, 718–724.

Chen, S., Akbar, S. M., Miyake, T., Abe, M., Al-Mahtab, M., Furukawa, S., et al. (2015). Diminished immune response to vaccinations in obesity: Role of myeloid-derived suppressor and other myeloid cells. *Obesity Research & Clinical Practice, 9*, 35–44.

Cheng, P., Corzo, C. A., Luetteke, N., Yu, B., Nagaraj, S., Bui, M. M., et al. (2008). Inhibition of dendritic cell differentiation and accumulation of myeloid-derived suppressor cells in cancer is regulated by S100A9 protein. *The Journal of Experimental Medicine, 205*, 2235–2249.

Cheng, P., Kumar, V., Liu, H., Youn, J. I., Fishman, M., Sherman, S., et al. (2014). Effects of notch signaling on regulation of myeloid cell differentiation in cancer. *Cancer Research, 74*, 141–152.

Chornoguz, O., Grmai, L., Sinha, P., Artemenko, K. A., Zubarev, R. A., & Ostrand-Rosenberg, S. (2011). Proteomic pathway analysis reveals inflammation increases myeloid-derived suppressor cell resistance to apoptosis. *Molecular & Cellular Proteomics, 10*, M110.002980.

Chou, H. S., Hsieh, C. C., Charles, R., Wang, L., Wagner, T., Fung, J. J., et al. (2012). Myeloid-derived suppressor cells protect islet transplants by B7-H1 mediated enhancement of T regulatory cells. *Transplantation, 93*, 272–282.

Corzo, C. A., Condamine, T., Lu, L., Cotter, M. J., Youn, J. I., Cheng, P., et al. (2010). HIF-1α regulates function and differentiation of myeloid-derived suppressor cells in the tumor microenvironment. *The Journal of Experimental Medicine, 207*, 2439–2453.

Corzo, C. A., Cotter, M. J., Cheng, P., Cheng, F., Kusmartsev, S., Sotomayor, E., et al. (2009). Mechanism regulating reactive oxygen species in tumor-induced myeloid-derived suppressor cells. *Journal of Immunology, 182*, 5693–5701.

Cui, T. X., Kryczek, I., Zhao, L., Zhao, E., Kuick, R., Roh, M. H., et al. (2013). Myeloid-derived suppressor cells enhance stemness of cancer cells by inducing microRNA101 and suppressing the corepressor CtBP2. *Immunity, 39*, 611–621.

Danelli, L., Frossi, B., Gri, G., Mion, F., Guarnotta, C., Bongiovanni, L., et al. (2015). Mast cells boost myeloid-derived suppressor cell activity and contribute to the development of tumor-favoring microenvironment. *Cancer Immunology Research, 3*, 85–95.

Delano, M. J., Scumpia, P. O., Weinstein, J. S., Coco, D., Nagaraj, S., Kelly-Scumpia, K. M., et al. (2007). MyD88-dependent expansion of an immature GR-1(+)CD11b(+) population induces T cell suppression and Th2 polarization in sepsis. *The Journal of Experimental Medicine, 204*, 1463–1474.

Diaz-Montero, C. M., Salem, M. L., Nishimura, M. I., Garrett-Mayer, E., Cole, D. J., & Montero, A. J. (2009). Increased circulating myeloid-derived suppressor cells correlate with clinical cancer stage, metastatic tumor burden, and doxorubicin-cyclophosphamide chemotherapy. *Cancer Immunology, Immunotherapy, 58*, 49–59.

Dolcetti, L., Peranzoni, E., Ugel, S., Marigo, I., Fernandez Gomez, A., Mesa, C., et al. (2010). Hierarchy of immunosuppressive strength among myeloid-derived suppressor cell subsets is determined by GM-CSF. *European Journal of Immunology, 40*, 22–35.

Dumitru, C. A., Moses, K., Trellakis, S., Lang, S., & Brandau, S. (2012). Neutrophils and granulocytic myeloid-derived suppressor cells: Immunophenotyping, cell biology and clinical relevance in human oncology. *Cancer Immunology, Immunotherapy, 61*, 1155–1167.

Dunn, G. P., Bruce, A. T., Ikeda, H., Old, L. J., & Schreiber, R. D. (2002). Cancer immunoediting: From immunosurveillance to tumor escape. *Nature Immunology, 3*, 991–998.

El Gazzar, M., & McCall, C. E. (2012). MicroRNAs regulatory networks in myeloid lineage development and differentiation: Regulators of the regulators. *Immunology and Cell Biology, 90*, 587–593.

Elkabets, M., Ribeiro, V. S., Dinarello, C. A., Ostrand-Rosenberg, S., Di Santo, J. P., Apte, R. N., et al. (2010). IL-1beta regulates a novel myeloid-derived suppressor cell subset that impairs NK cell development and function. *European Journal of Immunology, 40*, 3347–3357.

Eruslanov, E., Daurkin, I., Ortiz, J., Vieweg, J., & Kusmartsev, S. (2010). Pivotal advance: Tumor-mediated induction of myeloid-derived suppressor cells and M2-polarized macrophages by altering intracellular PGE_2 catabolism in myeloid cells. *Journal of Leukocyte Biology, 88*, 839–848.

Eruslanov, E., Neuberger, M., Daurkin, I., Perrin, G. Q., Algood, C., Dahm, P., et al. (2012). Circulating and tumor-infiltrating myeloid cell subsets in patients with bladder cancer. *International Journal of Cancer, 130*, 1109–1119.

Espagnolle, N., Barron, P., Mandron, M., Blanc, I., Bonnin, J., Agnel, M., et al. (2014). Specific inhibition of the VEGFR-3 tyrosine kinase by SAR131675 reduces peripheral and tumor associated immunosuppressive myeloid cells. *Cancers, 6*, 472–490.

Ezernitchi, A. V., Vaknin, I., Cohen-Daniel, L., Levy, O., Manaster, E., Halabi, A., et al. (2006). TCR zeta down-regulation under chronic inflammation is mediated by myeloid suppressor cells differentially distributed between various lymphatic organs. *Journal of Immunology, 177*, 4763–4772.

Farren, M. R., Carlson, L. M., & Lee, K. P. (2010). Tumor-mediated inhibition of dendritic cell differentiation is mediated by down regulation of protein kinase C beta II expression. *Immunologic Research, 46*, 165–176.

Fletcher, M., Ramirez, M. E., Sierra, R. A., Raber, P., Thevenot, P., Al-Khami, A. A., et al. (2015). L-Arginine depletion blunts antitumor T-cell responses by inducing myeloid-derived suppressor cells. *Cancer Research, 75*, 275–283.

Forghani, P., Khorramizadeh, M. R., & Waller, E. K. (2014). Silibinin inhibits accumulation of myeloid-derived suppressor cells and tumor growth of murine breast cancer. *Cancer Medicine, 3*, 215–224.

Fridlender, Z. G., Sun, J., Kim, S., Kapoor, V., Cheng, G., Ling, L., et al. (2009). Polarization of tumor-associated neutrophil phenotype by TGF-beta: "N1" versus "N2" TAN. *Cancer Cell, 16*, 183–194.

Fukumura, D., Kashiwagi, S., & Jain, R. K. (2006). The role of nitric oxide in tumour progression. *Nature Reviews. Cancer, 6*, 521–534.

Gabitass, R. F., Annels, N. E., Stocken, D. D., Pandha, H. A., & Middleton, G. W. (2011). Elevated myeloid-derived suppressor cells in pancreatic, esophageal and gastric cancer are an independent prognostic factor and are associated with significant elevation of the Th2 cytokine interleukin-13. *Cancer Immunology, Immunotherapy, 60*, 1419–1430.

Gabriele, L., Phung, J., Fukumoto, J., Segal, D., Wang, I. M., Giannakakou, P., et al. (1999). Regulation of apoptosis in myeloid cells by interferon consensus sequence-binding protein. *The Journal of Experimental Medicine, 190*, 411–421.

Gabrilovich, D. I., Bronte, V., Chen, S. H., Colombo, M. P., Ochoa, A., Ostrand-Rosenberg, S., et al. (2007). The terminology issue for myeloid-derived suppressor cells. *Cancer Research, 67*, 425, author reply 426.

Gabrilovich, D., Ishida, T., Oyama, T., Ran, S., Kravtsov, V., Nadaf, S., et al. (1998). Vascular endothelial growth factor inhibits the development of dendritic cells and dramatically affects the differentiation of multiple hematopoietic lineages in vivo. *Blood, 92*, 4150–4166.

Gabrilovich, D. I., Velders, M. P., Sotomayor, E. M., & Kast, W. M. (2001). Mechanism of immune dysfunction in cancer mediated by immature Gr-1+ myeloid cells. *Journal of Immunology, 166*, 5398–5406.

Garrity, T., Pandit, R., Wright, M. A., Benefield, J., Keni, S., & Young, M. R. (1997). Increased presence of CD34+ cells in the peripheral blood of head and neck cancer patients and their differentiation into dendritic cells. *International Journal of Cancer, 73*, 663–669.

Gehad, A. E., Lichtman, M. K., Schmults, C. D., Teague, J. E., Calarese, A. W., Jiang, Y., et al. (2012). Nitric oxide-producing myeloid-derived suppressor cells inhibit vascular E-selectin expression in human squamous cell carcinomas. *The Journal of Investigative Dermatology, 132*, 2642–2651.

Gleason, M. K., Ross, J. A., Warlick, E. D., Lund, T. C., Verneris, M. R., Wiernik, A., et al. (2014). CD16xCD33 bispecific killer cell engager (BiKE) activates NK cells against primary MDS and MDSC CD33+ targets. *Blood, 123*, 3016–3026.

Goñi, O., Alcaide, P., & Fresno, M. (2002). Immunosuppression during acute Trypanosoma cruzi infection: Involvement of Ly6G (Gr1(+))CD11b(+)immature myeloid suppressor cells. *International Immunology, 14*, 1125–1134.

Grizzle, W. E., Xu, X., Zhang, S., Stockard, C. R., Liu, C., Yu, S., et al. (2007). Age-related increase of tumor susceptibility is associated with myeloid-derived suppressor cell mediated suppression of T cell cytotoxicity in recombinant inbred BXD12 mice. *Mechanisms of Ageing and Development, 128*, 672–680.

Haile, L. A., von Wasielewski, R., Gamrekelashvili, J., Krüger, C., Bachmann, O., Westendorf, A. M., et al. (2008). Myeloid-derived suppressor cells in inflammatory bowel disease: A new immunoregulatory pathway. *Gastroenterology, 135*, 871–881, 881.e1–5.

Hanson, E. M., Clements, V. K., Sinha, P., Ilkovitch, D., & Ostrand-Rosenberg, S. (2009). Myeloid-derived suppressor cells down-regulate L-selectin expression on CD4+ and CD8+ T cells. *Journal of Immunology, 183*, 937–944.

He, D., Li, H., Yusuf, N., Elmets, C. A., Li, J., Mountz, J. D., et al. (2010). IL-17 promotes tumor development through the induction of tumor promoting microenvironments at tumor sites and myeloid-derived suppressor cells. *Journal of Immunology, 184*, 2281–2288.

Highfill, S. L., Rodriguez, P. C., Zhou, Q., Goetz, C. A., Koehn, B. H., Veenstra, R., et al. (2010). Bone marrow myeloid-derived suppressor cells (MDSCs) inhibit graft-versus-host disease (GVHD) via an arginase-1-dependent mechanism that is up-regulated by interleukin-13. *Blood, 116*, 5738–5747.

Hix, L. M., Karavitis, J., Khan, M. W., Shi, Y. H., Khazaie, K., & Zhang, M. (2013). Tumor STAT1 transcription factor activity enhances breast tumor growth and immune suppression mediated by myeloid-derived suppressor cells. *The Journal of Biological Chemistry, 288*, 11676–11688.

Hoechst, B., Ormandy, L. A., Ballmaier, M., Lehner, F., Kruger, C., Manns, M. P., et al. (2008). A new population of myeloid-derived suppressor cells in hepatocellular carcinoma patients induces CD4(+)CD25(+)Foxp3(+) T cells. *Gastroenterology, 135*, 234–243.

Horlad, H., Fujiwara, Y., Takemura, K., Ohnishi, K., Ikeda, T., Tsukamoto, H., et al. (2013). Corosolic acid impairs tumor development and lung metastasis by inhibiting the immunosuppressive activity of myeloid-derived suppressor cells. *Molecular Nutrition & Food Research, 57*, 1046–1054.

Hu, X., Bardhan, K., Paschall, A. V., Yang, D., Waller, J. L., Park, M. A., et al. (2013). Deregulation of apoptotic factors Bcl-xL and Bax confers apoptotic resistance to myeloid-derived suppressor cells and contributes to their persistence in cancer. *The Journal of Biological Chemistry, 288*, 19103–19115.

Huang, B., Pan, P. Y., Li, Q., Sato, A. I., Levy, D. E., Bromberg, J., et al. (2006). Gr-1+CD115+ immature myeloid suppressor cells mediate the development of tumor-induced T regulatory cells and T-cell anergy in tumor-bearing host. *Cancer Research, 66*, 1123–1131.

Huang, A., Zhang, B., Wang, B., Zhang, F., Fan, K. X., & Guo, Y. J. (2013). Increased CD14(+)HLA-DR (-/low) myeloid-derived suppressor cells correlate with extrathoracic metastasis and poor response to chemotherapy in non-small cell lung cancer patients. *Cancer Immunology, Immunotherapy, 62*, 1439–1451.

Iclozan, C., Antonia, S., Chiappori, A., Chen, D. T., & Gabrilovich, D. (2013). Therapeutic regulation of myeloid-derived suppressor cells and immune response to cancer vaccine in patients with extensive stage small cell lung cancer. *Cancer Immunology, Immunotherapy, 62*, 909–918.

Ilkovitch, D., & Lopez, D. M. (2009). The liver is a site for tumor-induced myeloid-derived suppressor cell accumulation and immunosuppression. *Cancer Research, 69*, 5514–5521.

Ioannou, M., Alissafi, T., Lazaridis, I., Deraos, G., Matsoukas, J., Gravanis, A., et al. (2012). Crucial role of granulocytic myeloid-derived suppressor cells in the regulation of central nervous system autoimmune disease. *Journal of Immunology, 188*, 1136–1146.

Jablonska, J., Leschner, S., Westphal, K., Lienenklaus, S., & Weiss, S. (2010). Neutrophils responsive to endogenous IFN-beta regulate tumor angiogenesis and growth in a mouse tumor model. *The Journal of Clinical Investigation, 120*, 1151–1164.

Karin, M. (2006). Nuclear factor-kappaB in cancer development and progression. *Nature, 441*, 431–436.

Kim, K., Skora, A. D., Li, Z., Liu, Q., Tam, A. J., Blosser, R. L., et al. (2014). Eradication of metastatic mouse cancers resistant to immune checkpoint blockade by suppression of myeloid-derived cells. *Proceedings of the National Academy of Sciences of the United States of America*, *111*, 11774–11779.

Kimura, T., McKolanis, J. R., Dzubinski, L. A., Islam, K., Potter, D. M., Salazar, A. M., et al. (2013). MUC1 vaccine for individuals with advanced adenoma of the colon: A cancer immunoprevention feasibility study. *Cancer Prevention Research (Philadelphia, PA)*, *6*, 18–26.

Köstlin, N., Kugel, H., Spring, B., Leiber, A., Marmé, A., Henes, M., et al. (2014). Granulocytic myeloid derived suppressor cells expand in human pregnancy and modulate T-cell responses. *European Journal of Immunology*, *44*, 2582–2591.

Kowanetz, M., Wu, X., Lee, J., Tan, M., Hagenbeek, T., Qu, X., et al. (2010). Granulocyte-colony stimulating factor promotes lung metastasis through mobilization of Ly6G+Ly6C+ granulocytes. *Proceedings of the National Academy of Sciences of the United States of America*, *107*, 21248–21255.

Kujawski, M., Kortylewski, M., Lee, H., Herrmann, A., Kay, H., & Yu, H. (2008). Stat3 mediates myeloid cell-dependent tumor angiogenesis in mice. *The Journal of Clinical Investigation*, *118*, 3367–3377.

Kusmartsev, S., Eruslanov, E., Kübler, H., Tseng, T., Sakai, Y., Su, Z., et al. (2008). Oxidative stress regulates expression of VEGFR1 in myeloid cells: Link to tumor-induced immune suppression in renal cell carcinoma. *Journal of Immunology*, *181*, 346–353.

Kusmartsev, S., & Gabrilovich, D. I. (2005). STAT1 signaling regulates tumor-associated macrophage-mediated T cell deletion. *Journal of Immunology*, *174*, 4880–4891.

Levring, T. B., Hansen, A. K., Nielsen, B. L., Kongsbak, M., von Essen, M. R., Woetmann, A., et al. (2012). Activated human CD4+ T cells express transporters for both cysteine and cystine. *Scientific Reports*, *2*, 266.

Li, W., Wu, K., Zhao, E., Shi, L., Li, R., Zhang, P., et al. (2013). HMGB1 recruits myeloid derived suppressor cells to promote peritoneal dissemination of colon cancer after resection. *Biochemical and Biophysical Research Communications*, *436*, 156–161.

Li, L., Zhang, J., Diao, W., Wang, D., Wei, Y., Zhang, C. Y., et al. (2014). MicroRNA-155 and MicroRNA-21 promote the expansion of functional myeloid-derived suppressor cells. *Journal of Immunology*, *192*, 1034–1043.

Lieschke, G. J., Grail, D., Hodgson, G., Metcalf, D., Stanley, E., Cheers, C., et al. (1994). Mice lacking granulocyte colony-stimulating factor have chronic neutropenia, granulocyte and macrophage progenitor cell deficiency, and impaired neutrophil mobilization. *Blood*, *84*, 1737–1746.

Lin, Y., Gustafson, M. P., Bulur, P. A., Gastineau, D. A., Witzig, T. E., & Dietz, A. B. (2011). Immunosuppressive CD14+HLA-DR(low)/- monocytes in B-cell non-Hodgkin lymphoma. *Blood*, *117*, 872–881.

Liu, Y., Lai, L., Chen, Q., Song, Y., Xu, S., Ma, F., et al. (2012). MicroRNA-494 is required for the accumulation and functions of tumor-expanded myeloid-derived suppressor cells via targeting of PTEN. *Journal of Immunology*, *188*, 5500–5510.

Liu, C., Yu, S., Kappes, J., Wang, J., Grizzle, W. E., Zinn, K. R., et al. (2007). Expansion of spleen myeloid suppressor cells represses NK cell cytotoxicity in tumor-bearing host. *Blood*, *109*, 4336–4342.

Liu, Q., Zhang, M., Jiang, X., Zhang, Z., Dai, L., Min, S., et al. (2011). miR-223 suppresses differentiation of tumor-induced $CD11b^+$ $Gr1^+$ myeloid-derived suppressor cells from bone marrow cells. *International Journal of Cancer*, *129*, 2662–2673.

Lu, T., & Gabrilovich, D. I. (2012). Molecular pathways: Tumor-infiltrating myeloid cells and reactive oxygen species in regulation of tumor microenvironment. *Clinical Cancer Research*, *18*, 4877–4882.

Lu, T., Ramakrishnan, R., Altiok, S., Youn, J. I., Cheng, P., Celis, E., et al. (2011). Tumor-infiltrating myeloid cells induce tumor cell resistance to cytotoxic T cells in mice. *The Journal of Clinical Investigation, 121*, 4015–4029.

MacDonald, K. P., Rowe, V., Clouston, A. D., Welply, J. K., Kuns, R. D., Ferrara, J. L., et al. (2005). Cytokine expanded myeloid precursors function as regulatory antigen-presenting cells and promote tolerance through IL-10-producing regulatory T cells. *Journal of Immunology, 174*, 1841–1850.

Makarenkova, V. P., Bansal, V., Matta, B. M., Perez, L. A., & Ochoa, J. B. (2006). CD11b+/Gr-1+ myeloid suppressor cells cause T cell dysfunction after traumatic stress. *Journal of Immunology, 176*, 2085–2094.

Mao, Y., Sarhan, D., Steven, A., Seliger, B., Kiessling, R., & Lundqvist, A. (2014). Inhibition of tumor-derived prostaglandin-e2 blocks the induction of myeloid-derived suppressor cells and recovers natural killer cell activity. *Clinical Cancer Research, 20*, 4096–4106.

Marigo, I., Bosio, E., Solito, S., Mesa, C., Fernandez, A., Dolcetti, L., et al. (2010). Tumor-induced tolerance and immune suppression depend on the C/EBPbeta transcription factor. *Immunity, 32*, 790–802.

Markiewski, M. M., DeAngelis, R. A., Benencia, F., Ricklin-Lichtsteiner, S. K., Koutoulaki, A., Gerard, C., et al. (2008). Modulation of the antitumor immune response by complement. *Nature Immunology, 9*, 1225–1235.

Martin, R. K., Saleem, S. J., Folgosa, L., Zellner, H. B., Damle, S. R., Nguyen, G. K., et al. (2014). Mast cell histamine promotes the immunoregulatory activity of myeloid-derived suppressor cells. *Journal of Leukocyte Biology, 96*, 151–159.

Mazzoni, A., Bronte, V., Visintin, A., Spitzer, J. H., Apolloni, E., Serafini, P., et al. (2002). Myeloid suppressor lines inhibit T cell responses by an NO-dependent mechanism. *Journal of Immunology, 168*, 689–695.

Melani, C., Chiodoni, C., Forni, G., & Colombo, M. P. (2003). Myeloid cell expansion elicited by the progression of spontaneous mammary carcinomas in c-erbB-2 transgenic BALB/c mice suppresses immune reactivity. *Blood, 102*, 2138–2145.

Melani, C., Sangaletti, S., Barazzetta, F. M., Werb, Z., & Colombo, M. P. (2007). Amino-biphosphonate-mediated MMP-9 inhibition breaks the tumor-bone marrow axis responsible for myeloid-derived suppressor cell expansion and macrophage infiltration in tumor stroma. *Cancer Research, 67*, 11438–11446.

Mikyskova, R., Indrova, M., Vlkova, V., Bieblova, J., Simova, J., Parackova, Z., et al. (2014). DNA demethylating agent 5-azacytidine inhibits myeloid-derived suppressor cells induced by tumor growth and cyclophosphamide treatment. *Journal of Leukocyte Biology, 95*, 743–753.

Molon, B., Ugel, S., Del Pozzo, F., Soldani, C., Zilio, S., Avella, D., et al. (2011). Chemokine nitration prevents intratumoral infiltration of antigen-specific T cells. *The Journal of Experimental Medicine, 208*, 1949–1962.

Montero, A. J., Diaz-Montero, C. M., Kyriakopoulos, C. E., Bronte, V., & Mandruzzato, S. (2012). Myeloid-derived suppressor cells in cancer patients: a clinical perspective. *Journal of Immunotherapy, 35*, 107–115.

Morales, J. K., Kmieciak, M., Knutson, K. L., Bear, H. D., & Manjili, M. H. (2010). GM-CSF is one of the main breast tumor-derived soluble factors involved in the differentiation of CD11b-Gr1- bone marrow progenitor cells into myeloid-derived suppressor cells. *Breast Cancer Research and Treatment, 123*, 39–49.

Mostafa, M. H., Sheweita, S. A., & O'Connor, P. J. (1999). Relationship between schistosomiasis and bladder cancer. *Clinical Microbiology Reviews, 12*, 97–111.

Movahedi, K., Guilliams, M., Van den Bossche, J., Van den Bergh, R., Gysemans, C., Beschin, A., et al. (2008). Identification of discrete tumor-induced myeloid-derived suppressor cell subpopulations with distinct T cell-suppressive activity. *Blood, 111*, 4233–4244.

Mucha, J., Majchrzak, K., Taciak, B., Hellmen, E., & Krol, M. (2014). MDSCs mediate angiogenesis and predispose canine mammary tumor cells for metastasis via IL-28/IL-28RA (IFN-lambda) signaling. *PLoS One*, *9*, e103249.

Mundy-Bosse, B. L., Thornton, L. M., Yang, H. C., Andersen, B. L., & Carson, W. E. (2011). Psychological stress is associated with altered levels of myeloid-derived suppressor cells in breast cancer patients. *Cellular Immunology*, *270*, 80–87.

Munn, D. H., Sharma, M. D., Baban, B., Harding, H. P., Zhang, Y., Ron, D., et al. (2005). GCN2 kinase in T cells mediates proliferative arrest and anergy induction in response to indoleamine 2,3-dioxygenase. *Immunity*, *22*, 633–642.

Nefedova, Y., Cheng, P., Gilkes, D., Blaskovich, M., Beg, A. A., Sebti, S. M., et al. (2005). Activation of dendritic cells via inhibition of Jak2/STAT3 signaling. *Journal of Immunology*, *175*, 4338–4346.

Nefedova, Y., Huang, M., Kusmartsev, S., Bhattacharya, R., Cheng, P., Salup, R., et al. (2004). Hyperactivation of STAT3 is involved in abnormal differentiation of dendritic cells in cancer. *Journal of Immunology*, *172*, 464–474.

Noman, M. Z., Desantis, G., Janji, B., Hasmim, M., Karray, S., Dessen, P., et al. (2014). PD-L1 is a novel direct target of HIF-1alpha, and its blockade under hypoxia enhanced MDSC-mediated T cell activation. *The Journal of Experimental Medicine*, *211*, 781–790.

Obermajer, N., Muthuswamy, R., Lesnock, J., Edwards, R. P., & Kalinski, P. (2011). Positive feedback between PGE2 and COX2 redirects the differentiation of human dendritic cells toward stable myeloid-derived suppressor cells. *Blood*, *118*, 5498–5505.

Okazaki, T., Ebihara, S., Asada, M., Kanda, A., Sasaki, H., & Yamaya, M. (2006). Granulocyte colony-stimulating factor promotes tumor angiogenesis via increasing circulating endothelial progenitor cells and Gr1+CD11b+ cells in cancer animal models. *International Immunology*, *18*, 1–9.

Ortiz, M. L., Kumar, V., Martner, A., Mony, S., Donthireddy, L., Condamine, T., et al. (2015). Immature myeloid cells directly contribute to skin tumor development by recruiting IL-17-producing CD4+ T cells. *The Journal of Experimental Medicine*, *212*, 351–367.

Ostrand-Rosenberg, S., & Sinha, P. (2009). Myeloid-derived suppressor cells: Linking inflammation and cancer. *Journal of Immunology*, *182*, 4499–4506.

OuYang, L. Y., Wu, X. J., Ye, S. B., Zhang, R. X., Li, Z. L., Liao, W., et al. (2015). Tumor-induced myeloid-derived suppressor cells promote tumor progression through oxidative metabolism in human colorectal cancer. *Journal of Translational Medicine*, *13*, 47.

Pan, P. Y., Ma, G., Weber, K. J., Ozao-Choy, J., Wang, G., Yin, B., et al. (2010). Immune stimulatory receptor CD40 is required for T-cell suppression and T regulatory cell activation mediated by myeloid-derived suppressor cells in cancer. *Cancer Research*, *70*, 99–108.

Panka, D. J., Liu, Q., Geissler, A. K., & Mier, J. W. (2013). Effects of HDM2 antagonism on sunitinib resistance, p53 activation, SDF-1 induction, and tumor infiltration by CD11b+/Gr-1+ myeloid derived suppressor cells. *Molecular Cancer*, *12*, 17.

Parker, K., Sinha, P., Horn, L., Clements, V., & Ostrand-Rosenberg, S. (2014). HMGB1 enhances immune suppression by facilitating the differentiation and suppressive activity of myeloid-derived suppressor cells. *Cancer Research*, *74*, 5723–5733.

Porembka, M. R., Mitchem, J. B., Belt, B. A., Hsieh, C. S., Lee, H. M., Herndon, J., et al. (2012). Pancreatic adenocarcinoma induces bone marrow mobilization of myeloid-derived suppressor cells which promote primary tumor growth. *Cancer Immunology, Immunotherapy*, *61*, 1373–1385.

Punturieri, A., Szabo, E., Croxton, T. L., Shapiro, S. D., & Dubinett, S. M. (2009). Lung cancer and chronic obstructive pulmonary disease: Needs and opportunities for integrated research. *Journal of the National Cancer Institute*, *101*, 554–559.

Raber, P. L., Thevenot, P., Sierra, R., Wyczechowska, D., Halle, D., Ramirez, M. E., et al. (2014). Subpopulations of myeloid-derived suppressor cells impair T cell responses through independent nitric oxide-related pathways. *International Journal of Cancer, 134*, 2853–2864.

Rodriguez, P. C., Ernstoff, M. S., Hernandez, C., Atkins, M., Zabaleta, J., Sierra, R., et al. (2009). Arginase I-producing myeloid-derived suppressor cells in renal cell carcinoma are a subpopulation of activated granulocytes. *Cancer Research, 69*, 1553–1560.

Rodriguez, P. C., Hernandez, C. P., Morrow, K., Sierra, R., Zabaleta, J., Wyczechowska, D. D., et al. (2010). L-Arginine deprivation regulates cyclin D3 mRNA stability in human T cells by controlling HuR expression. *Journal of Immunology, 185*, 5198–5204.

Rodriguez, P. C., Hernandez, C. P., Quiceno, D., Dubinett, S. M., Zabaleta, J., Ochoa, J. B., et al. (2005). Arginase I in myeloid suppressor cells is induced by COX-2 in lung carcinoma. *The Journal of Experimental Medicine, 202*, 931–939.

Rodriguez, P. C., Quiceno, D. G., Zabaleta, J., Ortiz, B., Zea, A. H., Piazuelo, M. B., et al. (2004). Arginase I production in the tumor microenvironment by mature myeloid cells inhibits T-cell receptor expression and antigen-specific T-cell responses. *Cancer Research, 64*, 5839–5849.

Rodriguez, P. C., Zea, A. H., Culotta, K. S., Zabaleta, J., Ochoa, J. B., & Ochoa, A. C. (2002). Regulation of T cell receptor CD3zeta chain expression by L-arginine. *The Journal of Biological Chemistry, 277*, 21123–21129.

Sakamaki, I., Kwak, L. W., Cha, S. C., Yi, Q., Lerman, B., Chen, J., et al. (2014). Lenalidomide enhances the protective effect of a therapeutic vaccine and reverses immune suppression in mice bearing established lymphomas. *Leukemia, 28*, 329–337.

Saleem, S. J., Martin, R. K., Morales, J. K., Sturgill, J. L., Gibb, D. R., Graham, L., et al. (2012). Cutting edge: Mast cells critically augment myeloid-derived suppressor cell activity. *Journal of Immunology, 189*, 511–515.

Santhanam, L., Lim, H. K., Miriel, V., Brown, T., Patel, M., Balanson, S., et al. (2007). Inducible NO synthase dependent S-nitrosylation and activation of arginase1 contribute to age-related endothelial dysfunction. *Circulation Research, 101*, 692–702.

Santilli, G., Piotrowska, I., Cantilena, S., Chayka, O., D'Alicarnasso, M., Morgenstern, D. A., et al. (2013). Polyphenon [corrected] E enhances the antitumor immune response in neuroblastoma by inactivating myeloid suppressor cells. *Clinical Cancer Research, 19*, 1116–1125.

Schilling, B., Sucker, A., Griewank, K., Zhao, F., Weide, B., Gorgens, A., et al. (2013). Vemurafenib reverses immunosuppression by myeloid derived suppressor cells. *International Journal of Cancer, 133*, 1653–1663.

Schmielau, J., & Finn, O. J. (2001). Activated granulocytes and granulocyte-derived hydrogen peroxide are the underlying mechanism of suppression of t-cell function in advanced cancer patients. *Cancer Research, 61*, 4756–4760.

Serafini, P. (2013). Myeloid derived suppressor cells in physiological and pathological conditions: The good, the bad, and the ugly. *Immunologic Research, 57*, 172–184.

Serafini, P., Carbley, R., Noonan, K. A., Tan, G., Bronte, V., & Borrello, I. (2004). High-dose granulocyte-macrophage colony-stimulating factor-producing vaccines impair the immune response through the recruitment of myeloid suppressor cells. *Cancer Research, 64*, 6337–6343.

Serafini, P., Mgebroff, S., Noonan, K., & Borrello, I. (2008). Myeloid-derived suppressor cells promote cross-tolerance in B-cell lymphoma by expanding regulatory T cells. *Cancer Research, 68*, 5439–5449.

Shacter, E., & Weitzman, S. A. (2002). Chronic inflammation and cancer. *Oncology (Williston Park), 16*, 217–226, 229; discussion 230–232.

Shen, P., Wang, A., He, M., Wang, Q., & Zheng, S. (2014). Increased circulating Lin(-/low) CD33(+) HLA-DR(-) myeloid-derived suppressor cells in hepatocellular carcinoma patients. *Hepatology Research*, *44*, 639–650.

Sica, A., & Mantovani, A. (2012). Macrophage plasticity and polarization: In vivo veritas. *The Journal of Clinical Investigation*, *122*, 787–795.

Sinha, P., Chornoguz, O., Clements, V. K., Artemenko, K. A., Zubarev, R. A., & Ostrand-Rosenberg, S. (2011). Myeloid-derived suppressor cells express the death receptor Fas and apoptose in response to T cell-expressed FasL. *Blood*, *117*, 5381–5390.

Sinha, P., Clements, V. K., Bunt, S. K., Albelda, S. M., & Ostrand-Rosenberg, S. (2007). Cross-talk between myeloid-derived suppressor cells and macrophages subverts tumor immunity toward a type 2 response. *Journal of Immunology*, *179*, 977–983.

Sinha, P., Clements, V. K., Fulton, A. M., & Ostrand-Rosenberg, S. (2007). Prostaglandin E2 promotes tumor progression by inducing myeloid-derived suppressor cells. *Cancer Research*, *67*, 4507–4513.

Sinha, P., Clements, V. K., & Ostrand-Rosenberg, S. (2005a). Interleukin-13-regulated M2 macrophages in combination with myeloid suppressor cells block immune surveillance against metastasis. *Cancer Research*, *65*, 11743–11751.

Sinha, P., Clements, V. K., & Ostrand-Rosenberg, S. (2005b). Reduction of myeloid-derived suppressor cells and induction of M1 macrophages facilitate the rejection of established metastatic disease. *Journal of Immunology*, *174*, 636–645.

Sinha, P., Okoro, C., Foell, D., Freeze, H. H., Ostrand-Rosenberg, S., & Srikrishna, G. (2008). Proinflammatory S100 proteins regulate the accumulation of myeloid-derived suppressor cells. *Journal of Immunology*, *181*, 4666–4675.

Sinha, P., & Ostrand-Rosenberg, S. (2013). Myeloid-derived suppressor cell function is reduced by Withaferin A, a potent and abundant component of Withania somnifera root extract. *Cancer Immunology, Immunotherapy*, *62*, 1663–1673.

Sinha, P., Parker, K. H., Horn, L., & Ostrand-Rosenberg, S. (2012). Tumor-induced myeloid-derived suppressor cell function is independent of IFN-γ and IL-4Rα. *European Journal of Immunology*, *42*, 2052–2059.

Sionov, R. V., Fridlender, Z. G., & Granot, Z. (2014). The multifaceted roles neutrophils play in the tumor microenvironment. *Cancer Microenvironment*.

Smith, C., Chang, M. Y., Parker, K. H., Beury, D. W., DuHadaway, J. B., Flick, H. E., et al. (2012). IDO is a nodal pathogenic driver of lung cancer and metastasis development. *Cancer Discovery*, *2*, 722–735.

Song, X., Krelin, Y., Dvorkin, T., Bjorkdahl, O., Segal, S., Dinarello, C. A., et al. (2005). CD11b+/Gr-1+ immature myeloid cells mediate suppression of T cells in mice bearing tumors of IL-1beta-secreting cells. *Journal of Immunology*, *175*, 8200–8208.

Song, C., Yuan, Y., Wang, X. M., Li, D., Zhang, G. M., Huang, B., et al. (2014). Passive transfer of tumour-derived MDSCs inhibits asthma-related airway inflammation. *Scandinavian Journal of Immunology*, *79*, 98–104.

Srivastava, M. K., Bosch, J. J., Thompson, J. A., Ksander, B. R., Edelman, M. J., & Ostrand-Rosenberg, S. (2008). Lung cancer patients' CD4(+) T cells are activated in vitro by MHC II cell-based vaccines despite the presence of myeloid-derived suppressor cells. *Cancer Immunology, Immunotherapy*, *57*, 1493–1504.

Srivastava, M. K., Sinha, P., Clements, V. K., Rodriguez, P., & Ostrand-Rosenberg, S. (2010). Myeloid-derived suppressor cells inhibit T-cell activation by depleting cystine and cysteine. *Cancer Research*, *70*, 68–77.

Stewart, T. J., Liewehr, D. J., Steinberg, S. M., Greeneltch, K. M., & Abrams, S. I. (2009). Modulating the expression of IFN regulatory factor 8 alters the protumorigenic behavior of CD11b+Gr-1+ myeloid cells. *Journal of Immunology*, *183*, 117–128.

Strober, S. (1984). Natural suppressor (NS) cells, neonatal tolerance, and total lymphoid irradiation: Exploring obscure relationships. *Annual Review of Immunology*, *2*, 219–237.

Terabe, M., Matsui, S., Park, J. M., Mamura, M., Noben-Trauth, N., Donaldson, D. D., et al. (2003). Transforming growth factor-beta production and myeloid cells are an effector mechanism through which CD1d-restricted T cells block cytotoxic T lymphocyte-mediated tumor immunosurveillance: Abrogation prevents tumor recurrence. *The Journal of Experimental Medicine, 198*, 1741–1752.

Thevenot, P. T., Sierra, R. A., Raber, P. L., Al-Khami, A. A., Trillo-Tinoco, J., Zarreii, P., et al. (2014). The stress-response sensor chop regulates the function and accumulation of myeloid-derived suppressor cells in tumors. *Immunity, 41*, 389–401.

Tu, S., Bhagat, G., Cui, G., Takaishi, S., Kurt-Jones, E. A., Rickman, B., et al. (2008). Overexpression of interleukin-1beta induces gastric inflammation and cancer and mobilizes myeloid-derived suppressor cells in mice. *Cancer Cell, 14*, 408–419.

Vakkila, J., & Lotze, M. T. (2004). Inflammation and necrosis promote tumour growth. *Nature Reviews. Immunology, 4*, 641–648.

Venereau, E., Casalgrandi, M., Schiraldi, M., Antoine, D. J., Cattaneo, A., De Marchis, F., et al. (2012). Mutually exclusive redox forms of HMGB1 promote cell recruitment or proinflammatory cytokine release. *The Journal of Experimental Medicine, 209*, 1519–1528.

Verschoor, C. P., Johnstone, J., Millar, J., Dorrington, M. G., Habibagahi, M., Lelic, A., et al. (2013). Blood CD33(+)HLA-DR(-) myeloid-derived suppressor cells are increased with age and a history of cancer. *Journal of Leukocyte Biology, 93*, 633–637.

Voisin, M. B., Buzoni-Gatel, D., Bout, D., & Velge-Roussel, F. (2004). Both expansion of regulatory GR1+ CD11b+ myeloid cells and anergy of T lymphocytes participate in hyporesponsiveness of the lung-associated immune system during acute toxoplasmosis. *Infection and Immunity, 72*, 5487–5492.

Vuk-Pavlović, S., Bulur, P. A., Lin, Y., Qin, R., Szumlanski, C. L., Zhao, X., et al. (2010). Immunosuppressive CD14+HLA-DRlow/- monocytes in prostate cancer. *Prostate, 70*, 443–455.

Waight, J. D., Netherby, C., Hensen, M. L., Miller, A., Hu, Q., Liu, S., et al. (2013). Myeloid-derived suppressor cell development is regulated by a STAT/IRF-8 axis. *The Journal of Clinical Investigation, 123*, 4464–4478.

Wang, L., Chang, E. W., Wong, S. C., Ong, S. M., Chong, D. Q., & Ling, K. L. (2013). Increased myeloid-derived suppressor cells in gastric cancer correlate with cancer stage and plasma S100A8/A9 proinflammatory proteins. *Journal of Immunology, 190*, 794–804.

Wang, R., & Green, D. R. (2012). Metabolic checkpoints in activated T cells. *Nature Immunology, 13*, 907–915.

Wang, L., Yi, T., Kortylewski, M., Pardoll, D. M., Zeng, D., & Yu, H. (2009). IL-17 can promote tumor growth through an IL-6-Stat3 signaling pathway. *The Journal of Experimental Medicine, 206*, 1457–1464.

Weed, D. T., Vella, J. L., Reis, I. M., De la Fuente, A. C., Gomez, C., Sargi, Z., et al. (2015). Tadalafil reduces myeloid-derived suppressor cells and regulatory T cells and promotes tumor immunity in patients with head and neck squamous cell carcinoma. *Clinical Cancer Research, 21*, 39–48.

Wesolowski, R., Markowitz, J., & Carson, W. E., 3rd. (2013). Myeloid derived suppressor cells—A new therapeutic target in the treatment of cancer. *Journal for Immunotherapy of Cancer, 1*, 10.

Wu, S., Rhee, K. J., Albesiano, E., Rabizadeh, S., Wu, X., Yen, H. R., et al. (2009). A human colonic commensal promotes colon tumorigenesis via activation of T helper type 17 T cell responses. *Nature Medicine, 15*, 1016–1022.

Wu, J., Zhang, R., Tang, N., Gong, Z., Zhou, J., Chen, Y., et al. (2015). Dopamine inhibits the function of Gr-1+CD115+ myeloid-derived suppressor cells through D1-like receptors and enhances anti-tumor immunity. *Journal of Leukocyte Biology, 97*, 191–200.

Xia, S., Sha, H., Yang, L., Ji, Y., Ostrand-Rosenberg, S., & Qi, L. (2011). Gr-1 + CD11b+ myeloid-derived suppressor cells suppress inflammation and promote insulin sensitivity in obesity. *The Journal of Biological Chemistry*, *286*, 23591–23599.

Xin, H., Zhang, C., Herrmann, A., Du, Y., Figlin, R., & Yu, H. (2009). Sunitinib inhibition of Stat3 induces renal cell carcinoma tumor cell apoptosis and reduces immunosuppressive cells. *Cancer Research*, *69*, 2506–2513.

Yazawa, T., Shibata, M., Gonda, K., Machida, T., Suzuki, S., Kenjo, A., et al. (2013). Increased IL-17 production correlates with immunosuppression involving myeloid-derived suppressor cells and nutritional impairment in patients with various gastrointestinal cancers. *Molecular and Clinical Oncology*, *1*, 675–679.

Ye, J., Livergood, R. S., & Peng, G. (2013). The role and regulation of human Th17 cells in tumor immunity. *The American Journal of Pathology*, *182*, 10–20.

Yin, Y., Huang, X., Lynn, K. D., & Thorpe, P. E. (2013). Phosphatidylserine-targeting antibody induces M1 macrophage polarization and promotes myeloid-derived suppressor cell differentiation. *Cancer Immunology Research*, *1*, 256–268.

Yin, B., Ma, G., Yen, C. Y., Zhou, Z., Wang, G. X., Divino, C. M., et al. (2010). Myeloid-derived suppressor cells prevent type 1 diabetes in murine models. *Journal of Immunology*, *185*, 5828–5834.

Youn, J. I., Collazo, M., Shalova, I. N., Biswas, S. K., & Gabrilovich, D. I. (2012). Characterization of the nature of granulocytic myeloid-derived suppressor cells in tumor-bearing mice. *Journal of Leukocyte Biology*, *91*, 167–181.

Youn, J. I., Nagaraj, S., Collazo, M., & Gabrilovich, D. I. (2008). Subsets of myeloid-derived suppressor cells in tumor-bearing mice. *Journal of Immunology*, *181*, 5791–5802.

Young, M. R., Petruzzelli, G. J., Kolesiak, K., Achille, N., Lathers, D. M., & Gabrilovich, D. I. (2001). Human squamous cell carcinomas of the head and neck chemoattract immune suppressive CD34(+) progenitor cells. *Human Immunology*, *62*, 332–341.

Yu, J., Du, W., Yan, F., Wang, Y., Li, H., Cao, S., et al. (2013). Myeloid-derived suppressor cells suppress antitumor immune responses through IDO expression and correlate with lymph node metastasis in patients with breast cancer. *Journal of Immunology*, *190*, 3783–3797.

Yuan, H., Cai, P., Li, Q., Wang, W., Sun, Y., Xu, Q., et al. (2014). Axitinib augments antitumor activity in renal cell carcinoma via STAT3-dependent reversal of myeloid-derived suppressor cell accumulation. *Biomedicine & Pharmacotherapy*, *68*, 751–756.

Zea, A. H., Rodriguez, P. C., Atkins, M. B., Hernandez, C., Signoretti, S., Zabaleta, J., et al. (2005). Arginase-producing myeloid suppressor cells in renal cell carcinoma patients: A mechanism of tumor evasion. *Cancer Research*, *65*, 3044–3048.

Zea, A. H., Rodriguez, P. C., Culotta, K. S., Hernandez, C. P., DeSalvo, J., Ochoa, J. B., et al. (2004). L-Arginine modulates CD3zeta expression and T cell function in activated human T lymphocytes. *Cellular Immunology*, *232*, 21–31.

Zhang, M., Liu, Q., Mi, S., Liang, X., Zhang, Z., Su, X., et al. (2011). Both miR-17-5p and miR-20a alleviate suppressive potential of myeloid-derived suppressor cells by modulating STAT3 expression. *Journal of Immunology*, *186*, 4716–4724.

Zhang, Y. L., Luan, B., Wang, X. F., Qiao, J. Y., Song, L., Lei, R. R., et al. (2013). Peripheral blood MDSCs, IL-10 and IL-12 in children with asthma and their importance in asthma development. *PLoS One*, *8*, e63775.

Zhang, B., Wang, Z., Wu, L., Zhang, M., Li, W., Ding, J., et al. (2013). Circulating and tumor-infiltrating myeloid-derived suppressor cells in patients with colorectal carcinoma. *PLoS One*, *8*, e57114.

Zhu, B., Bando, Y., Xiao, S., Yang, K., Anderson, A. C., Kuchroo, V. K., et al. (2007). CD11b+Ly-6C(hi) suppressive monocytes in experimental autoimmune encephalomyelitis. *Journal of Immunology*, *179*, 5228–5237.

Zitvogel, L., Apetoh, L., Ghiringhelli, F., & Kroemer, G. (2008). Immunological aspects of cancer chemotherapy. *Nature Reviews. Immunology*, *8*, 59–73.

Zong, W. X., & Thompson, C. B. (2006). Necrotic death as a cell fate. *Genes & Development*, *20*, 1–15.

Zoso, A., Mazza, E. M., Bicciato, S., Mandruzzato, S., Bronte, V., Serafini, P., et al. (2014). Human fibrocytic myeloid-derived suppressor cells express IDO and promote tolerance via Treg-cell expansion. *European Journal of Immunology*, *44*, 3307–3319.

CHAPTER FOUR

Phagocytes as Corrupted Policemen in Cancer-Related Inflammation

Eduardo Bonavita[*,1], **Maria Rosaria Galdiero**[*,†,1], **Sebastien Jaillon**[*,1], **Alberto Mantovani**[*,‡,2]

*IRCCS Istituto Clinico Humanitas, Rozzano, Italy
†Division of Clinical Immunology and Allergy, University of Naples Federico II, Naples, Italy
‡Humanits University, Rozzano, Italy
[2]Corresponding author: e-mail address: alberto.mantovani@humanitasresearch.it

Contents

Abstract

Inflammation is a key component of the tumor microenvironment. Tumor-associated macrophages (TAMs) and tumor-associated neutrophils (TANs) are prototypic inflammatory cells in cancer-related inflammation. Macrophages provide a first line of resistance against infectious agents but in the ecological niche of cancer behave as corrupted policemen. TAMs promote tumor growth and metastasis by direct interactions with cancer cells, including cancer stem cells, as well as by promoting angiogenesis and tissue remodeling and suppressing effective adaptive immunity. In addition,

[1] E.B., M.R.G., and S.J. have equally contributed to this review and are in alphabetical order. Specifically, E.B. contributed to the field of macrophage and complement and M.R.G. and S.J. to the neutrophils section.

Advances in Cancer Research, Volume 128
ISSN 0065-230X
http://dx.doi.org/10.1016/bs.acr.2015.04.013

the efficacy of chemotherapy, radiotherapy, and checkpoint blockade inhibitors is profoundly affected by regulation of TAMs. In particular, TAMs can protect and rescue tumor cells from cytotoxic therapy by orchestrating a misguided tissue repair response. Following extensive preclinical studies, there is now proof of concept that targeting tumor-promoting macrophages by diverse strategies (e.g., Trabectedin, anti-colony-stimulating factor-1 receptor antibodies) can result in antitumor activity in human cancer and further studies are ongoing. Neutrophils have long been overlooked as a minor component of the tumor microenvironment, but there is evidence for an important role of TANs in tumor progression. Targeting phagocytes (TAMs and TANs) as corrupted policemen in cancer may pave the way to innovative therapeutic strategies complementing cytoreductive therapies and immunotherapy.

1. INTRODUCTION

Epidemiological, genetic, and experimental evidence demonstrate that chronic nonresolving inflammation can increase cancer risk and promotes cancer progression (Coussens, Zitvogel, & Palucka, 2013; Mantovani & Allavena, 2015; Mantovani, Allavena, Sica, & Balkwill, 2008). Tumor-promoting inflammation is now recognized as a key component of cancer (Hanahan & Weinberg, 2011). A link between chronic inflammation and cancer has long been suspected, but only recently the cellular and molecular mechanisms have in part been disclosed.

Epidemiological studies indicate that the risk of carcinogenesis increases under conditions of persistent nonresolving inflammation. Estimate suggests that chronic infections are at the basis of 15–20% of all cancers developed. Examples include viral infections with hepatitis B and C for liver cancer, papilloma virus for cervix carcinoma; bacterial infections, such as *Helicobacter pylori* for gastric cancer or lymphoma; parasites, such as Schistosoma for bladder cancer.

Chronic inflammation can also be triggered by noninfectious agents including irritants such as tobacco smoke, asbestos, silica, gastric reflux, chronic inflammatory disorders of the gastrointestinal tract, and autoimmune diseases can promote cancer development and metabolic dysfunctions, obesity in particular, are associated with a state of low-grade inflammation and increased cancer risk. Long-term use of nonsteroidal antiinflammatory drugs aspirin in particular reduces the risk of carcinogenesis and tumor progression.

Another line of evidence is provided by the composition of the tumor microenvironment, where inflammatory leukocytes and many inflammatory mediators (cytokines, chemokines, enzymes) are present. Inflammatory cells and mediators are an essential constituent of the tumor microenvironment (Coussens et al., 2013; Hanahan & Weinberg, 2011; Mantovani et al., 2008). Cells of the monocyte–macrophage lineage are major components of the host cell infiltrate of tumors that can reach up to 50% of the total mass. The analysis of the function of leukocyte infiltrate has paved the way to the dissection of tumor-promoting inflammatory mechanisms in cancer (De Palma & Lewis, 2013; Mantovani, Bottazzi, Colotta, Sozzani, & Ruco, 1992; Mantovani, Sozzani, Locati, Allavena, & Sica, 2002; Noy & Pollard, 2014). Indeed, the observation of leukocyte infiltration in tumors was first made by the German pathologist Rudolf Virchow in the nineteenth century, who postulated that cancer may arise in chronically inflamed tissues (Balkwill & Mantovani, 2001; Mantovani et al., 1992).

Not all the tumors have an underlying cause of infection or chronic inflammation, but also in these tumors a reactive inflammatory microenvironment and inflammatory cell infiltration have been described. Inflammation, in these cases, is triggered by the activation of oncogenes (e.g., Ras, Myc, BRAF) and/or the inactivation of tumor-suppressor genes (e.g., p53, PTEN), that in addition to promote cell proliferation, also stimulate the transcription of inflammatory genes, including cytokines and chemokines that recruit circulating leukocytes to the tumor tissues and further fuel the inflammatory response. Several lines of evidence indicate that macrophages have the potential to kill tumor cells and to elicit tumor-destructive reactions. Tumor-associated macrophages (TAMs) are drivers of tumor progression in established tumors, promoting cancer cell proliferation and survival, angiogenesis and lymphoangiogenesis, skewing and taming effective T-cell responses. There is also evidence that inflammatory cells may mediate tumor initiation and promote genetic instability (Mantovani et al., 2008; Noy & Pollard, 2014). Thus, extrinsic causes of inflammation (infections, irritants) and intrinsic causes (oncogene-activated inflammatory response in cancer cells) both concur to build up an inflammatory tumor microenvironment (Mantovani & Allavena, 2015; Mantovani et al., 2008). Here, we will review the role of phagocytes (macrophages and neutrophils) in tumor progression and their connection with humoral innate immunity, prompted by recent evidence (Bonavita et al., 2015).

2. ORIGIN AND FUNCTIONS OF TAMs

Tissue-resident macrophages, characterized in mice by the expression of the chemokine receptor CX3CR1, protect tissues and maintain homeostasis, whereas inflammatory macrophages, characterized by the expression of CCR2, are recruited at inflammatory sites and contribute to the inflammatory response. Mouse-resident macrophages (Kupffer cells in liver, microglia in brain, Langerhans cells in the skin, and alveolar macrophages in lung) develop in the embryo (Gomez Perdiguero et al., 2015). During this process, progenitors colonize peripheral tissues and differentiate into resident macrophages which will self-maintain throughout life (De Kleer et al., 2014). On the other hand, inflammatory macrophages derive from adult bone marrow-derived monocytes. However, resident macrophages in the gut, heart, and dermis originally derive from the yolk sac, but during adult life are replenished by bone marrow progenitors (Bain et al., 2014; McGovern et al., 2014; Molawi et al., 2014; Wynn et al., 2013). In tumors, TAMs mainly originate from bone marrow monocytes (Franklin et al., 2014; Mantovani et al., 1992; Noy & Pollard, 2014; Shand et al., 2014). In some mouse tumors, local proliferation does occur (Bottazzi et al., 1990; Tymoszuk et al., 2014), but recent evidence suggests that, in general, recruitment of circulating monocytes is essential for TAMs accumulation (Franklin et al., 2014; Noy & Pollard, 2014). Chemokines (e.g., CCL2, CCL5, and CXCL12) and the growth factor CSF-1 (M-CSF) play a major role in monocyte infiltration in tumors. Recently, components of the Complement cascade have also been described to play a role in macrophage recruitment (e.g., Bonavita et al., 2015). Incoming blood monocytes preferentially localize in hypoxic or necrotic areas within tumor stroma; they are profoundly influenced by the tumor environment and rapidly differentiate into tumor-conditioned macrophages. Among chemokines, CCL5/RANTES, CXCL12/SDF-1, and CXC3L1/fractalkine, for instance, were found in neoplastic tissues and contribute to macrophage recruitment and tumor promotion (Balkwill, 2004; Bottazzi et al., 1983; Mantovani et al., 2004; Reed et al., 2012; Ueno et al., 2000). In addition to chemokines and growth factors, noncanonical chemotactic peptides also produced by stromal and tumor cells, such as vascular endothelial growth factor (VEGF), transforming growth factor-beta (TGF-β), basic fibroblast growth factor (bFGF), macrophage colony-stimulating factor (M-CSF/CSF-1), urokinase plasminogen activator (uPa), the antimicrobial peptide β-defensin-3, and the lectin Reg3β (Allavena & Mantovani, 2012; Bierie & Moses, 2010; Gironella et al., 2013; Jin et al., 2010; Lin, Gouon-Evans, Nguyen, & Pollard, 2002; Linde et al., 2012; Reed et al., 2012; Zhang, Sud, Mizutani, Gyetko, & Pienta, 2011), caused monocyte recruitment and macrophage differentiation. CXC chemokines (CXCL8, CXCL1,

CXCL2, CXCL3, CXCL5), known for their role in neutrophil recruitment in both physiological and pathological conditions and involved in cancer progression, are also produced in tumor-associated inflammation. This favors tumor angiogenesis and metastasis (Keeley, Mehrad, & Strieter, 2010; Lazennec & Richmond, 2010; Mantovani, Cassatella, Costantini, & Jaillon, 2011).

Plasticity and diversity are key properties of cells of the monocyte–macrophage lineage (Biswas & Mantovani, 2010; Mosser & Edwards, 2008; Sica & Mantovani, 2012). In primary tumors and in metastatic sites, TAMs are involved in complex bidirectional interactions with tumor cells; cancer stem cells (CSCs); fibroblasts; mesenchymal stem cells; endothelial cells; and T, B, and NK cells. Macrophages can undergo polarized classical M1 activation in response to interferon-γ (IFN-γ) and Lipopolysaccharide (LPS), or alternative M2 activation driven by IL-4 or IL-13. M1- and M2-polarized macrophages are extremes of a continuum in a universe of functional states. The molecular mechanisms and functional properties of polarized macrophages have recently been reviewed (Mantovani & Allavena, 2015; Murray et al., 2014). In many mouse and human tumors, TAMs have a frank M2 phenotype or properties which are to some extent shared with M2-polarized cells. In general, TAMs promote tumor growth and metastasis, angiogenesis, and subversion of effective antitumor immunity (Biswas & Mantovani, 2010; Coussens et al., 2013; Sica & Mantovani, 2012). Signals derived from tumors and host cells shape the functional phenotype of TAMs. In different tumor and tissue contexts, these functional determinants include hypoxia, cytokines (e.g., TGF-β and CSF-1), and metabolic products of cancer cells (e.g., lactic acid); IL-4 and IL-13 produced by Th2 cells; and IL-10 produced by Treg cells, B cells, and immune complexes (Colegio et al., 2014; Coussens et al., 2013; De Palma & Lewis, 2013; Mantovani & Allavena, 2015; Mantovani et al., 2008; Noy & Pollard, 2014; Ruffell, Affara, & Coussens, 2012; Sica & Mantovani, 2012). Within the cancer tissue, there can be microanatomical diversity of TAMs function with accumulation of M2-like cells in hypoxic areas (Movahedi et al., 2010). Moreover, inflammatory components and pathways of orchestration differ in tumors originating in distinct anatomical sites (Ruffell et al., 2012).

There is strong evidence that macrophages can be "reprogrammed" by some immunological stimuli, such as IFN-γ or IFN-α, from immunosuppressive M2 macrophages into immunostimulatory cells (De Palma & Lewis, 2013; Duluc et al., 2009). At the clinical level, it has been reported that IFN-γ-driven intratumoral microenvironment exhibits superior prognostic effect compared with an IFN-α-driven microenvironment in patients with colon carcinoma. This gives a successful proof of principle that complex cytokine interaction networks can be found and dissected in human tissues (Grenz et al., 2013). Moreover, a Th1-dominated tumor micromilieu is strongly associated with a positive prognosis in CRC (Camus et al., 2009; Galon et al., 2006; Naschberger et al., 2008). Several lines of evidence indicate that macrophages infiltrating the tumor take part in the inflammatory process, favoring tumor formation and progression and a M2-like phenotype for TAMs has been reported in several studies (Biswas et al., 2006). The M2-like phenotype can be induced by the tumor cells. Katara et al. reported that vacuolar ATPase (V-ATPase) produced by tumor cells can promote tumor survival and growth. In particular, cancer tissues and cells overexpress the a2 isoform of V-ATPase (a2V). The relevance of the a2V role has been tested in *in vitro* studies, exposing macrophages to the cleaved N-terminal domain of a2V. In these conditions, macrophages express and secrete TAM-associated molecules such as mannose receptor-1, arginase-1, interleukin-10, TGF-β, MMP-9, and VEGF (Katara et al., 2014). A member of the TGF-β family has recently been reported to promote M2-like polarization of TAMs and to inhibit IL-12 (Wang et al., 2014).

During tumor growth and progression, functions of TAMs include extracellular matrix remodeling, promotion of tumor cell invasion and metastasis, angiogenesis, lymphangiogenesis, and immune suppression (Mantovani et al., 2002). In fact, TAMs produce a number of proteolytic molecules, such as plasmin, urokinase-type plasminogen activator, cathepsin B, and matrix metalloproteases (MMPs) which may directly remodel the extra cellular matrix (ECM) (Gocheva et al., 2010; Nagakawa, Aoki, Kasuya, Tsuchida, & Koyanagi, 2002; Wang et al., 2011). The role of MMPs in tumor progression has been suggested by their capacity to degrade the basement membrane to activate growth factors and to enhance angiogenesis (Huang et al., 2002; Stetler-Stevenson & Yu, 2001; Wang, So, Reierstad, & Fishman, 2005). Invasiveness of cancer cells is facilitated by TAMs expression of nonproteolytic molecules. For instance, expression of chemokines that bind CXCR2 was increased in macrophages exposed to conditioned media from mammary epithelial cells containing FGF receptor 1-induced soluble factors. In turn, these chemokines induced migration of primary and tumoral mammary epithelial cells (Bohrer & Schwertfeger, 2012). In mice injected subcutaneously with pancreatic cancer cells, expression of scavenger-receptor A in hematopoietic cells, consistent with its expression on macrophages, was required for cancer metastasis (Neyen et al., 2013). In glioma stem-like cells, the expression of MMP-9 promoted by macrophages-derived TGF-β1 increased the invasiveness of tumor cells (Ye et al., 2012). Finally, tumor-derived versican V1 enhanced the expression of the antimicrobial peptide hCAP18/LL37 in macrophages, which in turn contributed to ovarian tumor cell proliferation and invasion (Li et al., 2013).

Macrophages have been described to be associated with the metastatic potential of several tumors (Lin, Li, Tadashi, & Dong, 2011; Qing et al., 2012). In classical experiments of Gorelik and coworkers, it was described that transfer of thioglycollate-elicited peritoneal macrophages in mice increased by up to 100-fold the number of metastatic lung nodules induced by the intravenous injection of melanoma or Lewis lung carcinoma tumor cells (Gorelik, Wiltrout, Brunda, Holden, & Herberman, 1982). In a mouse model of breast cancer, IL-4-treated macrophages upregulated the expression of cysteine protease cathepsin B, which promoted lung metastasis (Vasiljeva et al., 2006). Moreover, M2-polarizing cytokines or tumor cell-conditioned media cause macrophages expression of a truncated fibronectin isoform, namely migration-stimulating factor, that is a potent chemotactic factor for tumor cells (Solinas et al., 2010). Depletion studies in experimental animals cause reduced incidence of metastasis, giving further support to the prometastatic function of TAMs (DeNardo et al., 2009; Joyce & Pollard, 2009).

TAMs are associated with tumor angiogenesis and lymphangiogenesis: TAMs express mediators such as TGF-β, VEGF-A, VEGF-C, PDGF, MMP-9, thymidine phosphorylase, and chemokines (e.g., CXCL8/IL-8) which are directly or indirectly involved in new vessel formation and sprouting (Granata et al., 2010; Hotchkiss et al., 2003; Murdoch, Giannoudis, & Lewis, 2004; Schmidt & Carmeliet, 2010; Schoppmann, Horvat, & Birner, 2002). TAMs-derived MMP-9 induces the release of heparin-bound growth factors, particularly VEGF-A, crucial for the angiogenic switch (Ebrahem et al., 2010). VEGF-recruited monocytes improve their performance as angiogenic cells (Avraham-Davidi et al., 2013). Recruited monocytes derive from the pool of circulating Ly6Chi monocytes that undergo phenotypic and functional changes upon entry in the VEGF-rich environment. These recruited monocytes acquire enhanced proangiogenic capabilities and, importantly, a markedly increased capacity to remodel existing blood vessels.

In the tumor microenvironment, low-oxygen tension increases the expression levels of Hypoxia-inducible factor (HIF) -1 and HIF-2, which trigger a proangiogenic program in macrophages characterized by high expression levels of VEGF, bFGF, CXCL8/IL-8, and glycolytic enzymes (Murdoch et al., 2004). In the tumor microenvironment, local hypoxia causes high levels of adenosine that stimulate angiogenic and lymphangiogenic factors released by human (Granata et al., 2010). Casazza and coworkers recently reported that the Sema3A/neuropilin-1 signaling axis controls TAMs localization into hypoxic tumor areas. If TAMs are confined inside normoxic regions by blunting the Sema3A/neuropilin-1 pathway, antitumor immunity is restored and angiogenesis abated, and consequently tumor growth and metastasis are inhibited. Thus, cancer cell-derived Sema3A, not VEGF, is responsible for TAMs entry into hypoxic niches through neuropilin-1 signaling, where TAMs escape antitumor immunity and promote vascularization (Casazza et al., 2013). Modulating TAMs localization and thus their phenotype can be a new approach to guide TAMs activities against cancer. Moreover, Laoui et al. reported that hypoxia is not a major driver of the TAMs subset differentiation found in tumor infiltrate, namely $CD11b^{hi}F4/80^{hi}Ly6C^{lo}$ $MHC\text{-}II^{lo}$ or $MHC\text{-}II^{hi}$ TAMs, both of which derived from tumor-infiltrating Ly6Chi monocytes, but rather specifically fine-tunes the phenotype of M2-like $MHC\text{-}II^{lo}$ TAMs, that as a consequence contain higher mRNA levels for hypoxia-regulated genes than their $MHC\text{-}II^{hi}$ counterparts (Laoui et al., 2014).

TAMs also express immunosuppressive potential, secreting or expressing a wide range of molecules, such as TGF-β, iNOS, arginase-1, IDO, and IL-10, known for their immunosuppressive role (Hagemann et al., 2006; Mantovani & Sica, 2010; Sica et al., 2000; Zhao et al., 2012). In murine models of breast cancer, TAMs suppress T-cell functions through their metabolic activities, expressing arginase-1 or iNOS (Bronte & Zanovello, 2005; Chang, Liao, & Kuo, 2001; Doedens et al., 2010; Movahedi et al., 2010). However and particularly in humans, TAMs-mediated T-cell suppression may also occur irrespective of L-arginine metabolism (Kryczek et al., 2006). For instance, TAMs have been shown to express the immunosuppressive molecule B7-H1 in hepatocellular carcinoma (HCC), B7-H4 in ovarian and lung cancer, and B7-H3 in lung cancer (Chen et al., 2012, 2013; Kryczek et al., 2006; Kuang et al., 2009). In addition, TAMs have the capacity to induce the expression of these molecules on cancer cell surface, thus providing a novel mechanism by which cancer cells escape the immune surveillance (Chen et al., 2013).

3. MACROPHAGES IN COMPLEMENT-MEDIATED, PTX3-REGULATED TUMOR PROMOTION

The physiological functions of the Complement system include defence against microbial infections, and disposal of immune complexes and products of inflammatory injury (Ricklin & Lambris, 2013). The Complement system also controls different immunological and inflammatory processes. The latter include enhancement of humoral immunity, regulation of adaptive immunity, apoptotic cell clearance, angiogenesis, cellular regeneration, and growth (Ricklin, Hajishengallis, Yang, & Lambris, 2010). The interaction of Complement components with receptors present on macrophages leads to modulation of cytokine production and induction of inflammatory responses. The myelomonocytic cell lineage expresses Complement receptors which mediate pathogen phagocytosis (e.g., C1qR (s), CR1, CR3, CR4, and CRIg) or induce inflammatory responses (e.g., C3aR, C5aR1, and C5aR2; Bohlson, O'Conner, Hulsebus, Ho, & Fraser, 2014; Fig. 1). C3a and C5a mediate macrophage activation through different signaling mechanisms. For instance, C3a activates NLRP3 inflammasome

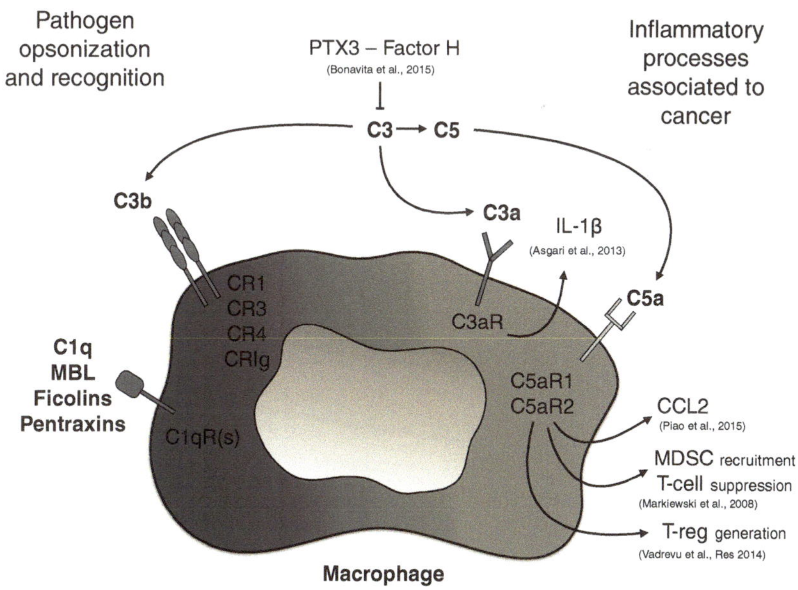

Figure 1 Macrophages and the interplay with humoral innate immunity in the regulation of inflammation and cancer. For explanation, see text. (See the color plate.)

increasing ATP release and favoring IL-1β production (Asgari et al., 2013). C5a has been correlated with IL-6 induction and development of inflammatory Th17 response (Fang, Zhang, Miwa, & Song, 2009).

During neoplastic transformation, tumor cells can acquire new morphological changes that render them susceptible to Complement attack. The high number of genetic alterations associated with carcinogenesis dramatically changes the composition of the cell membrane. For example, an altered glycosylation is considered a hallmark of cancer cells (Hanahan & Weinberg, 2011), and progression of epithelial cells from a normal to malignant phenotype is associated with an aberrant metabolism of membrane phospholipids affecting signal transduction pathways (Pio, Corrales, & Lambris, 2014). However, in comparison to normal counterpart, tumor cells have also been shown to express higher levels of membrane-bound regulatory proteins and soluble Complement inhibitors, including CD21, CD35, CD46, CD55, CD59, and Factor H, which could be responsible of hindered Complement cytotoxicity (Bellone et al., 2012; Gelderman, Tomlinson, Ross, & Gorter, 2004; Hörl et al., 2013).

Although no formal evidence supports the existence of an effective immune surveillance mediated by Complement during carcinogenesis, changes in the composition of cell membrane may target tumor cells for Complement recognition. Several observations support Complement-mediated recognition of malignant cells and Complement activation in many cancers. Elevated levels of C3a are present in the ascitic fluid of patients with ovarian cancer (Bjorge et al., 2005). C3c and C4 levels are elevated in lung cancer patients and their concentration is directly correlated with tumor volume (Ajona et al., 2013, 2015). The lectin pathway of Complement is more activated in colorectal cancer patients in comparison to healthy individuals, and systemic levels of MASP-2 have been reported to be an independent prognostic marker for poor survival (Ytting, Jarle Christensen, Thiel, Jensenius, & Nielsen, 2005). The activation of the classical pathway of Complement has also been found in patients affected by mucosa-associated lymphoid tissue lymphoma (Bu, Zheng, Wang, & Yu, 2007). Moreover, Complement-dependent cytotoxicity was necessary for immunotherapeutic response to rituximab in central nervous system (CNS) lymphomas (Kadoch et al., 2014) and chronic lymphocytic leukemia (Middleton et al., 2015).

In recent years, many studies have identified new and unexpected roles for Complement activation within the tumor microenvironment challenging the classical view of the Complement system as an anticancer mechanism (Bonavita et al., 2015) Complement elements can promote growth of transplanted tumors in the context of chronic inflammation (Markiewski et al., 2008). Notably, mice deficient in C3 or C5aR show decreased tumor growth in models of transplantable tumors, in comparison to wild-type mice, suggesting that the Complement system somehow promotes tumor growth (Rutkowski, Sughrue, Kane, Mills, & Parsa, 2010). In line with this view, several studies have demonstrated a protumorigenic role for activated Complement components in all stages of carcinogenesis. The genetic abrogation of C3 significantly reduced tumor incidence in models of 3-methylcholanthrene- and 7,12-dimethylbenz [a] anthracene/terephthalic acid (DMBA/TPA)-induced carcinogenesis (Bonavita et al., 2015). Moreover C3 deficiency was associated with reduced tumor macrophages infiltration (Bonavita et al., 2015). Complement activation promoted azoxymethane/dextran sodium sulphate (AOM/DSS)-induced carcinogenesis in IL-1β/IL-17A-dependent manner and C3-deficient mice developed significantly less colonic lesions (Ning et al., 2015). Complement can suppress antitumoral immunity via C5a that is a potent chemoattractant for myeloid-derived suppressor cells (MDSCs), which inhibit cytotoxic T limphocytes (CTL) (Markiewski et al., 2008). In a preclinical model of breast cancer, C5aR engagement facilitated metastasis by suppressing effectors CD8 and CD4 T-cell responses in the lungs (Vadrevu et al., 2014). In addition, C5a favored liver metastasis by promoting tumor inflammation. Indeed, genetic deficiency of C5aR leads to impaired production of CCL2 (Piao et al., 2015). Finally, data obtained studying pathologies not related to cancer raise the possibility that Complement proteins may enhance Epithelial–mesenchymal transition (EMT), provide chemotactic stimuli (i.e., C5a and C3a; Pasinetti et al., 1996), and induce production of growth factors (i.e., VEGF and TGF-β; Nozaki et al., 2006), which prime and encourage tumor invasion and migration (Christofori, 2006).

Although several lines of evidence sustain a protumoral role for Complement, this system can play different roles in different tumor contexts. For instance, C3 deficiency did not affect tumor incidence in a model of skin carcinogenesis driven by HPV16 (de Visser, Korets, & Coussens, 2004), or even promoted tumor formation in the case of Her2/neu breast tumors (Bandini et al., 2013). Collectively, these data suggest that Complement activation has a dual role in cancer: it has the potential to kill cancer cells, but Complement elements can modulate macrophage functions promoting cancer-related inflammation and tumor progression.

Modulation of Complement activation is a common feature of pentraxins. The short pentraxins C-reactive protein (CRP) and serum amyloid P component recognize different Complement components.

The interaction between CRP and C1q leads to the formation of C3 convertase and thus to the activation of the classical pathway (Sjoberg, Trouw, McGrath, Hack, & Blom, 2006). Surface-bound CRP inhibits alternative pathway amplification through a specific interaction with Factor H, the main soluble regulator of this pathway. In addition, CRP and SAP bind C4b-binding protein (C4BP), a soluble regulator of the classical and lectin pathways (Inforzato et al., 2013).

Similarly, the prototype of long pentraxins PTX3 has a dual role in Complement activation. The first protein identified as PTX3 ligand was C1q, the activator of the classical pathway (Bottazzi et al., 1997). The interaction between PTX3 and the globular head of C1q occurs in a calcium-dependent manner and depending on the way it is presented leads either to activation or inhibition of the Complement cascade (Doni et al., 2012). PTX3 has also been shown to interact with three members of the lectin pathway, namely ficolin-1, ficolin-2, and mannose-binding lectin (MBL; Gout et al., 2011). PTX3 enhances ficolin-1, ficolin-2, and MBL-dependent Complement deposition on the surface of *Aspergillus fumigatus* and *Candida albicans*, respectively, favoring Complement-mediated innate immune responses (Ma et al., 2013). In addition, the formation of a complex ficolin-1/PTX3 on the surface of apoptotic cell facilitated the clearance of apoptotic cells down-regulating in parallel the release of IL-8 by macrophages (Ma et al., 2013). Finally, PTX3 interacts with Factor H, favoring its deposition on PTX3-coated surface and limiting an exacerbated activation of the Complement cascade (Deban et al., 2008). In atypical hemolytic uremic syndrome, mutations observed in Factor H reduced the interaction with PTX3 and lead to enhanced inflammation and Complement-mediated damage (Okemefuna, Nan, Miller, Gor, & Perkins, 2010). PTX3 has also been shown to interact with C4BP, which inhibits Complement activation by acting as a cofactor for factor I in the cleavage and inactivation of C4b (Braunschweig & Jozsi, 2011). This interaction promoted the recruitment of C4BP on late-apoptotic cells and extracellular matrix, suggesting negative modulation of local Complement activation that would otherwise lead to inflammation and tissue damage.

In a model of 3-methylcholanthrene-induced carcinogenesis, PTX3 deficiency was associated to increased susceptibility to cancer, higher proinflammatory mediator release (i.e., CCL2), and gene instability. Tumor tissues from PTX3-deficient mice were characterized by significantly higher C3 deposition in comparison to wild-type tumors because of defective Factor H recruitment. Deficiency of C3 in PTX3 gene-targeted mice was sufficient to rescue the increased susceptibility to tumor growth and macrophage recruitment. Higher tumor incidence in PTX3-deficient mice was also associated with increased C5a levels and the pharmacological blocking of C5aR *in vivo* reduced tumor frequency (Bonavita et al., 2015). Thus, PTX3 deficiency unleashes unrestrained Complement activation with production of C5a, CCL2, and enhanced recruitment of tumor-promoting macrophages. These results indicate that an essential component of the humoral arm of innate immunity and regulator of Complement activation acts as an extrinsic oncosuppressor by acting at the level of Complement-mediated, macrophage-sustained, tumor-promoting inflammation.

4. THE YIN YANG OF TAMs IN ANTICANCER THERAPY

The evidence and consensus about the role of TAMs in tumor-promoting inflammation (Hanahan & Weinberg, 2011) raise the issue of their involvement in current treatment modalities and of their potential as therapeutic targets. In general, two main approaches have been used: direct depletion of macrophages or inhibition of monocyte recruitment and restimulation of their cytotoxic function (reeducation of TAMs; Beatty et al., 2011; Edwards & Emens, 2010; Germano et al., 2013; Mantovani & Allavena, 2015; Rozel et al., 2009; Xin et al., 2009). As mentioned above, cancer cell-centered therapeutic strategies and immunotherapy profoundly influence the function of TAMs by directly modulating their function or by affecting components of the tumor microenvironment (e.g., effective adaptive immune responses). In turn, TAMs can contribute to the ultimate efficacy of anticancer strategies or retain and amplify their tumor-promoting function by orchestrating a misdirected tissue repair response. The role of TAMs in anticancer therapy has recently been reviewed (Mantovani & Allavena, 2015). Evidence suggests that in conventional cytotoxic therapeutic strategies (chemotherapy and radiotherapy), TAMs can have a dual role. Chemotherapy and radiotherapy can elicit a misdirected macrophage-orchestrated tissue repair response and thus rescue and protect tumor cells including CSCs. On the other hand, TAMs can contribute to the antitumor activity of selected anticancer drugs and low-dose radiotherapy (Mantovani & Allavena, 2015). Moreover, TAMs may play a role in targeted therapies and in checkpoint blockade inhibiting antibodies (Mantovani & Allavena, 2015). Finally, following extensive preclinical testing, there is now proof of principle that targeting TAMs can have antitumor activity in human tumors (Germano et al., 2013). In particular, there is evidence that Trabectedin, approved for clinical use in Europe for sarcomas and ovarian carcinoma, acts at least in part by depleting tumor-promoting monocytes (Germano et al., 2013).

5. NEUTROPHILS AND CANCER

Neutrophils represent the most abundant leukocyte subpopulation in human peripheral blood and play a primary role in host defence against pathogens during the earliest phases of the inflammatory responses. The role of neutrophils in tumor development has long been underestimated due to their short half-life and terminally differentiated phenotype. In the last decade, the advent of new technical tools allowed to better characterize these cells, thus challenging this limited classical point of view. Indeed, evidences propose emerging roles for neutrophils in coordinating many aspects of the inflammatory response and tumor development. Similarly to TAMs, tumor-associated neutrophils (TANs) can exert both antitumoral and protumoral functions and experimental animal models suggest that neutrophils are characterized by a surprising plasticity (Fridlender et al., 2009; Mantovani, 2009; Fig. 2).

5.1 Neutrophil Recruitment and Their Prognostic Significance in Tumors

Within the tumor microenvironment, a number of CXC chemokines (e.g., CXCL1, CXCL2, CXCL3, CXCL5, CXCL8), known for their neutrophil

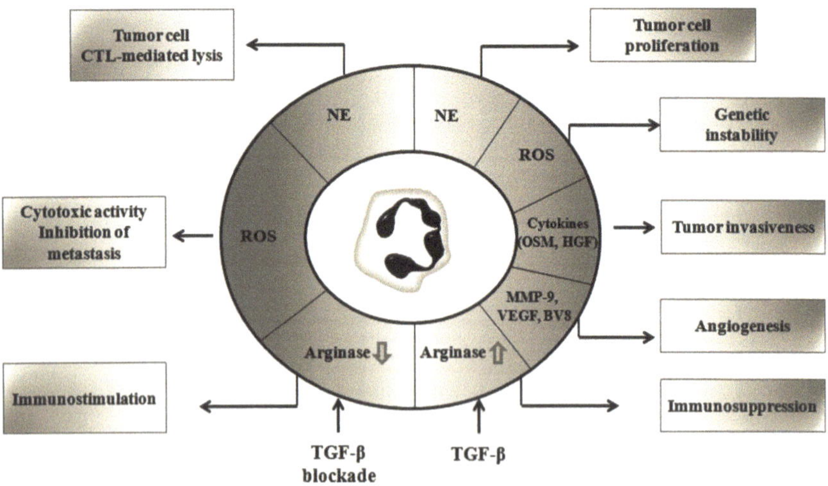

Figure 2 Neutrophils potentially impact key aspects of cancer. For explanation, see text. (See the color plate.)

chemoattractant properties, are produced by tumor and stromal cells and have been related to cancer initiation, to the promotion of tumor angiogenesis, and metastasis (Keeley et al., 2010; Lazennec & Richmond, 2010; Mantovani et al., 2011). For example, evidence derived from murine models described an important role for the CXCR2 signaling pathway in lung and pancreatic cancer promotion (Ijichi et al., 2011; Keane, Belperio, Xue, Burdick, & Strieter, 2004). In various murine models of cancers (inflammation-associated skin cancer, colitis-associated or spontaneous intestinal cancer), CXCR2 abrogation or neutrophil depletion inhibited both inflammation-induced and spontaneous carcinogenesis (Jamieson et al., 2012). Moreover, in a murine model of graft tumor, CXCL17 promoted the recruitment of myeloid $CD11b^{+}Gr1^{+}F4/80^{-}$ cells within the tumor, favoring tumor growth, angiogenesis, and metastatic behavior (Matsui et al., 2012). In humans, HCC cells and head and neck squamous cell carcinoma (HNSCC) cell lines recruited neutrophils in a CXCR2-dependent manner through the production of CXCL8 (Kuang et al., 2011) and macrophage-inhibiting factor (MIF; Dumitru et al., 2011; Trellakis, Farjah, et al., 2011). Moreover, in a wide cohort of HCC tumors, correlations between increased CXCL5 expression, neutrophil infiltration, and poor patients' survival were found (Zhou et al., 2012). In addition, in a murine model of lung cancer determined by K-ras activation and p53 abrogation, TAM and TAN precursors relocated from the spleen to the tumor and splenectomy significantly reduced the infiltration of myeloid cells within the tumor (Cortez-Retamozo et al., 2012). In addition, Angiotensin II was identified as a pivotal factor in the amplification of hematopoietic self-renewal (Cortez-Retamozo et al., 2013).

Various epidemiological evidences described a negative correlation between TANs and patient clinical outcome in metastatic and localized renal cell carcinoma, bronchioloalveolar carcinoma, HCC, colorectal cancer, and head and neck cancer (Donskov, 2013; Jensen et al., 2009; Kuang et al., 2011; Rao et al., 2012; Trellakis, Bruderek, et al., 2011; Wislez et al., 2003). Moreover, higher tumor-infiltrating neutrophil density was associated with higher histological grade in glioma (Fossati et al., 1999) and more aggressive pancreatic cancer (Reid et al., 2011). In contrast, the association between neutrophil infiltration and patients' clinical outcome remains controversial for some tumor types, such as gastric and colorectal cancer (Caruso et al., 2002; Hirt et al., 2013). These controversial evidences may be due to variability in the methods used to identify neutrophils within tumors (e.g., immunohistochemistry, hematoxylin–eosin staining), as well as the choice of patient datasets and outcomes.

5.2 Neutrophils in Tumor Initiation and Progression

The association between neutrophil-derived reactive oxygen species (ROS) and carcinogenesis has been described already 30 years ago (Weitzman, Weitberg, Clark, & Stossel, 1985). Accordingly, neutrophil-derived ROS and related products, such as myeloperoxidase-mediated HOCl, induced genetic instability, an emerging hallmark of cancer, due to DNA point mutations (Gungor et al., 2010; Hanahan & Weinberg, 2011).

Neutrophil-derived granule proteins can also play dual roles in tumor progression. For instance, neutrophil elastase (NE) can favor tumor cell proliferation via the alteration of the platelet-derived growth factor receptor (PDGFR) intracellular signaling and epithelial-to-mesenchymal transition (Grosse-Steffen et al., 2012; Houghton et al., 2010). In contrast, NE can be taken up by cancer cells, leading to alteration of self-antigens and activation of a CTL-mediated antitumor response (Mittendorf et al., 2012).

Neutrophils also produce a number of cytokines, which play important roles in cancer (Tecchio, Scapini, Pizzolo, & Cassatella, 2013). For instance, stimulated neutrophils secrete Oncostatin M, which stimulates cancer cells to produce VEGF, thus enhancing tumor cell invasive behavior (Queen, Ryan, Holzer, Keller-Peck, & Jorcyk, 2005). In addition, neutrophil-derived hepatocyte growth factor (HGF) promoted the invasive behavior of cholangiocellular and hepatocellular cell lines *in vitro* (Imai et al., 2005). In bronchoalveolar carcinoma patients, an association between neutrophil infiltration, poor patients' prognosis, and levels of HGF in bronchoalveolar lavage fluid was described (Wislez et al., 2003). In HNSCC patients, a correlation between tumor-infiltrating neutrophils and the expression of CORTACTIN, a protein involved in cellular migration, was found (Dumitru et al., 2013). Moreover, tumor-infiltrating neutrophils and CORTACTIN were associated with poor patients' outcome (Dumitru et al., 2013). In contrast, neutrophil-derived molecules can also display antitumoral functions. For instance, neutrophils are an important source of TNF-related apoptosis-inducing ligand (TRAIL), which displays antitumoral activities (Cassatella, 2006; Hewish, Lord, Martin, Cunningham, & Ashworth, 2010). Indeed, *Mycobacterium bovis* Bacillus Calmette–Guerin (BCG) induced the release of TRAIL from neutrophils, suggesting a role for neutrophils in mediating the anticancer effects of BCG in bladder cancer (Kemp et al., 2005). Moreover, neutrophil-derived TRAIL promoted apoptosis of leukemic cells in chronic myeloid leukemia patients (Tanaka, Ito, Kyo, & Kimura, 2007; Tecchio et al., 2004). In addition, in lung cancer patients, TANs present an activated phenotype, characterized by high expression levels of proinflammatory mediators (i.e., CCL2, CCL3, CXCL8). These activated TANs efficiently stimulate T-cell proliferation and IFN-γ release through a cell contact-dependent manner (Eruslanov et al., 2014). This cross-talk enhanced the expression of costimulatory molecules in neutrophils, sustaining a positive-feedback loop and supporting an antitumoral role for TANs in early stages of human lung cancers (Eruslanov et al., 2014).

5.3 Neutrophils in Tumor Progression: Angiogenesis and Metastatic Behavior Modulation

Neutrophils play a dual role in modulating angiogenesis and metastatic behavior of tumors. Neutrophils express various angiogenic factors, such as VEGF-A, which is also the main mediator of the CXCL1-induced angiogenic activity (Scapini et al., 2004). In murine models of subcutaneous melanoma and fibrosarcoma, in the absence of IFN-β, TANs acquired proangiogenic features, such as increased expression of CXCR4, VEGF-A, and MMP-9 (Jablonska, Leschner, Westphal, Lienenklaus, & Weiss, 2010). MMP-9 is a well-known proangiogenic factor, inducing the release of the active form of VEGF-A from the ECM (Nozawa, Chiu, & Hanahan, 2006).

Bv8 (also known as prokineticin-2) is known to promote neutrophil mobilization and angiogenesis. In a tumor xenograft model, G-CSF induced the expression of Bv8 in neutrophils and blocking Bv8 impaired neutrophil recruitment, tumor growth, and angiogenesis (Shojaei et al., 2007). Interestingly, tumors resistant to anti-VEGF therapy displayed high neutrophil infiltration, and resistance to anti-VEGF treatment was due to G-CSF-induced Bv8 expression. Indeed, blocking G-CSF or Bv8 impaired tumor growth and angiogenesis (Shojaei, Singh, Thompson, & Ferrara, 2008; Shojaei et al., 2009). In contrast, neutrophils also display antiangiogenic properties. For instance, NE itself degraded VEGF and FGF-2 and *in vitro*-generated angiostatin-like fragments from plasminogen, which suppressed VEGF- and FGF-2-mediated angiogenesis (Ai et al., 2007; Scapini et al., 2002). Neutrophils play many roles in modifying the tumor metastatic behavior. Melanoma-derived CXCL8 increased the expression of β_2-integrin on neutrophils, which engaged ICAM-1 expressed on melanoma cells, thus favoring the interaction between neutrophils and melanoma cells. This dangerous interaction allowed melanoma cells to transit across the endothelium, giving rise to distant metastasis (Huh, Liang, Sharma, Dong, & Robertson, 2010). In addition, neutrophil extracellular traps were able to capture circulating tumor cells and promoted their engraftment to distant organ sites (Cools-Lartigue et al., 2013). In contrast, in an *in vivo* model of breast cancer, under the influence of G-CSF and tumor-derived CCL2, neutrophils accumulated in the premetastatic lung and inhibited metastatic engraftment through the release of H_2O_2. Accordingly, following neutrophil depletion, the metastatic load was significantly enhanced (Granot et al., 2011). Recently, a role for type I IFN signaling in reducing the metastatic load has been described. More in detail, in a model of breast cancer, *Ifnar1*-deficient mice displayed an increased metastatic load together with increased neutrophil infiltration in the premetastatic lung, compared to the wild-type mice. *Ifnar1*$^{-/-}$ neutrophils displayed altered killing activity and increased CXCR2 expression, responsible for their homing in the premetastatic lungs (Wu et al., 2015).

5.4 Neutrophil Plasticity and Heterogeneity in Cancer

In contrast with the classical point of view, neutrophils appear as cells endowed with unsuspected plasticity. In murine models of mesothelioma and lung cancer, neutrophils acquired a protumoral phenotype under the influence of TGF-β (Fridlender et al., 2009). Accordingly, neutrophils recruited in TGF-β-blocking conditions displayed increased antitumor cytotoxic activity, high expression of TNF-α, CCL3, and ICAM-1, and low levels of arginase-1, a well-known T-cell inhibitory factor. TGF-β neutralization also enhanced a T-cell mediated antitumor response, in which neutrophils played a role as effector cells (Fridlender et al., 2009). In contrast, type I interferon signaling has been involved in the acquisition of an antitumoral phenotype in neutrophils. Therefore, in mice lacking type I IFN signals, neutrophils displayed proangiogenic and prometastatic features (Jablonska et al., 2010; Wu et al., 2015). Thus, similarly to the Th1–Th2 and M1–M2 paradigms, a new paradigm has been proposed in which neutrophils can be polarized toward an antitumor N1 or a protumor N2 phenotype in response to signals derived from the microenvironment.

5.5 Neutrophils, TANs, and MDSCs

During cancer development, a heterogeneous population of myeloid cells appears in peripheral blood of tumor-bearing mice and cancer patients. These cells, namely MDSCs, display immunosuppressive and cancer-promoting properties and are divided into monocytic (Mo-MDSCs) and granulocytic (G-MDSCs) cells, on the basis of distinct morphological and phenotypical aspects (Youn & Gabrilovich, 2010).

The distinction between G-MDSCs and TANs is not so clear. Indeed, neutrophils and G-MDSCs display the same membrane markers (CD11b, Gr1, and Ly6G), similar morphology, and immunosuppressive properties via arginase-1 production (Gabrilovich, Ostrand-Rosenberg, & Bronte, 2012). Accordingly and recently, in a murine model of breast cancer, atypical $CD11b^{+}Ly6G^{+}Rb1^{low}$ neutrophils appeared during tumor progression in peripheral tissues, but not in the primary tumors. This neutrophil subpopulation suppressed T-cell-mediated immune response through the production of ROS. Hematopoietic stem cell differentiation toward the myeloid lineage in bone marrow was found to be driven by tumor-derived G-CSF (Casbon et al., 2015).

In patients with renal cancer, a subset of activated neutrophils in peripheral blood was identified, able to induce T-cell immunosuppression through the production of arginase-1 (Rodriguez et al., 2009; Schmielau & Finn, 2001). Therefore, in this view, these activated neutrophils were considered as G-MDSCs due to their immunosuppressive phenotype. In contrast, MDSCs have been also referred as immature neutrophils (Solito et al., 2011; Trellakis, Farjah, et al., 2011). Indeed, in a genetic conditional lung adenocarcinoma model, TAN precursors physically relocated from spleen to tumors and, since MDSCs accumulated in the spleen of tumor-bearing animals, TAN activities were at least in part attributed to MDSCs (Cortez-Retamozo et al., 2012). Accordingly, G-MDSCs acquired phenotypical and functional aspects of neutrophils, under the influence of GM-CSF, supporting the theory by which G-MDSCs are immature neutrophils (Youn, Collazo, Shalova, Biswas, & Gabrilovich, 2012). Immature neutrophilic MDSCs have also been described in peripheral blood of cancer patients and correlated with poor clinical outcome (Trellakis, Farjah, et al., 2011).

In contrast with these evidences, Fridlender and colleagues performed a transcriptomic analysis on peripheral neutrophils, TANs, and G-MDSCs in tumor-bearing mice, and found that TANs and G-MDSCs are distinct populations of cells and that naïve neutrophils and G-MDSCs are more closely related to each other than to TANs (Fridlender et al., 2012). Accordingly and quite recently, a heterogeneous population of low-density neutrophils (LDNs) has been identified in peripheral blood of tumor-bearing mice and cancer patients (Sagiv et al., 2015). Compared to mature high-density neutrophils (HDNs), LDNs displayed reduced chemotactic activity, phagocytosis, and oxidative burst as well as lower expression of chemokines (i.e., CXCL1, CXCL2, CXCL10) and chemokine receptors (i.e., CXCR2). From the functional point of view, LDNs impaired $CD8^+$ T-cell proliferation. Thus, in contrast to HDNs, LDNs displayed protumoral activities, which were mainly driven by TGF-β. In addition, within LDNs, two populations of neutrophils were identified, which displayed similar immunosuppressive properties, but different maturation stages. Thus, finally, three distinct populations of neutrophils can be distinguished. The first one consists of HDNs, previously referred as N1 neutrophils, which displayed a mature phenotype together with cytotoxic and antitumor activities. The second and third populations are found within LDNs and consist of immature cells, previously described as G-MDSCs and mature cells, previously described as N2 neutrophils, both sharing immunosuppressive and tumor-promoting functions (Sagiv et al., 2015). Therefore, this increasing body of evidence emphasizes the high versatility of neutrophils in different pathophysiological settings and paves the way for new therapeutic approaches based on their multifaceted biological aspects.

6. CONCLUDING REMARKS

Cells of the myelomonocytic lineage have emerged as a key feature of cancer-related inflammation. They are important players both in the extrinsic pathway connecting inflammation and cancer, consisting of inflammatory conditions which predispose to cancerogenesis, and of the oncogene-driven tumorigenesis process. Macrophage and neutrophils are a major source of humoral fluid-phase pattern recognition molecules such as the long pentraxin PTX3, and their recruitment and function is regulated by the humoral arm of innate immunity. Recent work has highlighted (Bonavita et al., 2015) that Complement and its regulation by PTX3 are an important component of the inflammatory microenvironment and that PTX3 acts as a *bona fide* cancer suppressor gene in mouse and human tumors. There is evidence that targeting TAMs has antitumor activity in human cancer and these preclinical and clinical results are likely to pave the way to innovative therapeutic strategies.

ACKNOWLEDGMENT

Supported by Associazione Italiana per la Ricerca sul Cancro and Italian Ministry of Health.

REFERENCES

Ai, S., Cheng, X. W., Inoue, A., Nakamura, K., Okumura, K., Iguchi, A., et al. (2007). Angiogenic activity of bFGF and VEGF suppressed by proteolytic cleavage by neutrophil elastase. *Biochemical and Biophysical Research Communications, 364*, 395–401.

Ajona, D., Pajares, M. J., Corrales, L., Perez-Gracia, J. L., Agorreta, J., Lozano, M. D., et al. (2013). Investigation of complement activation product C4d as a diagnostic and prognostic biomarker for lung cancer. *Journal of the National Cancer Institute, 105*, 1385–1393.

Ajona, D., Razquin, C., Pastor, M. D., Pajares, M. J., Garcia, J., Cardenal, F., et al. (2015). Elevated levels of the complement activation product C4d in bronchial fluids for the diagnosis of lung cancer. *PloS One, 10*, e0119878.

Allavena, P., & Mantovani, A. (2012). Immunology in the clinic review series; focus on cancer: Tumour-associated macrophages: Undisputed stars of the inflammatory tumour microenvironment. *Clinical and Experimental Immunology, 167*, 195–205.

Asgari, E., Le Friec, G., Yamamoto, H., Perucha, E., Sacks, S. S., Köhl, J., et al. (2013). C3a modulates IL-1β secretion in human monocytes by regulating ATP efflux and subsequent NLRP3 inflammasome activation. *Blood, 122*, 3473–3481.

Avraham-Davidi, I., Yona, S., Grunewald, M., Landsman, L., Cochain, C., Silvestre, J. S., et al. (2013). On-site education of VEGF-recruited monocytes improves their performance as angiogenic and arteriogenic accessory cells. *The Journal of Experimental Medicine, 210*, 2611–2625.

Bain, C. C., Bravo-Blas, A., Scott, C. L., Gomez Perdiguero, E., Geissmann, F., Henri, S., et al. (2014). *Nature Immunology, 15*, 929–937.

Balkwill, F. (2004). Cancer and the chemokine network. *Nature Reviews. Cancer, 4*, 540–550.

Balkwill, F., & Mantovani, A. (2001). Inflammation and cancer: Back to Virchow? *Lancet, 357*, 539–545.

Bandini, S., Curcio, C., Macagno, M., Quaglino, E., Arigoni, M., Lanzardo, S., et al. (2013). Early onset and enhanced growth of autochthonous mammary carcinomas in C3-deficient Her2/neu transgenic mice. *Oncoimmunology, 2*, e26137.

Beatty, G. L., Chiorean, E. G., Fishman, M. P., Saboury, B., Teitelbaum, U. R., Sun, W., et al. (2011). CD40 agonists alter tumor stroma and show efficacy against pancreatic carcinoma in mice and humans. *Science, 331*, 1612–1616.

Bellone, S., Roque, D., Cocco, E., Gasparrini, S., Bortolomai, I., Buza, N., et al. (2012). Downregulation of membrane complement inhibitors CD55 and CD59 by siRNA sensitises uterine serous carcinoma overexpressing Her2/neu to complement and antibody-dependent cell cytotoxicity in vitro: Implications for trastuzumab-based immunotherapy. *British Journal of Cancer, 106*, 1543–1550.

Bierie, B., & Moses, H. L. (2010). Transforming growth factor beta (TGF-beta) and inflammation in cancer. *Cytokine & Growth Factor Reviews, 21*, 49–59.

Biswas, S. K., Gangi, L., Paul, S., Schioppa, T., Saccani, A., Sironi, M., et al. (2006). A distinct and unique transcriptional program expressed by tumor-associated macrophages (defective NF-kappaB and enhanced IRF-3/STAT1 activation). *Blood, 107*, 2112–2122.

Biswas, S. K., & Mantovani, A. (2010). Macrophage plasticity and interaction with lymphocyte subsets: Cancer as a paradigm. *Nature Immunology, 11*, 889–896.

Bjorge, L., Hakulinen, J., Vintermyr, O. K., Jarva, H., Jensen, T. S., Iversen, O. E., et al. (2005). Ascitic complement system in ovarian cancer. *British Journal of Cancer, 92*, 895–905.

Bohlson, S. S., O'Conner, S. D., Hulsebus, H. J., Ho, M.-M., & Fraser, D. A. (2014). Complement, C1q, and C1q-related molecules regulate macrophage polarization. *Frontiers in Immunology, 5*, 402.

Bohrer, L. R., & Schwertfeger, K. L. (2012). Macrophages promote fibroblast growth factor receptor-driven tumor cell migration and invasion in a CXCR2-dependent manner. *Molecular Cancer Research: MCR, 10*, 1294–1305.

Bonavita, E., Gentile, S., Rubino, M., Maina, V., Papait, R., Kunderfranco, P., et al. (2015). PTX3 is an extrinsic oncosuppressor regulating complement-dependent inflammation in cancer. *Cell*, *160*, 700–714.

Bottazzi, B., Erba, E., Nobili, N., Fazioli, F., Rambaldi, A., & Mantovani, A. (1990). A paracrine circuit in the regulation of the proliferation of macrophages infiltrating murine sarcomas. *Journal of Immunology*, *144*, 2409–2412.

Bottazzi, B., Polentarutti, N., Acero, R., Balsari, A., Boraschi, D., Ghezzi, P., et al. (1983). Regulation of the macrophage content of neoplasms by chemoattractants. *Science*, *220*, 210–212.

Bottazzi, B., Vouret-Craviari, V., Bastone, A., De Gioia, L., Matteucci, C., Peri, G., et al. (1997). Multimer formation and ligand recognition by the long pentraxin PTX3. Similarities and differences with the short pentraxins C-reactive protein and serum amyloid P component. *The Journal of Biological Chemistry*, *272*, 32817–32823.

Braunschweig, A., & Jozsi, M. (2011). Human pentraxin 3 binds to the complement regulator c4b-binding protein. *PloS One*, *6*, e23991.

Bronte, V., & Zanovello, P. (2005). Regulation of immune responses by L-arginine metabolism. *Nature Reviews. Immunology*, *5*, 641–654.

Bu, X., Zheng, Z., Wang, C., & Yu, Y. (2007). Significance of C4d deposition in the follicular lymphoma and MALT lymphoma and their relationship with follicular dendritic cells. *Pathology, Research and Practice*, *203*, 163–167.

Camus, M., Tosolini, M., Mlecnik, B., Pages, F., Kirilovsky, A., Berger, A., et al. (2009). Coordination of intratumoral immune reaction and human colorectal cancer recurrence. *Cancer Research*, *69*, 2685–2693.

Caruso, R. A., Bellocco, R., Pagano, M., Bertoli, G., Rigoli, L., & Inferrera, C. (2002). Prognostic value of intratumoral neutrophils in advanced gastric carcinoma in a high-risk area in northern Italy. *Modern Pathology: An Official Journal of the United States and Canadian Academy of Pathology, Inc*, *15*, 831–837.

Casazza, A., Laoui, D., Wenes, M., Rizzolio, S., Bassani, N., Mambretti, M., et al. (2013). Impeding macrophage entry into hypoxic tumor areas by Sema3A/Nrp1 signaling blockade inhibits angiogenesis and restores antitumor immunity. *Cancer Cell*, *24*, 695–709.

Casbon, A. J., Reynaud, D., Park, C., Khuc, E., Gan, D. D., Schepers, K., et al. (2015). Invasive breast cancer reprograms early myeloid differentiation in the bone marrow to generate immunosuppressive neutrophils. *Proceedings of the National Academy of Sciences of the United States of America*, *112*, E566–E575.

Cassatella, M. A. (2006). On the production of TNF-related apoptosis-inducing ligand (TRAIL/Apo-2L) by human neutrophils. *Journal of Leukocyte Biology*, *79*, 1140–1149.

Chang, C. I., Liao, J. C., & Kuo, L. (2001). Macrophage arginase promotes tumor cell growth and suppresses nitric oxide-mediated tumor cytotoxicity. *Cancer Research*, *61*, 1100–1106.

Chen, C., Qu, Q. X., Shen, Y., Mu, C. Y., Zhu, Y. B., Zhang, X. G., et al. (2012). Induced expression of B7-H4 on the surface of lung cancer cell by the tumor-associated macrophages: A potential mechanism of immune escape. *Cancer Letters*, *317*, 99–105.

Chen, C., Shen, Y., Qu, Q. X., Chen, X. Q., Zhang, X. G., & Huang, J. A. (2013). Induced expression of B7-H3 on the lung cancer cells and macrophages suppresses T-cell mediating anti-tumor immune response. *Experimental Cell Research*, *319*, 96–102.

Christofori, G. (2006). New signals from the invasive front. *Nature*, *441*, 444–450.

Colegio, O. R., Chu, N. Q., Szabo, A. L., Chu, T., Rhebergen, A. M., Jairam, V., et al. (2014). Functional polarization of tumour-associated macrophages by tumour-derived lactic acid. *Nature*, *513*, 559–563.

Cools-Lartigue, J., Spicer, J., McDonald, B., Gowing, S., Chow, S., Giannias, B., et al. (2013). Neutrophil extracellular traps sequester circulating tumor cells and promote metastasis. *The Journal of Clinical Investigation, 123*, 3446–3458.

Cortez-Retamozo, V., Etzrodt, M., Newton, A., Rauch, P. J., Chudnovskiy, A., Berger, C., et al. (2012). Origins of tumor-associated macrophages and neutrophils. *Proceedings of the National Academy of Sciences of the United States of America, 109*, 2491–2496.

Cortez-Retamozo, V., Etzrodt, M., Newton, A., Ryan, R., Pucci, F., Sio, S. W., et al. (2013). Angiotensin II drives the production of tumor-promoting macrophages. *Immunity, 38*, 296–308.

Coussens, L. M., Zitvogel, L., & Palucka, A. K. (2013). Neutralizing tumor-promoting chronic inflammation: A magic bullet? *Science, 339*, 286–291.

De Palma, M., & Lewis, C. E. (2013). Macrophage regulation of tumor responses to anticancer therapies. *Cancer Cell, 23*, 277–286.

de Visser, K. E., Korets, L. V., & Coussens, L. M. (2004). Early neoplastic progression is complement independent. *Neoplasia, 6*, 768–776.

Deban, L., Jarva, H., Lehtinen, M. J., Bottazzi, B., Bastone, A., Doni, A., et al. (2008). Binding of the long pentraxin PTX3 to factor H: Interacting domains and function in the regulation of complement activation. *Journal of Immunology, 181*, 8433–8440.

De Kleer, I., Willems, F., Lambrecht, B., & Goriely, S. (2014). *Frontiers in Immunology, 5*, 423.

DeNardo, D. G., Barreto, J. B., Andreu, P., Vasquez, L., Tawfik, D., Kolhatkar, N., et al. (2009). CD4(+) T cells regulate pulmonary metastasis of mammary carcinomas by enhancing protumor properties of macrophages. *Cancer Cell, 16*, 91–102.

Doedens, A. L., Stockmann, C., Rubinstein, M. P., Liao, D., Zhang, N., DeNardo, D. G., et al. (2010). Macrophage expression of hypoxia-inducible factor-1 alpha suppresses T-cell function and promotes tumor progression. *Cancer Research, 70*, 7465–7475.

Doni, A., Garlanda, C., Bottazzi, B., Meri, S., Garred, P., & Mantovani, A. (2012). Interactions of the humoral pattern recognition molecule PTX3 with the complement system. *Immunobiology, 217*, 1122–1128.

Donskov, F. (2013). Immunomonitoring and prognostic relevance of neutrophils in clinical trials. *Seminars in Cancer Biology, 23*, 200–207.

Duluc, D., Corvaisier, M., Blanchard, S., Catala, L., Descamps, P., Gamelin, E., et al. (2009). Interferon-gamma reverses the immunosuppressive and protumoral properties and prevents the generation of human tumor-associated macrophages. *International Journal of Cancer. Journal International du Cancer, 125*, 367–373.

Dumitru, C. A., Bankfalvi, A., Gu, X., Eberhardt, W. E., Zeidler, R., Lang, S., et al. (2013). Neutrophils activate tumoral CORTACTIN to enhance progression of orohypopharynx carcinoma. *Frontiers in Immunology, 4*, 33.

Dumitru, C. A., Gholaman, H., Trellakis, S., Bruderek, K., Dominas, N., Gu, X., et al. (2011). Tumor-derived macrophage migration inhibitory factor modulates the biology of head and neck cancer cells via neutrophil activation. *International Journal of Cancer Journal International du Cancer, 129*, 859–869.

Ebrahem, Q., Chaurasia, S. S., Vasanji, A., Qi, J. H., Klenotic, P. A., Cutler, A., et al. (2010). Cross-talk between vascular endothelial growth factor and matrix metalloproteinases in the induction of neovascularization in vivo. *The American Journal of Pathology, 176*, 496–503.

Edwards, J. P., & Emens, L. A. (2010). The multikinase inhibitor sorafenib reverses the suppression of IL-12 and enhancement of IL-10 by PGE(2) in murine macrophages. *International Immunopharmacology, 10*, 1220–1228.

Eruslanov, E. B., Bhojnagarwala, P. S., Quatromoni, J. G., Stephen, T. L., Ranganathan, A., Deshpande, C., et al. (2014). Tumor-associated neutrophils stimulate T cell responses in early-stage human lung cancer. *The Journal of Clinical Investigation, 124*, 5466–5480.

Fang, C., Zhang, X., Miwa, T., & Song, W.-C. (2009). Complement promotes the development of inflammatory T-helper 17 cells through synergistic interaction with Toll-like receptor signaling and interleukin-6 production. *Blood*, *114*, 1005–1015.
Fossati, G., Ricevuti, G., Edwards, S. W., Walker, C., Dalton, A., & Rossi, M. L. (1999). Neutrophil infiltration into human gliomas. *Acta Neuropathologica*, *98*, 349–354.
Franklin, R. A., Liao, W., Sarkar, A., Kim, M. V., Bivona, M. R., Liu, K., et al. (2014). The cellular and molecular origin of tumor-associated macrophages. *Science*, *344*, 921–925.
Fridlender, Z. G., Sun, J., Kim, S., Kapoor, V., Cheng, G., Ling, L., et al. (2009). Polarization of tumor-associated neutrophil phenotype by TGF-beta: "N1" versus "N2" TAN. *Cancer Cell*, *16*, 183–194.
Fridlender, Z. G., Sun, J., Mishalian, I., Singhal, S., Cheng, G., Kapoor, V., et al. (2012). Transcriptomic analysis comparing tumor-associated neutrophils with granulocytic myeloid-derived suppressor cells and normal neutrophils. *PloS One*, 7, e31524.
Gabrilovich, D. I., Ostrand-Rosenberg, S., & Bronte, V. (2012). Coordinated regulation of myeloid cells by tumours. *Nature Reviews. Immunology*, *12*, 253–268.
Galon, J., Costes, A., Sanchez-Cabo, F., Kirilovsky, A., Mlecnik, B., Lagorce-Pages, C., et al. (2006). Type, density, and location of immune cells within human colorectal tumors predict clinical outcome. *Science*, *313*, 1960–1964.
Gelderman, K. A., Tomlinson, S., Ross, G. D., & Gorter, A. (2004). Complement function in mAb-mediated cancer immunotherapy. *Trends in Immunology*, *25*, 158–164.
Germano, G., Frapolli, R., Belgiovine, C., Anselmo, A., Pesce, S., Liguori, M., et al. (2013). Role of macrophage targeting in the anti-tumor activity of Trabectedin. *Cancer Cell*, *23*, 249–262.
Gironella, M., Calvo, C., Fernandez, A., Closa, D., Iovanna, J. L., Rosello-Catafau, J., et al. (2013). Reg3beta deficiency impairs pancreatic tumor growth by skewing macrophage polarization. *Cancer Research*, *73*, 5682–5694.
Gocheva, V., Wang, H. W., Gadea, B. B., Shree, T., Hunter, K. E., Garfall, A. L., et al. (2010). IL-4 induces cathepsin protease activity in tumor-associated macrophages to promote cancer growth and invasion. *Genes & Development*, *24*, 241–255.
Gomez Perdiguero, E., Klapproth, K., Schulz, C., Busch, K., Azzoni, E., Crozet, L., et al. (2015). *Nature*, *518*, 547–551.
Gorelik, E., Wiltrout, R. H., Brunda, M. J., Holden, H. T., & Herberman, R. B. (1982). Augmentation of metastasis formation by thioglycollate-elicited macrophages. *International Journal of Cancer. Journal International du Cancer*, *29*, 575–581.
Gout, E., Moriscot, C., Doni, A., Dumestre-Perard, C., Lacroix, M., Perard, J., et al. (2011). M-ficolin interacts with the long pentraxin PTX3: A novel case of cross-talk between soluble pattern-recognition molecules. *Journal of Immunology*, *186*, 5815–5822.
Granata, F., Frattini, A., Loffredo, S., Staiano, R. I., Petraroli, A., Ribatti, D., et al. (2010). Production of vascular endothelial growth factors from human lung macrophages induced by group IIA and group X secreted phospholipases A2. *Journal of Immunology*, *184*, 5232–5241.
Granot, Z., Henke, E., Comen, E. A., King, T. A., Norton, L., & Benezra, R. (2011). Tumor entrained neutrophils inhibit seeding in the premetastatic lung. *Cancer Cell*, *20*, 300–314.
Grenz, S., Naschberger, E., Merkel, S., Britzen-Laurent, N., Schaal, U., Konrad, A., et al. (2013). IFN-gamma-driven intratumoral microenvironment exhibits superior prognostic effect compared with an IFN-alpha-driven microenvironment in patients with colon carcinoma. *The American Journal of Pathology*, *183*, 1897–1909.
Grosse-Steffen, T., Giese, T., Giese, N., Longerich, T., Schirmacher, P., Hansch, G. M., et al. (2012). Epithelial-to-mesenchymal transition in pancreatic ductal adenocarcinoma

and pancreatic tumor cell lines: The role of neutrophils and neutrophil-derived elastase. *Clinical & Developmental Immunology*, *2012*, 720768.

Gungor, N., Knaapen, A. M., Munnia, A., Peluso, M., Haenen, G. R., Chiu, R. K., et al. (2010). Genotoxic effects of neutrophils and hypochlorous acid. *Mutagenesis*, *25*, 149–154.

Hagemann, T., Wilson, J., Burke, F., Kulbe, H., Li, N. F., Pluddemann, A., et al. (2006). Ovarian cancer cells polarize macrophages toward a tumor-associated phenotype. *Journal of Immunology*, *176*, 5023–5032.

Hanahan, D., & Weinberg, R. A. (2011). Hallmarks of cancer: The next generation. *Cell*, *144*, 646–674.

Hewish, M., Lord, C. J., Martin, S. A., Cunningham, D., & Ashworth, A. (2010). Mismatch repair deficient colorectal cancer in the era of personalized treatment. *Nature Reviews. Clinical Oncology*, *7*, 197–208.

Hirt, C., Eppenberger-Castori, S., Sconocchia, G., Iezzi, G., Tornillo, L., Terracciano, L., et al. (2013). Colorectal carcinoma infiltration by myeloperoxidase-expressing neutrophil granulocytes is associated with favorable prognosis. *Oncoimmunology*, *2*, e25990.

Hörl, S., Bánki, Z., Huber, G., Ejaz, A., Windisch, D., Muellauer, B., et al. (2013). Reduction of complement factor H binding to CLL cells improves the induction of rituximab-mediated complement-dependent cytotoxicity. *Leukemia*, *27*, 2200–2208.

Hotchkiss, K. A., Ashton, A. W., Klein, R. S., Lenzi, M. L., Zhu, G. H., & Schwartz, E. L. (2003). Mechanisms by which tumor cells and monocytes expressing the angiogenic factor thymidine phosphorylase mediate human endothelial cell migration. *Cancer Research*, *63*, 527–533.

Houghton, A. M., Rzymkiewicz, D. M., Ji, H., Gregory, A. D., Egea, E. E., Metz, H. E., et al. (2010). Neutrophil elastase-mediated degradation of IRS-1 accelerates lung tumor growth. *Nature Medicine*, *16*, 219–223.

Huang, S., Van Arsdall, M., Tedjarati, S., McCarty, M., Wu, W., Langley, R., et al. (2002). Contributions of stromal metalloproteinase-9 to angiogenesis and growth of human ovarian carcinoma in mice. *Journal of the National Cancer Institute*, *94*, 1134–1142.

Huh, S. J., Liang, S., Sharma, A., Dong, C., & Robertson, G. P. (2010). Transiently entrapped circulating tumor cells interact with neutrophils to facilitate lung metastasis development. *Cancer Research*, *70*, 6071–6082.

Ijichi, H., Chytil, A., Gorska, A. E., Aakre, M. E., Bierie, B., Tada, M., et al. (2011). Inhibiting Cxcr2 disrupts tumor-stromal interactions and improves survival in a mouse model of pancreatic ductal adenocarcinoma. *The Journal of Clinical Investigation*, *121*, 4106–4117.

Imai, Y., Kubota, Y., Yamamoto, S., Tsuji, K., Shimatani, M., Shibatani, N., et al. (2005). Neutrophils enhance invasion activity of human cholangiocellular carcinoma and hepatocellular carcinoma cells: An in vitro study. *Journal of Gastroenterology and Hepatology*, *20*, 287–293.

Inforzato, A., Doni, A., Barajon, I., Leone, R., Garlanda, C., Bottazzi, B., et al. (2013). PTX3 as a paradigm for the interaction of pentraxins with the complement system. *Seminars in Immunology*, *25*, 79–85.

Jablonska, J., Leschner, S., Westphal, K., Lienenklaus, S., & Weiss, S. (2010). Neutrophils responsive to endogenous IFN-beta regulate tumor angiogenesis and growth in a mouse tumor model. *The Journal of Clinical Investigation*, *120*, 1151–1164.

Jamieson, T., Clarke, M., Steele, C. W., Samuel, M. S., Neumann, J., Jung, A., et al. (2012). Inhibition of CXCR2 profoundly suppresses inflammation-driven and spontaneous tumorigenesis. *The Journal of Clinical Investigation*, *122*, 3127–3144.

Jensen, H. K., Donskov, F., Marcussen, N., Nordsmark, M., Lundbeck, F., & von der Maase, H. (2009). Presence of intratumoral neutrophils is an independent prognostic factor in localized renal cell carcinoma. *Journal of Clinical Oncology: Official Journal of the American Society of Clinical Oncology, 27*, 4709–4717.

Jin, G., Kawsar, H. I., Hirsch, S. A., Zeng, C., Jia, X., Feng, Z., et al. (2010). An antimicrobial peptide regulates tumor-associated macrophage trafficking via the chemokine receptor CCR2, a model for tumorigenesis. *PloS One, 5*, e10993.

Joyce, J. A., & Pollard, J. W. (2009). Microenvironmental regulation of metastasis. *Nature Reviews. Cancer, 9*, 239–252.

Kadoch, C., Li, J., Wong, V. S., Chen, L., Cha, S., Munster, P., et al. (2014). Complement activation and intraventricular rituximab distribution in recurrent central nervous system lymphoma. *Clinical Cancer Research: An Official Journal of the American Association for Cancer Research, 20*, 1029–1041.

Katara, G. K., Jaiswal, M. K., Kulshrestha, A., Kolli, B., Gilman-Sachs, A., & Beaman, K. D. (2014). Tumor-associated vacuolar ATPase subunit promotes tumorigenic characteristics in macrophages. *Oncogene, 33*, 5649–5654.

Keane, M. P., Belperio, J. A., Xue, Y. Y., Burdick, M. D., & Strieter, R. M. (2004). Depletion of CXCR2 inhibits tumor growth and angiogenesis in a murine model of lung cancer. *Journal of Immunology, 172*, 2853–2860.

Keeley, E. C., Mehrad, B., & Strieter, R. M. (2010). CXC chemokines in cancer angiogenesis and metastases. *Advances in Cancer Research, 106*, 91–111.

Kemp, T. J., Ludwig, A. T., Earel, J. K., Moore, J. M., Vanoosten, R. L., Moses, B., et al. (2005). Neutrophil stimulation with Mycobacterium bovis bacillus Calmette-Guerin (BCG) results in the release of functional soluble TRAIL/Apo-2L. *Blood, 106*, 3474–3482.

Kryczek, I., Zou, L., Rodriguez, P., Zhu, G., Wei, S., Mottram, P., et al. (2006). B7-H4 expression identifies a novel suppressive macrophage population in human ovarian carcinoma. *The Journal of Experimental Medicine, 203*, 871–881.

Kuang, D. M., Zhao, Q., Peng, C., Xu, J., Zhang, J. P., Wu, C., et al. (2009). Activated monocytes in peritumoral stroma of hepatocellular carcinoma foster immune privilege and disease progression through PD-L1. *The Journal of Experimental Medicine, 206*, 1327–1337.

Kuang, D. M., Zhao, Q., Wu, Y., Peng, C., Wang, J., Xu, Z., et al. (2011). Peritumoral neutrophils link inflammatory response to disease progression by fostering angiogenesis in hepatocellular carcinoma. *Journal of Hepatology, 54*, 948–955.

Laoui, D., Van Overmeire, E., Di Conza, G., Aldeni, C., Keirsse, J., Morias, Y., et al. (2014). Tumor hypoxia does not drive differentiation of tumor-associated macrophages but rather fine-tunes the M2-like macrophage population. *Cancer Research, 74*, 24–30.

Lazennec, G., & Richmond, A. (2010). Chemokines and chemokine receptors: New insights into cancer-related inflammation. *Trends in Molecular Medicine, 16*, 133–144.

Li, D., Wang, X., Wu, J. L., Quan, W. Q., Ma, L., Yang, F., et al. (2013). Tumor-produced versican V1 enhances hCAP18/LL-37 expression in macrophages through activation of TLR2 and vitamin D3 signaling to promote ovarian cancer progression in vitro. *PloS One, 8*, e56616.

Lin, E. Y., Gouon-Evans, V., Nguyen, A. V., & Pollard, J. W. (2002). The macrophage growth factor CSF-1 in mammary gland development and tumor progression. *Journal of Mammary Gland Biology and Neoplasia, 7*, 147–162.

Lin, J. Y., Li, X. Y., Tadashi, N., & Dong, P. (2011). Clinical significance of tumor-associated macrophage infiltration in supraglottic laryngeal carcinoma. *Chinese Journal of Cancer, 30*, 280–286.

Linde, N., Lederle, W., Depner, S., van Rooijen, N., Gutschalk, C. M., & Mueller, M. M. (2012). Vascular endothelial growth factor-induced skin carcinogenesis depends on recruitment and alternative activation of macrophages. *The Journal of Pathology, 227*, 17–28.

Ma, Y. J., Doni, A., Romani, L., Jurgensen, H. J., Behrendt, N., Mantovani, A., et al. (2013). Ficolin-1-PTX3 complex formation promotes clearance of altered self-cells and modulates IL-8 production. *Journal of Immunology*, *191*, 1324–1333.

Mantovani, A. (2009). The yin-yang of tumor-associated neutrophils. *Cancer Cell*, *16*, 173–174.

Mantovani, A., & Allavena, P. (2015). The interaction of anticancer therapies with tumor-associated macrophages. *The Journal of Experimental Medicine*, *212*, 435–445. http://dx.doi.org/10.1084/jem.20150295.

Mantovani, A., Allavena, P., Sica, A., & Balkwill, F. (2008). Cancer-related inflammation. *Nature*, *454*, 436–444.

Mantovani, A., Allavena, P., Sozzani, S., Vecchi, A., Locati, M., & Sica, A. (2004). Chemokines in the recruitment and shaping of the leukocyte infiltrate of tumors. *Seminars in Cancer Biology*, *14*, 155–160.

Mantovani, A., Bottazzi, B., Colotta, F., Sozzani, S., & Ruco, L. (1992). The origin and function of tumor-associated macrophages. *Immunology Today*, *13*, 265–270.

Mantovani, A., Cassatella, M. A., Costantini, C., & Jaillon, S. (2011). Neutrophils in the activation and regulation of innate and adaptive immunity. *Nature Reviews. Immunology*, *11*, 519–531.

Mantovani, A., & Sica, A. (2010). Macrophages, innate immunity and cancer: Balance, tolerance, and diversity. *Current Opinion in Immunology*, *22*, 231–237.

Mantovani, A., Sozzani, S., Locati, M., Allavena, P., & Sica, A. (2002). Macrophage polarization: Tumor-associated macrophages as a paradigm for polarized M2 mononuclear phagocytes. *Trends in Immunology*, *23*, 549–555.

Markiewski, M. M., DeAngelis, R. A., Benencia, F., Ricklin-Lichtsteiner, S. K., Koutoulaki, A., Gerard, C., et al. (2008). Modulation of the antitumor immune response by complement. *Nature Immunology*, *9*, 1225–1235.

Matsui, A., Yokoo, H., Negishi, Y., Endo-Takahashi, Y., Chun, N. A., Kadouchi, I., et al. (2012). CXCL17 expression by tumor cells recruits CD11b+Gr1 high F4/80-cells and promotes tumor progression. *PloS One*, *7*, e44080.

McGovern, N., Schlitzer, A., Gunawan, M., Jardine, L., Shin, A., Poyner, E.,V., et al. (2014). *Immunity*, *41*, 465–477.

Middleton, O., Cosimo, E., Dobbin, E., McCaig, A. M., Clarke, C., Brant, A. M., et al. (2015). Complement deficiencies limit CD20 monoclonal antibody treatment efficacy in CLL. *Leukemia*, *29*, 107–114.

Mittendorf, E. A., Alatrash, G., Qiao, N., Wu, Y., Sukhumalchandra, P., St John, L. S., et al. (2012). Breast cancer cell uptake of the inflammatory mediator neutrophil elastase triggers an anticancer adaptive immune response. *Cancer Research*, *72*, 3153–3162.

Molawi, K., Wolf, Y., Kandalla, P. K., Favret, J., Hagemeyer, N., Frenzel, K., et al. (2014). *The Journal of Experimental Medicine*, *211*, 2151–2158.

Mosser, D. M., & Edwards, J. P. (2008). Exploring the full spectrum of macrophage activation. *Nature Reviews Immunology*, *8*, 958–969.

Movahedi, K., Laoui, D., Gysemans, C., Baeten, M., Stange, G., Van den Bossche, J., et al. (2010). Different tumor microenvironments contain functionally distinct subsets of macrophages derived from Ly6C(high) monocytes. *Cancer Research*, *70*, 5728–5739.

Murdoch, C., Giannoudis, A., & Lewis, C. E. (2004). Mechanisms regulating the recruitment of macrophages into hypoxic areas of tumors and other ischemic tissues. *Blood*, *104*, 2224–2234.

Murray, P. J., Allen, J. E., Biswas, S. K., Fisher, E. A., Gilroy, D. W., Goerdt, S., et al. (2014). Macrophage activation and polarization: Nomenclature and experimental guidelines. *Immunity*, *41*, 14–20.

Nagakawa, Y., Aoki, T., Kasuya, K., Tsuchida, A., & Koyanagi, Y. (2002). Histologic features of venous invasion, expression of vascular endothelial growth factor and matrix metalloproteinase-2 and matrix metalloproteinase-9, and the relation with liver metastasis in pancreatic cancer. *Pancreas*, *24*, 169–178.

Naschberger, E., Croner, R. S., Merkel, S., Dimmler, A., Tripal, P., Amann, K. U., et al. (2008). Angiostatic immune reaction in colorectal carcinoma: Impact on survival and perspectives for antiangiogenic therapy. *International Journal of Cancer. Journal International du Cancer*, *123*, 2120–2129.

Neyen, C., Pluddemann, A., Mukhopadhyay, S., Maniati, E., Bossard, M., Gordon, S., et al. (2013). Macrophage scavenger receptor a promotes tumor progression in murine models of ovarian and pancreatic cancer. *Journal of Immunology*, *190*, 3798–3805.

Ning, C., Li, Y. Y., Wang, Y., Han, G. C., Wang, R. X., Xiao, H., et al. (2015). Complement activation promotes colitis-associated carcinogenesis through activating intestinal IL-1β/IL-17A axis. *Mucosal Immunology*. http://dx.doi.org/10.1038/mi.2015.18, 2015 March 4.

Noy, R., & Pollard, J. W. (2014). Tumor-associated macrophages: From mechanisms to therapy. *Immunity*, *41*, 49–61.

Nozaki, M., Raisler, B. J., Sakurai, E., Sarma, J. V., Barnum, S. R., Lambris, J. D., et al. (2006). Drusen complement components C3a and C5a promote choroidal neovascularization. *Proceedings of the National Academy of Sciences of the United States of America*, *103*, 2328–2333.

Nozawa, H., Chiu, C., & Hanahan, D. (2006). Infiltrating neutrophils mediate the initial angiogenic switch in a mouse model of multistage carcinogenesis. *Proceedings of the National Academy of Sciences of the United States of America*, *103*, 12493–12498.

Okemefuna, A. I., Nan, R., Miller, A., Gor, J., & Perkins, S. J. (2010). Complement factor H binds at two independent sites to C-reactive protein in acute phase concentrations. *The Journal of Biological Chemistry*, *285*, 1053–1065.

Pasinetti, G. M., Tocco, G., Sakhi, S., Musleh, W. D., DeSimoni, M. G., Mascarucci, P., et al. (1996). Hereditary deficiencies in complement C5 are associated with intensified neurodegenerative responses that implicate new roles for the C-system in neuronal and astrocytic functions. *Neurobiology of Disease*, *3*, 197–204.

Piao, C., Cai, L., Qiu, S., Jia, L., Song, W., & Du, J. (2015). Complement 5a enhances hepatic metastases of colon cancer via monocyte chemoattractant protein-1-mediated inflammatory cell infiltration. *Journal of Biological Chemistry*, *290*, 10667–10676, 2015 March 4, pii: jbc.M114.612622.

Pio, R., Corrales, L., & Lambris, J. (2014). The role of complement in tumor growth. In C. Koumenis, E. Hammond, & A. Giaccia (Eds.), *Tumor microenvironment and cellular stress* (pp. 229–262). New York: Springer.

Qing, W., Fang, W. Y., Ye, L., Shen, L. Y., Zhang, X. F., Fei, X. C., et al. (2012). Density of tumor-associated macrophages correlates with lymph node metastasis in papillary thyroid carcinoma. *Thyroid: Official Journal of the American Thyroid Association*, *22*, 905–910.

Queen, M. M., Ryan, R. E., Holzer, R. G., Keller-Peck, C. R., & Jorcyk, C. L. (2005). Breast cancer cells stimulate neutrophils to produce oncostatin M: Potential implications for tumor progression. *Cancer Research*, *65*, 8896–8904.

Rao, H. L., Chen, J. W., Li, M., Xiao, Y. B., Fu, J., Zeng, Y. X., et al. (2012). Increased intratumoral neutrophil in colorectal carcinomas correlates closely with malignant phenotype and predicts patients' adverse prognosis. *PloS One*, *7*, e30806.

Reed, J. R., Stone, M. D., Beadnell, T. C., Ryu, Y., Griffin, T. J., & Schwertfeger, K. L. (2012). Fibroblast growth factor receptor 1 activation in mammary tumor cells promotes macrophage recruitment in a CX3CL1-dependent manner. *PloS One*, *7*, e45877.

Reid, M. D., Basturk, O., Thirabanjasak, D., Hruban, R. H., Klimstra, D. S., Bagci, P., et al. (2011). Tumor-infiltrating neutrophils in pancreatic neoplasia. *Modern Pathology: An Official Journal of the United States and Canadian Academy of Pathology, Inc*. *24*, 1612–1619.

Ricklin, D., Hajishengallis, G., Yang, K., & Lambris, J. D. (2010). Complement: A key system for immune surveillance and homeostasis. *Nature Immunology, 11*, 785–797.
Ricklin, D., & Lambris, J. D. (2013). Complement in immune and inflammatory disorders: Pathophysiological mechanisms. *Journal of Immunology, 190*, 3831–3838.
Rodriguez, P. C., Ernstoff, M. S., Hernandez, C., Atkins, M., Zabaleta, J., Sierra, R., et al. (2009). Arginase I-producing myeloid-derived suppressor cells in renal cell carcinoma are a subpopulation of activated granulocytes. *Cancer Research, 69*, 1553–1560.
Rozel, S., Galban, C. J., Nicolay, K., Lee, K. C., Sud, S., Neeley, C., et al. (2009). Synergy between anti-CCL2 and docetaxel as determined by DW-MRI in a metastatic bone cancer model. *Journal of Cellular Biochemistry, 107*, 58–64.
Ruffell, B., Affara, N. I., & Coussens, L. M. (2012). Differential macrophage programming in the tumor microenvironment. *Trends in Immunology, 33*, 119–126.
Rutkowski, M. J., Sughrue, M. E., Kane, A. J., Mills, S. A., & Parsa, A. T. (2010). Cancer and the complement cascade. *Molecular Cancer Research: MCR, 8*, 1453–1465.
Sagiv, J. Y., Michaeli, J., Assi, S., Mishalian, I., Kisos, H., Levy, L., et al. (2015). Phenotypic diversity and plasticity in circulating neutrophil subpopulations in cancer. *Cell Reports, 10*, 562–573.
Scapini, P., Morini, M., Tecchio, C., Minghelli, S., Di Carlo, E., Tanghetti, E., et al. (2004). CXCL1/macrophage inflammatory protein-2-induced angiogenesis in vivo is mediated by neutrophil-derived vascular endothelial growth factor-A. *Journal of Immunology, 172*, 5034–5040.
Scapini, P., Nesi, L., Morini, M., Tanghetti, E., Belleri, M., Noonan, D., et al. (2002). Generation of biologically active angiostatin kringle 1–3 by activated human neutrophils. *Journal of Immunology, 168*, 5798–5804.
Schmidt, T., & Carmeliet, P. (2010). Blood-vessel formation: Bridges that guide and unite. *Nature, 465*, 697–699.
Schmielau, J., & Finn, O. J. (2001). Activated granulocytes and granulocyte-derived hydrogen peroxide are the underlying mechanism of suppression of t-cell function in advanced cancer patients. *Cancer Research, 61*, 4756–4760.
Schoppmann, S. F., Horvat, R., & Birner, P. (2002). Lymphatic vessels and lymphangiogenesis in female cancer: Mechanisms, clinical impact and possible implications for anti-lymphangiogenic therapies (Review). *Oncology Reports, 9*, 455–460.
Shand, F. H. W., Ueha, S., Otsuji, M., Koid, S. S., Shichino, S., Tsukui, T., et al. (2014). *Proceedings of the National Academy of Sciences, 111*, 7771–7776.
Shojaei, F., Singh, M., Thompson, J. D., & Ferrara, N. (2008). Role of Bv8 in neutrophil-dependent angiogenesis in a transgenic model of cancer progression. *Proceedings of the National Academy of Sciences of the United States of America, 105*, 2640–2645.
Shojaei, F., Wu, X., Qu, X., Kowanetz, M., Yu, L., Tan, M., et al. (2009). G-CSF-initiated myeloid cell mobilization and angiogenesis mediate tumor refractoriness to anti-VEGF therapy in mouse models. *Proceedings of the National Academy of Sciences of the United States of America, 106*, 6742–6747.
Shojaei, F., Wu, X., Zhong, C., Yu, L., Liang, X. H., Yao, J., et al. (2007). Bv8 regulates myeloid-cell-dependent tumour angiogenesis. *Nature, 450*, 825–831.
Sica, A., & Mantovani, A. (2012). Macrophage plasticity and polarization: In vivo veritas. *The Journal of Clinical Investigation, 122*, 787–795.
Sica, A., Saccani, A., Bottazzi, B., Polentarutti, N., Vecchi, A., van Damme, J., et al. (2000). Autocrine production of IL-10 mediates defective IL-12 production and NF-kappa B activation in tumor-associated macrophages. *Journal of Immunology, 164*, 762–767.
Sjoberg, A. P., Trouw, L. A., McGrath, F. D., Hack, C. E., & Blom, A. M. (2006). Regulation of complement activation by C-reactive protein: Targeting of the inhibitory activity of C4b-binding protein. *Journal of Immunology, 176*, 7612–7620.

Solinas, G., Schiarea, S., Liguori, M., Fabbri, M., Pesce, S., Zammataro, L., et al. (2010). Tumor-conditioned macrophages secrete migration-stimulating factor: A new marker for M2-polarization, influencing tumor cell motility. *Journal of Immunology, 185*, 642–652.

Solito, S., Falisi, E., Diaz-Montero, C. M., Doni, A., Pinton, L., Rosato, A., et al. (2011). A human promyelocytic-like population is responsible for the immune suppression mediated by myeloid-derived suppressor cells. *Blood, 118*, 2254–2265.

Stetler-Stevenson, W. G., & Yu, A. E. (2001). Proteases in invasion: Matrix metalloproteinases. *Seminars in Cancer Biology, 11*, 143–152.

Tanaka, H., Ito, T., Kyo, T., & Kimura, A. (2007). Treatment with IFNalpha in vivo up-regulates serum-soluble TNF-related apoptosis inducing ligand (sTRAIL) levels and TRAIL mRNA expressions in neutrophils in chronic myelogenous leukemia patients. *European Journal of Haematology, 78*, 389–398.

Tecchio, C., Huber, V., Scapini, P., Calzetti, F., Margotto, D., Todeschini, G., et al. (2004). IFNalpha-stimulated neutrophils and monocytes release a soluble form of TNF-related apoptosis-inducing ligand (TRAIL/Apo-2 ligand) displaying apoptotic activity on leukemic cells. *Blood, 103*, 3837–3844.

Tecchio, C., Scapini, P., Pizzolo, G., & Cassatella, M. A. (2013). On the cytokines produced by human neutrophils in tumors. *Seminars in Cancer Biology, 23*, 159–170.

Trellakis, S., Bruderek, K., Dumitru, C. A., Gholaman, H., Gu, X., Bankfalvi, A., et al. (2011). Polymorphonuclear granulocytes in human head and neck cancer: Enhanced inflammatory activity, modulation by cancer cells and expansion in advanced disease. *International Journal of Cancer. Journal International du Cancer, 129*, 2183–2193.

Trellakis, S., Farjah, H., Bruderek, K., Dumitru, C. A., Hoffmann, T. K., Lang, S., et al. (2011). Peripheral blood neutrophil granulocytes from patients with head and neck squamous cell carcinoma functionally differ from their counterparts in healthy donors. *International Journal of Immunopathology and Pharmacology, 24*, 683–693.

Tymoszuk, P., Evens, H., Marzola, V., Wachowicz, K., Wasmer, M. H., Datta, S., et al. (2014). In situ proliferation contributes to accumulation of tumor-associated macrophages in spontaneous mammary tumors. *European Journal of Immunology, 44*, 2247–2262.

Ueno, T., Toi, M., Saji, H., Muta, M., Bando, H., Kuroi, K., et al. (2000). Significance of macrophage chemoattractant protein-1 in macrophage recruitment, angiogenesis, and survival in human breast cancer. *Clinical Cancer Research, 8*, 3282–3289.

Vadrevu, S. K., Chintala, N. K., Sharma, S. K., Sharma, P., Cleveland, C., Riediger, L., et al. (2014). Complement C5a receptor facilitates cancer metastasis by altering T-cell responses in the metastatic niche. *Cancer Research, 74*, 3454–3465.

Vasiljeva, O., Papazoglou, A., Kruger, A., Brodoefel, H., Korovin, M., Deussing, J., et al. (2006). Tumor cell-derived and macrophage-derived cathepsin B promotes progression and lung metastasis of mammary cancer. *Cancer Research, 66*, 5242–5250.

Wang, F. Q., So, J., Reierstad, S., & Fishman, D. A. (2005). Matrilysin (MMP-7) promotes invasion of ovarian cancer cells by activation of progelatinase. *International Journal of Cancer. Journal International du Cancer, 114*, 19–31.

Wang, X. F., Wang, H. S., Zhang, F., Guo, Q., Wang, H., Wang, K. F., et al. (2014). Nodal promotes the generation of M2-like macrophages and downregulates the expression of IL-12. *European Journal of Immunology, 44*, 173–183.

Wang, R., Zhang, J., Chen, S., Lu, M., Luo, X., Yao, S., et al. (2011). Tumor-associated macrophages provide a suitable microenvironment for non-small lung cancer invasion and progression. *Lung Cancer, 74*, 188–196.

Weitzman, S. A., Weitberg, A. B., Clark, E. P., & Stossel, T. P. (1985). Phagocytes as carcinogens: Malignant transformation produced by human neutrophils. *Science (New York, N.Y.), 227*, 1231–1233.

Wislez, M., Rabbe, N., Marchal, J., Milleron, B., Crestani, B., Mayaud, C., et al. (2003). Hepatocyte growth factor production by neutrophils infiltrating bronchioloalveolar subtype pulmonary adenocarcinoma: Role in tumor progression and death. *Cancer Research, 63*, 1405–1412.

Wu, C. F., Andzinski, L., Kasnitz, N., Kroger, A., Klawonn, F., Lienenklaus, S., et al. (2015). The lack of type I interferon induces neutrophil-mediated pre-metastatic niche formation in the mouse lung. *International Journal of Cancer. Journal International du Cancer.* http://dx.doi.org/10.1002/ijc.29444.

Wynn, T. A., Chawla, A., & Pollard, J. W. (2013). *Nature, 496*, 445–455.

Xin, H., Zhang, C., Herrmann, A., Du, Y., Figlin, R., & Yu, H. (2009). Sunitinib inhibition of Stat3 induces renal cell carcinoma tumor cell apoptosis and reduces immunosuppressive cells. *Cancer Research, 69*, 2506–2513.

Ye, X. Z., Xu, S. L., Xin, Y. H., Yu, S. C., Ping, Y. F., Chen, L., et al. (2012). Tumor-associated microglia/macrophages enhance the invasion of glioma stem-like cells via TGF-beta1 signaling pathway. *Journal of Immunology, 189*, 444–453.

Youn, J. I., Collazo, M., Shalova, I. N., Biswas, S. K., & Gabrilovich, D. I. (2012). Characterization of the nature of granulocytic myeloid-derived suppressor cells in tumor-bearing mice. *Journal of Leukocyte Biology, 91*, 167–181.

Youn, J. I., & Gabrilovich, D. I. (2010). The biology of myeloid-derived suppressor cells: The blessing and the curse of morphological and functional heterogeneity. *European Journal of Immunology, 40*, 2969–2975.

Ytting, H., Jarle Christensen, I., Thiel, S., Jensenius, J. C., & Nielsen, H. J. (2005). Serum mannan-binding lectin-associated serine protease 2 levels in colorectal cancer: Relation to recurrence and mortality. *Clinical Cancer Research, 11*, 1441–1446.

Zhang, J., Sud, S., Mizutani, K., Gyetko, M. R., & Pienta, K. J. (2011). Activation of urokinase plasminogen activator and its receptor axis is essential for macrophage infiltration in a prostate cancer mouse model. *Neoplasia, 13*, 23–30.

Zhao, Q., Kuang, D. M., Wu, Y., Xiao, X., Li, X. F., Li, T. J., et al. (2012). Activated CD69+ T cells foster immune privilege by regulating IDO expression in tumor-associated macrophages. *Journal of Immunology, 188*, 1117–1124.

Zhou, S. L., Dai, Z., Zhou, Z. J., Wang, X. Y., Yang, G. H., Wang, Z., et al. (2012). Overexpression of CXCL5 mediates neutrophil infiltration and indicates poor prognosis for hepatocellular carcinoma. *Hepatology, 56*, 2242–2254.

CHAPTER FIVE

Tumor-Elicited Inflammation and Colorectal Cancer

Kepeng Wang, Michael Karin[1]
Departments of Pharmacology and Pathology, Laboratory of Gene Regulation and Signal Transduction, School of Medicine, University of California, San Diego, California, USA
[1]Corresponding author: e-mail address: karinoffice@ucsd.edu

Contents

Abstract

The link between chronic inflammation and cancer has long been suspected, due to the pioneering work of Rudolf Virchow over 150 years ago. Yet the causal relationship between inflammation and cancer was only deciphered in the past decade or so, using animal models of various cancers. Up to 20% of all human cancers result from chronic inflammation and persistent infections. Proinflammatory cytokines and tumor-infiltrating myeloid and immune cells play critical roles in almost every developmental stages of inflammation-induced cancers, from initiation, promotion, and progression to malignant metastasis. However, even in cancers with no preceding inflammation, inflammatory cells infiltrate tumor stroma and contribute to cancer development. Such "tumor-elicited inflammation" further emphasizes the importance of inflammation in different types of cancers, including that of the colon. In this review, we summarize our current knowledge of the function and induction mechanisms of inflammatory cytokines during colorectal cancer development, and hope to provide insight into the development of novel anticancer therapies by modulating tumor-elicited inflammation.

Advances in Cancer Research, Volume 128
ISSN 0065-230X
http://dx.doi.org/10.1016/bs.acr.2015.04.014

1. INTRODUCTION

Colorectal cancer (CRC) is one of the major malignancies in humans and the third leading cause of cancer-related deaths in the United States (Siegel, Desantis, & Jemal, 2014; Siegel, Ma, Zou, & Jemal, 2014). More than one million new cases of CRC are diagnosed worldwide each year (Tenesa & Dunlop, 2009). Only a small fraction of human CRC is genetically predisposed, including familial adenomatous polyposis, hereditary nonpolyposis colorectal cancer (Lynch syndrome), hamartomatous polyposis syndrome, and other, more rare, disorders (Rustgi, 2007). The largest fraction of CRC cases has been linked to environmental and nonhereditary events. Among them, chronic inflammation is a significant risk factor for CRC development (Feagins, Souza, & Spechler, 2009). Patients who suffer from inflammatory bowel diseases (IBD) have a high risk of developing colitis-associated CRC (CAC) and have high mortality from the disease (Feagins et al., 2009; Lakatos & Lakatos, 2008). More importantly, in the majority of patients who did not show signs of IBD pathogenesis prior to CRC onset, tumor-associated inflammation is evident in clinical samples and has been shown to drive cancer development in the gut, suggesting a fundamental role for inflammation in both CAC and sporadic CRC development (Grivennikov, Greten, & Karin, 2010).

Various mouse models of CRC have been developed to mimic human CRC progression and provide insights into the interaction of stromal and tumor cells in a physiologically relevant setting. Two of the most widely used models include the AOM/DSS model of CAC and the sporadic CRC model based on genetic ablation/mutation of the *Apc* tumor suppressor gene (Moser et al., 1993; Rosenberg, Giardina, & Tanaka, 2009; Tanaka et al., 2003). Recent studies using mouse models of CAC and sporadic CRC have demonstrated the importance of chronic inflammation in CRC development and elucidated the mechanisms of inflammation-driven carcinogenesis in the gut. Of particular importance is the function of pro- and anti-inflammatory cytokines in this process, including that of tumor-necrosis factor (TNF), transforming growth factor-β (TGF-β), IL-6, IL-10, IL-17, IL-21, IL-22, IL-23, and their family members (Fig. 1). The following sections will summarize the roles of these cytokines in CRC, induction mechanisms of tumor-elicited inflammation, and potential therapeutic options for human CRCs.

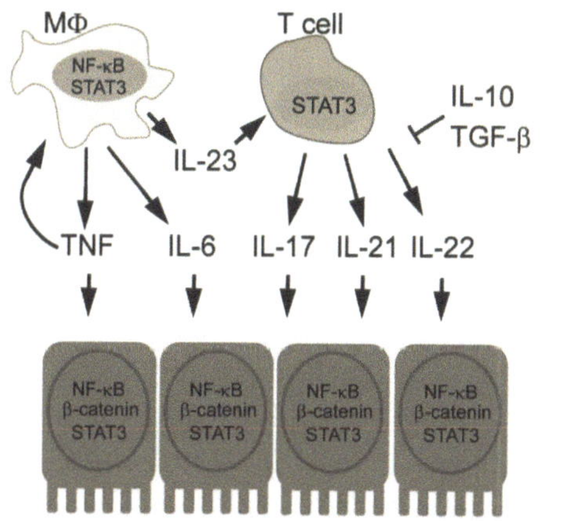

Figure 1 Cytokines and colorectal cancer development. Tumor-infiltrating myeloid cells and lymphocytes produce inflammatory cytokines including TNF, IL-6, IL-17, IL-21, IL-22, and IL-23. TNF activates NF-κB in myeloid cells and stimulates tumor-associated inflammation. IL-23 signals to T lymphocytes to stimulate the production of IL-17 and IL-22. TNF, IL-6, IL-17, IL-21, and IL-22 activate STAT3 and NF-κB signaling in transformed colonic epithelial cells and promote their survival and proliferation. IL-10 and TGF-β limit the development of colorectal cancer by ameliorating tumor-associated inflammation. (See the color plate.)

2. CYTOKINES IN CRC DEVELOPMENT

2.1 Tumor-Necrosis Factor

TNF belongs to a large family of cytokines with diverse and important roles in immune responses, hematopoiesis, and morphogenesis. TNF family proteins have also been implicated in tumorigenesis, transplant rejection, septic shock, viral replication, bone resorption, rheumatoid arthritis, and diabetes (Aggarwal, 2003). TNF was initially discovered in the finding that bacterial infection, or the injection of bacterial products (LPS as an example), resulted in tumor regression (Aggarwal, 2003). Scientists later found that bacterial products induce the production of a secreted factor, which in turn promotes hemorrhagic necrosis of tumors by inducing systemic hypotension, collapse of tumor vasculature, and tumor cell anorexia and cell death, hence the name "tumor-necrosis factor" (Aggarwal, 2003; Algire, Legallais, & Anderson, 1952; Carswell et al., 1975; Williamson, Carswell, Rubin, Prendergast, & Old, 1983). Despite its name, TNF is now commonly regarded as a tumor promoter that stimulates the proliferation, invasion, and metastasis of tumor cells (Aggarwal, 2003; Balkwill, 2006).

Through the activation of NF-κB, TNF supports the survival of cancer cells, and induces the expression of various genes that are involved in invasion and metastasis, including adhesion molecules, urokinase plasminogen activator, matrix metalloproteinase 9 (MMP9), cyclo-oxygenase 2 (COX-2), and vascular endothelial growth factor (VEGF) (Aggarwal, 2003; Balkwill, 2006). Mice deficient in TNF are resistant to chemically induced skin cancer (Moore et al., 1999). Compared to wild-type control, *Tnf*$^{-/-}$ mice developed significantly fewer skin tumors when treated with DMPA/TPA or with repeated doses of DMPA (Moore et al., 1999). Both TNF receptors (TNFR1 and TNFR2) mediate the protumorigenic function of TNF in skin cancer induction, though TNFR1 seems to play a major role in this process (Arnott et al., 2004). TNF signaling through TNFR1 also promotes oval cell proliferation and liver tumorigenesis induced by a choline-deficient, ethionine-supplemented diet (Knight et al., 2000).

The role of TNF in CRC development was illustrated in the AOM/DSS model of mouse CAC, as expression of TNF is elevated in mouse colon following AOM/DSS treatment (Popivanova et al., 2008). At the same time, TNF receptor-expressing leukocytes infiltrate lamina propria and submucosal regions of the colon (Popivanova et al., 2008). Ablation of TNFR1 resulted in reduced mucosal damage, macrophage and neutrophil recruitment, and tumor formation in mouse colon, suggesting a tumor-promoting role of TNF in CAC (Popivanova et al., 2008). Importantly, blockage of TNF signaling in hematopoietic cells also resulted in reduced colonic tumorigenesis, suggesting that TNF signaling recruits myeloid cells into colonic tissue and promotes chronic inflammation and tumor formation in the colon (Popivanova et al., 2008). Etanercept, a specific antagonist of TNF, inhibits CAC induction in mice by limiting TNF-induced infiltration of neutrophils and macrophages (Popivanova et al., 2008). In addition to primary tumor development in the colon, TNF also promotes CRC metastasis (Kitakata et al., 2002). TNF expression is elevated around the central and portal veins of the liver following intrasplenic injection of colon cancer cells. Ablation of host TNFR1 attenuated the induction of VCAM-1 on sinusoidal endothelial cells in the liver and subsequently decreased liver metastasis of injected colon cancer cells (Kitakata et al., 2002).

2.2 Interleukin-10

Interleukin-10 (IL-10) is an important anti-inflammatory cytokine (Fiorentino, Zlotnik, Mosmann, Howard, & O'Garra, 1991; Fiorentino, Zlotnik, Vieira, et al., 1991). Ablation of IL-10 in mice results in spontaneous and severe colitis and the development of colonic tumors in some hosts (Berg et al., 1996; Davidson et al., 1996). By 6 months of age, about 60% of IL-10 knockout mice exhibit adenocarcinomas in their large intestine (Berg et al., 1996). Administration of IL-10 to newly weaned mice prevented the induction of colitis, whereas treatment in adult mice only stopped disease progression (Berg et al., 1996). IL-10 is produced in large amounts by T cells and regulatory T cells (Treg) in normal colon and colonic tumors (Davidson et al., 1996; Dennis et al., 2013). Ablation of IL-10 in T cells resulted in an effect similar to whole body IL-10 deficiency, with increased tumor number and size (Davidson et al., 1996; Dennis et al., 2013). Mice receiving antibiotic treatment to deplete gut bacteria showed reduced inflammation and tumorigenesis in the colon under the condition of IL-10 ablation, suggesting that IL-10 limits bacteria-driving, cancer-promoting inflammation in the colon (Dennis et al., 2013). Through the production of IL-10, Treg cells inhibit cancer-associated inflammation in the colon (Erdman, Poutahidis, et al., 2003; Erdman, Rao, et al., 2003; Erdman et al., 2005; Gounaris et al., 2009). Ablation of IL-10 also resulted in increased expression of proinflammatory enzyme COX-2, whose ablation reduced spontaneous intestinal tumorigenesis in mice harboring mutant *Apc* tumor suppressor gene (Arico et al., 2002; Chen et al., 2003; Oshima et al., 1996; Shattuck-Brandt et al., 2000). Adoptive transfer of IL-10-expressing Treg cells led to increased tumor cell apoptosis and decreased expression of COX-2, and tumor regression in Apc^{Min} mice (Erdman et al., 2005). However, the protection against intestinal tumorigenesis by Treg cells is gradually lost as these cells expand in colonic tumors, switching from the production of IL-10 to IL-17 and becoming tumor-promoting (Gounaris et al., 2009), suggesting that IL-10 plays a critical role in preventing tumor-promoting chronic inflammation. Targeted delivery of IL-10 to precancerous sites may prove useful as adjuvant therapy in limiting the degree of tumor-associated inflammation. Indeed, in a recent study, Chung et al. showed that orally delivered IL-10 microparticles ameliorated local and systemic disease and enhanced survival of Apc^{Min} mice (Chung et al., 2014). IL-10 administration resulted in the reversal of pathogenic IL-17-producing $FoxP3^+/ROR\gamma t^+$ cells into regular Treg cells (Chung et al., 2014). It remains to be tested if such treatment is effective against CRC in humans.

2.3 Transforming Growth Factor-β

The TGF-β family of proteins is comprised of secreted molecules with unique and pluripotent immune modulatory functions (Letterio & Roberts, 1998).

TGF-β signaling is transduced by a heteromeric receptor complex composed of TGFβRI and TGFβRII, both of which are serine/threonine kinases and are essential for TGF-β signal transduction (Attisano & Wrana, 2002; Heldin, Miyazono, & ten Dijke, 1997; Massague, Attisano, & Wrana, 1994). Activation TGF-β receptor complex leads to phosphorylation of SMAD proteins, which subsequently dimerize with SMAD4, translocate to the nucleus, and initiate the transcription of TGF-β-targeted genes (Attisano & Wrana, 2002; Heldin et al., 1997; Massague & Chen, 2000). Inhibitory SMADs serve as negative regulators for TGF-β signaling by blocking the activation of pathway-restricted SMADs (Attisano & Wrana, 2002; Heldin et al., 1997; Massague & Chen, 2000).

Alterations in TGF-β signaling have been discovered in human CRCs, suggesting the cytokine has a role in cancer development. For instance, inactivating mutations in TGFβRII were frequently found in human patients with CRC, suggesting a tumor-suppressing role of TGF-β signaling in the colon (Grady et al., 1999; Markowitz et al., 1995). Targeted disruption of SMAD3, a mediator protein for TGF-β signaling, led to uncontrolled immune cell activation, chronic intestinal inflammation, and development of neoplastic lesions in mouse colon (Yang et al., 1999).

Mechanistic insight into the role of TGF-β in CRC development came from cell-based and genetic models of CRC. TGF-β inhibits proliferation and induces apoptosis in transformed epithelial cells, pointing to a direct tumor-suppressing mechanism (Markowitz & Roberts, 1996; Moses, Yang, & Pietenpol, 1990; Wang, Eshleman, Willson, & Markowitz, 1995). Other studies suggested that TGF-β plays a role in regulating chronic inflammation that contributes to tumorigenesis in the colon. In a model of AOM/DSS-induced CAC in mice, TGF-β was found to suppress the development of colonic tumors by regulating the production of IL-6 by T lymphocytes (Becker et al., 2004). Consistent with human clinical data, transformed epithelial cells in neoplastic lesions in mouse colon induced by AOM/DSS treatment express reduced level of TGFβRI (Becker et al., 2004). TGF-β is produced by both T lymphocytes and tumor epithelial cells. Overexpression of TGF-β in T cells resulted in marked reduction in tumor development in mouse colon following AOM/DSS treatment. On the other hand, overexpression of a dominant-negative form of TGFβRII in T lymphocytes resulted in increased tumor size and number compared to wild-type controls, suggesting that TGF-β inhibits colitis-induced CRC at least in part by signaling to T lymphocytes that infiltrate the tumor microenvironment (Becker et al., 2004). T cells deficient in

TGF-β signaling produce increased amount of IL-6, which in turn signals on tumor epithelial cells to promote tumor cell growth and survival by activating STAT3 (Becker et al., 2004; Bollrath et al., 2009; Grivennikov et al., 2009). TGF-β also signals to stromal fibroblasts to inhibit cancer initiation and promotion (Bhowmick, Neilson, & Moses, 2004). Targeted ablation of a receptor for TGF-β in tumor-associated fibroblasts resulted in increased production of HGF by fibroblasts and development of intraepithelial neoplasia in prostate and invasive squamous cell carcinoma of the forestomach (Bhowmick, Chytil, et al., 2004).

Despite its role in limiting early tumor growth, TGF-β promotes cancer progression and metastasis by signaling to both tumor and stromal cells and is thus considered a double-edged sword for cancer development (Akhurst & Derynck, 2001; Derynck, Akhurst, & Balmain, 2001). On tumor cells, TGF-β was shown to induce "epithelial-mesenchymal transition," which is thought to contribute to cancer invasion and metastasis (Kimelman & Kirschner, 1987; Thiery, 2003; Xu, Lamouille, & Derynck, 2009). Tumor cells that express mesenchymal markers become isolated, motile, and resistant to anoikis (apoptosis induced by lack of cell attachment) and therefore have a greater tendency to be invasive and metastatic than tumor cells expressing only epithelial markers (Lamouille, Xu, & Derynck, 2014; Xu et al., 2009). In addition to the direct cancer-driving role, TGF-β signaling on stromal cells increases the efficiency of organ colonization by CRC cells, whereas mice treated with a pharmacological inhibitor of TGFβRI are resilient to metastasis formation (Calon et al., 2012). Such indirect prometastatic function of TGF-β was attributed to its role in promoting the production of IL-11 by fibroblasts. IL-11, in turn, signals on tumor cells and activates STAT3, which promotes the survival of metastatic cells (Calon et al., 2012).

2.4 IL-6 and IL-11

In the AOM/DSS model of CAC, IL-6 is expressed by T lymphocytes, dendritic cells, and transformed epithelial cells within the tumor microenvironment and is controlled by NF-κB signaling (Becker et al., 2004; Grivennikov et al., 2009). Antibody-mediated neutralization of IL-6R resulted in reduced tumorigenesis in mice (Becker et al., 2004). Soluble IL-6 receptor-mediated trans-signaling on tumor epithelial cells activates STAT3 signaling and promotes tumor cell proliferation (Becker et al., 2004). Consistent with this notion, genetic ablation of IL-6 in mice resulted in reduced CAC tumorigenesis (Grivennikov et al., 2009). Through the activation of STAT3, IL-6 promotes both survival and proliferation of normal and transformed intestinal epithelial cells (Grivennikov et al., 2009). Targeted ablation of STAT3 significantly impedes colitis-promoted tumorigenesis in mouse colon (Bollrath et al., 2009; Grivennikov et al., 2009). On the other hand, forced activation of STAT3 signaling by the expression of hyperactive gp130 transgene led to increased tumorigenesis in the colon (Bollrath et al., 2009). Of note, STAT3 mediates signaling from multiple cytokines other than IL-6, including IL-11, IL-21, and IL-22, all of which play roles in CRC development (Bollrath et al., 2009; Huber et al., 2012; Jauch et al., 2011; Kirchberger et al., 2013; Kryczek et al., 2014; Putoczki et al., 2013; Stolfi et al., 2011). In addition to CAC, IL-6 also promotes colonic tumorigenesis in mouse models of spontaneous CRC (Baltgalvis et al., 2008; Putoczki et al., 2013; Wang et al., 2014). Ablation of IL-6 resulted in reduced tumor number in mouse colon, though the effect is less profound compared to its family member IL-11 (Grivennikov, 2013; Putoczki et al., 2013; Wang et al., 2014).

IL-11 is a member of the IL-6 family that signals through a receptor complex containing its unique IL-11R and common gp130 proteins (Hilton et al., 1994; Yin et al., 1993). Similar to IL-6, IL-11 mainly activates STAT3 signaling. In human gastrointestinal cancers, IL-11 shows a stronger correlation with STAT3 activation than IL-6, indicating that IL-11 is the dominant inducing factor for STAT3-promoted tumorigenesis (Putoczki et al., 2013). Using mouse models of gastrointestinal cancers, Putoczki et al. showed that IL-11 plays a more prominent role than IL-6 in promoting the progression of sporadic and inflammation-associated colon and gastric cancers. Pharmacological inhibition of IL-11 signaling reduced STAT3 activation and tumor cell proliferation, and resulted in decreased tumor growth and invasion (Putoczki et al., 2013). Anti-IL-11 treatment for human gastrointestinal malignancy remains to be tested clinically, but may prove beneficial to human patients in the future.

2.5 IL-21

IL-21 is a member of the class I cytokine that signals through IL-21R and the common γ chain (Ozaki, Kikly, Michalovich, Young, & Leonard, 2000; Parrish-Novak et al., 2000). IL-21 augments Th2 function and is important for B cell development (Cao et al., 2015; Ozaki et al., 2002, 2004; Pesce et al., 2006). IL-21 is produced by Th17 cells and acts in an autocrine manner to boost Th17 differentiation (Korn et al., 2007; Nurieva et al., 2007).

Expression of IL-21 is elevated in patients with CAC, suggesting a potential protumorigenic role for the cytokine (Stolfi et al., 2011). Recent studies employing mouse model of CAC showed that IL-21 promotes inflammation-associated CRC development (Jauch et al., 2011; Stolfi et al., 2011). Expression of IL-21 was augmented in mouse colon under DSS-induced chronic colitis (Jauch et al., 2011; Stolfi et al., 2011), and mice lacking IL-21 showed reduced colitis and decreased formation of colonic tumors under the treatment of AOM and DSS. Ablation of IL-21 resulted in increased expression of IFNγ and reduced levels of IL-6 and IL-17 in colon tumors, consistent with an anti-tumorigenesis role of IFNγ and a tumor-promoting role of IL-6 and IL-17 in the intestine (Jauch et al., 2011; Stolfi et al., 2011). IL-21 promotes the development of CAC in part through the activation of STAT3 in tumor cells, which supports both tumor cell survival and growth (Jauch et al., 2011; Stolfi et al., 2011). So far, it is not clear if IL-21 mainly promotes CAC development by directly activating STAT3 in transformed cells, or by modulating the portfolio of inflammatory cytokines in the tumor microenvironment. Nonetheless, antibody-mediated neutralization of IL-21 during the last cycle of DSS treatment decreased colon inflammation and tumorigenesis, calling for the potential testing of such treatments in human CRC (Stolfi et al., 2011).

2.6 IL-22

IL-22 is a member of the IL-10 family that has an important role during antimicrobial defense and intestinal epithelial repair (Backert et al., 2014; Dumoutier, Lejeune, Colau, & Renauld, 2001; Zindl et al., 2013). IL-22 signals through a heterodimeric receptor complex comprised of a unique IL-22R1 subunit, and an IL-10R2 subunit that it shares with other IL-10 family members (Kotenko et al., 2001; Xie et al., 2000). The primary intracellular mediator of IL-22 signaling is STAT3. IL-22 also activates NF-κB, mitogen-activated protein kinases (MAPK), and PI3K/Akt signaling pathways (Lim & Savan, 2014; Sabat, Ouyang, & Wolk, 2014).

IL-22 promotes the development of CRC through the activation of STAT3 (Harrison, 2013; Lim & Savan, 2014). Expression level of IL-22 is elevated in human ulcerative colitis and CAC (Yu et al., 2013). Serum IL-22 is elevated in chemoresistant patients with CRC, whereas IL-22 administration to human CRC cell lines renders them chemoresistant (Wu et al., 2013). In human CRC, IL-22 is mainly produced by $CD4^+$ T cells that migrate to the colonic tumor microenvironment under the regulation of CCL20/CCR6 chemokine signaling (Kryczek et al., 2014). In the AOM/DSS model of mouse CAC, mice deficient in IL-22 developed fewer tumors, whereas mice deficient in IL-22BP, a naturally secreted inhibitor for IL-22 signaling, developed more tumors (Huber et al., 2012). IL-22BP is expressed at high levels by dendritic cells in healthy colon. Damage in intestinal mucosa resulted in activation of NLRP3 or NLRP6 inflammasomes and the production of IL-18, which signals to downregulate IL-22BP. The reduction in the IL-22BP/IL-22 ratio leads to the engagement of IL-22 to its cognate receptor complex and activation of STAT3 signaling in transformed intestinal epithelial cells (Huber et al., 2012). Similarly, in a model of bacteria-induced colon cancer, innate lymphoid cell (iLC)-derived IL-22 drives the development of colonic dysplasia and cancer (Kirchberger et al., 2013). Importantly, when treated with a neutralizing antibody against IL-22, dysplasia-bearing mice showed reduced severity of colitis and cancer development, suggesting that IL-22 is required for the maintenance and progression of CAC (Kirchberger et al., 2013). The expression of IL-22R1 is restricted to intestinal epithelial cells, indicating that IL-22 signals directly on transformed enterocytes to promote cancer development (Kirchberger et al., 2013). Indeed, a recent study showed that IL-22 activates STAT3 in colon cancer cells and induces the expression of the histone 3 lysine 79 (H3K79) methyltransferase DOT1L, which in turn upregulates cancer stem cell marker proteins NANOG, SOX2, and Pou5F1, resulting in increased cancer stemness and tumorigenic potential (Kryczek et al., 2014). Patients with high DOT1L expression and H3K79me2 in their CRC tissues have poor prognosis, illustrating the importance of IL-22-driven colon cancer stemness (Kryczek et al., 2014).

2.7 IL-23 and IL-17 Axis of Inflammation

Two inflammatory cytokines, IL-23 and IL-17A, produced by myeloid cells and different lymphocyte subsets, were found to play important pathogenic functions in several inflammation-related cancers. In CRC, elevated expression of IL-23, IL-23 receptor (IL-23R), and IL-17A has been linked to adverse prognostic outcome and rapid progression to metastatic disease (Tosolini et al., 2011). In mouse models of colorectal tumorigenesis, genetic or pharmacological inhibition of these cytokines attenuates tumor development and malignant progression (Chae et al., 2010; Grivennikov et al., 2012; Langowski et al., 2006; Wang et al., 2014; Wu et al., 2009).

IL-23 is a heterodimeric cytokine composed of a common p40 subunit that it shares with its relative, IL-12, and a unique p19 subunit (Oppmann et al., 2000; Trinchieri, Pflanz, & Kastelein, 2003; Vignali & Kuchroo, 2012). IL-23 binds to a heterodimeric IL-23R, whose engagement leads to activation of STAT3 and other signaling pathways (Oppmann et al., 2000; Parham et al., 2002; Trinchieri et al., 2003; Vignali & Kuchroo, 2012). IL-23 is mainly produced by activated M1 macrophages in response to engagement of Toll-like receptors (TLRs), which act to induce its expression through the NF-κB and STAT3 transcription factors (Carmody, Ruan, Liou, & Chen, 2007; Kortylewski et al., 2009; Roses et al., 2008). IL-23 plays an important role in expression of another cytokine, IL-17A, by phenotypically stabilizing and inducing the expansion of IL-17-producing T helper cells (Th17 cells), or through activation of iLCs and γδ T cells together with IL-1 (Cua & Tato, 2010; Harrington et al., 2005; Langrish et al., 2005; Park et al., 2005).

IL-17A (traditionally known as IL-17) is the first discovered and best characterized member in its family, which is composed of IL-17A, B, C, D, E, and F (Dungan & Mills, 2011). IL-17A and F are the family's closest members, and both bind to IL-17 receptors A (IL-17RA) and C, whose engagement leads to activation of MAPKs, NF-κB, and C/EBP signaling pathways through the adaptor proteins Act1 and TRAF6 (Iwakura, Ishigame, Saijo, & Nakae, 2011; Reynolds, Angkasekwinai, & Dong, 2010). IL-17A and F are produced by Th17 cells, γδT cells, NKT cells, and other types of iLCs (Reynolds et al., 2010; Sutton, Mielke, & Mills, 2012; Zou & Restifo, 2010). Although IL-23 and IL-17 have traditionally been studied for their roles in host defense, autoimmunity, and chronic inflammatory diseases, elevated expression of these cytokines and their receptors has also been detected in various human cancers, including colon, ovarian, lung, breast, stomach, skin, liver, and head and neck (Langowski et al., 2006; Grivennikov et al., 2012; Li et al., 2012). Importantly, elevated expression of IL-23, IL-17, and IL-6 in stages 1–4 CRC has been linked to adverse prognosis and a more aggressive disease (Schetter et al., 2009). Another study described a Th17 gene signature, whose elevated expression in stages 1 and 2 early CRC predictes rapid progression to incurable metastatic disease (Tosolini et al., 2011).

While the human studies described earlier suggest that elevated IL-23 and IL-17 expression has an important pathogenic function in cancer, strong and conclusive evidence that these cytokines indeed have a causal role in tumor development and progression came from mouse studies. The first study to show a role for IL-23 in cancer development had used the mouse two-step skin carcinogenesis model based on treatment of mice with the carcinogen DMBA and the tumor promoter TPA (Langowski et al., 2006). That study has shown that IL-23 promotes the development of skin cancer by inducing the expression of MMP9 and other genes involved in angiogenesis while reducing the infiltration of $CD8^+$ T cells into skin tumors (Langowski et al., 2006). Subsequent studies have shown that IL-17A also supports the development of skin cancer by activating STAT3 in tumor and stromal cells and promoting the infiltration of myeloid cells into the tumor microenvironment (He et al., 2012; Wang, Yi, Zhang, Pardoll, & Yu, 2010). IL-17 also supports cancer development in mouse pancreas (McAllister et al., 2014) and prostate (Zhang et al., 2012, 2014) and drives metastasis of lung cancer cells (Li et al., 2012).

A much deeper understanding of the relationship between IL-23 and IL-17 in cancer and the mechanisms that control their expression has been gained from studies of colorectal tumorigenesis in mice. Using the Apc^{Min} model of spontaneous colorectal tumorigenesis, Wu and colleagues have shown that infection of mice with the human enterotoxigenic bacterium *Bacteroides fragilis* (ETBF) triggers colitis and accelerates tumor development that is dependent on the induction of IL-17A expression (Wu et al., 2009). Neutralization of IL-17A with a specific antibody prevented the ETBF-induced acceleration of colorectal tumor development (Wu et al., 2009). IL-17A is also important for the development of CAC induced by administration of the procarcinogen AOM and the irritant DSS (Hyun et al., 2012; Tanaka et al., 2003; Tong et al., 2012). Although IL-17A and IL-17F belong to the same family and signal through the same receptors and effector mechanisms, IL-17F plays a role opposite to IL-17A and protects mice from CAC induction (Tong et al., 2012). The divergent roles of IL-17A and F cytokines in CAC may be explained by their distinct roles in autoimmune and chemically induced inflammation, which is a critical step in CAC induction (Yang et al., 2008). Other studies have shown that genetic ablation of either IL-17A or IL-17F results in attenuation of tumor development in Apc^{Min} mice (Chae & Bothwell, 2011; Chae et al., 2010).

However, the Apc^{Min} mouse does not provide the most accurate model for CRC as most tumors in these mice are microadenomas that develop in the small intestine rather than the distal colon. A more accurate model of CRC is provided by the so-called CPC-APC mouse, in which one allele of the *Apc* tumor suppressor gene is deleted in the colon and loss of the second allele through loss-of-heterozygocity results in development of large colonic adenomas that can progress to invasive carcinomas (Hinoi et al., 2007). Using this model, we found that colonic adenomas exhibit substantial upregulation of IL-23 and IL-17 expression relative to adjacent nontumor tissue (Grivennikov et al., 2012). The major site of IL-23 expression in colorectal tumors of CPC-APC mice are CD11b^{+} tumor-associated macrophages (TAM), whereas IL-17 is expressed in Th17 cells, γδ T cells, and iLC (Grivennikov et al., 2012). Disruption of either the *Il23a* or *Il23r* genes inhibited tumor development by 2.5- to 3-fold, mostly due to a decrease in tumor cell proliferation, rather than an increase in tumor cell apoptosis (Grivennikov et al., 2012). In addition, ablation of either IL-23p19 or IL-23R inhibited adenoma to carcinoma progression. Biochemical analysis indicated that the blockade of IL-23 signaling resulted in inhibition of STAT3 activation in tumor epithelial cells but had no effect on activation of β-catenin, which is driven by the loss of *Apc* (Grivennikov et al., 2012). Although IL-23R engagement can lead to STAT3 activation, there was no evidence that IL-23R is expressed on tumor epithelial cells. Furthermore, adoptive transfer experiments indicated that IL-23R signals to stimulate tumor development in hematopoietic-derived cells, which unlike epithelial cells, express high levels of this receptor. Indeed, IL-23 was found to control the tumoral expression of IL-17A, and ablation of IL-17RA also inhibited tumor development and progression, suggesting the operation of a protumorigenic cytokine cascade in which IL-23 controls IL-17A expression and IL-17A stimulates tumor development through engagement of IL-17RA (Grivennikov et al., 2012).

Unlike IL-23R, which is not expressed in tumor epithelial cells, IL-17RA is expressed both in tumor epithelial cells and various hematopoietic cell types. A recent study showed that IL-17 directly signals on transformed enterocytes to promote CRC development (Wang et al., 2014). IL-17RA engagement activates NF-κB and ERK signaling in intestinal epithelial cell and tumor cells, and promotes cell proliferation. Targeted ablation of IL-17RA in colon epithelial cells led to marked decrease in colonic tumorigenesis, pointing to a direct oncogenic mechanism of IL-17 in CRC (Wang et al., 2014). IL-17 also contributes to the activation of STAT3 in tumor cells in an indirect manner, in part by upregulating the production of IL-6. The increase in IL-17 expression was evident during early CRC development when only microscopic aberrant crypt foci (ACF) were found, and ablation of its receptor resulted in attenuated outgrowth of ACF to adenoma in mice, suggesting that IL-17 is critical for early-stage CRC development (Wang et al., 2014). Treatment in mice harboring established colon tumors with 5-fluorouracil (5-FU) resulted in further increased expression of tumoral IL-17A, whereas addition of anti-IL-17A monoclonal antibody to the treatment scheme showed a synergistic effect against sporadic CRC in mice (Wang et al., 2014).

3. COMMENSAL FLORA, BARRIER DEFECT, AND TUMOR-ELICITED INFLAMMATION

Most, if not all, solid tumors harbor inflammatory infiltrates in the tumor stroma. Recent studies in CRC development have revealed the mechanisms by which tumor-associated inflammation is induced and propagated and point to commensal flora as important players in CRC (Fig. 2; Grivennikov et al., 2010, 2012).

CRC-promoting IL-23 is expressed in TAMs but not in normal lamina propria macrophages, indicating that tumor-specific factor drives IL-23 production (Grivennikov et al., 2012). Adoptive transfer experiments revealed that IL-23 expression in TAM depends on expression of TLR2, 4, and 9 and their signaling adaptor MyD88, whose ablation prevents CRC development in mice (Grivennikov et al., 2012; Rakoff-Nahoum & Medzhitov, 2007; Salcedo et al., 2010). Most likely, engagement of these TLRs leads to MyD88-dependent NF-κB signaling and transcriptional activation of both the p40 and p19 genes. Supporting a role for TLRs in induction of IL-23 expression in TAMs, treatment of CPC-APC mice with a cocktail of broad spectrum antibiotics that leads to a 99.9% decrease in the colonic commensal bacterial population results in decreased IL-23 and IL-17 expression and a reduction in colorectal tumor load in wild-type, but not in IL-23R-deficient, mice (Grivennikov et al., 2012). These results strongly suggest that colonic commensal bacteria or their disintegration products are responsible for tumoral IL-23 induction.

How do colonic bacteria lead to specific induction of IL-23 only within TAM and not in normal lamina propria macrophages? The answer lies in the observation that tumor-bearing CPC-APC mice exhibit a marked increase in colonic barrier permeability. Introduction of fluorescent-labeled LPS into experimentally generated colonic loops of tumor-bearing mice revealed specific penetration of LPS into the tumors but not into the normal colonic epithelium (Grivennikov et al., 2012). Furthermore, within the tumors, most of the LPS signal was located right next to TAMs. These findings suggested that specific deterioration of the intestinal epithelial barrier is found only in

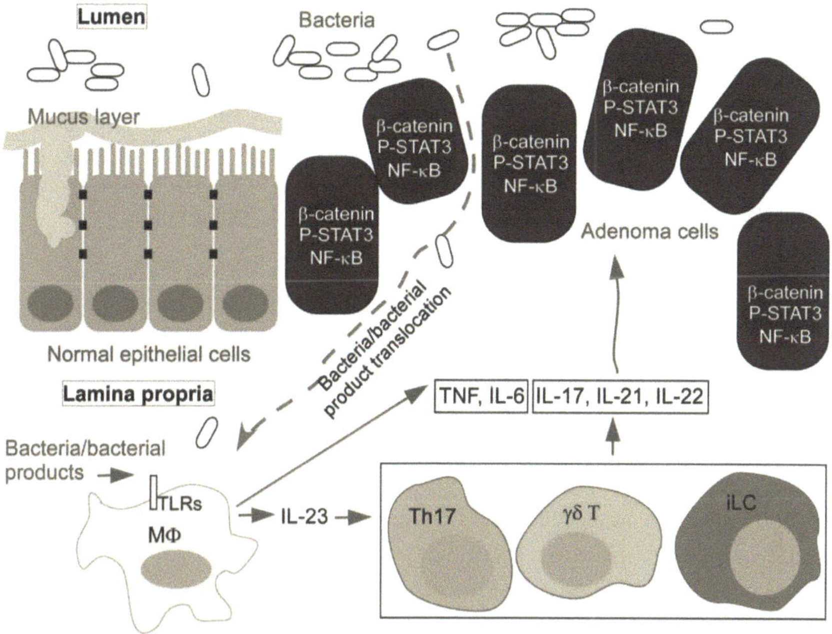

Figure 2 Commensal microflora, barrier loss, and tumor-elicited inflammation in colorectal cancer. Normal intestinal epithelium is covered by a mucus layer produced by Goblet cells. Enterocytes also form tight junctions that control paracellular translocation of ions and molecules, and prevent translocation of commensal bacteria and their products into the lamina propria. Loss of *Apc* and activation of β-catenin induce adenoma formation in the intestine. Adenoma cells fail to produce mucus and form an effective intercellular junctional structure. As a consequence, gut bacteria and/or their products translocate into tumor stroma and activate tumor-associated macrophages to produce inflammatory cytokines including IL-23, which in turn signals to Th17 cells and other IL-17-producing cells. Inflammatory cytokines signal on adenoma cells and activate NF-κB and STAT3 to promote tumor survival and proliferation. (See the color plate.)

tumor areas. Indeed, colorectal tumors in CPC-APC mice were found to be devoid of mucin-producing goblet cells, and as a result, are not coated by the mucin layer that coats the normal colonic epithelium and prevents access of commensal microbes. Consistent with this notion, mice lacking Muc2 protein develop spontaneous colitis followed by CAC (Van der Sluis et al., 2006; Velcich et al., 2002). In addition, colorectal tumors were found to be devoid of junctional-adhesion-molecule (JAM) expression and show other defects in tight junction formation. Importantly, absence of mucin coating, JAM deficiency, and tight junction defects were also observed in human CRCs (Grivennikov et al., 2012). Furthermore, in both mouse and human colorectal tumors, these defects are detected rather early in the tumorigenic pathway, at the adenoma stage or even earlier. In addition to the barrier defects, both human and mouse early adenomas exhibit upregulation of both IL-23 and IL-17 and occasional presence of bacterial 16S RNA (Grivennikov et al., 2012).

4. CONCLUDING REMARKS AND THERAPEUTIC OUTLOOK

The mouse studies reviewed earlier clearly indicate that tumor-associated inflammation, manifested by inflammatory cytokines including TNF, IL-6, IL-11, IL-17, IL-21, IL-22, and IL-23, and limited by TGFβ and IL-10, is of great importance in the pathogenesis of CRC and may be instrumental in other cancers as well. These studies also suggest that agents that inhibit inflammatory cytokine production, receptor binding, or receptor signaling may prove to be efficacious in the treatment or even prevention of CRC, one of the most common malignancies in the developed world and the third leading cause of cancer deaths. Such drugs are expected to be more effective in those patients whose tumors express these cytokines at high levels, especially in patients with CRC stage 1/2 that is highly positive for the IL-23-Th17 signature and suffer from poor prognosis (Tosolini et al., 2011). Several types of agents should be considered for clinical development. These include anti-TNF monoclonal antibody that has been shown to be effective in the treatment for human rheumatoid arthritis, psoriatic arthritis, and IBD (Bongartz et al., 2006; Palladino, Bahjat, Theodorakis, & Moldawer, 2003), humanized anti-IL-6R antibody used against rheumatoid arthritis, systemic juvenile idiopathic arthritis, and Castleman's disease (Kishimoto, 2010), and IL-23 and IL-17A antibodies already found to be effective and nontoxic in the treatment of various chronic inflammatory conditions such as rheumatoid arthritis, ankylosing spondylitis, IBD, and psoriasis (Burakoff et al., 2006; Cottone, Orlando, & Renna, 2010; Miossec & Kolls, 2012; Sandborn et al., 2008; Terzic, Grivennikov, Karin, & Karin, 2010). In addition to antibody-mediated treatment, several small-molecule inhibitors of Th17 differentiation were described (Huh et al., 2011; Huh & Littman, 2012; Solt et al., 2011) and among them, RORγt antagonists are likely to inhibit IL-17 expression not only in Th17 cells but also in iLC. Such agents, however, need to be evaluated for safety and efficacy in both small animal models and humans before their use in cancer treatment and prevention can be considered. Another class of agents that merits consideration are molecules capable of restoring barrier function, thus possibly inhibiting the induction of IL-23 within TAMs. However, such molecules remain to be identified and tested in the CPC-APC mouse model described earlier. Importantly, it is unlikely that any such agent will be able to exert an antitumor effect on its own, and their use should only be considered in conjunction with more conventional chemotherapeutic drugs, such as 5-fluorouracil, oxaliplatin, anti-VEGF, and anti-EGF receptor antibodies (Andre et al., 2004; Ferrara, Hillan, Gerber, & Novotny, 2004; Yang, Jia, Corvalan, Wang, & Davis, 2001), which have already proven effective in the treatment of CRC.

REFERENCES

Aggarwal, B. B. (2003). Signalling pathways of the TNF superfamily: A double-edged sword. *Nature Reviews. Immunology, 3*, 745–756.

Akhurst, R. J., & Derynck, R. (2001). TGF-beta signaling in cancer—A double-edged sword. *Trends in Cell Biology, 11*, S44–S51.

Algire, G. H., Legallais, F. Y., & Anderson, B. F. (1952). Vascular reactions of normal and malignant tissues *in vivo*. V. The role of hypotension in the action of a bacterial polysaccharide on tumors. *Journal of the National Cancer Institute, 12*, 1279–1295.

Andre, T., Boni, C., Mounedji-Boudiaf, L., Navarro, M., Tabernero, J., Hickish, T., et al. (2004). Oxaliplatin, fluorouracil, and leucovorin as adjuvant treatment for colon cancer. *The New England Journal of Medicine, 350*, 2343–2351.

Arico, S., Pattingre, S., Bauvy, C., Gane, P., Barbat, A., Codogno, P., et al. (2002). Celecoxib induces apoptosis by inhibiting 3-phosphoinositide-dependent protein kinase-1 activity in the human colon cancer HT-29 cell line. *The Journal of Biological Chemistry, 277*, 27613–27621.

Arnott, C. H., Scott, K. A., Moore, R. J., Robinson, S. C., Thompson, R. G., & Balkwill, F. R. (2004). Expression of both TNF-alpha receptor subtypes is essential for optimal skin tumour development. *Oncogene, 23*, 1902–1910.

Attisano, L., & Wrana, J. L. (2002). Signal transduction by the TGF-beta superfamily. *Science, 296*, 1646–1647.

Backert, I., Koralov, S. B., Wirtz, S., Kitowski, V., Billmeier, U., Martini, E., et al. (2014). STAT3 activation in Th17 and Th22 cells controls IL-22-mediated epithelial host defense during infectious colitis. *Journal of Immunology, 193*, 3779–3791.

Balkwill, F. (2006). TNF-alpha in promotion and progression of cancer. *Cancer Metastasis Reviews, 25*, 409–416.

Baltgalvis, K. A., Berger, F. G., Pena, M. M., Davis, J. M., Muga, S. J., & Carson, J. A. (2008). Interleukin-6 and cachexia in ApcMin/+ mice. *American Journal of Physiology, Regulatory, Integrative and Comparative Physiology, 294*, R393–R401.

Becker, C., Fantini, M. C., Schramm, C., Lehr, H. A., Wirtz, S., Nikolaev, A., et al. (2004). TGF-beta suppresses tumor progression in colon cancer by inhibition of IL-6 trans-signaling. *Immunity, 21*, 491–501.

Berg, D. J., Davidson, N., Kuhn, R., Muller, W., Menon, S., Holland, G., et al. (1996). Enterocolitis and colon cancer in interleukin-10-deficient mice are associated with aberrant cytokine production and CD4(+) TH1-like responses. *The Journal of Clinical Investigation, 98*, 1010–1020.

Bhowmick, N. A., Chytil, A., Plieth, D., Gorska, A. E., Dumont, N., Shappell, S., et al. (2004). TGF-beta signaling in fibroblasts modulates the oncogenic potential of adjacent epithelia. *Science, 303*, 848–851.

Bhowmick, N. A., Neilson, E. G., & Moses, H. L. (2004). Stromal fibroblasts in cancer initiation and progression. *Nature, 432*, 332–337.

Bollrath, J., Phesse, T. J., von Burstin, V. A., Putoczki, T., Bennecke, M., Bateman, T., et al. (2009). gp130-mediated Stat3 activation in enterocytes regulates cell survival and cell-cycle progression during colitis-associated tumorigenesis. *Cancer Cell*, *15*, 91–102.

Bongartz, T., Sutton, A. J., Sweeting, M. J., Buchan, I., Matteson, E. L., & Montori, V. (2006). Anti-TNF antibody therapy in rheumatoid arthritis and the risk of serious infections and malignancies: Systematic review and meta-analysis of rare harmful effects in randomized controlled trials. *JAMA*, *295*, 2275–2285.

Burakoff, R., Barish, C. F., Riff, D., Pruitt, R., Chey, W. Y., Farraye, F. A., et al. (2006). A phase 1/2A trial of STA 5326, an oral interleukin-12/23 inhibitor, in patients with active moderate to severe Crohn's disease. *Inflammatory Bowel Diseases*, *12*, 558–565.

Calon, A., Espinet, E., Palomo-Ponce, S., Tauriello, D. V., Iglesias, M., Cespedes, M. V., et al. (2012). Dependency of colorectal cancer on a TGF-beta-driven program in stromal cells for metastasis initiation. *Cancer Cell*, *22*, 571–584.

Cao, A. T., Yao, S., Gong, B., Nurieva, R. I., Elson, C. O., & Cong, Y. (2015). Interleukin (IL)-21 promotes intestinal IgA response to microbiota. *Mucosal Immunology*. http://dx.doi.org/10.1038/mi.2014.134. [Epub ahead of print].

Carmody, R. J., Ruan, Q., Liou, H. C., & Chen, Y. H. (2007). Essential roles of c-Rel in TLR-induced IL-23 p19 gene expression in dendritic cells. *Journal of Immunology (Baltimore, Md: 1950)*, *178*, 186–191.

Carswell, E. A., Old, L. J., Kassel, R. L., Green, S., Fiore, N., & Williamson, B. (1975). An endotoxin-induced serum factor that causes necrosis of tumors. *Proceedings of the National Academy of Sciences of the United States of America*, *72*, 3666–3670.

Chae, W. J., & Bothwell, A. L. (2011). IL-17F deficiency inhibits small intestinal tumorigenesis in ApcMin/+ mice. *Biochemical and Biophysical Research Communications*, *414*, 31–36.

Chae, W. J., Gibson, T. F., Zelterman, D., Hao, L., Henegariu, O., & Bothwell, A. L. (2010). Ablation of IL-17A abrogates progression of spontaneous intestinal tumorigenesis. *Proceedings of the National Academy of Sciences of the United States of America*, *107*, 5540–5544.

Chen, W. S., Liu, J. H., Wei, S. J., Liu, J. M., Hong, C. Y., & Yang, W. K. (2003). Colon cancer cells with high invasive potential are susceptible to induction of apoptosis by a selective COX-2 inhibitor. *Cancer Science*, *94*, 253–258.

Chung, A. Y., Li, Q., Blair, S. J., De Jesus, M., Dennis, K. L., LeVea, C., et al. (2014). Oral interleukin-10 alleviates polyposis via neutralization of pathogenic T-regulatory cells. *Cancer Research*, *74*, 5377–5385.

Cottone, M., Orlando, A., & Renna, S. (2010). Investigational agents for Crohn's disease. *Expert Opinion on Investigational Drugs*, *19*, 1147–1159.

Cua, D. J., & Tato, C. M. (2010). Innate IL-17-producing cells: The sentinels of the immune system. *Nature reviews Immunology*, *10*, 479–489.

Davidson, N. J., Leach, M. W., Fort, M. M., Thompson-Snipes, L., Kuhn, R., Muller, W., et al. (1996). T helper cell 1-type CD4+ T cells, but not B cells, mediate colitis in interleukin 10-deficient mice. *The Journal of Experimental Medicine*, *184*, 241–251.

Dennis, K. L., Wang, Y., Blatner, N. R., Wang, S., Saadalla, A., Trudeau, E., et al. (2013). Adenomatous polyps are driven by microbe-instigated focal inflammation and are controlled by IL-10-producing T cells. *Cancer Research*, *73*, 5905–5913.

Derynck, R., Akhurst, R. J., & Balmain, A. (2001). TGF-beta signaling in tumor suppression and cancer progression. *Nature Genetics*, *29*, 117–129.

Dumoutier, L., Lejeune, D., Colau, D., & Renauld, J. C. (2001). Cloning and characterization of IL-22 binding protein, a natural antagonist of IL-10-related T cell-derived inducible factor/IL-22. *Journal of Immunology*, *166*, 7090–7095.

Dungan, L. S., & Mills, K. H. (2011). Caspase-1-processed IL-1 family cytokines play a vital role in driving innate IL-17. *Cytokine*, *56*, 126–132.

Erdman, S. E., Poutahidis, T., Tomczak, M., Rogers, A. B., Cormier, K., Plank, B., et al. (2003). CD4+ CD25+ regulatory T lymphocytes inhibit microbially induced colon cancer in Rag2-deficient mice. *The American Journal of Pathology*, *162*, 691–702.

Erdman, S. E., Rao, V. P., Poutahidis, T., Ihrig, M. M., Ge, Z., Feng, Y., et al. (2003). CD4 (+)CD25(+) regulatory lymphocytes require interleukin 10 to interrupt colon carcinogenesis in mice. *Cancer Research*, *63*, 6042–6050.

Erdman, S. E., Sohn, J. J., Rao, V. P., Nambiar, P. R., Ge, Z., Fox, J. G., et al. (2005). CD4 + CD25 + regulatory lymphocytes induce regression of intestinal tumors in ApcMin/+ mice. *Cancer Research*, *65*, 3998–4004.

Feagins, L. A., Souza, R. F., & Spechler, S. J. (2009). Carcinogenesis in IBD: Potential targets for the prevention of colorectal cancer. *Nature Reviews. Gastroenterology & Hepatology*, *6*, 297–305.

Ferrara, N., Hillan, K. J., Gerber, H. P., & Novotny, W. (2004). Discovery and development of bevacizumab, an anti-VEGF antibody for treating cancer. *Nature Reviews. Drug Discovery*, *3*, 391–400.

Fiorentino, D. F., Zlotnik, A., Mosmann, T. R., Howard, M., & O'Garra, A. (1991). IL-10 inhibits cytokine production by activated macrophages. *Journal of Immunology*, *147*, 3815–3822.

Fiorentino, D. F., Zlotnik, A., Vieira, P., Mosmann, T. R., Howard, M., Moore, K. W., et al. (1991). IL-10 acts on the antigen-presenting cell to inhibit cytokine production by Th1 cells. *Journal of Immunology*, *146*, 3444–3451.

Gounaris, E., Blatner, N. R., Dennis, K., Magnusson, F., Gurish, M. F., Strom, T. B., et al. (2009). T-regulatory cells shift from a protective anti-inflammatory to a cancer-promoting proinflammatory phenotype in polyposis. *Cancer Research*, *69*, 5490–5497.

Grady, W. M., Myeroff, L. L., Swinler, S. E., Rajput, A., Thiagalingam, S., Lutterbaugh, J. D., et al. (1999). Mutational inactivation of transforming growth factor beta receptor type II in microsatellite stable colon cancers. *Cancer Research*, *59*, 320–324.

Grivennikov, S. I. (2013). IL-11: A prominent pro-tumorigenic member of the IL-6 family. *Cancer Cell*, *24*, 145–147.

Grivennikov, S. I., Greten, F. R., & Karin, M. (2010). Immunity, inflammation, and cancer. *Cell*, *140*, 883–899.

Grivennikov, S., Karin, E., Terzic, J., Mucida, D., Yu, G. Y., Vallabhapurapu, S., et al. (2009). IL-6 and Stat3 are required for survival of intestinal epithelial cells and development of colitis-associated cancer. *Cancer Cell*, *15*, 103–113.

Grivennikov, S. I., Wang, K., Mucida, D., Stewart, C. A., Schnabl, B., Jauch, D., et al. (2012). Adenoma-linked barrier defects and microbial products drive IL-23/IL-17-mediated tumour growth. *Nature*, *491*, 254–258.

Harrington, L. E., Hatton, R. D., Mangan, P. R., Turner, H., Murphy, T. L., Murphy, K. M., et al. (2005). Interleukin 17-producing CD4+ effector T cells develop via a lineage distinct from the T helper type 1 and 2 lineages. *Nature immunology*, *6*, 1123–1132.

Harrison, C. (2013). Cancer: IL-22: Linking inflammation and cancer. *Nature Reviews. Drug Discovery*, *12*, 504.

He, D., Li, H., Yusuf, N., Elmets, C. A., Athar, M., Katiyar, S. K., et al. (2012). IL-17 mediated inflammation promotes tumor growth and progression in the skin. *PloS One*, 7, e32126.

Heldin, C. H., Miyazono, K., & ten Dijke, P. (1997). TGF-beta signalling from cell membrane to nucleus through SMAD proteins. *Nature*, *390*, 465–471.

Hilton, D. J., Hilton, A. A., Raicevic, A., Rakar, S., Harrison-Smith, M., Gough, N. M., et al. (1994). Cloning of a murine IL-11 receptor alpha-chain; requirement for gp130 for high affinity binding and signal transduction. *The EMBO Journal*, *13*, 4765–4775.

Hinoi, T., Akyol, A., Theisen, B. K., Ferguson, D. O., Greenson, J. K., Williams, B. O., et al. (2007). Mouse model of colonic adenoma-carcinoma progression based on somatic Apc inactivation. *Cancer Research, 67*, 9721–9730.

Huber, S., Gagliani, N., Zenewicz, L. A., Huber, F. J., Bosurgi, L., Hu, B., et al. (2012). IL-22BP is regulated by the inflammasome and modulates tumorigenesis in the intestine. *Nature, 491*, 259–263.

Huh, J. R., Leung, M. W., Huang, P., Ryan, D. A., Krout, M. R., Malapaka, R. R., et al. (2011). Digoxin and its derivatives suppress TH17 cell differentiation by antagonizing RORgammat activity. *Nature, 472*, 486–490.

Huh, J. R., & Littman, D. R. (2012). Small molecule inhibitors of RORgammat: Targeting Th17 cells and other applications. *European Journal of Immunology, 42*, 2232–2237.

Hyun, Y. S., Han, D. S., Lee, A. R., Eun, C. S., Youn, J., & Kim, H. Y. (2012). Role of IL-17A in the development of colitis-associated cancer. *Carcinogenesis, 33*, 931–936.

Iwakura, Y., Ishigame, H., Saijo, S., & Nakae, S. (2011). Functional specialization of interleukin-17 family members. *Immunity, 34*, 149–162.

Jauch, D., Martin, M., Schiechl, G., Kesselring, R., Schlitt, H. J., Geissler, E. K., et al. (2011). Interleukin 21 controls tumour growth and tumour immunosurveillance in colitis-associated tumorigenesis in mice. *Gut, 60*, 1678–1686.

Kimelman, D., & Kirschner, M. (1987). Synergistic induction of mesoderm by FGF and TGF-beta and the identification of an mRNA coding for FGF in the early Xenopus embryo. *Cell, 51*, 869–877.

Kirchberger, S., Royston, D. J., Boulard, O., Thornton, E., Franchini, F., Szabady, R. L., et al. (2013). Innate lymphoid cells sustain colon cancer through production of interleukin-22 in a mouse model. *The Journal of Experimental Medicine, 210*, 917–931.

Kishimoto, T. (2010). IL-6: From its discovery to clinical applications. *International Immunology, 22*, 347–352.

Kitakata, H., Nemoto-Sasaki, Y., Takahashi, Y., Kondo, T., Mai, M., & Mukaida, N. (2002). Essential roles of tumor necrosis factor receptor p55 in liver metastasis of intrasplenic administration of colon 26 cells. *Cancer Research, 62*, 6682–6687.

Knight, B., Yeoh, G. C., Husk, K. L., Ly, T., Abraham, L. J., Yu, C., et al. (2000). Impaired preneoplastic changes and liver tumor formation in tumor necrosis factor receptor type 1 knockout mice. *The Journal of Experimental Medicine, 192*, 1809–1818.

Korn, T., Bettelli, E., Gao, W., Awasthi, A., Jager, A., Strom, T. B., et al. (2007). IL-21 initiates an alternative pathway to induce proinflammatory T(H)17 cells. *Nature, 448*, 484–487.

Kortylewski, M., Xin, H., Kujawski, M., Lee, H., Liu, Y., Harris, T., et al. (2009). Regulation of the IL-23 and IL-12 balance by Stat3 signaling in the tumor microenvironment. *Cancer cell, 15*, 114–123.

Kotenko, S. V., Izotova, L. S., Mirochnitchenko, O. V., Esterova, E., Dickensheets, H., Donnelly, R. P., et al. (2001). Identification of the functional interleukin-22 (IL-22) receptor complex: The IL-10R2 chain (IL-10Rbeta) is a common chain of both the IL-10 and IL-22 (IL-10-related T cell-derived inducible factor, IL-TIF) receptor complexes. *The Journal of Biological Chemistry, 276*, 2725–2732.

Kryczek, I., Lin, Y., Nagarsheth, N., Peng, D., Zhao, L., Zhao, E., et al. (2014). IL-22(+)CD4(+) T cells promote colorectal cancer stemness via STAT3 transcription factor activation and induction of the methyltransferase DOT1L. *Immunity, 40*, 772–784.

Lakatos, P. L., & Lakatos, L. (2008). Risk for colorectal cancer in ulcerative colitis: Changes, causes and management strategies. *World Journal of Gastroenterology, 14*, 3937–3947.

Lamouille, S., Xu, J., & Derynck, R. (2014). Molecular mechanisms of epithelial-mesenchymal transition. *Nature Reviews. Molecular Cell Biology, 15*, 178–196.

Langowski, J. L., Zhang, X., Wu, L., Mattson, J. D., Chen, T., Smith, K., et al. (2006). IL-23 promotes tumour incidence and growth. *Nature*, *442*, 461–465.

Langrish, C. L., Chen, Y., Blumenschein, W. M., Mattson, J., Basham, B., Sedgwick, J. D., et al. (2005). IL-23 drives a pathogenic T cell population that induces autoimmune inflammation. *The Journal of experimental medicine*, *201*, 233–240.

Letterio, J. J., & Roberts, A. B. (1998). Regulation of immune responses by TGF-beta. *Annual Review of Immunology*, *16*, 137–161.

Li, Q., Han, Y., Fei, G., Guo, Z., Ren, T., & Liu, Z. (2012). IL-17 promoted metastasis of non-small-cell lung cancer cells. *Immunology Letters*, *148*, 144–150.

Lim, C., & Savan, R. (2014). The role of the IL-22/IL-22R1 axis in cancer. *Cytokine & Growth Factor Reviews*, *25*, 257–271.

Markowitz, S. D., & Roberts, A. B. (1996). Tumor suppressor activity of the TGF-beta pathway in human cancers. *Cytokine & Growth Factor Reviews*, 7, 93–102.

Markowitz, S., Wang, J., Myeroff, L., Parsons, R., Sun, L., Lutterbaugh, J., et al. (1995). Inactivation of the type II TGF-beta receptor in colon cancer cells with microsatellite instability. *Science*, *268*, 1336–1338.

Massague, J., Attisano, L., & Wrana, J. L. (1994). The TGF-beta family and its composite receptors. *Trends in Cell Biology*, *4*, 172–178.

Massague, J., & Chen, Y. G. (2000). Controlling TGF-beta signaling. *Genes & Development*, *14*, 627–644.

McAllister, F., Bailey, J. M., Alsina, J., Nirschl, C. J., Sharma, R., Fan, H., et al. (2014). Oncogenic kras activates a hematopoietic-to-epithelial IL-17 signaling axis in preinvasive pancreatic neoplasia. *Cancer Cell*, *25*, 621–637.

Miossec, P., & Kolls, J. K. (2012). Targeting IL-17 and TH17 cells in chronic inflammation. *Nature Reviews. Drug Discovery*, *11*, 763–776.

Moore, R. J., Owens, D. M., Stamp, G., Arnott, C., Burke, F., East, N., et al. (1999). Mice deficient in tumor necrosis factor-alpha are resistant to skin carcinogenesis. *Nature Medicine*, *5*, 828–831.

Moser, A. R., Mattes, E. M., Dove, W. F., Lindstrom, M. J., Haag, J. D., & Gould, M. N. (1993). ApcMin, a mutation in the murine Apc gene, predisposes to mammary carcinomas and focal alveolar hyperplasias. *Proceedings of the National Academy of Sciences of the United States of America*, *90*, 8977–8981.

Moses, H. L., Yang, E. Y., & Pietenpol, J. A. (1990). TGF-beta stimulation and inhibition of cell proliferation: New mechanistic insights. *Cell*, *63*, 245–247.

Nurieva, R., Yang, X. O., Martinez, G., Zhang, Y., Panopoulos, A. D., Ma, L., et al. (2007). Essential autocrine regulation by IL-21 in the generation of inflammatory T cells. *Nature*, *448*, 480–483.

Oppmann, B., Lesley, R., Blom, B., Timans, J. C., Xu, Y., Hunte, B., et al. (2000). Novel p19 protein engages IL-12p40 to form a cytokine, IL-23, with biological activities similar as well as distinct from IL-12. *Immunity*, *13*, 715–725.

Oshima, M., Dinchuk, J. E., Kargman, S. L., Oshima, H., Hancock, B., Kwong, E., et al. (1996). Suppression of intestinal polyposis in Apc delta716 knockout mice by inhibition of cyclooxygenase 2 (COX-2). *Cell*, *87*, 803–809.

Ozaki, K., Kikly, K., Michalovich, D., Young, P. R., & Leonard, W. J. (2000). Cloning of a type I cytokine receptor most related to the IL-2 receptor beta chain. *Proceedings of the National Academy of Sciences of the United States of America*, *97*, 11439–11444.

Ozaki, K., Spolski, R., Ettinger, R., Kim, H. P., Wang, G., Qi, C. F., et al. (2004). Regulation of B cell differentiation and plasma cell generation by IL-21, a novel inducer of blimp-1 and Bcl-6. *Journal of Immunology*, *173*, 5361–5371.

Ozaki, K., Spolski, R., Feng, C. G., Qi, C. F., Cheng, J., Sher, A., et al. (2002). A critical role for IL-21 in regulating immunoglobulin production. *Science*, *298*, 1630–1634.

Palladino, M. A., Bahjat, F. R., Theodorakis, E. A., & Moldawer, L. L. (2003). Anti-TNF-alpha therapies: The next generation. *Nature Reviews. Drug Discovery*, *2*, 736–746.

Parham, C., Chirica, M., Timans, J., Vaisberg, E., Travis, M., Cheung, J., et al. (2002). A receptor for the heterodimeric cytokine IL-23 is composed of IL-12Rbeta1 and a novel cytokine receptor subunit, IL-23R. *Journal of Immunology (Baltimore, Md: 1950)*, *168*, 5699–5708.

Park, H., Li, Z., Yang, X. O., Chang, S. H., Nurieva, R., Wang, Y. H., et al. (2005). A distinct lineage of CD4 T cells regulates tissue inflammation by producing interleukin 17. *Nature immunology*, *6*, 1133–1141.

Parrish-Novak, J., Dillon, S. R., Nelson, A., Hammond, A., Sprecher, C., Gross, J. A., et al. (2000). Interleukin 21 and its receptor are involved in NK cell expansion and regulation of lymphocyte function. *Nature*, *408*, 57–63.

Pesce, J., Kaviratne, M., Ramalingam, T. R., Thompson, R. W., Urban, J. F., Jr., Cheever, A. W., et al. (2006). The IL-21 receptor augments Th2 effector function and alternative macrophage activation. *The Journal of Clinical Investigation*, *116*, 2044–2055.

Popivanova, B. K., Kitamura, K., Wu, Y., Kondo, T., Kagaya, T., Kaneko, S., et al. (2008). Blocking TNF-alpha in mice reduces colorectal carcinogenesis associated with chronic colitis. *The Journal of Clinical Investigation*, *118*, 560–570.

Putoczki, T. L., Thiem, S., Loving, A., Busuttil, R. A., Wilson, N. J., Ziegler, P. K., et al. (2013). Interleukin-11 is the dominant IL-6 family cytokine during gastrointestinal tumorigenesis and can be targeted therapeutically. *Cancer Cell*, *24*, 257–271.

Rakoff-Nahoum, S., & Medzhitov, R. (2007). Regulation of spontaneous intestinal tumorigenesis through the adaptor protein MyD88. *Science*, *317*, 124–127.

Reynolds, J. M., Angkasekwinai, P., & Dong, C. (2010). IL-17 family member cytokines: Regulation and function in innate immunity. *Cytokine & Growth Factor Reviews*, *21*, 413–423.

Rosenberg, D. W., Giardina, C., & Tanaka, T. (2009). Mouse models for the study of colon carcinogenesis. *Carcinogenesis*, *30*, 183–196.

Roses, R. E., Xu, S., Xu, M., Koldovsky, U., Koski, G., & Czerniecki, B. J. (2008). Differential production of IL-23 and IL-12 by myeloid-derived dendritic cells in response to TLR agonists. *Journal of Immunology (Baltimore, Md: 1950)*, *181*, 5120–5127.

Rustgi, A. K. (2007). The genetics of hereditary colon cancer. *Genes & Development*, *21*, 2525–2538.

Sabat, R., Ouyang, W., & Wolk, K. (2014). Therapeutic opportunities of the IL-22-IL-22R1 system. *Nature Reviews. Drug Discovery*, *13*, 21–38.

Salcedo, R., Worschech, A., Cardone, M., Jones, Y., Gyulai, Z., Dai, R. M., et al. (2010). MyD88-mediated signaling prevents development of adenocarcinomas of the colon: Role of interleukin 18. *The Journal of Experimental Medicine*, *207*, 1625–1636.

Sandborn, W. J., Feagan, B. G., Fedorak, R. N., Scherl, E., Fleisher, M. R., Katz, S., et al. (2008). A randomized trial of ustekinumab, a human interleukin-12/23 monoclonal antibody, in patients with moderate-to-severe Crohn's disease. *Gastroenterology*, *135*, 1130–1141.

Schetter, A. J., Nguyen, G. H., Bowman, E. D., Mathe, E. A., Yuen, S. T., & Hawkes, J. E. (2009). Association of inflammation-related and microRNA gene expression with cancer-specific mortality of colon adenocarcinoma. *Clinical Cancer Research: An Official Journal of the American Association for Cancer Research*, *15*, 5878–5887.

Shattuck-Brandt, R. L., Varilek, G. W., Radhika, A., Yang, F., Washington, M. K., & DuBois, R. N. (2000). Cyclooxygenase 2 expression is increased in the stroma of colon carcinomas from IL-10(-/-) mice. *Gastroenterology*, *118*, 337–345.

Siegel, R., Desantis, C., & Jemal, A. (2014). Colorectal cancer statistics, 2014. *CA: A Cancer Journal for Clinicians*, *64*, 104–117.

Siegel, R., Ma, J., Zou, Z., & Jemal, A. (2014). Cancer statistics, 2014. *CA: A Cancer Journal for Clinicians, 64*, 9–29.

Solt, L. A., Kumar, N., Nuhant, P., Wang, Y., Lauer, J. L., Liu, J., et al. (2011). Suppression of TH17 differentiation and autoimmunity by a synthetic ROR ligand. *Nature, 472*, 491–494.

Stolfi, C., Rizzo, A., Franze, E., Rotondi, A., Fantini, M. C., Sarra, M., et al. (2011). Involvement of interleukin-21 in the regulation of colitis-associated colon cancer. *The Journal of Experimental Medicine, 208*, 2279–2290.

Sutton, C. E., Mielke, L. A., & Mills, K. H. (2012). IL-17-producing gammadelta T cells and innate lymphoid cells. *European Journal of Immunology, 42*, 2221–2231.

Tanaka, T., Kohno, H., Suzuki, R., Yamada, Y., Sugie, S., & Mori, H. (2003). A novel inflammation-related mouse colon carcinogenesis model induced by azoxymethane and dextran sodium sulfate. *Cancer Science, 94*, 965–973.

Tenesa, A., & Dunlop, M. G. (2009). New insights into the aetiology of colorectal cancer from genome-wide association studies. *Nature Reviews. Genetics, 10*, 353–358.

Terzic, J., Grivennikov, S., Karin, E., & Karin, M. (2010). Inflammation and colon cancer. *Gastroenterology, 138*, 2101-2114 e2105.

Thiery, J. P. (2003). Epithelial-mesenchymal transitions in development and pathologies. *Current Opinion in Cell Biology, 15*, 740–746.

Tong, Z., Yang, X. O., Yan, H., Liu, W., Niu, X., Shi, Y., et al. (2012). A protective role by interleukin-17 F in colon tumorigenesis. *PloS One, 7*, e34959.

Tosolini, M., Kirilovsky, A., Mlecnik, B., Fredriksen, T., Mauger, S., Bindea, G., et al. (2011). Clinical impact of different classes of infiltrating T cytotoxic and helper cells (Th1, th2, treg, th17) in patients with colorectal cancer. *Cancer Research, 71*, 1263–1271.

Trinchieri, G., Pflanz, S., & Kastelein, R. A. (2003). The IL-12 family of heterodimeric cytokines: New players in the regulation of T cell responses. *Immunity, 19*, 641–644.

Van der Sluis, M., De Koning, B. A., De Bruijn, A. C., Velcich, A., Meijerink, J. P., Van Goudoever, J. B., et al. (2006). Muc2-deficient mice spontaneously develop colitis, indicating that MUC2 is critical for colonic protection. *Gastroenterology, 131*, 117–129.

Velcich, A., Yang, W., Heyer, J., Fragale, A., Nicholas, C., Viani, S., et al. (2002). Colorectal cancer in mice genetically deficient in the mucin Muc2. *Science, 295*, 1726–1729.

Vignali, D. A., & Kuchroo, V. K. (2012). IL-12 family cytokines: Immunological playmakers. *Nature immunology, 13*, 722–728.

Wang, C. Y., Eshleman, J. R., Willson, J. K., & Markowitz, S. (1995). Both transforming growth factor-beta and substrate release are inducers of apoptosis in a human colon adenoma cell line. *Cancer Research, 55*, 5101–5105.

Wang, K., Kim, M. K., Di Caro, G., Wong, J., Shalapour, S., Wan, J., et al. (2014). Interleukin-17 receptor a signaling in transformed enterocytes promotes early colorectal tumorigenesis. *Immunity, 41*, 1052–1063.

Wang, L., Yi, T., Zhang, W., Pardoll, D. M., & Yu, H. (2010). IL-17 enhances tumor development in carcinogen-induced skin cancer. *Cancer Research, 70*, 10112–10120.

Williamson, B. D., Carswell, E. A., Rubin, B. Y., Prendergast, J. S., & Old, L. J. (1983). Human tumor necrosis factor produced by human B-cell lines: Synergistic cytotoxic interaction with human interferon. *Proceedings of the National Academy of Sciences of the United States of America, 80*, 5397–5401.

Wu, T., Cui, L., Liang, Z., Liu, C., Liu, Y., & Li, J. (2013). Elevated serum IL-22 levels correlate with chemoresistant condition of colorectal cancer. *Clinical Immunology, 147*, 38–39.

Wu, S., Rhee, K. J., Albesiano, E., Rabizadeh, S., Wu, X., Yen, H. R., et al. (2009). A human colonic commensal promotes colon tumorigenesis via activation of T helper type 17 T cell responses. *Nature Medicine, 15*, 1016–1022.

Xie, M. H., Aggarwal, S., Ho, W. H., Foster, J., Zhang, Z., Stinson, J., et al. (2000). Interleukin (IL)-22, a novel human cytokine that signals through the interferon receptor-related proteins CRF2-4 and IL-22R. *The Journal of Biological Chemistry*, *275*, 31335–31339.

Xu, J., Lamouille, S., & Derynck, R. (2009). TGF-beta-induced epithelial to mesenchymal transition. *Cell Research*, *19*, 156–172.

Yang, X. O., Chang, S. H., Park, H., Nurieva, R., Shah, B., Acero, L., et al. (2008). Regulation of inflammatory responses by IL-17 F. *The Journal of Experimental Medicine*, *205*, 1063–1075.

Yang, X. D., Jia, X. C., Corvalan, J. R., Wang, P., & Davis, C. G. (2001). Development of ABX-EGF, a fully human anti-EGF receptor monoclonal antibody, for cancer therapy. *Critical Reviews in Oncology/Hematology*, *38*, 17–23.

Yang, X., Letterio, J. J., Lechleider, R. J., Chen, L., Hayman, R., Gu, H., et al. (1999). Targeted disruption of SMAD3 results in impaired mucosal immunity and diminished T cell responsiveness to TGF-beta. *The EMBO Journal*, *18*, 1280–1291.

Yin, T., Taga, T., Tsang, M. L., Yasukawa, K., Kishimoto, T., & Yang, Y. C. (1993). Involvement of IL-6 signal transducer gp130 in IL-11-mediated signal transduction. *Journal of Immunology*, *151*, 2555–2561.

Yu, L. Z., Wang, H. Y., Yang, S. P., Yuan, Z. P., Xu, F. Y., Sun, C., et al. (2013). Expression of interleukin-22/STAT3 signaling pathway in ulcerative colitis and related carcinogenesis. *World Journal of Gastroenterology*, *19*, 2638–2649.

Zhang, Q., Liu, S., Ge, D., Xue, Y., Xiong, Z., Abdel-Mageed, A. B., et al. (2012). Interleukin-17 promotes formation and growth of prostate adenocarcinoma in mouse models. *Cancer Research*, *72*, 2589–2599.

Zhang, Q., Liu, S., Xiong, Z., Wang, A. R., Myers, L., Melamed, J., et al. (2014). Interleukin-17 promotes development of castration-resistant prostate cancer potentially through creating an immunotolerant and pro-angiogenic tumor microenvironment. *The Prostate*, *74*, 869–879.

Zindl, C. L., Lai, J. F., Lee, Y. K., Maynard, C. L., Harbour, S. N., Ouyang, W., et al. (2013). IL-22-producing neutrophils contribute to antimicrobial defense and restitution of colonic epithelial integrity during colitis. *Proceedings of the National Academy of Sciences of the United States of America*, *110*, 12768–12773.

Zou, W., & Restifo, N. P. (2010). T(H)17 cells in tumour immunity and immunotherapy. *Nature Reviews. Immunology*, *10*, 248–256.

CHAPTER SIX

Therapeutic Lymphoid Organogenesis in the Tumor Microenvironment

Aliyah M. Weinstein*, Walter J. Storkus*,†,‡,1

*Department of Immunology, University of Pittsburgh School of Medicine, Pittsburgh, Pennsylvania, USA
†Department of Dermatology, University of Pittsburgh School of Medicine, Pittsburgh, Pennsylvania, USA
‡University of Pittsburgh Cancer Institute, Pittsburgh, Pennsylvania, USA
[1]Corresponding author: e-mail address: storkuswj@upmc.edu

Contents

Abstract

The inflammatory status of the tumor microenvironment (TME) has been heavily investigated in recent years. Chemokine- and cytokine-signaling pathways such as CCR7, CXCR5, lymphotoxin, and IL-36, which are involved in the generation of secondary lymphoid organs and effector immune responses, are now recognized as having value both as prognostic factors and as immunomodulatory therapeutics in the context of cancer. Furthermore, when produced in the TME, these mediators have been shown to promote the recruitment of immune cells, including T cells, B cells, dendritic cells (DCs),

Advances in Cancer Research, Volume 128
ISSN 0065-230X
http://dx.doi.org/10.1016/bs.acr.2015.04.003

and other specialized immune cell subsets such as follicular DCs and T follicular helper cells, in association with the formation of "tertiary" lymphoid structures (TLSs) within or adjacent to sites of disease. Although TLSs are composed of a heterogeneous collection of immune cell types, whose composition differs based on cancer subtype, the qualitative presence of TLSs has been shown to represent a biomarker of good prognosis for cancer patients. A comprehensive understanding of the role each of these pathways plays within the TME may support the rational design of future immunotherapies to selectively promote/bolster TLS formation and function, leading to improved clinical outcomes across the vast range of solid cancer types.

1. INTRODUCTION

In recent years, a growing body of literature has established important roles for inflammatory immune cells in the etiology of a wide variety of diseases, including infectious virus-associated diseases, autoimmune diseases such as psoriasis and arthritis, and cancer. More recently, work in this field has expanded in an attempt to elucidate critical signaling pathways involved in initiating and fine tuning inflammatory immune cell activity within affected tissue sites. It has become clear that an array of chemokines (i.e., CXCL13, CCL19, CCL21, and members of the TNF family) and cytokines (i.e., IL-36R and LTβR agonists) play important roles in the recruitment, activation, and function of immune cells within inflamed/diseased tissue microenvironments. The orchestration of these factors culminates in the development of organized networks of innate and adaptive immune cells within the tumor microenvironment (TME) that have commonly been referred to as tertiary lymphoid structures (TLSs). In this chapter, we will attempt to provide a better understanding of these pathways in order to provide a foundation for the design of next-generation immunotherapies that will allow for the selective targeting of inflammatory pathways at the appropriate time and location during disease evolution in order to prevent, deter, or eradicate cancer *in vivo*.

2. DEVELOPMENT OF TLSs IN CHRONICALLY DISEASED TISSUES

Our understanding of the dynamics of how immune cells infiltrate and persist as an operational unit within the TME has evolved considerably over the past decade and now encompasses a paradigm in which TLSs develop at the periphery or within tumor lesions to limit disease progression or as a consequence of effective treatment intervention. TLSs are distinct from primary and secondary lymphoid organs as they do not form during embryonic development and instead can originate in any nonlymphoid tissue that has been subject to prolonged/chronic inflammation (Aloisi & Pujol-Borrell, 2006). TLSs express chemokines including CCL19, CCL21, and CXCL13 that recruit naive and effector $CD4^+$ and $CD8^+$ and memory $CD4^+$ T cells, B cells, and NK cells to sites of inflammation (Pimenta & Barnes, 2014). The primary cell populations found within TLSs are dendritic cells (DCs), B cells, and naive and memory T cells (Fridman, Pagès, Sautès-Fridman, & Galon, 2012). For example, lymphocytic infiltrates and an upregulation of associated chemokines have been observed in the affected tissues of individuals with chronic inflammatory diseases such as Sjögren syndrome, rheumatoid arthritis, multiple sclerosis, myasthenia gravis, and Hashimoto's thyroiditis (Pitzalis, Jones, Bombardieri, & Jones, 2014), as well as cancer.

2.1 TLSs: Organizational Structure

Interestingly, it has been observed that there is not a uniform distribution of TLSs within inflammatory peripheral tissue microenvironments. For instance, in the setting of oral squamous cell carcinoma, approximately one-third of tumors presenting with TLSs were missed when only one section of the tumor was evaluated by pathologists (Wirsing, Rikardsen, Steigen, Uhlin-Hansen, & Hadler-Olsen, 2014). In Merkel cell carcinoma, most tumor-infiltrating $CD8^+$ T cells and TLSs were located at the tumor periphery, with the presence of TLSs correlating with an increased $CD8^+$-to-$CD4^+$ T cell ratio at the cortex, but not in the center, of the tumor mass (Behr et al., 2014). Similarly, in breast cancer, TLSs are sometimes observed within the tumor core proximal to the stroma, and within an individual lymphoid structure, the number of lymphocytes decreased as a function of proximity to the center of the tumor, with the most actively proliferating lymphocytes localized to a small area adjacent to the stroma (Gu-Trantien et al., 2013). In other models of breast cancer, tumor-infiltrating lymphocytes (TILs) are observed within the tumor stroma but not embedded in the tumor tissue itself (Mahmoud et al., 2012). In metastatic colorectal cancer, B cell infiltrates (BILs) were localized to the outer edges of the tumor lesion (Meshcheryakova et al., 2014). These data suggest that the TME is architecturally heterogeneous with regard to the presence and localization of TILs/TLSs, and that diverse signals likely contribute to determining the anatomic locations in which TLSs are "seeded." In this regard, studies have shown that the same signals controlling lymphocyte recruitment to sites of inflammation may play drastically different roles under normoxic (characteristic of the tumor outer cortex) versus hypoxic (characteristic of the tumor core) conditions. For example, signaling via the CCL21/CCR7 axis has been shown to promote angiogenesis in inflammatory microenvironments (Pickens et al., 2012), and new blood vessel formation is one mechanism that facilitates both tumor growth and metastasis. In ovarian cancer, hypoxia induced an increase in intrinsic CCR7 expression by tumor cells, with CCL21 signaling in the hypoxic TME contributing to an upregulation of N-cadherin and the matrix metalloproteinase MMP-9, that are known to promote cell migration and invasiveness (Cheng et al., 2014). In patients with non-small cell lung cancer (NSCLC), a similar effect has been observed, as expression of MMP-1 and ADAM metallopeptidase with thrombospondin type 1 motif, 2 (ADAMTS2) in peripheral blood mononuclear cells was correlated with poor clinical outcome (Kossenkov et al., 2012).

The organizational structure of TLSs in tumors can vary substantially. While classical lymphoid structures are comprised of a B cell follicle intertwined with a network of follicular DCs, intratumoral BILs have been observed in which the B cells are heterogeneously "sprinkled" throughout the tissue instead of being localized within focused aggregates. This has been observed in human oral squamous cell carcinoma (Wirsing et al., 2014) and breast cancer (Mahmoud et al., 2012) tissues, and in tissue sections of murine MCA205 fibrosarcomas (Chen, Fabian, Taylor, & Storkus, 2013), in association with more beneficial disease outcomes. Thus, the establishment of higher order structure in TLSs in or near tumors *in vivo* may not be a critical factor to the development of effective antitumor immune response. It may only be required that the infiltrating effector cells and antigen (cross)-presenting cells interact productively within the TME.

3. TLSs IN CANCER: CLINICAL CORRELATES OF DISEASE PROGRESSION AND RESPONSE TO TREATMENT

In the cancer setting, the presence of TLSs in the TME correlates with increased disease-free survival in patients, with similar results obtained in murine tumor models (see Table 1). These structures allow for activation, expansion, and differentiation of tumor antigen-specific B and T cells within the tumor itself, leading to more effective antitumor immune response even in the absence of therapeutic intervention (De Chaisemartin et al., 2011;

Table 1 Presence and Prognostic Significance of TLSs in Cancer

Cancer Subtype	Location of TLSs	Inflammatory Infiltrates	Anti-Inflammatory Infiltrates	Predictive Outcome of TIL Presence	References
Melanoma	Peritumoral stroma; tumor core	B cells; T cells; $CD86^+$ DCs	N/A	Increased survival	DiLillo, Yanaba, and Tedder (2010), Messina et al. (2012)
Oral squamous cell carcinoma	Peritumoral stroma	B cells; follicular DCs	N/A	Increased survival	Wirsing et al. (2014)
Merkel cell carcinoma	Tumor periphery	$CD8^+$ T cells; B cells; APCs	N/A	Increased recurrence-free survival	Behr et al. (2014)
Lung cancer (NSCLC)	Tumor stroma	Mature DCs; follicular DCs; $CD62L^+$ and naive $CD4^+$ and $CD8^+$ T cells; B cells; follicular DCs	N/A	Increased survival	De Chaisemartin et al. (2011), Dieu-Nosjean et al. (2008); Germain et al. (2014), Goc, Fridman, Hammond, Sautès-Fridman, and Dieu-Nosjean (2014), Goc, Germain et al. (2014)
Metastatic colorectal cancer	Tumor periphery	$CD45^+$ T cells; $CD20^+$ B cells	N/A	Increased overall survival; decreased disease recurrence	Meshcheryakova et al. (2014)

Continued

Table 1 Presence and Prognostic Significance of TLSs in Cancer—cont'd

Cancer Subtype	Location of TLSs	Inflammatory Infiltrates	Anti-Inflammatory Infiltrates	Predictive Outcome of TIL Presence	References
Breast cancer	Proximal to/within tumor stroma	Lymphocytes; B cells; T cells; follicular DCs; plasma cells; Tfh	N/A	Decreased disease recurrence; increased response to chemotherapy	Alexe et al. (2007), Denkert et al. (2010), Gu-Trantien et al. (2013), Mahmoud et al. (2012)
Colorectal carcinoma	Tumor periphery	B cells; Type 1-polarized memory T cells; $CD8^+$ T cells; $CD45RO^+$ T cells	Tregs	Inflammatory cells: disease progression and recurrence; Tregs: positive prognosis	Fridman et al. (2011), Pimenta and Barnes (2014), Salama et al. (2008)
Head and neck cancer	Tumor stroma; tumor periphery; intratumorally	Macrophages; $CD4^+$ T cells; $CD8^+$ T cells	$FoxP3^+$ Tregs	Effector T cells: increased overall survival; Tregs: decreased local recurrence	Balermpas et al. (2013) Fridman et al. (2011)

Pimenta & Barnes, 2014). In melanoma, a 12-gene signature has been characterized that predicts both the presence of TLSs within a tumor and increased survival. This signature includes genes that encode for CCL19, CCL21, and CXCL13, as well as CCL4, CXCL9, CXCL10, and CXCL13 (Messina et al., 2012). In patients with oral squamous cell carcinoma, the presence of TLSs is associated with a decrease in tumor-associated death (Wirsing et al., 2014). In Merkel cell carcinoma, the presence of TLSs correlated with significantly increased recurrence-free survival compared with patients whose tumors did not contain TLSs (Behr et al., 2014). Even in patients with metastatic disease, particularly metastatic colorectal cancer, an increased number of discrete TLSs within the TME correlates with an increase in overall survival and a decrease in disease recurrence compared with patients presenting with less immune cell infiltrates. These groups can be stratified based on the presence of TLSs or the level of $CD45^+$ or $CD20^+$ tumor-infiltrating cells (Meshcheryakova et al., 2014), indicating that the interactions between B cells and other lymphocyte populations play a role in mediating antitumor immunity. This paradigm is also relevant in lung cancer, as patients with intratumoral TLSs have an increased likelihood of survival compared to those who do not (Dieu-Nosjean et al., 2008; Germain et al., 2014). In lung cancer, TLSs arise spontaneously and confer a beneficial phenotype to patients (De Chaisemartin et al., 2011). In these patients, both the density of mature DCs (Dieu-Nosjean et al., 2008) and follicular DCs (Germain et al., 2014) can be used as markers for increased survival. Tumors containing less mature DCs demonstrate a corresponding decrease in Type 1-polarized $CD4^+$ T cells (Dieu-Nosjean et al., 2008), suggesting that TLSs within the TME are crucial locations for generating effective Type 1 antitumor immune responses and that a diminished ability to prime a Type 1 response allows for tumor growth. Supporting this contention, in lung cancer, the presence of mature DCs within TLSs was a better predictor of patient survival than the presence of $CD8^+$ T cells in TLSs, with high densities of mature DCs also correlating with increased expression of genes related to Type 1 effector cell polarization and cytotoxicity in the TME (Goc, Fridman, Hammond, Sautès-Fridman, & Dieu-Nosjean, 2014; Goc, Germain et al., 2014). In primary $HER2^+$ breast cancer, infiltration of lymphocytes corresponded to a decrease in the recurrence rate of tumors and a more favorable patient outcome. This was marked by an increase in intratumoral levels of chemokines associated with the development of lymphoid structures—including CCR7, CCL19, CXCL9, CXCL10, CXCL13, and LIGHT—and levels of genes associated with lymphocytes—such as ZAP70, CD8, CD28, and Lck (Alexe et al., 2007). B cell infiltration also corresponded with a more favorable prognosis in breast cancer. The number of B cells found within the TME correlated with an increase in cancer-specific survival and disease-free survival in patients (Mahmoud et al., 2012). B cells in the TME undergo antigen-driven proliferation, somatic hypermutation, and affinity maturation within the tumor, and these cells colocalize with T cells, follicular DCs, and plasma cells into structures resembling tertiary lymphoid organs (Nzula, Going, & Stott, 2003). In a subsequent study of breast cancer patients, an additional marker of overall survival related to the presence of TLSs was determined to be the presence of T follicular helper (Tfh) cells, a subset of $CD4^+$ T cells that produces CXCL13 and recruits B cells to sites of inflammation (Gu-Trantien et al., 2013). In this study, the presence of CXCL13 was also positively correlated with IFN-γ expression, suggesting that Tfh cells play a role in initiating Type 1 immune responses. B cells have independently been shown to be required for the generation of antitumor CTL responses, especially in melanoma. Depletion of B cells before inoculation of B16 melanoma into mice led to an increase in primary tumor burden and in number of lung metastases, indicating that B cells are important for the initial immune response generated against a tumor. The increase in tumor growth was concurrent with a decrease in IFN-γ- and TNF-α-secreting T cells in the TME as well as with a decrease in the number of T cells found in the periphery and in the tumor-draining lymph node (DiLillo et al., 2010). Of note, it was also observed that the T cells present within tumors with high numbers of TILs were more likely to be Tfh cells or Type 1-polarized $CD4^+$ cells (Gu-Trantien et al., 2013). These data support the idea that orchestrated interactions between immune cell subtypes within the tumor are critical to the generation of protective antitumor immune responses. Interestingly, some tumors that arise in highly inflammatory microenvironments benefit from the infiltration of regulatory T cells (Tregs) as opposed to effector immune cells into the TME. In particular, in the cases of head and neck cancer and colorectal cancer, the presence of intratumoral Treg has been reported to convey good clinical prognosis (Fridman et al., 2011; Salama et al., 2008).

Furthermore, the presence and magnitude of TILs in the TME have been strongly associated with the effectiveness of a range of chemo- and immunotherapeutic agents. Many immunotherapy strategies currently being investigated in clinical trials involve immune checkpoint blockade, including the use of antibodies capable of inhibiting signaling through

CTLA-4 or PD-1 into T cells. Interestingly, it appears that these therapies may work, in part, via increasing the ability of newly arrived $CD8^+$ TILs to be primed and then mature into protective antitumor T effector cells. Priming of $CD8^+$ T cells in the tumor-draining lymph nodes or the trafficking of circulating T effector cells into the TME appears less important to clinical outcome than the priming of resident TILs after blockade of CTLA-4, PD-L1, or IDO (Spranger et al., 2014). Similarly, the presence of Tfh cells in breast cancer TME predicts for superior responsiveness to preoperative chemotherapy (Gu-Trantien et al., 2013). More broadly, the presence of TLS or CXCL9 expression in the TME of patients with breast cancer is a statistically significant predictor of a higher incidence of complete response to neoadjuvant chemotherapy (Denkert et al., 2010).

4. CUES FOR TLS DEVELOPMENT

While the precise sequence of signals that control TLS development has yet to be completely elucidated, especially in the context of the TME, certain signaling pathways classically known to recruit immune cells into inflammatory tissue microenvironments appear to be involved.

4.1 The Requirement for Lymphotoxin Signaling in the Evolution of TLSs in the TME

Lymphotoxin (LT)-α/-β signaling through the LTβR is required for the establishment and maintenance of lymphoid structures. LTα and LTβ are members of the TNF family and share common receptors and signaling pathways with other members of their family. The lymphotoxin ligands are expressed predominantly by immune cell subsets, while the receptors are found on epithelial cell populations. The receptor–ligand interactions promote the organization of immune cells and stromal cells within lymphoid structures (Schneider, Potter, & Ware, 2004). The LTα/LTβ subunits exert their biologic function by forming three distinct trimeric molecules, each with different receptor specificity. The homotrimer of lymphotoxin alpha, $LT\alpha_3$, is a secreted protein that signals through TNFR1, TNFR2, and HVEM (herpesvirus entry mediator) (Mauri et al., 1998; Schneider et al., 2004). Two membrane-bound heterotrimers can also form from the subunits: $LT\alpha_1\beta_2$ and $LT\alpha_2\beta_1$, with $LT\alpha_1\beta_2$ being the predominant form. $LT\alpha_1\beta_2$ signals through the lymphotoxin beta receptor, while $LT\alpha_2\beta_1$ is able to bind TNFR1 and TNFR2 but does not have a clear biologic role in signaling through these receptors (Schneider et al., 2004). The receptors

TNFR1 and TNFR2 have broad expression throughout the body. The LTβR is expressed by stromal cells, epithelial cells, monocytes, and DCs. HVEM is expressed by T cells, DCs, macrophages, and epithelial cells (Zhu & Fu, 2011; Table 2). Specifically, signaling through the LTβR is required for high endothelial venule (HEV) differentiation and for the formation of organized secondary lymphoid organs. Blockade of signaling through the LTβR results in decreased lymphocyte migration into lymph nodes in a model of collagen-induced arthritis (CIA), and this appears due to impaired expression of adhesion molecules PNAd and MAdCAM on HEVs (Browning et al., 2005). A similar decrease in lymphocyte trafficking is observed in Peyer's patches in the absence of LTβR-mediated signaling (Dohi et al., 2001). In the spleen, signaling through the LTβR is required for the segregation of B cells and T cells into distinct zones, and for the generation of follicular DCs and the formation of B cell follicles (Gonzalez, Mackay, Browning, Kosco-Vilbois, & Noelle, 1998). LTβR-associated signaling also plays a key role in TLS formation. In mice that constitutively express both LTα and LTβ in the pancreas, the T and B cell chemokines CCL19, CCL21, and CXCL13 were more predominantly expressed, L-selectin^{+} (aka CD62L^{+}; binds PNAd and MAdCAM) cells were more abundant, and T and B cell zones within the immune infiltrate were more pronounced than in mice only expressing LTα (Drayton, Ying, Lee, Lesslauer, & Ruddle, 2003). In the TME, PNAd and L-selectin expression is exclusively found within TLSs and not elsewhere in the stroma or the tumor tissue, and the two colocalize with each other (De Chaisemartin et al., 2011). L-selectin is important for the recruitment of central memory

Table 2 Lymphotoxin/LIGHT Receptors and Their Cell Expression Profiles

Receptor	Expression	Ligands	References
TNFR1	Widespread	TNF-α; LTα3; $LT\alpha_2\beta_1$	Schneider et al. (2004), Zhu and Fu (2011)
TNFR2	Widespread	TNF-α; LTα3; $LT\alpha_2\beta_1$	Schneider et al. (2004), Zhu and Fu (2011)
LTβR	Stromal cells; epithelial cells; monocytes; DCs	$LT\alpha_1\beta_2$; LIGHT	Mauri et al. (1998), Zhu and Fu (2011)
HVEM	T cells; DCs; macrophages; NK cells; epithelial cells	LIGHT; $LT\alpha_3$	Zhu and Fu (2011)

T cells (Jung, Rutishauser, Joshi, Haberman, & Kaech, 2010), in conjunction with CCL19 and CCL21 gradients that signal through CCR7 on these cells (Jung et al., 2010; Pimenta & Barnes, 2014). LTα/LTβ induce the production of CCL19, CCL21, and CXCL13 (Ansel et al., 2000). Specifically, lymphotoxin alpha is required for CCL19, CCL21, and CXCL13 expression, while LTβ is most critically required for CXCL13, but less so CCL19 or CCL21, expression (Wang et al., 2002). This appears to be a result of the differential receptor-binding ability of the lymphotoxins and the downstream signaling components being activated (Schneider et al., 2004). Such pathways appear to involve a positive-feedback loop in the spleen, where cells expressing the LTβR and CXCL13 recruit B cells, with activated B cells subsequently expressing $LT\alpha_1\beta_2$, begetting further expression of CXCL13 by stromal cells (Ansel et al., 2000). A similar biologic circuit has been shown to exist between $LT\alpha_1\beta_2$ and CCL19 and CCL21 in both secondary and tertiary lymphoid organs (Ansel et al., 2000; Luther et al., 2002). Blockade of signaling through the LTβR using a soluble decoy receptor blocks the recruitment of both B cells and $CD8^+$ T cells into lymphoid organs (Browning et al., 2005).

Surprisingly, tumor and stromal cells may also express and respond to signaling through the LTβR. Induction of this signaling pathway by the natural ligand $LT\alpha_1\beta_2$ or by cross-linking with LTβR-Ig can induce the secretion of the proinflammatory mediators IL-8 and CCL5 by both melanoma (A375) and fibroblast (WI38VA13) cell lines *in vitro* (Degli-Esposti et al., 1997). The effect of LTβR signaling on nonimmune cell subsets is predicted to have an additional role in promoting antitumor immunity in addition to the role of this signaling axis in the formation of TLSs.

4.2 EnLIGHTening Protective Immunity in TLSs

Both stromal and immune cell populations respond to LIGHT (also known as TNFSF-14). LIGHT, expressed by T cells, immature DCs, and macrophages (Zhu & Fu, 2011), is related to the lymphotoxins and is also able to signal through multiple receptors in the TNF superfamily, including the LTβR on stromal cells and HVEM (also known as TNFRSF-14; Mauri et al., 1998) on T cells. In regard to the generation of an immune response, LIGHT is required for $CD8^+$ but not $CD4^+$ T cell proliferation and differentiation (Tamada et al., 2002). Mice lacking LIGHT were shown to have impaired $CD8^+$ T cell responses to bacterial infection (Tamada et al., 2002), indicating a requirement for LIGHT in the generation of successful

Type 1 immune responses. Furthermore, LIGHT is able to synergize with IFN-γ to enhance the production of CXCL9, CXCL10, and CXCL11, which serve to recruit and polarize $CXCR3^+$ Type-1 immune responses (Miyagaki et al., 2012).

In the context of tumor immunology, expression of LIGHT appears to have a broadly beneficial role in reducing tumor burden and improving survival. In human breast cancer patients, LIGHT expression correlates with the generation of TLSs—specifically, *de novo* formation of lymph nodes—in the TME. Expression of LIGHT mRNA was five times greater in the newly formed lymph nodes than in normal lymph nodes isolated from the same patient (Gantsev et al., 2013), suggesting that LIGHT may be a driver in the formation of TLSs in the cancer setting. Introduction of LIGHT into the TME has been shown to promote the development of antitumor immunity in numerous models of cancer. Forced expression of LIGHT in a fibrosarcoma model ($Ag104L^d$) resulted in increased signaling through the LTβR on stromal cells in the TME, leading to upregulated expression of CCL21 and MAdCAM-1 by these cells. Treated tumors also exhibited increased $CD8^+$ T cell infiltration that ultimately led to the rejection of established disease (Yu et al., 2004, 2007). A similar result was observed in established primary melanoma (B16) and colon (MC38) cancers (Yu et al., 2007). Intratumoral vaccination with a recombinant adenovirus encoding the cDNA for LIGHT (Ad.LIGHT) is able to mount antitumor immune responses against B cell lymphoma (Hu et al., 2010), cervical cancer (Kanodia et al., 2010), and breast cancer (Yu et al., 2007). In this B cell lymphoma model, treatment with Ad.LIGHT induces expression of CCL21 and recruitment of T cells into the TME, increases overall survival from primary tumor challenge, and protects treated mice against normally lethal tumor rechallenge (Hu et al., 2010). When applied in combination with a HPV16-VRP vaccine in cervical cancer models, Ad.LIGHT is able to increase circulating levels of antitumor T cells, promote $CD8^+$ T cell infiltration into the TME, regulate tumor growth, and increase overall survival, when compared with vaccines alone (Kanodia et al., 2010). Ad.LIGHT injected into established murine 4T1 breast cancers results in diminished lung metastasis after surgical removal of the primary tumor (Yu et al., 2007). These results suggest that Ad.LIGHT is able to initiate a systemic, tumor antigen-specific immune response that is protective. Work evaluating treatment with mesenchymal stem cells engineered to overexpress LIGHT (MSC-L) has also been shown to inhibit tumor growth in both gastric (Zhu et al., 2013) and breast (Zou et al., 2012) cancer models. In the breast cancer model, the efficacy of MSC-L was dependent on the ability of lymphocytes to be recruited into the TME via LTβR-dependent signaling events (Zou et al., 2012). Interestingly, another study evaluating LIGHT/HVEM signaling determined that advanced stage gastric cancer patients expressed significantly lower levels of HVEM on the surface of their leukocytes, and higher serum levels of soluble HVEM shed from leukocytes when compared to healthy controls (Heo et al., 2012). Prior studies reported the presence of robust levels of soluble HVEM in the serum of patients with autoimmune diseases such as psoriasis, dermatitis, and arthritis (Jung et al., 2003), suggesting that soluble HVEM may represent a marker of ongoing chronic inflammatory conditions. In addition, low levels of HVEM have been shown to drive the generation of dominant Type-2-polarized immune responses in patients with cutaneous T cell lymphoma, in association with disease progression (Miyagaki et al., 2012). Low levels of LIGHT production in metastatic colorectal cancer lesions have been linked to a decreased number of intratumoral T cells compared to normal tissue (Qin, Upadhyay, Prabhakar, & Maker, 2013). This could support a mechanism of immunosuppression that could be reversed by introducing LIGHT into the system as an interventional strategy. In support of this possibility, forced expression of LIGHT in the mouse TRAMP-C2 model of prostate cancer overcomes Treg-mediated immunosuppression and synergizes with a biologic vaccination strategy (PSCA TriVax) to activate DCs and recruit effector T cells into the TME (Yan et al., 2015). In particular, this pancreatic tumor model expresses "self"-antigens, suggesting that LIGHT plays a role in the generation of autoimmune responses, which in the context of cancer may promote a reduction in tumor burden. HVEM, the receptor for LIGHT, is also able to bind BTLA, a molecule found on T effector cells that enhances their ability to be suppressed by Tregs (Tao, Wang, Murphy, Fraser, & Hancock, 2008). Thus, in the immunosuppressive TME, LIGHT may compete with BTLA for binding of HVEM, thereby limiting the ability of Tregs to suppress immune effector cells (Tao et al., 2008). Furthermore, LIGHT has the capacity to bind to decoy receptor 3 (DcR3), a soluble receptor that is expressed by many tumors, including esophagus, stomach, colorectal, pancreatic, lung, brain, renal, ovarian, blood, hepatocellular, and oral cancers (Lin & Hsieh, 2011). DcR3 is related to two other decoy receptors of the TNF family that bind but do not induce signaling upon binding their ligand. Since DcR3 sequesters LIGHT, an additional avenue of translational research aims to engineer a mutant LIGHT that is unable to bind DcR3 but retains its ability to signal through HVEM and LTβR in order to induce more potent antitumor immune responses. Of note, LIGHT that is unable to bind DcR3 is better able to induce the apoptotic death of tumor cells (Morishige et al., 2010), with its effects on immune cell subsets to be determined. LIGHT does appear to have detrimental effects in tumors that arise as a result of chronic inflammation. In livers affected with hepatitis or virally induced hepatocellular carcinoma, levels of LTA, LTB, LIGHT, and LTβR are increased, and chronic hepatitis in this model can be alleviated by treatment with LTβR-Ig, which serves as a sink for LTβR ligands (Haybaeck et al., 2009).

LIGHT has also been shown to play a role in NK cell involvement in antitumor immunity. NK cells constitutively express HVEM, and forced expression of LIGHT in the TME mediates recruitment of NK cells to the tumor from the periphery and activation of these cells, including secretion of IFN-γ. Strikingly, this study observed a requirement for both activated NK cells and IFN-γ in inducing an antitumor CTL response at later time points: peak NK cell infiltration was observed at 10 days post-tumor inoculation, while peak $CD8^+$ T cell levels occurred 22 days post-tumor inoculation. This unique role for NK cells in $CD8^+$ T cell activation is not observed in secondary lymphoid organs such as the spleen (Fan et al., 2006). NK cells have also been shown to induce the maturation of DCs using a similar pathway. Upon recognition of target cells, NK cells upregulate their cell surface expression of LIGHT. LIGHT-expressing NK cells were able to induce upregulation of CD86 on the surface of autologous DCs in a cytokine-independent manner (Holmes et al., 2014). Thus in addition to playing a role in the recruitment of lymphocytes to the TME, LIGHT appears to also have a direct role in priming antitumor immune responses, pointing to LIGHT as a potential therapeutic agent to be explored in the clinic.

4.3 The Importance of CCR7 Agonists for TLS Evolution in the TME

CCL19 (i.e., EBV-induced molecule 1 ligand chemokine/ELC or MIP-3β) and CCL21 (i.e., secondary lymphoid chemokine/SLC) are constitutively expressed by stromal cells and serve to recruit $CCR7^+$ cells to sites of inflammation (Legler, Uetz-von Allmen, & Hauser, 2014). Within the immune repertoire, CCR7 is expressed on naive and memory T cells, B cells, DCs, and NK cells (Badr, Borhis, Treton, & Richard, 2005; Ohmatsu, Sugaya, Kadono, & Tamaki, 2007; Pimenta & Barnes, 2014). In a mouse model involving the forced expression of CCL19, CCL21a, or CCL21b in peripheral tissues, each single chemokine was sufficient to induce immune cell infiltration into the pancreas (Chen, Vassileva, et al., 2002; Luther et al., 2002), but not into the skin or the central nervous system (Chen, Leach, et al., 2002; Chen, Vassileva, et al., 2002). CCL19/CCL21-induced infiltrated tissue contained HEV and organized networks of stromal cells (Luther et al., 2002), consistent with the TLS paradigm. Some cancers have evolved mechanisms to antagonize the host-protective effects of CCR7-mediated immune cell chemotaxis. HPV-induced cervical cancer manipulates its local microenvironment by secreting IL-6, which inhibits NFκB and CCR7 expression by mature DCs and instead upregulates the protumorigenic MMP-9 metalloproteinase. Such effects are reversible as a consequence of treatment with neutralizing anti-IL-6 antibodies (Pahne-Zeppenfeld et al., 2014). However, CCR7 has also been reported to have detrimental effects in certain cancers. In hepatocellular carcinoma, signaling by both CCL19 and CCL21 promoted the proliferation and invasion of tumor cells, while CCRL1/CCX-CKR, a naturally occurring receptor sink for the CCR7 ligands, was able to mitigate these effects (Shi et al., 2015). CCRL1 is unable to induce intrinsic intracellular signaling pathways, but it mediates the internalization and degradation of CCL19 and disallows its agonism of CCR7 (Comerford, Milasta, Morrow, Milligan, & Nibbs, 2006). In melanoma, cells have been shown to express CCL19 and CCR7, and expression of CCR7 correlates with metastasis, especially to the liver (Dobner, Riechardt, Joussen, Englert, & Bechrakis, 2012). Thus in certain cases, it appears that tumor cells have established mechanisms to use the body's natural chemokine gradients to benefit their own survival. While in many instances their roles are considered as parallel or redundant, expression of CCL19 and CCL21 in different organs may be under the control of different signaling pathways. For example, blockade of signaling through the LTβR causes a decrease in CCL19, but not CCL21, levels in lymph nodes (Browning et al., 2005). These results suggest that signaling pathways involving these chemokines include both shared and differential components and that these differences may be organ-dependent.

Chemotaxis of (naive) B cells toward a CCL21 gradient is mediated in part by Type-1 IFN-α. Specifically, IFN-α is able to diminish the ligand-induced receptor internalization of CCR7 in the presence of CCL21, allowing for B cells in proinflammatory microenvironments to traffic more efficiently during the generation of antigen-specific humoral immune responses (Badr et al., 2005). In mice, three isoforms of CCL21 exist. CCL21a differs from CCL21b and CCL21c based on the presence of a serine instead of a leucine at position 65, whereas the exon sequences of CCL21b and CCL21c are identical and may represent splice variants (Nakano & Gunn, 2001). Humans express just one isoform of this protein, which contains a leucine at position 65 but performs the same functions as all three mouse isoforms. The tissue distribution of CCL21 varies between mouse and humans as well: in humans, CCL21 expression is found predominantly in lymphoid tissues (lymph node, spleen, and appendix), while in mice, CCL21 is more broadly expressed and is found at the highest levels in spleen and lung (Hedrick & Zlotnik, 1997). Within lymphoid structures, CCL21 is expressed by stromal cells and endothelial cells, especially those that make up HEV (Ohmatsu et al., 2007) and allow for the recruitment of CCR7-expressing immune cells toward a gradient. In melanomas treated with DCs engineered to express recombinant CCL21 (i.e., DC.CCL21), TLSs developed at the site of vaccination, and expression of IFN-γ by $CD4^+$ and $CD8^+$ T cells was observed, concurrent with a reduction in tumor burden in treated patients (Chen, Fabian, et al., 2013; Mulé, 2009). In this situation, generation of antitumor effector T cells takes place within the TLSs: DC.CCL21 (i.e., DCs transduced to express CCL21) do not migrate to the tumor-draining lymph node. Instead, naive T cells are recruited to the TME from the peripheral circulation and begin to express CD25 (IL-2Rα) within 24 h of organ-site arrival (Mulé, 2009). Interestingly, some tumors intrinsically express CCL21, in association with an immunosuppressed TME. This may be the result of CCL21 recruitment of $CCR7^+$ Tregs that can mitigate the clinical benefits of inflammatory immune effector cells (Schneider, Meingassner, Lipp, Moore, & Rot, 2007). In the setting of melanoma, tumor cell secretion of CCL21 promotes tumor immune escape through the production of TGF-β and the recruitment of Tregs and myeloid-derived suppressor cells (MDSCs; Zlotnik, Burkhardt, & Homey, 2011). A similar result has been observed in a pancreatic islet beta cell tumor model, in which forced overexpression of CCL21 in the tumor cells led to enhanced tumor progression and significantly higher numbers of Tregs found within the TME (Shields, Kourtis, Tomei, Roberts, & Swartz, 2010). This latter result was dependent on host tissue expression of CCR7. CCL21–CCR7 signaling has also been reported to have a proangiogenic effect. In a model of rheumatoid arthritis, a CCL21 gradient caused migration of $CCR7^+$ microvascular endothelial cells. CCL21 also leads to the secretion of proangiogenic factors, such as VEGF, Ang-1, and IL-8, by fibroblasts and macrophages. Neutralization of CCL21 or blockade of CCR7 abrogated microvascular endothelial cell migration *in vivo* (Pickens et al., 2012). Thus in the context of cancer, the proangiogenic capability of CCL21 signaling may mediate tumor progression, as *de novo* blood vessel formation is required for tumor growth and metastasis.

CCL19 is expressed by stromal cells in lymphoid organs, as well as by mature DCs (Sanchez-Sanchez, Riol-Blanco, & Rodriguez-Fernandez, 2006). Like CCL21, the transcription of CCL19 is regulated by two NFκB-binding sites and one interferon-stimulated response element in its promoter region. The inhibition of NFκB activation partially downregulates transcription of IFN-γ and CXCL10 by DCs (Pietila et al., 2006). However, CCL19 also stimulates the proliferation and metastasis of breast cancer cells, which can only be alleviated by interfering with CCR7 receptivity on tumor cells (Su et al., 2014). Increased levels of CCL19 and CCR7 are also known to be expressed by prostate cancer tissues, and signaling by CCL19 through CCR7 expressed on prostate cancer cells induces cell proliferation (Peng, Zhou, An, & Yang, 2015). CCR7 is expressed by gastric cancer cells, with higher levels of CCR7 expression associated with lymph node metastasis, higher stage tumor, and poor overall survival. Treatment of human gastric cancer cells with CCL19 induced the expression of MMP-9 and decreased levels of E-cadherin, consistent with a shift toward a prometastatic phenotype (Cheng, Guo, Yang, & Yang, 2015). In ovarian cancer, $CCR7^+$ tumor status was also correlated with advanced disease stage and with lymph node metastasis, and these clinical parameters were linked to increased expression of MMP-9 and N-cadherin (Cheng et al., 2014) that were subsequently determined to be dependent upon CCL19 signaling (Cheng et al., 2015).

Interestingly, however, in a metastatic melanoma model, coadministration of CCR7 at the time of adoptive T cell therapy resulted in increased survival, proliferation, and effector function of transferred T cells and led to prolonged survival of $CCR7^+$ T cell-treated mice compared to mice treated with transferred T cells alone (Thanarajasingam et al., 2007). In a lung cancer model, intratumoral injection of recombinant CCR7 led to complete tumor regression concurrent with trafficking of $CD4^+$ and $CD8^+$ T cells to the tumor and to the tumor-draining lymph node (Sharma et al., 2000). This effect was dependent upon T cell recruitment (Sharma et al., 2000) and the recruiting cytokines/chemokines CXCL9, CXCL10, and IFN-γ (Sharma et al., 2003). In the LoVo model of human colorectal cancer, treatment with recombinant CCL19 suppressed tumor growth *in vivo* concurrent with increased serum levels of IL-12 and IFN-γ via a T cell-independent mechanism that involved DC and NK cells

(Lu et al., 2015). Furthermore, results from nontumor models support a beneficial role for CCL21 in generating protective Type 1 immune responses. CCL21 can costimulate effector $CD4^+$ and $CD8^+$ T cells, induce T cell proliferation, and induce a Type 1 polarized immune response characterized by secretion of IFN-γ but not IL-4 or IL-5 (Flanagan, Moroziewicz, Kwak, Hörig, & Kaufman, 2004). When taken together, these results suggest a dual function for CCR7 and its ligands CCL19 and CCL21 in tumor immunity, as CCR7 signaling may promote the formation of TLSs and the recruitment and survival of immune effector cells in an inflammatory microenvironment, or the recruitment of suppressive immune cells such as Tregs and MDSCs and the secretion of regulatory cytokines, depending on context. The precise signals involved with determining the pro- versus antitumor impact of CCR7 and its ligands have not yet been elucidated.

DCs are also recruited to lymphoid organs and activated via CCR7 ligand gradients. After the acquisition of antigen in its local microenvironment and the provision of activation (danger or maturation) signals, DCs upregulate CCR7 on their surface and become competent to migrate in response to secondary lymph node chemokines, CCL19 or CCL21 (Ashour, Turnquist, Singh, Talmadge, & Solheim, 2007; Clatworthy et al., 2014). The ability of DCs to migrate in response to a CCR7 ligand gradient was found to be partially dependent on MMP-9 expression by the DCs (Clatworthy et al., 2014). Subcutaneous injection of CCL21 led to the recruitment of lymphocytic infiltrates into the skin at the site of injection 4 days later. CCL21 injection also led to an increased DC and T cell recruitment to the draining lymph node, and this recruitment also peaked 4 days postinjection (Ashour et al., 2007). In addition to recruiting DCs to sites of inflammation, CCL21 has the ability to boost the T cell priming function of DCs. Human DCs treated with recombinant CCL21 and subsequently peptide pulsed and cocultured with $CD8^+$ T cells were better able to stimulate IFN-γ release from the T cells than peptide-pulsed DCs that were not treated with CCL21. The T cells also expressed slightly elevated levels of perforin, granzyme B, and FasL. Interestingly, this benefit of CCL21 treatment required CXCL10 signaling during the T cell priming phase (Hong, Lee, Kim, & Lee, 2014).

4.4 The Importance of CXCR5 Agonists in TLS Evolution

CXCL13, also known as BLC, is critical for the formation of SLO and TLS. CXCR5 is expressed on the surface of B cells, and these cells migrate toward gradients of CXCL13 expressed by follicular DCs or stromal cells in lymphoid organs (Ohmatsu et al., 2007). Mice deficient in either CXCL13 or its receptor, CXCR5, lack structured lymphoid organs including lymph nodes, Peyer's patches, and spleen, which appears due to a lack of follicular DC networks that are required for the organization of recruited B cells into follicles/germinal centers (Ansel et al., 2000). CXCL13 is under the transcriptional control of LTβR-mediated signaling in all secondary lymphoid organs (Browning et al., 2005), and signaling by CXCL13 through CXCR5 leads to increased cell surface expression of $LT\alpha_1\beta_2$ (Ansel et al., 2000). Interestingly, the CCR7 ligands CCL19 and CCL21 also promote elevated expression of $LT\alpha_1\beta_2$ on the surface of B cells, though to a lesser extent than does CXCL13 (Ansel et al., 2000). In response to infection, DCs and $CD4^+$ T cells are able to upregulate CXCR5, and this promotes the recruitment of B cells to sites of immune priming in lymphoid organs (León et al., 2012). Forced expression of CXCL13 in nonlymphoid organs leads to the formation of lymphoid structures and the recruitment of immune cells into affected tissue sites (Luther, Lopez, Bai, Hanahan, & Cyster, 2000). Interestingly, CXCL13 expression within lymphoid organs appears to be required not only for B cell migration to lymphoid organs but also for antigen presentation to B cells at these sites (Coelho et al., 2013).

Like CCR7 ligand chemokines, CXCL13 appears to play multiple roles within the TME. Although this chemokine is crucial for the recruitment of immune cells into sites of inflammation, it can also mediate the invasion and metastasis of many types of cancer. Colon cancer cell lines commonly express the CXCR5 receptor and are able to proliferate and migrate in response to CXCL13 gradients in a CXCR5-dependent manner (Zhu et al., 2015). Interestingly, the migratory capacity of these colon cancer cells appears to be mediated downstream of CXCR5 signaling by the matrix metalloproteinase MMP-13 (Zhu et al., 2015), consistent with results observed in human colon cancer patients (Zucker & Vacirca, 2004). A similar result has been observed in prostate cancer, as primary prostate cancer tissues and prostate cancer cell lines both express CXCR5. After treatment with CXCL13, prostate cancer cell lines upregulate MMP-1, MMP-2, and MMP-9 and are able to migrate toward a CXCL13 gradient in a CXCR5-dependent manner (Singh et al., 2009). In the Myc-CaP and TRAMP prostate cancer models *in vivo*, CXCL13 is upregulated by myofibroblasts in the tumor stroma downstream of TGF-β in response to hypoxia, and this promotes metastasis and the development of more aggressive, hormone-independent tumors (Ammirante, Shalapour, Kang, Jamieson, &

Karin, 2014). Many subtypes of human lung cancers also express CXCR5. Specifically, adenocarcinomas and squamous cell carcinomas, but not healthy lung tissues, express CXCR5 (Singh, Gupta, Kloecker, Singh, & Lillard, 2014). Furthermore, patients with lung adenocarcinomas or squamous cell carcinomas present with increased serum levels of CXCL13 when compared to healthy patients, and CXCR5-expressing lung cancer cell lines are able to migrate toward a CXCL13 gradient *in vivo* (Singh et al., 2014). In colorectal cancer, both CXCR5 and CXCL13 may be upregulated in malignant compared to normal tissues, and patients with higher expression of CXCR5 and CXCL13 present with a lower 5-year overall survival and lower 5-year progression-free survival when compared to disease stage-matched patients whose tumors were negative for CXCR5 and CXCL13 (Qi et al., 2014). Some breast cancer patients have been shown to express elevated levels of CXCL13 in both the TME and systemically in the peripheral blood (Panse et al., 2008). In particular, patients with metastatic breast cancer present with significantly higher serum levels of CXCL13 when compared to normal controls and to patients whose tumors were resected, suggesting that CXCL13 may be a potential biomarker capable of detecting early metastatic disease in these patients (Panse et al., 2008). Both CXCR5 and CXCL13 have also been shown to be expressed by patients with infiltrating ductal carcinoma, and that their coexpression correlates with lymph node metastasis and an upregulation in expression of MMP-9 in these patients, supporting a role for the CXCR5–CXCL13 axis in promoting epithelial to mesenchymal transition of breast cancer cells (Biswas et al., 2014).

In a clinical trial, the presence of CXCL13 on TILs was associated with a lower occurrence of complete response to treatment in HER2-positive breast cancer patients (Denkert et al., 2014). However, other groups have reported a beneficial role for CXCL13 and CXCR5 in breast cancer. In particular, there was a positive correlation observed between high intratumoral CXCL13 or CXCR5 expression and increased disease-free survival in high-risk HER2-positive, estrogen receptor-low breast cancer patients (Razis et al., 2012). In hormone receptor-positive invasive ductal carcinoma, patients with grade I nontriple negative breast cancer presented with higher intratumoral levels of CXCL13 compared to patients with higher grade (grade II/III) or triple negative tumors (Pimenta et al., 2014). Interestingly, interferon regulatory factor 5 (IRF5), a regulator of CXCL13, is present in some but not all breast cancers, and media conditioned *in vitro* by IRF5-positive tumors is able to recruit B and T cells, while IRF5-negative tumor-conditioned media is not (Pimenta et al., 2014), suggesting that these tumors may secrete CXCL13 *in vivo*, generating a gradient to recruit lymphocytes into the TME. Thus in the cancer setting, increased CXCL13/CXCR5 expression—especially in patients with metastatic disease—may in fact represent a mechanism by which protective immune responses are actively recruited into disease sites.

Overall, work evaluating the role of chemokine signaling in the context of tumor progression suggests that chemokine/chemokine receptor expression may not be entirely beneficial or entirely harmful to the patient. Instead, expression may coordinately mediate immune cell recruitment into the TME as well as promote the metastasis of tumor cells, as many forms of tumor/tumor cell lines have been shown to express chemokines or chemokine receptors. Thus in the context of generating novel therapeutics to cancer, it will be important to balance the positive and the negative effects of enhancing or inhibiting signaling through these pathways. Specifically, it may be useful to stratify patients based on expression of chemokines/chemokine receptors in order to optimize the benefits of targeted (immuno) therapies.

5. THERAPEUTIC MANIPULATION OF TLSs IN CANCER PATIENTS: ESTABLISHING A PARADIGM FOR ANTITUMOR EFFICACY

Our own work in murine models suggests that forced overexpression of cDNA encoding the Type 1 transactivator Tbet within the TME is therapeutic in the cancer setting. In particular, we have shown that DCs engineered to (over)express Tbet (i.e., DC.Tbet) inhibit the growth of CMS4 (BALB/c) and MCA205 (C57BL/6) sarcomas *in vivo* after intratumoral injection, leading to the prolonged overall survival of treated tumor-bearing mice (Chen, Taylor, et al., 2013; Qu, Chen, Lowe, Storkus, & Taylor, 2012). This result is dependent upon the presence of host lymphocytes and NK cells, as RAG1$^{-/-}$ mice and mice depleted of either CD8^{+} T cells or NK cells were not protected from tumor growth by treatment with DC.Tbet (Chen, Taylor, et al., 2013). As T cells and NK cells must be able to traffic to the site of the tumor, it stands to reason that early chemokine signaling plays a key role in the mechanism by which intratumoral delivery of DC.Tbet leads to the recruitment of Type 1-polarized immune cells into the TME. In support of this hypothesis, DC.Tbet (but not control DCs) cells express increased transcript levels for numerous chemokines, including CCL1, CCL4, CCL8, CCL12,

CCL17, CCL25, CCL28, and CXCL12 (Chen, Taylor, et al., 2013). Furthermore, DC.Tbet treatment leads to an upregulation of CXCL9 and CXCL10 in the TME as late as 21 days post-tumor inoculation (Qu et al., 2012). As a set, these chemokines are attractants for T cells, B cells, and NK cells as well as for DCs and monocytes. These results provide a framework by which DC.Tbet promotes a rapid (hours) and sustained (days to weeks) chemokine response to actively recruit and retain immune cells in TLSs within the effectively treated TME.

6. IMPORTANCE OF IL-1 FAMILY MEMBER CYTOKINES IN ESTABLISHING THERAPEUTIC TLSs

The IL-36 family of cytokines is comprised by a recently identified IL-1 subfamily that supports the generation of proinflammatory immune responses. These cytokines share sequence similarities and three-dimensional structures with known IL-1 family members such as IL-1α and IL-1β and were in fact identified using genomics approaches to identify homologous sequences to IL-1 and IL-1Ra (Barton, Herbst, Bosisio, Higgins, & Nicklin, 2000; Busfield et al., 2000). The IL-36 subfamily consists of three agonists (IL-36α, IL-36-β, and IL-36γ, previously referred to as IL-1F6, 8, and 9, respectively) and one antagonist (IL-36Ra/IL-1F5) that signal through a heterodimeric receptor consisting of IL-1Rrp2, a unique receptor, and IL-1RAcP, a co-receptor shared with the IL-1 and IL-33 receptors. Like all IL-1 family members, the IL-36 agonists and IL-1F5 require processing before they become fully active biologically. Indeed, specific truncation of the N-terminus of each of these proteins results in a 10^3–10^5 fold increase in biologic activity when compared to unprocessed, full-length protein (Towne et al., 2011).

Similar to other IL-1 family members, the IL-36 family cytokines lack a signal sequence that directs classical secretion from the cell (Busfield et al., 2000). Instead, both the cleavage and secretion of the IL-36 cytokines occur through a pathway that is also involved in the secretion of IL-1β and IL-18, i.e., pyroptosis. This is a proinflammatory form of cell death that is distinct from apoptosis and requires the processing of the proforms of these cytokines by the noncanonical inflammasome, with the participation of caspase-1 (Lian, Milora, Manupipatpong, & Jensen, 2012; Van de Veerdonk, Netea, Dinarello, & Joosten, 2011). The cytokines themselves are not involved in activating the cell death pathway; instead, recognition of pathogens or danger signals through Toll-like receptors and NOD-like receptors on antigen-presenting cells activate caspase-1, with the secondary release of these proinflammatory cytokines from producer cells undergoing pyroptosis propagating Type-1 immune responses (Bergsbaken, Fink, & Cookson, 2009). In immune cells, IL-36 expression is also induced downstream of IL-18 and Tbet (Bachmann, Scheiermann, Härdle, Pfeilschifter, & Mühl, 2012); in epithelial cells, IL-36 is classified as an alarmin and is induced by cathelicidins such as LL37 (Li et al., 2014). Once released from cells, the IL-36 cytokines have effects on many IL-36R$^+$ cell types throughout the body. In addition to expression on immune cells, in humans, predominant IL-36R expression occurs in the skin, while in mice, receptor expression is more broadly distributed throughout organs including the prostate, esophagus, uterus, seminal vesicle, and paw (Towne et al., 2011). Numerous immune cell subsets also express the IL-36R. In mice, these subsets include DCs, CD4$^+$ T cells, macrophages, and neutrophils but not B cells (Vigne et al., 2011). CD8$^+$ T cell expression of IL-36R is equivocal, with reports either supporting the presence or lack of expression on these immune effector cells (Vigne et al., 2011; Weinstein et al., unpublished). In humans, the receptor has been reported to be expressed by antigen-presenting cells (Foster et al., 2014; Mutamba, Allison, Mahida, Barrow, & Foster, 2012) but not neutrophils, T cells, or B cells (Foster et al., 2014).

Despite speciation in the range of cell types expressing the IL-36 receptor (i.e., between mice and humans), IL-36 ligands appear to induce similar immune responses in both species. Downstream effectors of IL-36 signaling include NFκB, MAPK, ERK1/2, and Jnk. This leads to secretion of IL-6, IL-8, and GM-CSF by IL-36-treated mouse and human transformed cell lines (Towne et al., 2011). Interestingly, in a mouse model of fibrosarcoma (MC57-SIY), NFκB signaling is required in both CD4$^+$ and CD8$^+$ T cells for priming of a Type 1 immune response (as measured by secretion of IFN-γ and TNF-α, and specific lysis of target cells) and control of tumor growth (Barnes et al., 2015). This suggests a possible mechanism by which signaling through the IL-36 receptor via NFκB may promote antitumor immunity.

Among primary cells, IL-36 induces the activation and maturation of human and mouse DCs. In response to treatment with IL-36 agonists, murine DCs upregulate CD80, CD86, and MHCII (Vigne et al., 2011), and human DCs upregulate CD83, CD86, and HLA-DR. Furthermore, IL-36 signaling leads to increased secretion of IL-1β and IL-6 by human DCs (Foster et al., 2014) and IL-1β, IL-6, and IL-12 by mouse DCs (Vigne et al., 2011), strong indications that IL-36 plays a critical role in promoting states of both acute and chronic inflammation. Reports conflict as to which subsets of human DCs express the IL-36 receptor. However, transcript analyses and functional assays suggest that both human plasmacytoid (Mutamba et al., 2012) and myeloid (Foster et al., 2014) DCs may express high levels of IL-36R mRNA and increase proinflammatory cytokine secretion (pDC: IFN-α; mDC: IL-1β, IL-6) in response to signaling through the IL-36 receptor.

Naive murine $CD4^+$ T cells constitutively express the IL-36 receptor and mature in response to IL-36 signaling. In particular, IL-36 (but not other IL-1 family members or IL-12) specifically induces IL-2 secretion and the proliferation of naive $CD4^+$ T cells (Vigne et al., 2012). Treatment of $CD4^+$ T cells with recombinant IL-36β in the presence of antigen leads to the secretion of proinflammatory cytokines/chemokines and the induction of a canonical Type-1 effector cell phenotype characterized by expression of Tbet and secretion of IFN-γ (Vigne et al., 2012). In the presence of IL-12, IL-36 can induce secretion of IFN-γ by $CD4^+$ T cells (Vigne et al., 2012). However, the local cytokine milieu plays a role in conditioning the cellular response to IL-36R agonism. In the absence of IL-12, signaling through the IL-36 receptor instead leads to transcription of GATA3 and secretion of IL-4 in T cells (Vigne et al., 2012). Notably, mice deficient in expression of IL-36R exhibit impaired IFN-γ, IL-6, TNF-α, and nitrite responses to bacterial challenge (Vigne et al., 2012), suggesting that IL-36 plays a crucial role in the initiation of adaptive immunity *in vivo*. It is worth noting that IL-36R expression is lost in Th1-, Th2-, and Th17-polarized $CD4^+$ T cells after they have matured (Vigne et al., 2012).

Although human T cells do not express the IL-36R (Foster et al., 2014), DCs treated with rhIL-36 induce effects on the responding human T cell repertoire that appear similar to those induced directly on murine T cells by rmIL-36. For example, IL-36α-treated DCs enhance allogeneic $CD3^+$ T cell proliferation to a degree greater than mitogen-activated T cells (Mutamba et al., 2012), with human T cells expanded with IL-36-conditioned DCs also secreting increased levels of IFN-γ (Mutamba et al., 2012). Human T cells primed in the presence of IL-36 are likely to be Type 1 polarized, since IL-36β treatment of DCs leads to their secretion of IL-12 and IL-18, which then prompt the transcriptional activation of Tbet in responder T cells (Mutamba et al., 2012).

6.1 IL-36 as an Early Inflammatory Mediator of Lymphoid Organogenesis in Tissues, Including Cancer

In the context of disease, IL-36 family cytokines have been implicated in the pathogenesis of several autoimmune diseases. Most notably, IL-36 signaling plays a major role in skin autoimmune diseases such as psoriasis and dermatitis. Pustular psoriasis may arise from DITRA, a deficiency in the IL-36R antagonist IL-1F5 (Renert-Yuval et al., 2014). A murine model of this disease is characterized by massive immune cell infiltrate into skin lesions of IL-1F5-deficient mice. This infiltrate consists of $CD45^+$ lymphocytes, neutrophils, and macrophages that are recruited into the diseased skin in an IL-36R-dependent manner (Tortola et al., 2012). Mutations in IL-1F5 have also been observed in patients presenting with acute generalized exanthematous pustulosis, a drug-induced side effect that presents with skin lesions containing robust lymphocytic infiltrates (Nakai, Sugiura, Akiyama, & Katoh, 2015; Navarini et al., 2013). It has been hypothesized that individuals with loss-of-function mutations in IL-1F5 are more likely to develop lesional skin diseases. Similar immune infiltrates have been observed in patients presenting with pustular psoriasis, although in this disease setting, the dominant driver of pathogenesis appears to be locoregional overexpression of IL-36R agonist cytokines that leads to increased activation of MAPK and NFκB signaling in lesional skin (He et al., 2013).

The role of IL-36R agonists in the pathogenesis of arthritis remains contentious. Clinical reports suggest that patients with psoriatic arthritis and rheumatoid arthritis express elevated levels of IL-36α in their synovial lining when compared to patients with osteoarthritis, with IL-36α expression correlated with increased production of IL-6 and IL-8 in the affected joints (Frey et al., 2013). Expression of both the IL-36R and IL-36α is increased in the human TNF transgenic mouse model of inflammatory arthritis (*hTNFtg*) concurrent with lymphocytic infiltration into the joints; however, blockade of signaling through the IL-36 receptor using an antagonist antibody did not relieve inflammation (Derer et al., 2014). A similar result was observed in a CIA model (Lamacchia et al., 2013). Thus, in arthritis, IL-36 is likely a contributing factor in disease pathogenesis, but not necessarily a dominant driver as it is in skin autoimmune conditions.

Notably, IL-36 is a downstream target of Tbet (Bachmann et al., 2012), with a positive-feedback loop allowing for IL-36 to induce secondary transcription of Tbet as well (Vigne et al., 2011). In human myeloid cells, silencing of Tbet by siRNA decreased expression of IL-36γ, and expression of IL-36γ by DCs was also dependent upon IL-18/IL-18R signaling via MAPK- and NFκB-dependent pathways. Specifically, the promoter region of IL-36γ contains both Tbet and NFκB-binding sites, with IL-18 signaling inducing Tbet binding to the IL-36γ promoter (Bachmann et al., 2012). Tbet is also expressed in both human and murine DCs, where it has been shown to be critical to DC1 functional polarization and the ability of these

Antigen Presenting Cell (APCs) to activate Type-1 T cell responses *in vivo* (Lugo-Villarino, Maldonado-Lopez, Possemato, Penaranda, & Glimcher, 2003). Interestingly, DC.Tbet generated from $CCR7^{-/-}$ hosts appeared most effective in preventing tumor growth, strongly suggesting that their preferred biology was manifest in the TME and not the TDLN (Chen, Taylor, et al., 2013). Indeed, the antitumor efficacy of intra-tumoral (i.t.)-delivered DC.Tbet appears critically dependent upon TIL recruitment, activation, expansion, and differentiation within the TME. In this context, IL-36 has been shown to bolster T cell proliferation and cytokine secretion, including secretion of IFN-γ (Vigne et al., 2011). Furthermore, CCL1 and CXCL10—chemokines observed to be upregulated by DC.Tbet cells—are known to be upregulated by wild-type DCs after stimulation with IL-36R agonists (Vigne et al., 2011). Thus, we believe that IL-36 is a key early mediator of TLS development in inflamed tissues and that purposeful instigation of IL-36 delivery or production in the TME (via administration of DC.Tbet or an equivalent modality) will have the potential to evolve both humoral and cellular immunity that is protective and/or therapeutic to the cancer-bearing host.

Consistent with the observation that overexpression of IL-36 in tissues correlates with increased immune cell infiltration, results from our laboratory suggest that IL-36 plays a role in the induction of chemokines that can rapidly recruit T and B cells into the inflammatory microenvironment of therapeutically managed tumors. In contrast to concerns for pathologic autoimmunity resulting from such immune infiltrates in psoriasis and arthritis models, this is a highly preferred biologic outcome in the context of cancer.

7. CONCLUSIONS AND FUTURE DIRECTIONS FOR CLINICAL TRANSLATION

Chemokine expression within the TME and the development of TLSs can often, but not always, represent a positive prognostic marker in patients with solid tumors. Due to the differential requirements for effector and regulatory immune cell subsets within the TME of a diverse array of cancer types, immunotherapies designed to promote the recruitment of immune cells into the TME, or those targeting chemokine pathways, must be evaluated on an empirical "case-by-case" basis. Examples of controversial effects of TLSs include the positive effect of TLS presence in metastatic, but not primary, colorectal carcinoma, or the benefit of both Treg and effector T cell infiltration in head and neck cancer (Balermpas et al., 2013;

Fridman et al., 2011), which traditionally arises as a result of prolonged inflammation at the site of disease. Future avenues of research must elucidate whether the presence or absence of certain chemokines, cytokines, or cell populations within the TLSs can predict a patient's ability to mount a successful antitumor immune response secondary to treatment. Although trends in the prognostic value of TLSs are seen within cancer subtypes, it is likely that a better method of stratifying patients for immunotherapy will be to evaluate the specific immune cell infiltrates and chemokines expressed at the time of diagnosis, in order to determine whether enhancing or suppressing the immune response therapeutically is the best course of treatment.

Therapeutic agents targeting TLS-relevant chemokine pathways have thus far been evaluated in mouse tumor models, with forced expression of LIGHT or CCL21 both mediating beneficial therapeutic outcomes against a variety of solid tumors. Further analyses of the pathways involved in beneficial immune responses within the TME have identified additional immunomodulatory agents that may prove to be clinically important targets of immunotherapy. One such chemokine is IL-36, a proinflammatory member of the IL-1 family and potent inducer of NFκB activation in IL-36R$^+$ responder cells and an apparent orchestrator of TLS development in the TME of tumor-bearing mice treated with DC.Tbet cellular therapy *in vivo*. We are currently evaluating the ability of IL-36 to drive Type 1 antitumor immune responses and TLS formation *in vivo*, when used as a single agent or in the context of combination immunotherapies (i.e., vaccines and adoptive T cell transfer).

In summary, recent advances in our understanding of chemokine and cytokine pathways and their role in the generation of lymphoid organs have allowed for a greater appreciation of the dynamic cross talk between immune cell types that occurs within TLSs that form in or proximal to the TME. This paradigm provides a set of biologic endpoints that should be achieved in order to render improved clinical benefit as a consequence of (immuno)therapeutic intervention in cancer patients. Specifically, intratumoral delivery or promotion of TLS-facilitating factors, applied as single agents via viral vectors or transduced cells (i.e., DCs) or direct injection of recombinant proteins into accessible tumor lesions, may allow for the preferential manipulation of protective-over-regulatory TILs within tumor-associated TLSs. Under such conditions, TLS-primed/expanded antitumor immune effector cells may confer systemic clinical benefits (i.e., locoregional treatment of a single lesion may beget circulating immune-mediated regulation of disseminated disease) with minimal anticipated off-target toxicities.

ACKNOWLEDGMENT

The authors wish to thank Drs. Jennifer Taylor and Ronald Fecek for their thoughtful review of this manuscript.

REFERENCES

Alexe, G., Dalgin, G. S., Scanfeld, D., Tamayo, P., Mesirov, J. P., DeLisi, C., et al. (2007). High expression of lymphocyte-associated genes in node-negative HER2+ breast cancers correlates with lower recurrence rates. *Cancer Research*, *67*(22), 10669–10676. http://dx.doi.org/10.1158/0008-5472.CAN-07-0539.

Aloisi, F., & Pujol-Borrell, R. (2006). Lymphoid neogenesis in chronic inflammatory diseases. *Nature Reviews. Immunology*, *6*(3), 205–217. http://dx.doi.org/10.1038/nri1786.

Ammirante, M., Shalapour, S., Kang, Y., Jamieson, C. A. M., & Karin, M. (2014). Tissue injury and hypoxia promote malignant progression of prostate cancer by inducing CXCL13 expression in tumor myofibroblasts. *Proceedings of the National Academy of Sciences of the United States of America*, *111*(41), 14776–14781. http://dx.doi.org/10.1073/pnas.1416498111.

Ansel, K. M., Ngo, V. N., Hyman, P. L., Luther, S. A., Förster, R., Sedgwick, J. D., et al. (2000). A chemokine-driven positive feedback loop organizes lymphoid follicles. *Nature*, *406*(6793), 309–314. http://dx.doi.org/10.1038/35018581.

Ashour, A. E., Turnquist, H. R., Singh, R. K., Talmadge, J. E., & Solheim, J. C. (2007). CCL21-induced immune cell infiltration. *International Immunopharmacology*, 7(2), 272–276. http://dx.doi.org/10.1016/j.intimp.2006.10.004.

Bachmann, M., Scheiermann, P., Härdle, L., Pfeilschifter, J., & Mühl, H. (2012). IL-36γ/IL-1F9, an innate T-bet target in myeloid cells. *The Journal of Biological Chemistry*, *287*(50), 41684–41696. http://dx.doi.org/10.1074/jbc.M112.385443.

Badr, G., Borhis, G., Treton, D., & Richard, Y. (2005). IFN{alpha} enhances human B-cell chemotaxis by modulating ligand-induced chemokine receptor signaling and internalization. *International Immunology*, *17*(4), 459–467. http://dx.doi.org/10.1093/intimm/dxh227.

Balermpas, P., Michel, Y., Wagenblast, J., Seitz, O., Weiss, C., Rödel, F., et al. (2013). Tumour-infiltrating lymphocytes predict response to definitive chemoradiotherapy in head and neck cancer. *British Journal of Cancer*, *110*(2), 501–509. http://dx.doi.org/10.1038/bjc.2013.640.

Barnes, S. E., Wang, Y., Chen, L., Molinero, L. L., Gajewski, T. F., Evaristo, C., et al. (2015). T cell-NF-κB activation is required for tumor control *in vivo*. *Journal for Immunotherapy of Cancer*, *3*(1), 1. http://dx.doi.org/10.1186/s40425-014-0045-x.

Barton, J. L., Herbst, R., Bosisio, D., Higgins, L., & Nicklin, M. J. (2000). A tissue specific IL-1 receptor antagonist homolog from the IL-1 cluster lacks IL-1, IL-1ra, IL-18 and IL-18 antagonist activities. *European Journal of Immunology*, *30*(11), 3299–3308. http://dx.doi.org/10.1002/1521-4141(200011)30:11<3299::AID-IMMU3299>3.0.CO;2-S.

Behr, D. S., Peitsch, W. K., Hametner, C., Lasitschka, F., Houben, R., Schönhaar, K., et al. (2014). Prognostic value of immune cell infiltration, tertiary lymphoid structures and PD-L1 expression in Merkel cell carcinomas. *International Journal of Clinical and Experimental Pathology*, 7(11), 7610–7621. Retrieved from http://www.pubmedcentral.nih.gov/articlerender.fcgi?artid=4270630&tool=pmcentrez&rendertype=abstra.

Bergsbaken, T., Fink, S. L., & Cookson, B. T. (2009). Pyroptosis: Host cell death and inflammation. *Nature Reviews. Microbiology*, 7(2), 99–109. http://dx.doi.org/10.1038/nrmicro2070.

Biswas, S., Sengupta, S., Roy Chowdhury, S., Jana, S., Mandal, G., Mandal, P. K., et al. (2014). CXCL13-CXCR5 co-expression regulates epithelial to mesenchymal transition of breast cancer cells during lymph node metastasis. *Breast Cancer Research and Treatment*, *143*(2), 265–276. http://dx.doi.org/10.1007/s10549-013-2811-8.

Browning, J. L., Allaire, N., Ngam-Ek, A., Notidis, E., Hunt, J., Perrin, S., et al. (2005). Lymphotoxin-beta receptor signaling is required for the homeostatic control of HEV differentiation and function. *Immunity*, *23*(5), 539–550. http://dx.doi.org/10.1016/j.immuni.2005.10.002.

Busfield, S. J., Comrack, C. A., Yu, G., Chickering, T. W., Smutko, J. S., Zhou, H., et al. (2000). Identification and gene organization of three novel members of the IL-1 family on human chromosome 2. *Genomics*, *66*(2), 213–216. http://dx.doi.org/10.1006/geno.2000.6184.

Chen, L., Fabian, K. L., Taylor, J. L., & Storkus, W. J. (2013). Therapeutic use of dendritic cells to promote the extranodal priming of anti-tumor immunity. *Frontiers in Immunology*, *4*, 388. http://dx.doi.org/10.3389/fimmu.2013.00388.

Chen, S.-C., Leach, M. W., Chen, Y., Cai, X.-Y., Sullivan, L., Wiekowski, M., et al. (2002). Central nervous system inflammation and neurological disease in transgenic mice expressing the CC chemokine CCL21 in oligodendrocytes. *The Journal of Immunology*, *168*(3), 1009–1017. http://dx.doi.org/10.4049/jimmunol.168.3.1009.

Chen, L., Taylor, J. L., Sabins, N. C., Lowe, D. B., Qu, Y., You, Z., et al. (2013). Extranodal induction of therapeutic immunity in the tumor microenvironment after intratumoral delivery of Tbet gene-modified dendritic cells. *Cancer Gene Therapy*, *20*(8), 469–477. http://dx.doi.org/10.1038/cgt.2013.42.

Chen, S.-C., Vassileva, G., Kinsley, D., Holzmann, S., Manfra, D., Wiekowski, M. T., et al. (2002). Ectopic expression of the murine chemokines CCL21a and CCL21b induces the formation of lymph node-like structures in pancreas, but not skin, of transgenic mice. *The Journal of Immunology*, *168*(3), 1001–1008. http://dx.doi.org/10.4049/jimmunol.168.3.1001.

Cheng, S., Guo, J., Yang, Q., & Yang, X. (2015). Crk-like adapter protein regulates CCL19/CCR7-mediated epithelial-to-mesenchymal transition via ERK signaling pathway in epithelial ovarian carcinomas. *Medical Oncology (Northwood, London, England)*, *32*(3), 47. http://dx.doi.org/10.1007/s12032-015-0494-1.

Cheng, S., Han, L., Guo, J., Yang, Q., Zhou, J., & Yang, X. (2014). The essential roles of CCR7 in epithelial-to-mesenchymal transition induced by hypoxia in epithelial ovarian carcinomas. *Tumour Biology: The Journal of the International Society for Oncodevelopmental Biology and Medicine*, *35*(12), 12293–12298. http://dx.doi.org/10.1007/s13277-014-2540-6.

Clatworthy, M. R., Aronin, C. E. P., Mathews, R. J., Morgan, N. Y., Smith, K. G. C., & Germain, R. N. (2014). Immune complexes stimulate CCR7-dependent dendritic cell migration to lymph nodes. *Nature Medicine*, *20*(12), 1458–1463. http://dx.doi.org/10.1038/nm.3709.

Coelho, F. M., Natale, D., Soriano, S. F., Hons, M., Swoger, J., Mayer, J., et al. (2013). Naive B-cell trafficking is shaped by local chemokine availability and LFA-1-independent stromal interactions. *Blood*, *121*(20), 4101–4109. http://dx.doi.org/10.1182/blood-2012-10-465336.

Comerford, I., Milasta, S., Morrow, V., Milligan, G., & Nibbs, R. (2006). The chemokine receptor CCX-CKR mediates effective scavenging of CCL19 *in vitro*. *European Journal of Immunology*, *36*(7), 1904–1916. http://dx.doi.org/10.1002/eji.200535716.

De Chaisemartin, L., Goc, J., Damotte, D., Validire, P., Magdeleinat, P., Alifano, M., et al. (2011). Characterization of chemokines and adhesion molecules associated with T cell presence in tertiary lymphoid structures in human lung cancer. *Cancer Research*, *71*(20), 6391–6399. http://dx.doi.org/10.1158/0008-5472.CAN-11-0952.

Degli-Esposti, M. A., Davis-Smith, T., Din, W. S., Smolak, P. J., Goodwin, R. G., & Smith, C. A. (1997). Activation of the lymphotoxin beta receptor by cross-linking induces chemokine production and growth arrest in A375 melanoma cells. *Journal of*

Immunology (Baltimore, Md: 1950), *158*(4), 1756–1762. Retrieved from http://www.jimmunol.org/content/158/4/1756.abstract.

Denkert, C., Loibl, S., Noske, A., Roller, M., Müller, B. M., Komor, M., et al. (2010). Tumor-associated lymphocytes as an independent predictor of response to neoadjuvant chemotherapy in breast cancer. *Journal of Clinical Oncology: Official Journal of the American Society of Clinical Oncology*, *28*(1), 105–113. http://dx.doi.org/10.1200/JCO.2009.23.7370.

Denkert, C., von Minckwitz, G., Brase, J. C., Sinn, B. V., Gade, S., Kronenwett, R., et al. (2014). Tumor-Infiltrating lymphocytes and response to neoadjuvant chemotherapy with or without carboplatin in human epidermal growth factor receptor 2-positive and triple-negative primary breast cancers. *Journal of Clinical Oncology: Official Journal of the American Society of Clinical Oncology, JCO*, *33*(9), 983–991. http://dx.doi.org/10.1200/JCO.2014.58.1967.

Derer, A., Groetsch, B., Harre, U., Böhm, C., Towne, J., Schett, G., et al. (2014). Blockade of IL-36 receptor signaling does not prevent from TNF-induced arthritis. *PLoS One*, *9*(8). http://dx.doi.org/10.1371/journal.pone.0101954, e101954.

Dieu-Nosjean, M.-C., Antoine, M., Danel, C., Heudes, D., Wislez, M., Poulot, V., et al. (2008). Long-term survival for patients with non-small-cell lung cancer with intratumoral lymphoid structures. *Journal of Clinical Oncology: Official Journal of the American Society of Clinical Oncology*, *26*(27), 4410–4417. http://dx.doi.org/10.1200/JCO.2007.15.0284.

DiLillo, D. J., Yanaba, K., & Tedder, T. F. (2010). B cells are required for optimal CD4+ and CD8+ T cell tumor immunity: Therapeutic B cell depletion enhances B16 melanoma growth in mice. *Journal of Immunology (Baltimore, Md: 1950)*, *184*(7), 4006–4016. http://dx.doi.org/10.4049/jimmunol.0903009.

Dobner, B. C., Riechardt, A. I., Joussen, A. M., Englert, S., & Bechrakis, N. E. (2012). Expression of haematogenous and lymphogenous chemokine receptors and their ligands on uveal melanoma in association with liver metastasis. *Acta Ophthalmologica*, *90*(8), e638–e644. http://dx.doi.org/10.1111/j.1755-3768.2012.02515.x.

Dohi, T., Rennert, P. D., Fujihashi, K., Kiyono, H., Shirai, Y., Kawamura, Y. I., et al. (2001). Elimination of colonic patches with lymphotoxin receptor-Ig prevents Th2 cell-type colitis. *The Journal of Immunology*, *167*(5), 2781–2790. http://dx.doi.org/10.4049/jimmunol.167.5.2781.

Drayton, D. L., Ying, X., Lee, J., Lesslauer, W., & Ruddle, N. H. (2003). Ectopic LT alpha beta directs lymphoid organ neogenesis with concomitant expression of peripheral node addressin and a HEV-restricted sulfotransferase. *The Journal of Experimental Medicine*, *197*(9), 1153–1163. http://dx.doi.org/10.1084/jem.20021761.

Fan, Z., Yu, P., Wang, Y., Wang, Y., Fu, M. L., Liu, W., et al. (2006). NK-cell activation by LIGHT triggers tumor-specific CD8+ T-cell immunity to reject established tumors. *Blood*, *107*(4), 1342–1351. http://dx.doi.org/10.1182/blood-2005-08-3485.

Flanagan, K., Moroziewicz, D., Kwak, H., Hörig, H., & Kaufman, H. L. (2004). The lymphoid chemokine CCL21 costimulates naive T cell expansion and Th1 polarization of non-regulatory CD4+ T cells. *Cellular Immunology*, *231*(1–2), 75–84. http://dx.doi.org/10.1016/j.cellimm.2004.12.006.

Foster, A. M., Baliwag, J., Chen, C. S., Guzman, A. M., Stoll, S. W., Gudjonsson, J. E., et al. (2014). IL-36 promotes myeloid cell infiltration, activation, and inflammatory activity in skin. *Journal of Immunology (Baltimore, Md: 1950)*, *192*(12), 6053–6061. http://dx.doi.org/10.4049/jimmunol.1301481.

Frey, S., Derer, A., Messbacher, M.-E., Baeten, D. L. P., Bugatti, S., Montecucco, C., et al. (2013). The novel cytokine interleukin-36α is expressed in psoriatic and rheumatoid arthritis synovium. *Annals of the Rheumatic Diseases*, *72*(9), 1569–1574. http://dx.doi.org/10.1136/annrheumdis-2012-202264.

Fridman, W. H., Galon, J., Dieu-Nosjean, M.-C., Cremer, I., Fisson, S., Damotte, D., et al. (2011). Immune infiltration in human cancer: Prognostic significance and disease control. *Current Topics in Microbiology and Immunology, 344*, 1–24. http://dx.doi.org/10.1007/82_2010_46.

Fridman, W. H., Pagès, F., Sautès-Fridman, C., & Galon, J. (2012). The immune contexture in human tumours: Impact on clinical outcome. *Nature Reviews. Cancer, 12*(4), 298–306. http://dx.doi.org/10.1038/nrc3245.

Gantsev, S. K., Umezawa, K., Islamgulov, D. V., Khusnutdinova, E. K., Ishmuratova, R. S., Frolova, V. Y., et al. (2013). The role of inflammatory chemokines in lymphoid neoorganogenesis in breast cancer. *Biomedicine & Pharmacotherapy = Biomédecine & Pharmacothérapie, 67*(5), 363–366. http://dx.doi.org/10.1016/j.biopha.2013.03.017.

Germain, C., Gnjatic, S., Tamzalit, F., Knockaert, S., Remark, R., Goc, J., et al. (2014). Presence of B cells in tertiary lymphoid structures is associated with a protective immunity in patients with lung cancer. *American Journal of Respiratory and Critical Care Medicine, 189*(7), 832–844. http://dx.doi.org/10.1164/rccm.201309-1611OC.

Goc, J., Fridman, W.-H., Hammond, S. A., Sautès-Fridman, C., & Dieu-Nosjean, M.-C. (2014). Tertiary lymphoid structures in human lung cancers, a new driver of antitumor immune responses. *Oncoimmunology, 3*, e28976. http://dx.doi.org/10.4161/onci.28976.

Goc, J., Germain, C., Vo-Bourgais, T. K. D., Lupo, A., Klein, C., Knockaert, S., et al. (2014). Dendritic cells in tumor-associated tertiary lymphoid structures signal a Th1 cytotoxic immune contexture and license the positive prognostic value of infiltrating CD8+ T cells. *Cancer Research, 74*(3), 705–715. http://dx.doi.org/10.1158/0008-5472.CAN-13-1342.

Gonzalez, M., Mackay, F., Browning, J. L., Kosco-Vilbois, M. H., & Noelle, R. J. (1998). The sequential role of lymphotoxin and B cells in the development of splenic follicles. *The Journal of Experimental Medicine, 187*(7), 997–1007. Retrieved from http://www.pubmedcentral.nih.gov/articlerender.fcgi?artid=2212214&tool=pmcentrez&rendertype=abstract.

Gu-Trantien, C., Loi, S., Garaud, S., Equeter, C., Libin, M., de Wind, A., et al. (2013). $CD4^+$ follicular helper T cell infiltration predicts breast cancer survival. *The Journal of Clinical Investigation, 123*(7), 2873–2892. http://dx.doi.org/10.1172/JCI67428.

Haybaeck, J., Zeller, N., Wolf, M. J., Weber, A., Wagner, U., Kurrer, M. O., et al. (2009). A lymphotoxin-driven pathway to hepatocellular carcinoma. *Cancer Cell, 16*(4), 295–308. http://dx.doi.org/10.1016/j.ccr.2009.08.021.

He, Q., Chen, H., Li, W., Wu, Y., Chen, S., Yue, Q., et al. (2013). IL-36 cytokine expression and its relationship with p38 MAPK and NF-κB pathways in psoriasis vulgaris skin lesions. *Journal of Huazhong University of Science and Technology. Medical Sciences = Hua Zhong Ke Ji Da Xue Xue Bao. Yi Xue Ying De Wen Ban = Huazhong Keji Daxue Xuebao. Yixue Yingdewen Ban, 33*(4), 594–599. http://dx.doi.org/10.1007/s11596-013-1164-1.

Hedrick, J. A., & Zlotnik, A. (1997). Identification and characterization of a novel beta chemokine containing six conserved cysteines. *Journal of Immunology (Baltimore, Md: 1950), 159*(4), 1589–1593. Retrieved from http://www.jimmunol.org/content/159/4/1589.abstract.

Heo, S.-K., Ju, S.-A., Kim, G. Y., Park, S.-M., Back, S. H., Park, N.-H., et al. (2012). The presence of high level soluble herpes virus entry mediator in sera of gastric cancer patients. *Experimental & Molecular Medicine, 44*(2), 149–158. http://dx.doi.org/10.3858/emm.2012.44.2.010.

Holmes, T. D., Wilson, E. B., Black, E. V. I., Benest, A. V., Vaz, C., Tan, B., et al. (2014). Licensed human natural killer cells aid dendritic cell maturation via TNFSF14/LIGHT. *Proceedings of the National Academy of Sciences of the United States of America, 111*(52), E5688–E5696. http://dx.doi.org/10.1073/pnas.1411072112.

Hong, C. Y., Lee, H.-J., Kim, H.-J., & Lee, J.-J. (2014). The lymphoid chemokine CCL21 enhances the cytotoxic T lymphocyte-inducing functions of dendritic cells. *Scandinavian Journal of Immunology*, *79*(3), 173–180. http://dx.doi.org/10.1111/sji.12145.

Hu, G., Liu, Y., Li, H., Zhao, D., Yang, L., Shen, J., et al. (2010). Adenovirus-mediated LIGHT gene modification in murine B-cell lymphoma elicits a potent antitumor effect. *Cellular & Molecular Immunology*, 7(4), 296–305. http://dx.doi.org/10.1038/cmi.2010.15.

Jung, H. W., La, S. J., Kim, J. Y., Heo, S. K., Kim, J. Y., Wang, S., et al. (2003). High levels of soluble herpes virus entry mediator in sera of patients with allergic and autoimmune diseases. *Experimental & Molecular Medicine*, *35*(6), 501–508. http://dx.doi.org/10.1038/emm.2003.65.

Jung, Y. W., Rutishauser, R. L., Joshi, N. S., Haberman, A. M., & Kaech, S. M. (2010). Differential localization of effector and memory CD8 T cell subsets in lymphoid organs during acute viral infection. *Journal of Immunology (Baltimore, Md: 1950)*, *185*(9), 5315–5325. http://dx.doi.org/10.4049/jimmunol.1001948.

Kanodia, S., Da Silva, D. M., Karamanukyan, T., Bogaert, L., Fu, Y.-X., & Kast, W. M. (2010). Expression of LIGHT/TNFSF14 combined with vaccination against human papillomavirus Type 16 E7 induces significant tumor regression. *Cancer Research*, *70*(10), 3955–3964. http://dx.doi.org/10.1158/0008-5472.CAN-09-3773.

Kossenkov, A. V., Dawany, N., Evans, T. L., Kucharczuk, J. C., Albelda, S. M., Showe, L. C., et al. (2012). Peripheral immune cell gene expression predicts survival of patients with non-small cell lung cancer. *PLoS One*, 7(3), e34392. http://dx.doi.org/10.1371/journal.pone.0034392.

Lamacchia, C., Palmer, G., Rodriguez, E., Martin, P., Vigne, S., Seemayer, C. A., et al. (2013). The severity of experimental arthritis is independent of IL-36 receptor signaling. *Arthritis Research & Therapy*, *15*(2), R38. http://dx.doi.org/10.1186/ar4192.

Legler, D. F., Uetz-von Allmen, E., & Hauser, M. A. (2014). CCR7: Roles in cancer cell dissemination, migration and metastasis formation. *The International Journal of Biochemistry & Cell Biology*, *54*, 78–82. http://dx.doi.org/10.1016/j.biocel.2014.07.002.

León, B., Ballesteros-Tato, A., Browning, J. L., Dunn, R., Randall, T. D., & Lund, F. E. (2012). Regulation of T(H)2 development by CXCR5+ dendritic cells and lymphotoxin-expressing B cells. *Nature Immunology*, *13*(7), 681–690. http://dx.doi.org/10.1038/ni.2309.

Li, N., Yamasaki, K., Saito, R., Fukushi-Takahashi, S., Shimada-Omori, R., Asano, M., et al. (2014). Alarmin function of cathelicidin antimicrobial peptide LL37 through IL-36γ induction in human epidermal keratinocytes. *Journal of Immunology (Baltimore, Md: 1950)*, *193*(10), 5140–5148. http://dx.doi.org/10.4049/jimmunol.1302574.

Lian, L.-H., Milora, K. A., Manupipatpong, K. K., & Jensen, L. E. (2012). The double-stranded RNA analogue polyinosinic-polycytidylic acid induces keratinocyte pyroptosis and release of IL-36γ. *The Journal of Investigative Dermatology*, *132*(5), 1346–1353. http://dx.doi.org/10.1038/jid.2011.482.

Lin, W.-W., & Hsieh, S.-L. (2011). Decoy receptor 3: A pleiotropic immunomodulator and biomarker for inflammatory diseases, autoimmune diseases and cancer. *Biochemical Pharmacology*, *81*(7), 838–847. http://dx.doi.org/10.1016/j.bcp.2011.01.011.

Lu, J., Ma, J., Cai, W., Wangpu, X., Feng, H., Zhao, J., et al. (2015). CC motif chemokine ligand 19 suppressed colorectal cancer *in vivo* accompanied by an increase in IL-12 and IFN-γ. *Biomedicine & Pharmacotherapy = Biomédecine & Pharmacothérapie*, *69*, 374–379. http://dx.doi.org/10.1016/j.biopha.2014.12.032.

Lugo-Villarino, G., Maldonado-Lopez, R., Possemato, R., Penaranda, C., & Glimcher, L. H. (2003). T-bet is required for optimal production of IFN-gamma and antigen-specific T cell activation by dendritic cells. *Proceedings of the National Academy of Sciences of the United States of America, 100*(13), 7749–7754. http://dx.doi.org/10.1073/pnas.1332767100.

Luther, S. A., Bidgol, A., Hargreaves, D. C., Schmidt, A., Xu, Y., Paniyadi, J., et al. (2002). Differing activities of homeostatic chemokines CCL19, CCL21, and CXCL12 in lymphocyte and dendritic cell recruitment and lymphoid neogenesis. *The Journal of Immunology, 169*(1), 424–433. http://dx.doi.org/10.4049/jimmunol.169.1.424.

Luther, S. A., Lopez, T., Bai, W., Hanahan, D., & Cyster, J. G. (2000). BLC expression in pancreatic islets causes B cell recruitment and lymphotoxin-dependent lymphoid neogenesis. *Immunity, 12*(5), 471–481. http://dx.doi.org/10.1016/S1074-7613(00)80199-5.

Mahmoud, S. M. A., Lee, A. H. S., Paish, E. C., Macmillan, R. D., Ellis, I. O., & Green, A. R. (2012). The prognostic significance of B lymphocytes in invasive carcinoma of the breast. *Breast Cancer Research and Treatment, 132*(2), 545–553. http://dx.doi.org/10.1007/s10549-011-1620-1.

Mauri, D. N., Ebner, R., Montgomery, R. I., Kochel, K. D., Cheung, T. C., Yu, G.-L., et al. (1998). LIGHT, a new member of the TNF superfamily, and lymphotoxin α are ligands for herpesvirus entry mediator. *Immunity, 8*(1), 21–30. http://dx.doi.org/10.1016/S1074-7613(00)80455-0.

Meshcheryakova, A., Tamandl, D., Bajna, E., Stift, J., Mittlboeck, M., Svoboda, M., et al. (2014). B cells and ectopic follicular structures: Novel players in anti-tumor programming with prognostic power for patients with metastatic colorectal cancer. *PLoS One, 9*(6), e99008. http://dx.doi.org/10.1371/journal.pone.0099008.

Messina, J. L., Fenstermacher, D. A., Eschrich, S., Qu, X., Berglund, A. E., Lloyd, M. C., et al. (2012). 12-Chemokine gene signature identifies lymph node-like structures in melanoma: Potential for patient selection for immunotherapy? *Scientific Reports, 2*, 765. http://dx.doi.org/10.1038/srep00765.

Miyagaki, T., Sugaya, M., Suga, H., Morimura, S., Ohmatsu, H., Fujita, H., et al. (2012). Low herpesvirus entry mediator (HVEM) expression on dermal fibroblasts contributes to a Th2-dominant microenvironment in advanced cutaneous T-cell lymphoma. *The Journal of Investigative Dermatology, 132*(4), 1280–1289. http://dx.doi.org/10.1038/jid.2011.470.

Morishige, T., Yoshioka, Y., Inakura, H., Tanabe, A., Yao, X., Tsunoda, S., et al. (2010). Creation of a LIGHT mutant with the capacity to evade the decoy receptor for cancer therapy. *Biomaterials, 31*(12), 3357–3363. http://dx.doi.org/10.1016/j.biomaterials.2010.01.022.

Mulé, J. J. (2009). Dendritic cell-based vaccines for pancreatic cancer and melanoma. *Annals of the New York Academy of Sciences, 1174*(1), 33–40. http://dx.doi.org/10.1111/j.1749-6632.2009.04936.x.

Mutamba, S., Allison, A., Mahida, Y., Barrow, P., & Foster, N. (2012). Expression of IL-1Rrp2 by human myelomonocytic cells is unique to DCs and facilitates DC maturation by IL-1F8 and IL-1F9. *European Journal of Immunology, 42*(3), 607–617. http://dx.doi.org/10.1002/eji.201142035.

Nakai, N., Sugiura, K., Akiyama, M., & Katoh, N. (2015). Acute generalized exanthematous pustulosis caused by dihydrocodeine phosphate in a patient with psoriasis vulgaris and a heterozygous IL36RN mutation. *JAMA Dermatology, 151*, 311–315. http://dx.doi.org/10.1001/jamadermatol.2014.3002.

Nakano, H., & Gunn, M. D. (2001). Gene duplications at the chemokine locus on mouse chromosome 4: Multiple strain-specific haplotypes and the deletion of secondary lymphoid-organ chemokine and ebi-1 ligand chemokine genes in the plt mutation. *The Journal of Immunology, 166*(1), 361–369. http://dx.doi.org/10.4049/jimmunol.166.1.361.

Navarini, A. A., Valeyrie-Allanore, L., Setta-Kaffetzi, N., Barker, J. N., Capon, F., Creamer, D., et al. (2013). Rare variations in IL36RN in severe adverse drug reactions manifesting as acute generalized exanthematous pustulosis. *The Journal of Investigative Dermatology*, *133*(7), 1904–1907. http://dx.doi.org/10.1038/jid.2013.44.

Nzula, S., Going, J. J., & Stott, D. I. (2003). Antigen-driven clonal proliferation, somatic hypermutation, and selection of B lymphocytes infiltrating human ductal breast carcinomas. *Cancer Research*, *63*(12), 3275–3280. Retrieved from http://cancerres.aacrjournals.org/content/63/12/3275.full.

Ohmatsu, H., Sugaya, M., Kadono, T., & Tamaki, K. (2007). CXCL13 and CCL21 are expressed in ectopic lymphoid follicles in cutaneous lymphoproliferative disorders. *The Journal of Investigative Dermatology*, *127*(10), 2466–2468. http://dx.doi.org/10.1038/sj.jid.5700873.

Pahne-Zeppenfeld, J., Schröer, N., Walch-Rückheim, B., Oldak, M., Gorter, A., Hegde, S., et al. (2014). Cervical cancer cell-derived interleukin-6 impairs CCR7-dependent migration of MMP-9-expressing dendritic cells. *International Journal of Cancer. Journal International Du Cancer*, *134*(9), 2061–2073. http://dx.doi.org/10.1002/ijc.28549.

Panse, J., Friedrichs, K., Marx, A., Hildebrandt, Y., Luetkens, T., Barrels, K., et al. (2008). Chemokine CXCL13 is overexpressed in the tumour tissue and in the peripheral blood of breast cancer patients. *British Journal of Cancer*, *99*(6), 930–938. http://dx.doi.org/10.1038/sj.bjc.6604621.

Peng, C., Zhou, K., An, S., & Yang, J. (2015). The effect of CCL19/CCR7 on the proliferation and migration of cell in prostate cancer. *Tumour Biology: The Journal of the International Society for Oncodevelopmental Biology and Medicine*, *36*(1), 329–335. http://dx.doi.org/10.1007/s13277-014-2642-1.

Pickens, S. R., Chamberlain, N. D., Volin, M. V., Pope, R. M., Talarico, N. E., Mandelin, A. M., et al. (2012). Role of the CCL21 and CCR7 pathways in rheumatoid arthritis angiogenesis. *Arthritis and Rheumatism*, *64*(8), 2471–2481. http://dx.doi.org/10.1002/art.34452.

Pietila, T. E., Veckman, V., Lehtonen, A., Lin, R., Hiscott, J., & Julkunen, I. (2006). Multiple NF- B and IFN regulatory factor family transcription factors regulate CCL19 gene expression in human monocyte-derived dendritic cells. *The Journal of Immunology*, *178*(1), 253–261. http://dx.doi.org/10.4049/jimmunol.178.1.253.

Pimenta, E. M., & Barnes, B. J. (2014). Role of tertiary lymphoid structures (TLS) in anti-tumor immunity: Potential tumor-induced cytokines/chemokines that regulate TLS formation in epithelial-derived cancers. *Cancers*, *6*(2), 969–997. http://dx.doi.org/10.3390/cancers6020969.

Pimenta, E. M., De, S., Weiss, R., Feng, D., Hall, K., Kilic, S., et al. (2014). IRF5 is a novel regulator of CXCL13 expression in breast cancer that regulates CXCR5(+) B- and T-cell trafficking to tumor-conditioned media. *Immunology and Cell Biology*, *92*, 331–339. http://dx.doi.org/10.1038/icb.2014.110.

Pitzalis, C., Jones, G. W., Bombardieri, M., & Jones, S. A. (2014). Ectopic lymphoid-like structures in infection, cancer and autoimmunity. *Nature Reviews. Immunology*, *14*(7), 447–462. http://dx.doi.org/10.1038/nri3700.

Qi, X.-W., Xia, S.-H., Yin, Y., Jin, L.-F., Pu, Y., Hua, D., et al. (2014). Expression features of CXCR5 and its ligand, CXCL13 associated with poor prognosis of advanced colorectal cancer. *European Review for Medical and Pharmacological Sciences*, *18*(13), 1916–1924. Retrieved February 21, 2015, from http://www.europeanreview.org/article/7571.

Qin, J. Z., Upadhyay, V., Prabhakar, B., & Maker, A. V. (2013). Shedding LIGHT (TNFSF14) on the tumor microenvironment of colorectal cancer liver metastases. *Journal of Translational Medicine*, *11*, 70. http://dx.doi.org/10.1186/1479-5876-11-70.

Qu, Y., Chen, L., Lowe, D. B., Storkus, W. J., & Taylor, J. L. (2012). Combined Tbet and IL12 gene therapy elicits and recruits superior antitumor immunity *in vivo*. *Molecular*

Therapy: The Journal of the American Society of Gene Therapy, *20*(3), 644–651. http://dx.doi.org/10.1038/mt.2011.283.

Razis, E., Kalogeras, K. T., Kotoula, V., Eleftheraki, A. G., Nikitas, N., Kronenwett, R., et al. (2012). Improved outcome of high-risk early HER2 positive breast cancer with high CXCL13-CXCR5 messenger RNA expression. *Clinical Breast Cancer*, *12*(3), 183–193. http://dx.doi.org/10.1016/j.clbc.2012.03.006.

Renert-Yuval, Y., Horev, L., Babay, S., Tams, S., Ramot, Y., Zlotogorski, A., et al. (2014). IL36RN mutation causing generalized pustular psoriasis in a Palestinian patient. *International Journal of Dermatology*, *53*(7), 866–868. http://dx.doi.org/10.1111/ijd.12525.

Salama, P., Phillips, M., Grieu, F., Morris, M., Zeps, N., Joseph, D., et al. (2008). Tumor-infiltrating FOXP3+ T regulatory cells show strong prognostic significance in colorectal cancer. *Journal of Clinical Oncology*, *27*(2), 186–192. http://dx.doi.org/10.1200/JCO.2008.18.7229.

Sanchez-Sanchez, N., Riol-Blanco, L., & Rodriguez-Fernandez, J. L. (2006). The multiple personalities of the chemokine receptor CCR7 in dendritic cells. *The Journal of Immunology*, *176*(9), 5153–5159. http://dx.doi.org/10.4049/jimmunol.176.9.5153.

Schneider, M. A., Meingassner, J. G., Lipp, M., Moore, H. D., & Rot, A. (2007). CCR7 is required for the *in vivo* function of CD4+ CD25+ regulatory T cells. *The Journal of Experimental Medicine*, *204*(4), 735–745. http://dx.doi.org/10.1084/jem.20061405.

Schneider, K., Potter, K. G., & Ware, C. F. (2004). Lymphotoxin and LIGHT signaling pathways and target genes. *Immunological Reviews*, *202*, 49–66. http://dx.doi.org/10.1111/j.0105-2896.2004.00206.x.

Sharma, S., Stolina, M., Luo, J., Strieter, R. M., Burdick, M., Zhu, L. X., et al. (2000). Secondary lymphoid tissue chemokine mediates T cell-dependent antitumor responses *in vivo*. *The Journal of Immunology*, *164*(9), 4558–4563. http://dx.doi.org/10.4049/jimmunol.164.9.4558.

Sharma, S., Yang, S.-C., Hillinger, S., Zhu, L. X., Huang, M., Batra, R. K., et al. (2003). SLC/CCL21-mediated anti-tumor responses require IFNgamma, MIG/CXCL9 and IP-10/CXCL10. *Molecular Cancer*, *2*, 22. Retrieved from http://www.pubmedcentral.nih.gov/articlerender.fcgi?artid=155639&tool=pmcentrez&rendertype=abstract.

Shi, J.-Y., Yang, L.-X., Wang, Z.-C., Wang, L.-Y., Zhou, J., Wang, X.-Y., et al. (2015). CC chemokine receptor-like 1 functions as a tumour suppressor by impairing CCR7-related chemotaxis in hepatocellular carcinoma. *The Journal of Pathology*, *235*(4), 546–558. http://dx.doi.org/10.1002/path.4450.

Shields, J. D., Kourtis, I. C., Tomei, A. A., Roberts, J. M., & Swartz, M. A. (2010). Induction of lymphoidlike stroma and immune escape by tumors that express the chemokine CCL21. *Science (New York, N.Y.)*, *328*(5979), 749–752. http://dx.doi.org/10.1126/science.1185837.

Singh, R., Gupta, P., Kloecker, G. H., Singh, S., & Lillard, J. W. (2014). Expression and clinical significance of CXCR5/CXCL13 in human non-small cell lung carcinoma. *International Journal of Oncology*, *45*(6), 2232–2240. http://dx.doi.org/10.3892/ijo.2014.2688.

Singh, S., Singh, R., Singh, U. P., Rai, S. N., Novakovic, K. R., Chung, L. W. K., et al. (2009). Clinical and biological significance of CXCR5 expressed by prostate cancer specimens and cell lines. *International Journal of Cancer. Journal International Du Cancer*, *125*(10), 2288–2295. http://dx.doi.org/10.1002/ijc.24574.

Spranger, S., Koblish, H. K., Horton, B., Scherle, P. A., Newton, R., & Gajewski, T. F. (2014). Mechanism of tumor rejection with doublets of CTLA-4, PD-1/PD-L1, or IDO blockade involves restored IL-2 production and proliferation of CD8(+) T cells directly within the tumor microenvironment. *Journal for Immunotherapy of Cancer*, *2*, 3. http://dx.doi.org/10.1186/2051-1426-2-3.

Su, M.-L., Chang, T.-M., Chiang, C.-H., Chang, H.-C., Hou, M.-F., Li, W.-S., et al. (2014). Inhibition of chemokine (C-C motif) receptor 7 sialylation suppresses CCL19-stimulated proliferation, invasion and anti-anoikis. *PLoS One*, *9*(6), e98823. http://dx.doi.org/10.1371/journal.pone.0098823.

Tamada, K., Ni, J., Zhu, G., Fiscella, M., Teng, B., van Deursen, J. M. A., et al. (2002). Cutting edge: Selective impairment of CD8+ T cell function in mice lacking the TNF superfamily member light. *The Journal of Immunology*, *168*(10), 4832–4835. http://dx.doi.org/10.4049/jimmunol.168.10.4832.

Tao, R., Wang, L., Murphy, K. M., Fraser, C. C., & Hancock, W. W. (2008). Regulatory T cell expression of herpesvirus entry mediator suppresses the function of B and T lymphocyte attenuator-positive effector T cells. *The Journal of Immunology*, *180*(10), 6649–6655. http://dx.doi.org/10.4049/jimmunol.180.10.6649.

Thanarajasingam, U., Sanz, L., Diaz, R., Qiao, J., Sanchez-Perez, L., Kottke, T., et al. (2007). Delivery of CCL21 to metastatic disease improves the efficacy of adoptive T-cell therapy. *Cancer Research*, *67*(1), 300–308. http://dx.doi.org/10.1158/0008-5472.CAN-06-1017.

Tortola, L., Rosenwald, E., Abel, B., Blumberg, H., Schäfer, M., Coyle, A. J., et al. (2012). Psoriasiform dermatitis is driven by IL-36-mediated DC-keratinocyte crosstalk. *The Journal of Clinical Investigation*, *122*(11), 3965–3976. http://dx.doi.org/10.1172/JCI63451.

Towne, J. E., Renshaw, B. R., Douangpanya, J., Lipsky, B. P., Shen, M., Gabel, C. A., et al. (2011). Interleukin-36 (IL-36) ligands require processing for full agonist (IL-36α, IL-36β, and IL-36γ) or antagonist (IL-36Ra) activity. *The Journal of Biological Chemistry*, *286*(49), 42594–42602. http://dx.doi.org/10.1074/jbc.M111.267922.

Van de Veerdonk, F. L., Netea, M. G., Dinarello, C. A., & Joosten, L. A. B. (2011). Inflammasome activation and IL-1β and IL-18 processing during infection. *Trends in Immunology*, *32*(3), 110–116. http://dx.doi.org/10.1016/j.it.2011.01.003.

Vigne, S., Palmer, G., Lamacchia, C., Martin, P., Talabot-Ayer, D., Rodriguez, E., et al. (2011). IL-36R ligands are potent regulators of dendritic and T cells. *Blood*, *118*(22), 5813–5823. http://dx.doi.org/10.1182/blood-2011-05-356873.

Vigne, S., Palmer, G., Martin, P., Lamacchia, C., Strebel, D., Rodriguez, E., et al. (2012). IL-36 signaling amplifies Th1 responses by enhancing proliferation and Th1 polarization of naive CD4+ T cells. *Blood*, *120*(17), 3478–3487. http://dx.doi.org/10.1182/blood-2012-06-439026.

Wang, J., Foster, A., Chin, R., Yu, P., Sun, Y., Wang, Y., et al. (2002). The complementation of lymphotoxin deficiency with LIGHT, a newly discovered TNF family member, for the restoration of secondary lymphoid structure and function. *European Journal of Immunology*, *32*(7), 1969–1979. http://dx.doi.org/10.1002/1521-4141(200207)32:7<1969::AID-IMMU1969>3.0.CO;2-M.

Wirsing, A. M., Rikardsen, O. G., Steigen, S. E., Uhlin-Hansen, L., & Hadler-Olsen, E. (2014). Characterisation and prognostic value of tertiary lymphoid structures in oral squamous cell carcinoma. *BMC Clinical Pathology*, *14*, 38. http://dx.doi.org/10.1186/1472-6890-14-38.

Yan, L., Da Silva, D. M., Verma, B., Gray, A., Brand, H. E., Skeate, J. G., et al. (2015). Forced LIGHT expression in prostate tumors overcomes Treg mediated immunosuppression and synergizes with a prostate tumor therapeutic vaccine by recruiting effector T lymphocytes. *The Prostate*, *75*(3), 280–291. http://dx.doi.org/10.1002/pros.22914.

Yu, P., Lee, Y., Liu, W., Chin, R. K., Wang, J., Wang, Y., et al. (2004). Priming of naive T cells inside tumors leads to eradication of established tumors. *Nature Immunology*, *5*(2), 141–149. http://dx.doi.org/10.1038/ni1029.

Yu, P., Lee, Y., Wang, Y., Liu, X., Auh, S., Gajewski, T. F., et al. (2007). Targeting the primary tumor to generate CTL for the effective eradication of spontaneous metastases.

Journal of Immunology (Baltimore, Md: 1950), *179*(3), 1960–1968. Retrieved from http://www.pubmedcentral.nih.gov/articlerender.fcgi?artid=2387226&tool=pmcentrez&rendertype=abstract.

Zhu, M., & Fu, Y.-X. (2011). The role of core TNF/LIGHT family members in lymph node homeostasis and remodeling. *Immunological Reviews*, *244*(1), 75–84. http://dx.doi.org/10.1111/j.1600-065X.2011.01061.x.

Zhu, X., Su, D., Xuan, S., Ma, G., Dai, Z., Liu, T., et al. (2013). Gene therapy of gastric cancer using LIGHT-secreting human umbilical cord blood-derived mesenchymal stem cells. *Gastric Cancer: Official Journal of the International Gastric Cancer Association and the Japanese Gastric Cancer Association*, *16*(2), 155–166. http://dx.doi.org/10.1007/s10120-012-0166-1.

Zhu, Z., Zhang, X., Guo, H., Fu, L., Pan, G., & Sun, Y. (2015). CXCL13-CXCR5 axis promotes the growth and invasion of colon cancer cells via PI3K/AKT pathway. *Molecular and Cellular Biochemistry*, *400*(1–2), 287–295. http://dx.doi.org/10.1007/s11010-014-2285-y.

Zlotnik, A., Burkhardt, A. M., & Homey, B. (2011). Homeostatic chemokine receptors and organ-specific metastasis. *Nature Reviews. Immunology*, *11*(9), 597–606. http://dx.doi.org/10.1038/nri3049.

Zou, W., Zheng, H., He, T.-C., Chang, J., Fu, Y.-X., & Fan, W. (2012). LIGHT delivery to tumors by mesenchymal stem cells mobilizes an effective antitumor immune response. *Cancer Research*, *72*(12), 2980–2989. http://dx.doi.org/10.1158/0008-5472.CAN-11-4216.

Zucker, S., & Vacirca, J. (2004). Role of matrix metalloproteinases (MMPs) in colorectal cancer. *Cancer and Metastasis Reviews*, *23*(1/2), 101–117. http://dx.doi.org/10.1023/A:1025867130437.

CHAPTER SEVEN

The Tumor Macroenvironment: Cancer-Promoting Networks Beyond Tumor Beds

Melanie R. Rutkowski, Nikolaos Svoronos, Alfredo Perales-Puchalt, Jose R. Conejo-Garcia[1]
Tumor Microenvironment and Metastasis Program, The Wistar Institute, Philadelphia, Pennsylvania, USA
[1]Corresponding author: e-mail address: jrconejo@Wistar.org

Contents

Abstract

During tumor progression, alterations within the systemic tumor environment, or macroenvironment, result in the promotion of tumor growth, tumor invasion to distal organs, and eventual metastatic disease. Distally produced hormones, commensal

Advances in Cancer Research, Volume 128
ISSN 0065-230X
http://dx.doi.org/10.1016/bs.acr.2015.04.011

microbiota residing within mucosal surfaces, myeloid cells and even the bone marrow impact the systemic immune system, tumor growth, and metastatic spread. Understanding the reciprocal interactions between the cells and soluble factors within the macroenvironment and the primary tumor will enable the design of specific therapies that have the potential to prevent dissemination and metastatic spread. This chapter will summarize recent findings detailing how the primary tumor and systemic tumor macroenvironment coordinate malignant progression.

ABBREVIATIONS

AR androgen receptor
ARG1 arginase
CRC colorectal cancer
DC dendritic cell
EPT estrogen–progesterone replacement therapy
ER estrogen receptor
MDSC myeloid-derived suppressor cell
PMN polymorphonuclear cell
ROS reactive oxygen species
SERM selective estrogen receptor modulator
TGFβ transforming growth factor beta
TIMP-1 tissue inhibitor of metalloproteinases 1
TLR toll-like receptor
TME tumor microenvironment
VEGF-A vascular endothelial growth factor

1. INTRODUCTION

Cancer is a systemic disease that affects multiple organs and systems in tumor-bearing hosts. In recent years, seminal mechanistic insight has been generated to understand the peculiarities of the tumor microenvironment (TME), which have resulted in novel therapeutic interventions. While much more work needs to address how multiple nontumor cell types and structures at tumor beds influence malignant progression, it is becoming increasingly clear that tumors release factors that drive the orchestration of an environment in the host that involves the crosstalk between multiple distal compartments, at places beyond tumor beds. Systemic alterations include changes in the functioning of the bone marrow, where especially myelopoiesis is heavily altered in the presence of a tumor. Distal hormonal signals and inflammatory mediators generated through interactions with commensal microorganisms also facilitate the formation of premetastatic niches where disseminated tumor cells home, lay dormant, and eventually develop into growing metastatic. Together, these inflammatory, tumor-promoting prometastatic networks, form a systemic "macroenvironment" in tumor-bearing hosts that influences both the function of distant tissues and the tumor itself. This chapter will focus on the role of immune cells and their products in the orchestration of this systemic "macroenvironment," which is critical for the progression of aggressive tumors and eventually for fatal outcomes.

2. INTERACTIONS BETWEEN THE TME AND THE BONE MARROW

2.1 Pathological Myelopoiesis Promotes Malignant Progression

The hematopoietic system has evolved to adjust the production of leukocytes to the presence of viral or bacterial infections. By increasing the production of leukocytes derived from the myeloid lineage, the host quickly generates myeloid effectors that are mobilized to the periphery from the bone marrow to fight pathogens (Takizawa, Boettcher, & Manz, 2012). These mechanisms of "emergency myelopoiesis" are co-opted by tumors for their own growth and dissemination. A common finding in advanced solid tumor-bearing hosts is that severe alterations of myelopoietic differentiation promote the expansion and accumulation of immature myeloid progenitors into the blood, lymph nodes, spleen, bone marrow, and tumor sites (Gabrilovich, Ostrand-Rosenberg, & Bronte, 2012; Ostrand-Rosenberg & Sinha, 2009). In cancer, unlike emergency myelopoiesis induced by acute infections, immature myeloid cells are also retained at early stages of differentiation by signals derived from the TME, which block the differentiation of immature precursors into lineage-committed leukocytes, further contributing to the accumulation of myeloid precursors. This impairs dendritic cell (DC)-mediated antigen presentation and macrophage-dependent cytotoxic (protective) activity.

Initially, immature myeloid cells mobilized in the presence of a tumor are not necessarily immunosuppressive, although they could play a role in tumor-promoting inflammation and neovascularization. As the tumor progress, however, immature myeloid cells constantly produced through expanded myelopoiesis are influenced by multiple tumor-derived factors that turn them into powerful suppressors of protective immune responses. These heterogeneous immature myeloid cells that are able to suppress antitumor T-cell responses through a variety of mechanisms are generically termed myeloid-derived suppressor cells (MDSCs), and in mice, are characterized by the coexpression of high levels of Gr1, along with CD11b. Under steady-state conditions, Gr-1^{+}CD11b^{+} cells comprise ~35% of bone marrow cells but only ~3% of splenocytes (Nagaraj & Gabrilovich, 2012). In certain advanced tumor models, however, they can represent more than 50% of total splenocytes, and ~12% of total cells in single-cell suspensions from dissociated human melanoma samples (Gros et al., 2012). They also accumulate in variable proportions at tumor beds where, besides promoting the suppression of tumor-specific immune responses, MDSCs drive angiogenesis (Yang et al., 2004) and interleukin (IL)-6-dependent tumor-promoting inflammation (Fukuda et al., 2011; Lesina et al., 2011). In addition, MDSCs mobilized from the bone marrow generate premetastatic niches that provide a favorable location for disseminated tumor cells to survive, expand and, by recruiting new myeloid cells, generate metastases that are eventually responsible for fatal outcomes (Kaplan, Rafii, & Lyden, 2006; Kaplan et al., 2005; Peinado et al., 2012; Psaila & Lyden, 2009).

MDSCs are therefore immature myeloid cells that acquire immunosuppressive activity through pathological activation in tumor-bearing hosts at places distal to the TME. As we will describe below, MDSCs play a critical role as systemic drivers of malignant progression.

2.2 Tumor-Derived Secreted Factors Promote the Expansion of Immunosuppressive MDSCs

MDSCs are induced by factors primarily produced in the TME, and in particular by inflammatory cytokines. Inflammatory mediators, such as IL-1β, IL-6, and PGE2, have been demonstrated to play a role in the mobilization of MDSCs in tumor-bearing mice (Bunt et al., 2007; Eruslanov, Daurkin, Ortiz, Vieweg, & Kusmartsev, 2010; Sinha, Clements, Fulton, & Ostrand-Rosenberg, 2007). In addition, immunosuppressive CD33^{+} leukocytes can be generated from human peripheral blood cells by incubation with granulocyte macrophage colony-stimulating factor (GM-CSF) and IL-6 (Lechner, Liebertz, & Epstein, 2010). Correspondingly, an important transcriptional pathway associated with both the expansion and the differentiation blockade of myeloid progenitors is mediated by STAT3. STAT3 activation by tumor-induced cytokines promotes the expansion of myeloid cells by upregulating both drivers of the cell cycle and antiapoptotic factors (Gabrilovich et al., 2012; Sander et al., 2010; Yu, Pardoll, & Jove, 2009).

Activated STAT3 also promotes the upregulation of C/EBPβ, which contributes to the acquisition of immunosuppressive activity (Marigo et al., 2010). In addition, STAT3 signaling in myeloid cells impairs DC and macrophage differentiation, at least in part by decreasing PKCβII (Farren et al., 2014; Nefedova et al., 2004). The combination of increased proliferation, decreased apoptosis, and impaired differentiation all contribute to the accumulation of immature myeloid leukocytes at bone marrow and lymphatic locations. STAT3 activation is not only caused by secreted inflammatory cytokines, as heat shock proteins contained within tumor-derived exosomes have been also shown to contribute to the mobilization of MDSCs in cancer through this mechanism (Chalmin et al., 2010).

STAT3 activation in myeloid cells also elicits an autocrine loop whereby S100A9 protein secretion is increased. S100A8/9 dimers bind to the receptor for advanced glycation end products (RAGE receptors) activating the NF-κB pathway (Sinha et al., 2008), further blocking the differentiation of these myeloid progenitors into macrophages and DCs (Cheng et al., 2008). In addition, S100A8/9 protein production in the TME promotes the recruitment of MDSCs to tumor beds and enhances their suppressive activity (Gabrilovich et al., 2012; Sinha et al., 2008).

3. SUBSETS OF MYELOID PRECURSORS PATHOLOGICALLY MOBILIZED IN TUMOR-BEARING HOSTS

While all MDSCs represent immature and pathologically activated myeloid cells, they include at least two main categories of precursors; granulocytes and macrophages/DCs. Thus, murine MDSCs were originally defined based on coexpression of CD11b and Gr-1 surface markers (Gabrilovich et al., 2007; Kusmartsev & Gabrilovich, 2002; Sinha et al., 2008). However, it became clear that this heterogeneous population could be subdivided into Ly-6C^{low}Ly-6G^{+} granulocytic/polymorphonuclear (PMN) MDSCs and Ly-6C^{hi}Ly-6G^{-} monocytic MDSCs (Dolcetti et al., 2010; Youn, Nagaraj, Collazo, & Gabrilovich, 2008).

The categorization of MDSCs in cancer patients is more complicated due to higher heterogeneity and differentiation from other myeloid subsets (e.g., *bona fide* neutrophils). Nevertheless, MDSCs are typically CD11b^{+}CD33^{+}HLA-DR$^{-/low}$ leukocytes that include a "monocytic" population with the capacity to differentiate into CD14^{+} cells and a CD15^{+} granulocytic type (Condamine et al., 2014; Gros et al., 2012;

Ostrand-Rosenberg & Sinha, 2009; Ramachandran et al., 2013). Immature myeloid cells in cancer patients are, however, quite heterogeneous in every tumor, and much remains to be learned about the phenotypic diversity of myeloid leukocytes in freshly processed human tumors due to the fact that granulocytic populations often die in the freeze/thawing process. In addition, because immature myeloid cells may not be intrinsically immunosuppressive at initial stages of tumor progression, the role of MDSCs in human tumors—resected as soon as they are detected—may not mirror the dramatic phenotypes identified in certain terminal transplantable tumors in mice.

Independently of additional subsets, granulocytic MDSCs outnumber monocytic MDSCs by a ratio of 3:1 (Youn et al., 2008). This reflects differences in the proportions of neutrophilic versus monocyte/macrophage precursors during myelopoiesis, but also the fact that typical myelopoiesis in cancer-bearing individuals is so corrupted that myelomonocytic precursors acquire the pathological capacity turning into granulocytes through epigenetic silencing of the retinoblastoma gene (Youn et al., 2013).

The two main subsets of MDSCs inhibit the protective activity of antitumor T cells through different mechanisms. Thus, the production of reactive oxygen species (ROS) is the main mechanism whereby granulocytic MDSCs suppress CD8 T-cell responses, which requires cell–cell contact (Corzo et al., 2009; Youn, Collazo, Shalova, Biswas, & Gabrilovich, 2012). In addition, granulocytic MDSCs are more active at generating immunosuppressive adenosine, a process that involves the sequential activity of the CD39 and CD73 ecto-enzymes (Ryzhov et al., 2011). In contrast, monocytic MDSCs primarily suppress through the generation of reactive nitrogen species (RNS) and the enzymatic activity of arginase (ARG1), which depletes the amino acid arginine, thus promoting T-cell unresponsiveness (Corzo et al., 2010; Gabrilovich et al., 2012).

4. LINEAGE-COMMITTED MYELOID POPULATIONS IN THE TME

Although tumor-derived factors hamper the differentiation of pathologically expanded immature myeloid progenitors into their lineage-committed cell types in tumor-bearing hosts, MDSCs contain precursors with the capacity to differentiate into macrophages, DCs, and granulocytes.

These myeloid cells are in fact the most abundant cell types identified in the microenvironment of most solid tumors. Tumor-derived MDSCs transferred into tumor-free syngeneic mice turn into immunocompetent macrophages and DCs (Gabrilovich et al., 2012; Narita, Wakita, Ohkur, Chamoto, & Nishimura, 2009). In contrast, MDSCs transferred into tumor-bearing hosts home to the TME where, under hypoxic conditions, turn primarily not only into immunosuppressive macrophages but also into DCs (~5% of them), with phenotypes that remain to be characterized in terms of immunosuppressive versus immunostimulatory potential (Corzo et al., 2010).

Monitoring the capacity of tumor-derived MDSCs for granulocytic differentiation is more challenging due to the short life and sensitive nature of neutrophils, but PMN/granulocytic MDSCs turn into *bona fide* neutrophils *in vitro* (Youn et al., 2012). The need to process fresh samples as soon as they are resected for the analysis of tumor-infiltrating neutrophils has limited our understanding of their activities in the TME. However, recent evidence indicates that neutrophils with an activated phenotype comprised 5–25% of cells isolated from freshly digested human lung tumors. Rather than impairing antitumor immunity, these cells were able to stimulate T-cell responses *in vitro* (Eruslanov et al., 2014). Whether this only reflects the nature of the myeloid cells that accumulate at tumor beds at relatively early stages of malignant progression (those that are resectable) remains unknown.

As aforementioned, macrophages are the most abundant leukocyte subset in the microenvironment of most tumors, at virtually any stage of malignant progression. Macrophages are known to promote angiogenesis through the production of vascular endothelial growth factor (VEGF-A) and by promoting tumor cell intravasation (Noy & Pollard, 2014). They are also, in general, driving immune privilege at tumor locations. Among the immunosuppressive mechanisms that macrophages promote in the TME, the secretion of IL-10 and transforming growth factor (TGF)-β1, the expression of PD-L1 on their surface and the production of ARG1 have all been shown to be significant (Noy & Pollard, 2014). From the therapeutic point of view, however, macrophages offer great potential because their tumor-promoting phenotype can be transformed into cytotoxic activities that are relevant for tumor shrinking. The potential of CD40 agonists, for instance, has been recently underscored in patients and preclinical models of pancreatic cancer, where macrophages (but not T cells) were responsible for objective clinical responses by altering the stroma (Beatty et al., 2011).

Besides macrophages, another cell type frequently identified in the microenvironment of epithelial malignancies includes DCs, both conventional and plasmacytoid (Chiba et al., 2012; Huarte et al., 2008; Scarlett et al., 2009, 2012; Wei et al., 2005). Because a continuum of differentiation and conflicting differentiation signals complicates the categorization of myeloid populations at tumor beds, the identification of *bona fide* DCs versus macrophage populations has been frequently challenged. In our hands, the most frequent leukocyte subset infiltrating ovarian carcinoma masses in mice and humans (but not in human tumor ascites or other tumor types) shows phenotypic attributes and functional activities of canonical DCs. In human solid ovarian tumors, for instance, $CD1c^{+}MHC\text{-}II^{+}CD19^{-}CD11c^{+}$ leukocytes outnumber $CD11c^{+}CD1c^{-}$ cells. These myeloid cells are able to suppress allogeneic T-cell responses in the absence of treatment (unpublished observations) and are therefore highly immunosuppressive. Corresponding surface determinants and suppressive functional activities of tumor-associated DCs have been identified in different ovarian cancer models of mice (Huarte et al., 2008; Scarlett et al., 2012). However, synergistic activation of CD40 and toll-like receptors (TLRs) or restoration of immunoregulatory miRNAs using synthetic reagents transforms them into an immunostimulatory cell type that is able to upregulate costimulatory molecules and effectively process and present antigens to T cells (Conejo-Garcia et al., 2004; Cubillos-Ruiz et al., 2010, 2012; Huarte et al., 2008; Rutkowski, Stephen, & Conejo-Garcia, 2012; Scarlett et al., 2009, 2012).

Further supporting the true dendritic nature of this abundant population, in both mouse and human tumors, we confirmed that they coexpress markers associated with the dendritic lineage. For instance, tumor-associated DCs express Zbtb46 mRNA levels at significantly higher levels than bone marrow-derived DCs in mice, where they also showed high expression of DNGR1/CLEC9A (Meredith et al., 2012; Schraml et al., 2013).

Independently of nomenclature, the identification of cells with the capacity to present antigens taken up in the TME has great potential for the design of therapeutic interventions that can both reverse immunosuppression and boost antitumor immunity *in vivo* and *in situ*.

5. METASTATIC SPREADING AND THE METASTATIC NICHE

Dissemination and metastatic growth of tumor cells accounts for the majority of cancer-related deaths, events that often occur before the primary mass is detected. Metastasis is a multistage process involving intrinsic changes to the tumor cells and exogenous soluble and cell-mediated factors that aid in extravasation of the primary tumor into the peripheral circulation, seeding and survival at distal sites, and eventual metastatic growth (Fig. 1). Long-term survival of disseminated tumor cells within the metastatic niche is facilitated by tumor-derived cytokines and immune cells that have been mobilized from the primary TME, or from the expression of tissue-specific cytokines and growth factors.

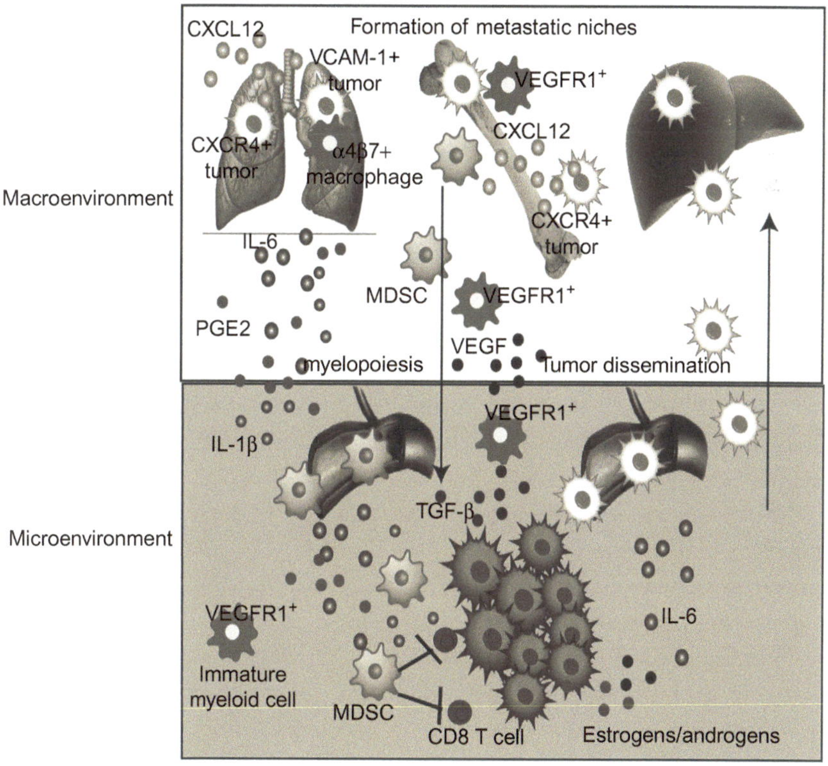

Figure 1 Crosstalk between the tumor macroenvironment and microenvironment results in dissemination and metastatic spread. CXCR4- and VCAM-1-expressing tumor cells are recruited out of the tumor microenvironment and into the macroenvironment due to high levels of CXCL12 expression in certain tissues. VCAM-1 helps tether tumor cells to tissue-associated macrophages which aide in the survival of tumor cells. VEGF R1-expressing immature myeloid cells are recruited out of the tumor environment by VEGF, TGFβ, and IL-6, where they home to distal organs to set up a premetastatic niche for disseminated tumor cells. MDSC and immature myeloid cells are recruited from the bone marrow into the tumor microenvironment to impair effective antitumor immunity and aide tumor growth and dissemination. (See the color plate.)

5.1 Tumor-Mediated Influence on the Premetastatic Niche: Preparation for Tumor Seeding at Distal Sites

The Lynden and Rafii laboratories helped to establish the concept of a premetastatic niche orchestrated by hematopoietic cells prior to the formation and seeding of metastases, facilitating the survival and outgrowth of disseminated tumor cells (Kaplan et al., 2006, 2005; Psaila & Lyden, 2009; Sceneay, Smyth, & Moller, 2013). The original studies identified a population of VEGFR1$^+$ immature myeloid cells and endothelial progenitors that were mobilized from the bone marrow in response to inflammatory signals that originated in the TME, such as VEGF-A, transforming growth factor beta (TGFβ), and placental growth factor (PlGF). Bone marrow-derived cells favorably homed to secondary organs, such as the lung, where proteins such as S100A8/9 and serum amyloid A3 (SAA3) are preferentially upregulated, resulting in the establishment of an environment favoring growth and survival of metastatic tumor cells.

In patients with advanced colorectal cancer (CRC), high systemic levels of tissue inhibitor of metalloproteinases (TIMP)-1 are predictive of poor outcome (Holten-Andersen et al., 2000) and more metastatic disease (Seubert et al., 2015). Using mouse models, Seubert et al. found that in tumor-bearing mice with high systemic levels of TIMP-1, CXCL12 was increased in the liver, resulting in the recruitment of CXCR4-expressing neutrophils that establish a premetastatic niche for disseminated CRC cells (Seubert et al., 2015).

More recently, the secretion of exosomes by tumor cells has also been shown to play an important role in the formation of premetastatic niches. Tumor-derived exosomes enhance vascular leakiness by inducing a vasculogenic phenotype in bone marrow progenitor cells, essentially "educating" the bone marrow to support tumor dissemination (Peinado et al., 2012). The role of immunosuppressive mediators (in addition to activators of myelopoiesis) potentially contained in these exosomes deserves further investigation. Additionally, understanding the significance of exosome release and metastasis for other cancer types could potentially uncover novel therapies that either inhibit the release of exosomes from primary tumors or target the proteins that enable metastatic growth.

Together, these studies have provided compelling data detailing mechanisms of tumor-induced metastatic spread and generation of the premetastatic niche in distal organs. However, the limitation to these studies is a lack of relevant preclinical animals that recapitulate the entire process of tumor dormancy and metastasis. Therefore, more clinical data are required to verify these events occur during the progression of malignant human disease (Keskinov & Shurin, 2015).

5.2 Tissue-Specific Properties in the Formation of Metastatic Niches

Metastatic cancers generally have a specific pattern of metastatic spread, with tropism for different tissues, indicating that tissue-specific factors may also be involved in the recruitment of disseminated tumor cells. Studies have shown that chemokine receptors, CXCR4 and CCR7, are overexpressed in metastatic breast cancer cells while the respective ligands, CXCL12 and CCL21, are most abundantly expressed in the sites most commonly associated with breast cancer dissemination, such as the lymph nodes, lung, bone marrow, and liver (Müller, Homey, Soto, Ge, & Catro, 2001). CXCL12 is also involved with inducing neovascular growth (Jin et al., 2006), which results in the outgrowth of dormant tumor cells residing within the perivascular niche (Ghajar et al., 2013). These studies demonstrate that cytokines and chemokines present within the local tissue milieu also facilitate tumor dissemination and metastatic growth, uncovering a mechanism that explains the tropism of certain tumors for specific organ sites.

Prosurvival and growth signals on tumor cells have also been shown to be mediated by adhesion between tissue-resident myeloid cells and disseminated tumor cells within each metastatic niche. For example, disseminated breast cancer cells in both the lungs and bone marrow utilize VCAM-1-mediated binding to integrins on tissue-resident myeloid cells to survive in distal sites. Aberrant VCAM-1 overexpression on breast tumor cells in the bone marrow promotes the recruitment and activation of osteoclast progenitors, accelerating growth of breast tumor cells within the bone marrow (Lu et al., 2011). In the lungs, another niche involved in breast tumor metastasis, metastasized VCAM-1 overexpressing breast tumor cells tether themselves to lung macrophages through binding of α4β1 integrins, resulting in the activation of prosurvival PI3K/AKT signaling (Chen, Zhang, & Massague, 2011). VCAM-1-mediated tumor-induced adhesion with myeloid cells in environments associated with metastatic spread may explain the high VCAM-1 expression in invasive breast tumor cell lines (Lu et al., 2011) and resected metastatic human tumor specimens (Minn, Gupta, Padua, & Bos, 2007).

Together, the primary TME and local tissue environment coordinate enrichment of prosurvival signals, allowing for survival of disseminated tumor cells. When disseminated tumor cells encounter these locations enriched in inflammatory and proangiogenic cells types, a niche is formed where tumor cells initiate the orchestration of a more complex tissue microenvironment where they will eventually form macroscopic masses. Targeted therapies inhibiting the soluble factors or cells that aide in supporting these events will provide novel treatment strategies for the control of highly metastatic cancers. For example, targeting the CXCL12/CXCR4 pathway has already been shown to reduce metastatic spread of prostate cancers (Wong, Kandagatla, Korz, & Chinni, 2014), the recurrence of glioblastomas (Tseng, Vasquez-Medrano, & Brown, 2011), dissemination of tumor cells and immunosuppression in ovarian cancer (Gil et al., 2014), and breast tumor metastasis (Gil, Seshadri, Komorowski, Abrams, & Kozbor, 2013).

6. ROLE OF THE MICROBIOTA IN TUMOR PROGRESSION

The skin, respiratory tract, genitourinary tract, and the gastrointestinal tract are colonized by billions of microorganisms, comprised of viruses, fungi, protozoan, and predominantly bacteria. Commensal microbiota provide a first line of defense against invading pathogens, maintain homeostasis at mucosal surfaces, and aid in digestion. However, the microbiota also have an important role in the development and function of the immune system (Arpaia et al., 2013; Chappert, Bouladoux, Naik, & Schwartz, 2013; Duan, Chung, Troy, & Kasper, 2010; Furusawa et al., 2013; Ivanov et al., 2008; Wei et al., 2010) as well as influencing the activation of innate immune cells within the periphery during pathogenic infection (Abt et al., 2012; Clarke et al., 2010; Ichinohe et al., 2011).

Dysbiosis is an altered balance in the composition of the microbiota, resulting in dysregulated immune function and excess inflammation. When this occurs within the intestines, a cascade of events is initiated that may eventually lead to malignant growth. Although the link between dysregulation of commensal microbiota and colonic inflammation and cancer has been well established (Arthur et al., 2012; Hu et al., 2013), until recently, very few studies had addressed the role of the microbiota for tumors occurring at distal extraintestinal locations.

6.1 Commensal Microbiota Are Required for Effective Antitumor Immune Responses for Extraintestinal Tumors

Two seminal studies demonstrated that the commensal microbiota were required for immune-mediated control of extraintestinal tumors (Iida et al., 2013; Viaud et al., 2013). In mice-bearing MC38 carcinoma, EL4 lymphoma, and B16 melanoma, the commensal microbiota were required for myeloid cell production of TNFα during intratumoral immunotherapy with CpG-oligodeoxynucleotides (CpG-ODN) and inhibition of IL-10 signaling (Iida et al., 2013), an immunotherapeutic combination that has been shown to reverse DC immune suppression within the TME (Vicari et al., 2002). Direct or indirect activation of DCs through TLR4-mediated interactions with the commensal microbiota primed the induction of TNFα production in response to TLR9 immunotherapy. The antitumor and immunogenic effects of oxaliplatin treatment were also dependent upon the commensal microbiota to induce the generation of ROS from myeloid cells (Iida et al., 2013).

Treatment using cyclophosphamide, an anticancer agent that elicits a therapeutic response by inducing an immunogenic cell death in tumor cells (Kroemer, Galluzzi, Kepp, & Zitvogel, 2012) was also shown to require the commensal microbiota (Viaud et al., 2013). Mechanistically, cyclophosphamide decreased the epithelial integrity of the intestinal mucosa, resulting in translocation of Gram-positive microbiota to secondary lymph organs and the conversion of IL-17-producing pathogenic Th1 CD4 T cells and enhancement of memory Th1 responses (Viaud et al., 2013).

These studies were among the first to demonstrate that the commensal microbiota were indispensable for the establishment of effective immune responses during immunotherapy and immunogenic chemotherapy of cancers occurring outside of the intestines. Commensal-mediated differences in immune responses to each therapy were not "one size fits all," indicating both treatment and context-dependent differences influenced priming and activation of the innate and adaptive immune system. These two studies also highlighted the role of specific microbial genera in controlling immune function. The *Lactobacillus* genus negatively correlated with TLR4-induced TNFα production, while *Ruminococcus* genera positively correlated with the production of TNFα and the priming of DCs (Iida et al., 2013). In cyclophosphamide-treated mice, *Lactobacilli* and segmented filamentous bacteria (SFB), or *Candidatus* Savagella (Thompson, Vier, Mikaelyan, Wienemann, & Brune,

2012), were shown to be positively associated with inducing pathogenic Th17 cells in peripheral lymph organs (Viaud et al., 2013).

6.2 The Role of Microbe-Induced Inflammation During Malignant Progression

Certain chemotherapies and cancer treatments suppress the immune system, creating a risk for individuals undergoing treatment to develop infections with opportunistic pathogens. Acute inflammation driven by infection with opportunistic pathogens has been suggested to promote metastasis to distal organ sites. Lipopolysaccharide (LPS) delivery or infection in the lungs enhances chemotaxis of CXCR4-expressing tumor cells due to the induction of ubiquitins in the pulmonary epithelium (Yan, Cai, & Xu, 2013), suggesting that treatment of cancer-bearing patients with antibiotics to prevent infection with opportunistic bacteria may result in a lower rate of metastasis. The caveat of this study is that certain antibiotics may eliminate commensal microbial species that facilitate antitumoral immune responses. The notion that acute inflammation, driven by pathogenic microorganisms, can drive metastasis or induce the formation of premetastatic niches warrants further studies and careful consideration of how treatment with antibiotics will alter the composition of the commensal microbiota in tumor-bearing hosts. Additionally, separate studies have demonstrated that inflammation induced by intratumoral injection of avirulent microorganisms, such as *Toxoplasma gondii*, induces a therapeutic benefit for the treatment of ovarian cancer and melanoma (Baird, Byrne, et al., 2013; Baird, Fox, et al., 2013), demonstrating that for certain cancers acute inflammation can be beneficial to the host.

The composition of the commensal microbiota is influenced by common genetic polymorphisms in pattern recognition receptors, resulting in systemic inflammation that affects the initiation and progression of tumors occurring outside of the intestinal tract. Homozygous and heterozygous carriers of a deleterious polymorphism in TLR5 ($TLR5^{R392X}$) (Hawn et al., 2003) have increased long-term survival after an initial ovarian cancer diagnosis, but a reduced survival when diagnosed with luminal breast cancer (Rutkowski et al., 2015). Rutkowski et al. demonstrated that TLR5-mediated interactions with commensal microbiota increased systemic levels of IL-6, resulting in the recruitment of MDSCs into the tumor environment, and the induction of galectin-1 expression in tumor-associated γδ T cells, abrogating effective antitumor immunity. IL-6-driven immune suppression was only observed in $TLR5^+$ animals bearing IL-6 responsive tumors (e.g., ovarian cancer, sarcoma), whereas IL-6 nonresponsive tumors (e.g., breast tumors) grew significantly slower compared to $TLR5^{-/-}$ mice (Rutkowski et al., 2015). Importantly, differences observed in tumor progression required the commensal microbiota, as antibiotic depletion eliminated all TLR5-mediated differences in tumor progression.

In the absence of TLR5 signaling, $TLR5^{-/-}$ mice maintained significant differences in the composition of major species of commensal microbiota, despite prolonged cohousing, commonly used to equilibrate differences in the microbiota (Ivanov et al., 2008). In the presence of a tumor, a significant increase in the systemic levels of IL-17 was observed in TLR5-deficient individuals, and in the absence of IL-6, tumor progression was driven by IL-17 (Rutkowski et al., 2015). This study helped to clarify the controversial role of IL-17 in tumor progression, suggesting that IL-17 has a tumor-promoting effect only in the absence of IL-6. Studies examining the role of these two cytokines in human cancers support this notion. In patients with ovarian cancer, high IL-17 levels associate with a positive prognosis (Kryczek et al., 2009), whereas in luminal breast cancer, tumors that have low levels of IL-6 (Hartman et al., 2013), IL-17 is associated with a poor prognosis (Chen et al., 2013). The production of IL-17 depends upon the commensal microbiota (Ivanov et al., 2008), demonstrating that these differences in tumor progression are driven by TLR5-mediated recognition of commensal microbes. This study implicated that common genetic polymorphisms in pattern recognition receptors, which are present at a high frequency within the general population (Casanova, Abel, & Quintana-Murci, 2011), have an important influence on tumor progression and survival outcome.

It is becoming increasingly clear that the microbiota influence systemic immunity during the progression of cancer (Fig. 2). What is now being appreciated is that differences in microbial composition result in systemic differences in the production of certain cytokines, such as TNFα, IL-6, and IL-17, which ultimately influence the immune environment and tumor growth. Genetic variation and the composition of the commensal microbiota will be important to consider for personalized treatment of cancer. Additionally, future studies that explore interventions that modify or reshape the microbiota with certain genera associated with the production of specific cytokines would enable the development of approaches that modify the systemic immune system to treat cancer.

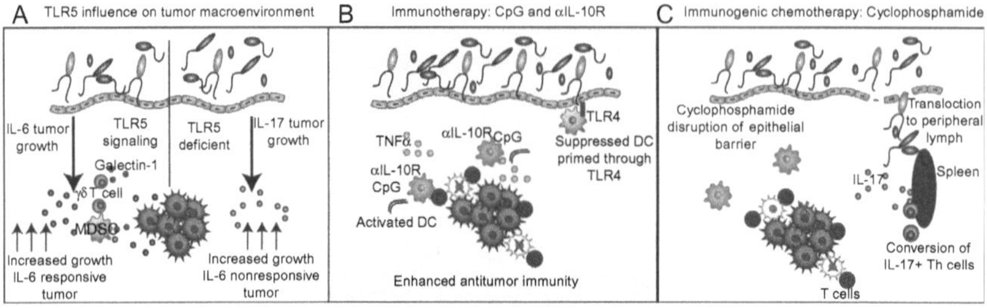

Figure 2 Commensal microbiota differentially influence the tumor environment and immunotherapy. (A) The influence of TLR5 expression on tumor progression. TLR5 responsive hosts have accelerated tumor progression in the presence of an IL-6 responsive tumor, resulting in increased levels of IL-6, increased recruitment of MDSCs into the tumor environment, and the induction of galectin-1 expression in tumor-associated γδ T cells. TLR5-deficient hosts have elevated levels of IL-17, which in the absence of IL-6 drives tumor progression. (B) Commensal microbiota are required for effective immunotherapy with CpG and anti-IL-10R antibody treatment to reverse the immune suppression of tumor-associated DCs. The commensal microbiota prime DCs through TLR4 interaction, resulting in the production of TNFα in response to the CpG treatment. This results in the conversion of suppressed DCs into immunostimulatory DCs, which elicit antitumor immunity. (C) The effects of cyclophosphamide are mediated through the microbiota. Cyclophosphamide disrupts the mucosal surface, allowing for bacterial translocation to distal lymph organs, such as the spleen. This results in the conversion of IL-17 producing Th cells, which enhance antitumor immune response. (See the color plate.)

7. DISTALLY PRODUCED HORMONES INFLUENCE TUMOR PROGRESSION

The endocrine system contributes significantly to the host macroenvironment by affecting a wide variety of biological functions, such as homeostasis, development, and inflammation. Hormonal changes, from either exogenous or endogenous sources, are associated with several diseases including certain cancers. In addition to having a direct impact on tumor cell growth for hormone-dependent cancers, hormones have been hypothesized to indirectly impact tumors by influencing host stromal responses. Currently, antihormonal therapies are used as adjuvant therapy only in hormone-dependent cancers, such as estrogen receptor (ER)-positive breast cancer (Burstein et al., 2014) and androgen receptor (AR)-positive prostate cancer (Loblaw et al., 2004); however, due to their pleiotropic effects on the host macroenvironment, endocrine therapies represent potential novel avenues for therapy in nonhormone-dependent cancers.

7.1 Estrogens and the Tumor Macroenvironment (Estrone, Estradiol, and Estriol)

Estrogens, produced mainly by the ovaries and adipose tissue in nongravid women, play a major role in female sexual development and health. Consequently, they have been implicated most strongly in the gynecological malignancies: breast, ovarian, and endometrial cancer. The Women's Health Initiative and Million Women Study found that women placed on combined estrogen–progesterone replacement therapy (EPT) are at an increased risk of breast cancer which is sustained approximately 3 years following termination of EPT (Beral, 2003; Rossouw et al., 2002). Additionally, elevated serum levels of estradiol in women without hormone therapy is associated with increased risk of ER-positive, but not ER-negative, breast cancer (Farhat et al., 2011). The Million Women Study found that women who were placed on postmenopausal estrogen replacement therapy were found to be at higher risk of developing ovarian cancer (Beral, Bull, Green, & Reeves, 2007), although this association is less clear when estrogen therapy is combined with progesterone (Anderson et al., 2003). Estrogen therapy alone is also known to increase the risk of endometrial cancer; however, this risk is mitigated when combined with progesterone (Weiderpass et al., 1999).

Canonically, estrogens directly regulate cell transcription via the steroid hormone receptors ERα and β (Nilsson et al., 2001). Upon ligand binding, ERs dimerize and translocate into the cell nucleus where they recognize estrogen response elements in gene promoters and enhancers. Depending on specific coregulators present within the nucleus, ER binding can activate or repress gene expression. ER can also form complexes with other transcription factors, such as AP-1 (Jakacka et al., 2001) and NF-κB (Galien & Garcia, 1997), thus directly affecting their activity in multiple cell types, including immune cells.

Estrogen signaling plays an important role in cancer by directly affecting ER-positive tumor cells. *In vitro* and *in vivo* studies using ER-positive breast tumor cells have shown that estradiol drives proliferation by inducing cell cycle progression via cyclin D1 (Hamelers, Van Schaik, Sussenbach, & Steenbergh, 2003). Treating breast cancer cells with the selective estrogen receptor modulator (SERM) tamoxifen results in cell cycle arrest and delayed tumor progression *in vivo* (Nunez et al., 2004). Clinically, SERMs used in ER-positive breast cancer patients have been shown to increase disease-free survival and decrease mortality (Swaby, Sharma, & Jordan, 2007). In ovarian cancer, the effect of estrogens on cell proliferation is less clear and seems to depend on the expression of the different ERs. ERα drives proliferation (Bossard et al., 2012) while ERβ and G protein-coupled estrogen receptor 1 (GPER) are inhibitory (Bossard et al., 2012; Ignatov et al., 2013). Consequently, ovarian clinical trials using antiestrogen therapy have failed to deliver the same benefits demonstrated in ER-positive breast cancer (Argenta et al., 2009). Endometrial tissue growth is driven by estrogen signaling (Groothuis, Dassen, Romano, & Punyadeera, 2007), which may be a major contributing factor in type 1 endometrial tumorigenesis. Because tamoxifen acts as an agonist in endometrial tissue (Diel, 2002), other antiestrogen therapies, such as aromatase inhibitors, have been used to treat premetastatic endometrial tumors; however, this antiestrogen therapy results in relatively low-response rates (Lindemann et al., 2014).

Due to the wide expression of ERs on cells comprising the tumor stroma, it has been hypothesized that estrogens can impact tumor growth independently of tumor cells. In a mouse xenograft model using ER-negative patient-derived tumor cells, it was shown that ERα-positive bone marrow cells were required for estrogen-triggered enhancement of tumor implantation and growth (Iyer et al., 2012). These cells appeared to contribute to the formation of tumor vasculature. Other studies have also implicated estrogen signaling in tumor vasculogenesis (George, Rajoria, Suriano, Mittleman, & Tiwari, 2012). In a model of liver cancer, estradiol was shown to suppress tumor growth by reducing IL-6 production by macrophages in response to chemical carcinogen-induced liver damage (Naugler et al., 2007).

7.2 Androgens in the Tumor Macroenvironment (Testosterone and Dihydrotestosterone)

Exposure to androgens has long been associated with prostate cancer (Herger & Sauer, 1947). Testosterone upon recognition by AR induces initiation and progression of prostate cancer by stimulating tumor cell proliferation and inhibiting apoptosis (Green, Mostaghel, & Nelson, 2012). Androgen deprivation therapy has been established as an effective treatment for advanced prostate cancer by inducing prostate cancer cell death (Feldman & Feldman, 2001). However, prostate cancer eventually recurs as castration resistant disease that relies upon alternative mechanisms for AR activation (Sharifi, 2013).

Besides direct effect on tumor cells, androgens have been shown to promote angiogenesis. Exposure to testosterone increased angiogenesis by selectively stimulating the AR in male endothelial cells *in vitro* and *in vivo* (Sieveking et al., 2010). This could further support progression and dissemination of cancer cells. High androgen levels may also help tumor promotion and progression by impairing the function of the antitumor immune response. Testosterone impairs Th1 differentiation by upregulation of Ptpn1 (Kissick et al., 2014). Furthermore, orchiectomy has been shown to increase intratumoral infiltration of M1 macrophages and CD8α T cells using a mouse model of thyroid cancer (Zhang et al., 2015).

7.3 Insulin and Insulin-Like Growth Factor-I in the Tumor Macroenvironment

Other hormones that impact tumor initiation and progression are insulin and insulin-like growth factor-I (IGF-I). Epidemiological studies found a higher overall risk of cancer in patients who were on insulin (Hemkens et al., 2009). Besides increasing IGF-I secretion, insulin has been implicated in tumorigenesis by accelerating tumor growth both *in vitro* and in mouse models of type 2 diabetes (Fierz, Novosyadlyy, Vijayakumar, Yakar, & LeRoith, 2010; Novosyadlyy et al., 2010; Zhang et al., 2010).

The role of IGF-I is clearly established in different types of cancer, such as breast, prostate, and colorectal (Chan et al., 1998; Hankinson et al., 1998; Ma et al., 1999). Patients with acromegaly have an increase in IGF-I secondary to a Growth Hormone hypersecretion, which is associated with an increased risk of CRC (Melmed, 2009). Decrease of IGF-I by caloric restriction or using a liver-specific IGF-I-deficient mice model results in protection against tumors, which can be reversed by the administration of IGF-I (Dunn et al., 1997; Wu, Yakar, Zhao, Hennighausen, & LeRoith, 2002; Wu et al., 2003).

8. CONCLUSIONS

Understanding of the intrinsic mutational or immunosuppressive events that result in malignant progression have aided in the development of targeted therapies that have enhanced the survival and quality of life for many patients with metastatic disease. Although many studies have uncovered mechanisms utilized by tumor cells to escape certain chemotherapies or immunotherapies, the systemic burden of cancer remains an indelible consequence for the outcome of current therapies. There is a trend toward utilizing large-scale screening techniques to choose drug combinations that exploit genetic differences in individual patient tumors to identify optimal drug sensitivity (Barretina et al., 2012; Garnett et al., 2012). However, utilizing large-scale genomic screening approaches have drawn criticism (Haibe-Kains et al., 2013) as there is no account for somatic genetic differences or systemic differences in immune or microbial composition that influence the bioactivity of the drug in humans.

Personalized cancer therapy will thus have to enter into a new era, where not only genetic and immune profiles of tumor cells will be considered, in addition to considering the factors that influence the tumor macroenvironment to effectively develop therapies that have maximal effectiveness with minimal toxicity. For example, inhibitors targeting the PI3K and MEK signaling pathways, pathways utilized by many cells within the body, can have unintended effects on malignant progression, due to their influence on the immune system or epithelial integrity of the mucosal surfaces. Cancer is an inflammatory disease, indicating that therapeutic combinations should be devised that not only target the tumor cell but also account for the influence of the macroenvironment in malignant progression and metastatic disease.

ACKNOWLEDGMENTS

This study was supported by R01CA157664, R01CA124515, R01CA178687, U54CA151662, P30CA10815, and Ovarian Cancer Research Fund (OCRF) Program Project Development awards. N.S. was supported by T32CA009171. A.P.P. was supported by the Ann Schreiber Mentored Investigator Award (OCRF).

REFERENCES

Abt, M. C., Osborne, L. C., Monticelli, L. A., Doering, T. A., Alenghat, T., Sonnenberg, G. F., et al. (2012). Commensal bacteria calibrate the activation threshold of innate antiviral immunity. *Immunity*, *37*, 158–170.

Anderson, G. L., Judd, H. L., Kaunitz, A. M., Barad, D. H., Beresford, S. A., Pettinger, M., et al. (2003). Effects of estrogen plus progestin on gynecologic cancers and associated diagnostic procedures: The Women's Health Initiative randomized trial. *JAMA*, *290*, 1739–1748.

Argenta, P. A., Thomas, S. G., Judson, P. L., Downs, L. S., Jr., Geller, M. A., Carson, L. F., et al. (2009). A phase II study of fulvestrant in the treatment of multiply-recurrent epithelial ovarian cancer. *Gynecologic Oncology*, *113*, 205–209.

Arpaia, N., Campbell, C., Fan, X., Dikiy, S., van der Veeken, J., Deroos, P., et al. (2013). Metabolites produced by commensal bacteria promote peripheral regulatory T-cell generation. *Nature*, *504*(7480), 451–455.

Arthur, J. C., Perez-Chanona, E., Mühlbauer, M., Tomkovich, S., Uronis, J. M., Fan, T.-J. J., et al. (2012). Intestinal inflammation targets cancer-inducing activity of the microbiota. *Science (New York, NY)*, *338*, 120–123.

Baird, J. R., Byrne, K. T., Lizotte, P. H., Toraya-Brown, S., Scarlett, U. K., Alexander, M. P., et al. (2013). Immune-mediated regression of established B16F10 melanoma by intratumoral injection of attenuated *Toxoplasma gondii* protects against rechallenge. *Journal of Immunology, 190*, 469–478.

Baird, J. R., Fox, B. A., Sanders, K. L., Lizotte, P. H., Cubillos-Ruiz, J. R., Scarlett, U. K., et al. (2013). Avirulent *Toxoplasma gondii* generates therapeutic antitumor immunity by reversing immunosuppression in the ovarian cancer microenvironment. *Cancer Research, 73*, 3842–3851.

Barretina, J., Caponigro, G., Stransky, N., Venkatesan, K., Margolin, A. A., Kim, S., et al. (2012). The Cancer Cell Line Encyclopedia enables predictive modelling of anticancer drug sensitivity. *Nature, 483*, 603–607.

Beatty, G. L., Chiorean, E. G., Fishman, M. P., Saboury, B., Teitelbaum, U. R., Sun, W., et al. (2011). CD40 agonists alter tumor stroma and show efficacy against pancreatic carcinoma in mice and humans. *Science, 331*, 1612–1616.

Beral, V. (2003). Breast cancer and hormone-replacement therapy in the Million Women Study. *Lancet, 362*, 419–427.

Beral, V., Bull, D., Green, J., & Reeves, G. (2007). Ovarian cancer and hormone replacement therapy in the Million Women Study. *Lancet, 369*, 1703–1710.

Bossard, C., Busson, M., Vindrieux, D., Gaudin, F., Machelon, V., Brigitte, M., et al. (2012). Potential role of estrogen receptor beta as a tumor suppressor of epithelial ovarian cancer. *PLoS One*, 7, e44787.

Bunt, S. K., Yang, L., Sinha, P., Clements, V. K., Leips, J., & Ostrand-Rosenberg, S. (2007). Reduced inflammation in the tumor microenvironment delays the accumulation of myeloid-derived suppressor cells and limits tumor progression. *Cancer Research, 67*, 10019–10026.

Burstein, H. J., Temin, S., Anderson, H., Buchholz, T. A., Davidson, N. E., Gelmon, K. E., et al. (2014). Adjuvant endocrine therapy for women with hormone receptor-positive breast cancer: American society of clinical oncology clinical practice guideline focused update. *Journal of Clinical Oncology, 32*, 2255–2269.

Casanova, J. L., Abel, L., & Quintana-Murci, L. (2011). Human TLRs and IL-1Rs in host defense: Natural insights from evolutionary, epidemiological, and clinical genetics. *Annual Review of Immunology, 29*, 447–491.

Chalmin, F., Ladoire, S., Mignot, G., Vincent, J., Bruchard, M., Remy-Martin, J. P., et al. (2010). Membrane-associated Hsp72 from tumor-derived exosomes mediates STAT3-dependent immunosuppressive function of mouse and human myeloid-derived suppressor cells. *The Journal of Clinical Investigation, 120*, 457–471.

Chan, J. M., Stampfer, M. J., Giovannucci, E., Gann, P. H., Ma, J., Wilkinson, P., et al. (1998). Plasma insulin-like growth factor-I and prostate cancer risk: A prospective study. *Science, 279*, 563–566.

Chappert, P., Bouladoux, N., Naik, S., & Schwartz, R. H. (2013). Specific gut commensal flora locally alters T cell tuning to endogenous ligands. *Immunity, 38*, 1198–1210.

Chen, W. C., Lai, Y. H., Chen, H. Y., Guo, H. R., Su, I. J., & Chen, H. H. (2013). Interleukin-17-producing cell infiltration in the breast cancer tumour microenvironment is a poor prognostic factor. *Histopathology, 63*, 225–233.

Chen, Q., Zhang, X. H., & Massague, J. (2011). Macrophage binding to receptor VCAM-1 transmits survival signals in breast cancer cells that invade the lungs. *Cancer Cell, 20*, 538–549.

Cheng, P., Corzo, C. A., Luetteke, N., Yu, B., Nagaraj, S., Bui, M. M., et al. (2008). Inhibition of dendritic cell differentiation and accumulation of myeloid-derived suppressor cells in cancer is regulated by S100A9 protein. *The Journal of Experimental Medicine, 205*, 2235–2249.

Chiba, S., Baghdadi, M., Akiba, H., Yoshiyama, H., Kinoshita, I., Dosaka-Akita, H., et al. (2012). Tumor-infiltrating DCs suppress nucleic acid-mediated innate immune responses through interactions between the receptor TIM-3 and the alarmin HMGB1. *Nature Immunology*, *13*, 832–842.

Clarke, T. B., Davis, K. M., Lysenko, E. S., Zhou, A. Y., Yu, Y., & Weiser, J. N. (2010). Recognition of peptidoglycan from the microbiota by Nod1 enhances systemic innate immunity. *Nature Medicine*, *16*, 228–231.

Condamine, T., Kumar, V., Ramachandran, I. R., Youn, J. I., Celis, E., Finnberg, N., et al. (2014). ER stress regulates myeloid-derived suppressor cell fate through TRAIL-R-mediated apoptosis. *The Journal of Clinical Investigation*, *124*, 2626–2639.

Conejo-Garcia, J. R., Benencia, F., Courreges, M. C., Kang, E., Mohamed-Hadley, A., Buckanovich, R. J., et al. (2004). Tumor-infiltrating dendritic cell precursors recruited by a beta-defensin contribute to vasculogenesis under the influence of VEGF-A. *Nature Medicine*, *10*, 950–958.

Corzo, C. A., Condamine, T., Lu, L., Cotter, M. J., Youn, J. I., Cheng, P., et al. (2010). HIF-1alpha regulates function and differentiation of myeloid-derived suppressor cells in the tumor microenvironment. *The Journal of Experimental Medicine*, *207*, 2439–2453.

Corzo, C. A., Cotter, M. J., Cheng, P., Cheng, F., Kusmartsev, S., Sotomayor, E., et al. (2009). Mechanism regulating reactive oxygen species in tumor-induced myeloid-derived suppressor cells. *Journal of Immunology*, *182*, 5693–5701.

Cubillos-Ruiz, J. R., Baird, J. R., Tesone, A. J., Rutkowski, M. R., Scarlett, U. K., Camposeco-Jacobs, A. L., et al. (2012). Reprogramming tumor-associated dendritic cells in vivo using microRNA mimetics triggers protective immunity against ovarian cancer. *Cancer Research*, *72*, 1683–1693.

Cubillos-Ruiz, J. R., Martinez, D., Scarlett, U. K., Rutkowski, M. R., Nesbeth, Y. C., Camposeco-Jacobs, A. L., et al. (2010). CD277 is a negative co-stimulatory molecule universally expressed by ovarian cancer microenvironmental cells. *Oncotarget*, *1*, 329–338.

Diel, P. (2002). Tissue-specific estrogenic response and molecular mechanisms. *Toxicology Letters*, *127*, 217–224.

Dolcetti, L., Peranzoni, E., Ugel, S., Marigo, I., Fernandez Gomez, A., Mesa, C., et al. (2010). Hierarchy of immunosuppressive strength among myeloid-derived suppressor cell subsets is determined by GM-CSF. *European Journal of Immunology*, *40*, 22–35.

Duan, J., Chung, H., Troy, E., & Kasper, D. L. (2010). Microbial colonization drives expansion of IL-1 receptor 1-expressing and IL-17-producing gamma/delta T cells. *Cell Host & Microbe*, *7*, 140–150.

Dunn, S. E., Kari, F. W., French, J., Leininger, J. R., Travlos, G., Wilson, R., et al. (1997). Dietary restriction reduces insulin-like growth factor I levels, which modulates apoptosis, cell proliferation, and tumor progression in p53-deficient mice. *Cancer Research*, *57*, 4667–4672.

Eruslanov, E. B., Bhojnagarwala, P. S., Quatromoni, J. G., Stephen, T. L., Ranganathan, A., Deshpande, C., et al. (2014). Tumor-associated neutrophils stimulate T cell responses in early-stage human lung cancer. *The Journal of Clinical Investigation*, *124*, 5466–5480.

Eruslanov, E., Daurkin, I., Ortiz, J., Vieweg, J., & Kusmartsev, S. (2010). Pivotal advance: Tumor-mediated induction of myeloid-derived suppressor cells and M2-polarized macrophages by altering intracellular PGE(2) catabolism in myeloid cells. *Journal of Leukocyte Biology*, *88*, 839–848.

Farhat, G. N., Cummings, S. R., Chlebowski, R. T., Parimi, N., Cauley, J. A., Rohan, T. E., et al. (2011). Sex hormone levels and risks of estrogen receptor-negative and estrogen receptor-positive breast cancers. *Journal of the National Cancer Institute*, *103*, 562–570.

Farren, M. R., Carlson, L. M., Netherby, C. S., Lindner, I., Li, P. K., Gabrilovich, D. I., et al. (2014). Tumor-induced STAT3 signaling in myeloid cells impairs dendritic cell generation by decreasing PKCbetaII abundance. *Science Signaling*, *7*, ra16.

Feldman, B. J., & Feldman, D. (2001). The development of androgen-independent prostate cancer. *Nature Reviews. Cancer*, *1*, 34–45.

Fierz, Y., Novosyadlyy, R., Vijayakumar, A., Yakar, S., & LeRoith, D. (2010). Insulin-sensitizing therapy attenuates type 2 diabetes-mediated mammary tumor progression. *Diabetes*, *59*, 686–693.

Fukuda, A., Wang, S. C., Morris, J. P. T., Folias, A. E., Liou, A., Kim, G. E., et al. (2011). Stat3 and MMP7 contribute to pancreatic ductal adenocarcinoma initiation and progression. *Cancer Cell*, *19*, 441–455.

Furusawa, Y., Obata, Y., Fukuda, S., Endo, T. A., Nakato, G., Takahashi, D., et al. (2013). Commensal microbe-derived butyrate induces the differentiation of colonic regulatory T cells. *Nature*, *504*(7480), 446–450.

Gabrilovich, D. I., Bronte, V., Chen, S. H., Colombo, M. P., Ochoa, A., Ostrand-Rosenberg, S., et al. (2007). The terminology issue for myeloid-derived suppressor cells. *Cancer Research*, *67*, 425, author reply 426.

Gabrilovich, D. I., Ostrand-Rosenberg, S., & Bronte, V. (2012). Coordinated regulation of myeloid cells by tumours. *Nature Reviews. Immunology*, *12*, 253–268.

Galien, R., & Garcia, T. (1997). Estrogen receptor impairs interleukin-6 expression by preventing protein binding on the NF-kappaB site. *Nucleic Acids Research*, *25*, 2424–2429.

Garnett, M. J., Edelman, E. J., Heidorn, S. J., Greenman, C. D., Dastur, A., Lau, K. W., et al. (2012). Systematic identification of genomic markers of drug sensitivity in cancer cells. *Nature*, *483*, 570–575.

George, A. L., Rajoria, S., Suriano, R., Mittleman, A., & Tiwari, R. K. (2012). Hypoxia and estrogen are functionally equivalent in breast cancer-endothelial cell interdependence. *Molecular Cancer*, *11*, 80.

Ghajar, C. M., Peinado, H. C., Mori, H., Matei, I. R., Evason, K. J., Brazier, H., et al. (2013). The perivascular niche regulates breast tumour dormancy. *Nature Cell Biology*, *15*, 807–817.

Gil, M., Komorowski, M. P., Seshadri, M., Rokita, H., McGray, A. J., Opyrchal, M., et al. (2014). CXCL12/CXCR4 blockade by oncolytic virotherapy inhibits ovarian cancer growth by decreasing immunosuppression and targeting cancer-initiating cells. *Journal of Immunology*, *193*, 5327–5337.

Gil, M., Seshadri, M., Komorowski, M. P., Abrams, S. I., & Kozbor, D. (2013). Targeting CXCL12/CXCR4 signaling with oncolytic virotherapy disrupts tumor vasculature and inhibits breast cancer metastases. *Proceedings of the National Academy of Sciences of the United States of America*, *110*, E1291–E1300.

Green, S. M., Mostaghel, E. A., & Nelson, P. S. (2012). Androgen action and metabolism in prostate cancer. *Molecular and Cellular Endocrinology*, *360*, 3–13.

Groothuis, P. G., Dassen, H. H., Romano, A., & Punyadeera, C. (2007). Estrogen and the endometrium: Lessons learned from gene expression profiling in rodents and human. *Human Reproduction Update*, *13*, 405–417.

Gros, A., Turcotte, S., Wunderlich, J. R., Ahmadzadeh, M., Dudley, M. E., & Rosenberg, S. A. (2012). Myeloid cells obtained from the blood but not from the tumor can suppress T-cell proliferation in patients with melanoma. *Clinical Cancer Research*, *18*, 5212–5223.

Haibe-Kains, B., El-Hachem, N., Birkbak, N. J., Jin, A. C., Beck, A. H., Aerts, H. J., et al. (2013). Inconsistency in large pharmacogenomic studies. *Nature*, *504*, 389–393.

Hamelers, I. H., Van Schaik, R. F., Sussenbach, J. S., & Steenbergh, P. H. (2003). 17beta-Estradiol responsiveness of MCF-7 laboratory strains is dependent on an autocrine signal activating the IGF type I receptor. *Cancer Cell International*, *3*, 10.

Hankinson, S. E., Willett, W. C., Colditz, G. A., Hunter, D. J., Michaud, D. S., Deroo, B., et al. (1998). Circulating concentrations of insulin-like growth factor-I and risk of breast cancer. *Lancet, 351*, 1393–1396.
Hartman, Z. C., Poage, G. M., den Hollander, P., Tsimelzon, A., Hill, J., Panupinthu, N., et al. (2013). Growth of triple-negative breast cancer cells relies upon coordinate autocrine expression of the proinflammatory cytokines IL-6 and IL-8. *Cancer Research, 73*, 3470–3480.
Hawn, T. R., Verbon, A., Lettinga, K. D., Zhao, L. P., Li, S. S., Laws, R. J., et al. (2003). A common dominant TLR5 stop codon polymorphism abolishes flagellin signaling and is associated with susceptibility to Legionnaires' disease. *The Journal of Experimental Medicine, 198*, 1563–1572.
Hemkens, L. G., Grouven, U., Bender, R., Gunster, C., Gutschmidt, S., Selke, G. W., et al. (2009). Risk of malignancies in patients with diabetes treated with human insulin or insulin analogues: A cohort study. *Diabetologia, 52*, 1732–1744.
Herger, C. C., & Sauer, H. R. (1947). A consideration of the effect of androgen control treatment of carcinoma of the prostate. *New York State Journal of Medicine, 47*, 494–501.
Holten-Andersen, M. N., Stephens, R. W., Nielsen, H. J., Murphy, G., Christensen, I. J., Stetler-Stevenson, W., et al. (2000). High preoperative plasma tissue inhibitor of metalloproteinase-1 levels are associated with short survival of patients with colorectal cancer. *Clinical Cancer Research, 6*, 4292–4299.
Hu, B., Elinav, E., Huber, S., Strowig, T., Hao, L., Hafemann, A., et al. (2013). Microbiota-induced activation of epithelial IL-6 signaling links inflammasome-driven inflammation with transmissible cancer. *Proceedings of the National Academy of Sciences of the United States of America, 110*, 9862–9867.
Huarte, E., Cubillos-Ruiz, J. R., Nesbeth, Y. C., Scarlett, U. K., Martinez, D. G., Buckanovich, R. J., et al. (2008). Depletion of dendritic cells delays ovarian cancer progression by boosting antitumor immunity. *Cancer Research, 68*, 7684–7691.
Ichinohe, T., Pang, I. K., Kumamoto, Y., Peaper, D. R., Ho, J. H., Murray, T. S., et al. (2011). Microbiota regulates immune defense against respiratory tract influenza A virus infection. *Proceedings of the National Academy of Sciences of the United States of America, 108*, 5354–5359.
Ignatov, T., Modl, S., Thulig, M., Weissenborn, C., Treeck, O., Ortmann, O., et al. (2013). GPER-1 acts as a tumor suppressor in ovarian cancer. *Journal of Ovarian Research, 6*, 51.
Iida, N., Dzutsev, A., Stewart, C. A., Smith, L., Bouladoux, N., Weingarten, R. A., et al. (2013). Commensal bacteria control cancer response to therapy by modulating the tumor microenvironment. *Science (New York, NY), 342*, 967–970.
Ivanov, I. I., Frutos, R. de L., Manel, N., Yoshinaga, K., Rifkin, D. B., Sartor, R. B., et al. (2008). Specific microbiota direct the differentiation of IL-17-producing T-helper cells in the mucosa of the small intestine. *Cell Host & Microbe, 4*, 337–349.
Iyer, V., Klebba, I., McCready, J., Arendt, L. M., Betancur-Boissel, M., Wu, M. F., et al. (2012). Estrogen promotes ER-negative tumor growth and angiogenesis through mobilization of bone marrow-derived monocytes. *Cancer Research, 72*, 2705–2713.
Jakacka, M., Ito, M., Weiss, J., Chien, P. Y., Gehm, B. D., & Jameson, J. L. (2001). Estrogen receptor binding to DNA is not required for its activity through the nonclassical AP1 pathway. *The Journal of Biological Chemistry, 276*, 13615–13621.
Jin, D. K., Shido, K., Kopp, H. G., Petit, I., Shmelkov, S. V., Young, L. M., et al. (2006). Cytokine-mediated deployment of SDF-1 induces revascularization through recruitment of CXCR4+ hemangiocytes. *Nature Medicine, 12*, 557–567.
Kaplan, R. N., Rafii, S., & Lyden, D. (2006). Preparing the "soil": The premetastatic niche. *Cancer Research, 66*, 11089–11093.

Kaplan, R. N., Riba, R. D., Zacharoulis, S., Bramley, A. H., Vincent, L., Costa, C., et al. (2005). VEGFR1-positive haematopoietic bone marrow progenitors initiate the pre-metastatic niche. *Nature*, *438*, 820–827.

Keskinov, A. A., & Shurin, M. R. (2015). Myeloid regulatory cells in tumor spreading and metastasis. *Immunobiology*, *220*, 236–242.

Kissick, H. T., Sanda, M. G., Dunn, L. K., Pellegrini, K. L., On, S. T., Noel, J. K., et al. (2014). Androgens alter T-cell immunity by inhibiting T-helper 1 differentiation. *Proceedings of the National Academy of Sciences of the United States of America*, *111*, 9887–9892.

Kroemer, G., Galluzzi, L., Kepp, O., & Zitvogel, L. (2012). Immunogenic cell death in cancer therapy. *Annual Review of Immunology*, *31*, 51–72.

Kryczek, I., Banerjee, M., Cheng, P., Vatan, L., Szeliga, W., Wei, S., et al. (2009). Phenotype, distribution, generation, and functional and clinical relevance of Th17 cells in the human tumor environments. *Blood*, *114*, 1141–1149.

Kusmartsev, S., & Gabrilovich, D. I. (2002). Immature myeloid cells and cancer-associated immune suppression. *Cancer Immunology, Immunotherapy*, *51*, 293–298.

Lechner, M. G., Liebertz, D. J., & Epstein, A. L. (2010). Characterization of cytokine-induced myeloid-derived suppressor cells from normal human peripheral blood mononuclear cells. *Journal of Immunology*, *185*, 2273–2284.

Lesina, M., Kurkowski, M. U., Ludes, K., Rose-John, S., Treiber, M., Kloppel, G., et al. (2011). Stat3/Socs3 activation by IL-6 transsignaling promotes progression of pancreatic intraepithelial neoplasia and development of pancreatic cancer. *Cancer Cell*, *19*, 456–469.

Lindemann, K., Malander, S., Christensen, R. D., Mirza, M. R., Kristensen, G. B., Aavall-Lundqvist, E., et al. (2014). Examestane in advanced or recurrent endometrial carcinoma: A prospective phase II study by the Nordic Society of Gynecologic Oncology (NSGO). *BMC Cancer*, *14*, 68.

Loblaw, D. A., Mendelson, D. S., Talcott, J. A., Virgo, K. S., Somerfield, M. R., Ben-Josef, E., et al. (2004). American Society of Clinical Oncology recommendations for the initial hormonal management of androgen-sensitive metastatic, recurrent, or progressive prostate cancer. *Journal of Clinical Oncology*, *22*, 2927–2941.

Lu, X., Mu, E., Wei, Y., Riethdorf, S., Yang, Q., Yuan, M., et al. (2011). VCAM-1 promotes osteolytic expansion of indolent bone micrometastasis of breast cancer by engaging alpha4beta1-positive osteoclast progenitors. *Cancer Cell*, *20*, 701–714.

Ma, J., Pollak, M. N., Giovannucci, E., Chan, J. M., Tao, Y., Hennekens, C. H., et al. (1999). Prospective study of colorectal cancer risk in men and plasma levels of insulin-like growth factor (IGF)-I and IGF-binding protein-3. *Journal of the National Cancer Institute*, *91*, 620–625.

Marigo, I., Bosio, E., Solito, S., Mesa, C., Fernandez, A., Dolcetti, L., et al. (2010). Tumor-induced tolerance and immune suppression depend on the C/EBPbeta transcription factor. *Immunity*, *32*, 790–802.

Melmed, S. (2009). Acromegaly pathogenesis and treatment. *The Journal of Clinical Investigation*, *119*, 3189–3202.

Meredith, M. M., Liu, K., Darrasse-Jeze, G., Kamphorst, A. O., Schreiber, H. A., Guermonprez, P., et al. (2012). Expression of the zinc finger transcription factor zDC (Zbtb46, Btbd4) defines the classical dendritic cell lineage. *The Journal of Experimental Medicine*, *209*, 1153–1165.

Minn, A. J., Gupta, G. P., Padua, D., & Bos, P. (2007). Lung metastasis genes couple breast tumor size and metastatic spread. *Proceedings of the National Academy of Sciences of the United States of America*, *104*, 6740–6745.

Müller, A., Homey, B., Soto, H., Ge, N., & Catron, D. (2001). Involvement of chemokine receptors in breast cancer metastasis. *Nature*, *410*(6824), 50–56.

Nagaraj, S., & Gabrilovich, D. I. (2012). Regulation of suppressive function of myeloid-derived suppressor cells by CD4+ T cells. *Seminars in Cancer Biology*, *22*, 282–288.

Narita, Y., Wakita, D., Ohkur, T., Chamoto, K., & Nishimura, T. (2009). Potential differentiation of tumor bearing mouse CD11b+Gr-1+ immature myeloid cells into both suppressor macrophages and immunostimulatory dendritic cells. *Biomedical Research*, *30*, 7–15.

Naugler, W. E., Sakurai, T., Kim, S., Maeda, S., Kim, K., Elsharkawy, A. M., et al. (2007). Gender disparity in liver cancer due to sex differences in MyD88-dependent IL-6 production. *Science*, *317*, 121–124.

Nefedova, Y., Huang, M., Kusmartsev, S., Bhattacharya, R., Cheng, P., Salup, R., et al. (2004). Hyperactivation of STAT3 is involved in abnormal differentiation of dendritic cells in cancer. *Journal of Immunology*, *172*, 464–474.

Nilsson, S., Makela, S., Treuter, E., Tujague, M., Thomsen, J., Andersson, G., et al. (2001). Mechanisms of estrogen action. *Physiological Reviews*, *81*, 1535–1565.

Novosyadlyy, R., Lann, D. E., Vijayakumar, A., Rowzee, A., Lazzarino, D. A., Fierz, Y., et al. (2010). Insulin-mediated acceleration of breast cancer development and progression in a nonobese model of type 2 diabetes. *Cancer Research*, *70*, 741–751.

Noy, R., & Pollard, J. W. (2014). Tumor-associated macrophages: From mechanisms to therapy. *Immunity*, *41*, 49–61.

Nunez, N. P., Jelovac, D., Macedo, L., Berrigan, D., Perkins, S. N., Hursting, S. D., et al. (2004). Effects of the antiestrogen tamoxifen and the aromatase inhibitor letrozole on serum hormones and bone characteristics in a preclinical tumor model for breast cancer. *Clinical Cancer Research*, *10*, 5375–5380.

Ostrand-Rosenberg, S., & Sinha, P. (2009). Myeloid-derived suppressor cells: Linking inflammation and cancer. *Journal of Immunology*, *182*, 4499–4506.

Peinado, H., Aleckovic, M., Lavotshkin, S., Matei, I., Costa-Silva, B., Moreno-Bueno, G., et al. (2012). Melanoma exosomes educate bone marrow progenitor cells toward a pro-metastatic phenotype through MET. *Nature Medicine*, *18*, 883–891.

Psaila, B., & Lyden, D. (2009). The metastatic niche: Adapting the foreign soil. *Nature Reviews. Cancer*, *9*, 285–293.

Ramachandran, I. R., Martner, A., Pisklakova, A., Condamine, T., Chase, T., Vogl, T., et al. (2013). Myeloid-derived suppressor cells regulate growth of multiple myeloma by inhibiting T cells in bone marrow. *Journal of Immunology*, *190*, 3815–3823.

Rossouw, J. E., Anderson, G. L., Prentice, R. L., LaCroix, A. Z., Kooperberg, C., Stefanick, M. L., et al. (2002). Risks and benefits of estrogen plus progestin in healthy postmenopausal women: Principal results from the Women's Health Initiative randomized controlled trial. *JAMA*, *288*, 321–333.

Rutkowski, M. R., Stephen, T. L., & Conejo-Garcia, J. R. (2012). Anti-tumor immunity: Myeloid leukocytes control the immune landscape. *Cellular Immunology*, *278*, 21–26.

Rutkowski, M. R., Stephen, T. L., Svoronos, N., Allegrezza, M. J., Tesone, A. J., Perales-Puchalt, A., et al. (2015). Microbially driven TLR5-dependent signaling governs distal malignant progression through tumor-promoting inflammation. *Cancer Cell*, *27*, 27–40.

Ryzhov, S., Novitskiy, S. V., Goldstein, A. E., Biktasova, A., Blackburn, M. R., Biaggioni, I., et al. (2011). Adenosinergic regulation of the expansion and immunosuppressive activity of CD11b+Gr1+ cells. *Journal of Immunology*, *187*, 6120–6129.

Sander, L. E., Sackett, S. D., Dierssen, U., Beraza, N., Linke, R. P., Muller, M., et al. (2010). Hepatic acute-phase proteins control innate immune responses during infection by promoting myeloid-derived suppressor cell function. *The Journal of Experimental Medicine*, *207*, 1453–1464.

Scarlett, U. K., Cubillos-Ruiz, J. R., Nesbeth, Y. C., Martinez, D. G., Engle, X., Gewirtz, A. T., et al. (2009). In situ stimulation of CD40 and toll-like receptor 3

transforms ovarian cancer-infiltrating dendritic cells from immunosuppressive to immunostimulatory cells. *Cancer Research*, *69*, 7329–7337.
Scarlett, U. K., Rutkowski, M. R., Rauwerdink, A. M., Fields, J., Escovar-Fadul, X., Baird, J., et al. (2012). Ovarian cancer progression is controlled by phenotypic changes in dendritic cells. *The Journal of Experimental Medicine*, *209*, 495–506.
Sceneay, J., Smyth, M. J., & Moller, A. (2013). The pre-metastatic niche: Finding common ground. *Cancer Metastasis Reviews*, *32*, 449–464.
Schraml, B. U., van Blijswijk, J., Zelenay, S., Whitney, P. G., Filby, A., Acton, S. E., et al. (2013). Genetic tracing via DNGR-1 expression history defines dendritic cells as a hematopoietic lineage. *Cell*, *154*, 843–858.
Seubert, B., Grunwald, B., Kobuch, J., Cui, H., Schelter, F., Schaten, S., et al. (2015). Tissue inhibitor of metalloproteinases (TIMP)-1 creates a premetastatic niche in the liver through SDF-1/CXCR4-dependent neutrophil recruitment in mice. *Hepatology*, *61*, 238–248.
Sharifi, N. (2013). Mechanisms of androgen receptor activation in castration-resistant prostate cancer. *Endocrinology*, *154*, 4010–4017.
Sieveking, D. P., Lim, P., Chow, R. W., Dunn, L. L., Bao, S., McGrath, K. C., et al. (2010). A sex-specific role for androgens in angiogenesis. *The Journal of Experimental Medicine*, *207*, 345–352.
Sinha, P., Clements, V. K., Fulton, A. M., & Ostrand-Rosenberg, S. (2007). Prostaglandin E2 promotes tumor progression by inducing myeloid-derived suppressor cells. *Cancer Research*, *67*, 4507–4513.
Sinha, P., Okoro, C., Foell, D., Freeze, H. H., Ostrand-Rosenberg, S., & Srikrishna, G. (2008). Proinflammatory S100 proteins regulate the accumulation of myeloid-derived suppressor cells. *Journal of Immunology*, *181*, 4666–4675.
Swaby, R. F., Sharma, C. G., & Jordan, V. C. (2007). SERMs for the treatment and prevention of breast cancer. *Reviews in Endocrine & Metabolic Disorders*, *8*, 229–239.
Takizawa, H., Boettcher, S., & Manz, M. G. (2012). Demand-adapted regulation of early hematopoiesis in infection and inflammation. *Blood*, *119*, 2991–3002.
Thompson, C. L., Vier, R., Mikaelyan, A., Wienemann, T., & Brune, A. (2012). 'Candidatus Arthromitus' revised: Segmented filamentous bacteria in arthropod guts are members of Lachnospiraceae. *Environmental Microbiology*, *14*, 1454–1465.
Tseng, D., Vasquez-Medrano, D. A., & Brown, J. M. (2011). Targeting SDF-1/CXCR4 to inhibit tumour vasculature for treatment of glioblastomas. *British Journal of Cancer*, *104*, 1805–1809.
Viaud, S., Saccheri, F., Mignot, G., Yamazaki, T., Daillère, R., Hannani, D., et al. (2013). The intestinal microbiota modulates the anticancer immune effects of cyclophosphamide. *Science (New York, NY)*, *342*, 971–976.
Vicari, A. P., Chiodoni, C., Vaure, C., Ait-Yahia, S., Dercamp, C., Matsos, F., et al. (2002). Reversal of tumor-induced dendritic cell paralysis by CpG immunostimulatory oligonucleotide and anti-interleukin 10 receptor antibody. *The Journal of Experimental Medicine*, *196*, 541–549.
Wei, S., Kryczek, I., Zou, L., Daniel, B., Cheng, P., Mottram, P., et al. (2005). Plasmacytoid dendritic cells induce CD8+ regulatory T cells in human ovarian carcinoma. *Cancer Research*, *65*, 5020–5026.
Wei, B., Wingender, G., Fujiwara, D., Chen, D. Y., McPherson, M., Brewer, S., et al. (2010). Commensal microbiota and CD8+ T cells shape the formation of invariant NKT cells. *Journal of Immunology (Baltimore, Md: 1950)*, *184*, 1218–1226.
Weiderpass, E., Adami, H. O., Baron, J. A., Magnusson, C., Bergstrom, R., Lindgren, A., et al. (1999). Risk of endometrial cancer following estrogen replacement with and without progestins. *Journal of the National Cancer Institute*, *91*, 1131–1137.
Wong, D., Kandagatla, P., Korz, W., & Chinni, S. R. (2014). Targeting CXCR4 with CTCE-9908 inhibits prostate tumor metastasis. *BMC Urology*, *14*, 12.

Wu, Y., Cui, K., Miyoshi, K., Hennighausen, L., Green, J. E., Setser, J., et al. (2003). Reduced circulating insulin-like growth factor I levels delay the onset of chemically and genetically induced mammary tumors. *Cancer Research*, *63*, 4384–4388.

Wu, Y., Yakar, S., Zhao, L., Hennighausen, L., & LeRoith, D. (2002). Circulating insulin-like growth factor-I levels regulate colon cancer growth and metastasis. *Cancer Research*, *62*, 1030–1035.

Yan, L., Cai, Q., & Xu, Y. (2013). The ubiquitin-CXCR4 axis plays an important role in acute lung infection-enhanced lung tumor metastasis. *Clinical Cancer Research*, *19*, 4706–4716.

Yang, L., DeBusk, L. M., Fukuda, K., Fingleton, B., Green-Jarvis, B., Shyr, Y., et al. (2004). Expansion of myeloid immune suppressor Gr+CD11b+ cells in tumor-bearing host directly promotes tumor angiogenesis. *Cancer Cell*, *6*, 409–421.

Youn, J. I., Collazo, M., Shalova, I. N., Biswas, S. K., & Gabrilovich, D. I. (2012). Characterization of the nature of granulocytic myeloid-derived suppressor cells in tumor-bearing mice. *Journal of Leukocyte Biology*, *91*, 167–181.

Youn, J. I., Kumar, V., Collazo, M., Nefedova, Y., Condamine, T., Cheng, P., et al. (2013). Epigenetic silencing of retinoblastoma gene regulates pathologic differentiation of myeloid cells in cancer. *Nature Immunology*, *14*, 211–220.

Youn, J. I., Nagaraj, S., Collazo, M., & Gabrilovich, D. I. (2008). Subsets of myeloid-derived suppressor cells in tumor-bearing mice. *Journal of Immunology*, *181*, 5791–5802.

Yu, H., Pardoll, D., & Jove, R. (2009). STATs in cancer inflammation and immunity: A leading role for STAT3. *Nature Reviews. Cancer*, *9*, 798–809.

Zhang, H., Fagan, D. H., Zeng, X., Freeman, K. T., Sachdev, D., & Yee, D. (2010). Inhibition of cancer cell proliferation and metastasis by insulin receptor downregulation. *Oncogene*, *29*, 2517–2527.

Zhang, L. J., Xiong, Y., Nilubol, N., He, M., Bommareddi, S., Zhu, X., et al. (2015). Testosterone regulates thyroid cancer progression by modifying tumor suppressor-genes and tumor immunity. *Carcinogenesis*, *36*(4), 420–428.

CHAPTER EIGHT

Control of CD8 T-Cell Infiltration into Tumors by Vasculature and Microenvironment

J. David Peske, Amber B. Woods, Victor H. Engelhard[1]
Department of Microbiology, Immunology, and Cancer Biology, Carter Immunology Center, University of Virginia School of Medicine, Charlottesville, Virginia, USA
[1]Corresponding author: e-mail address: vhe@virginia.edu

Contents

Abstract

CD8 T-cells are a critical brake on the initial development of tumors. In established tumors, the presence of CD8 T-cells is correlated with a positive patient prognosis, although immunosuppressive mechanisms limit their effectiveness and they are rarely curative without manipulation. Cancer immunotherapies aim to shift the balance back to dominant antitumor immunity through antibody blockade of immunosuppressive signaling pathways, vaccination, and adoptive transfer of activated or engineered T-cells. These approaches have yielded striking responses in small subsets of patients with solid tumors, most notably those with melanoma. Importantly, the subset of patients who respond to vaccination or immunosuppression blockade therapies are

Advances in Cancer Research, Volume 128
ISSN 0065-230X
http://dx.doi.org/10.1016/bs.acr.2015.05.001

those with CD8 T-cells present in the tumor prior to initiating therapy. While current adoptive cell therapy approaches can be dramatically effective, they require infusion of extremely large numbers of T-cells, but the number that actually infiltrates the tumor is very small. Thus, poor representation of CD8 T-cells in tumors is a fundamental hurdle to successful immunotherapy, over and above the well-established barrier of immunosuppression. In this review, we discuss the factors that determine whether immune cells are present in tumors, with a focus on the representation of cytotoxic CD8 T-cells. We emphasize the critically important role of tumor-associated vasculature as a gateway that enables the active infiltration of both effector and naïve CD8 T-cells that exert antitumor activity. We also discuss strategies to enhance the gateway function and extend the effectiveness of immunotherapies to a broader set of cancer patients.

ABBREVIATIONS

DC dendritic cell
ESL E-selectin ligand
HEV high endothelial venules
IFNγ interferon-γ
IP intraperitoneal
IV intravenous
LN lymph node
PNAd peripheral node addressin
PSL P-selectin ligand
SC subcutaneous
TLS tertiary lymphoid structure
TNFα tumor necrosis factor-alpha
Treg regulatory T-cell
VEGF vascular endothelial growth factor

1. PROGNOSTIC SIGNIFICANCE OF IMMUNE CELL REPRESENTATION IN TUMORS

A role for the immune system in cancer regression was suggested in the late-nineteenth century by William Coley, who observed that spontaneous remission of tumors sometimes occurred in patients who contracted acute bacterial infections. He subsequently developed a mixture of bacterial toxins that he believed activated the immune system and reported they were effective and even curative for some patients (Coley, 1893). Still, his method was controversial, and with the advent of chemo- and radiotherapy, fell out of favor (Wiemann & Starnes, 1994). It was not until the late-twentieth century that the importance of the immune system in tumor control was firmly established. In seminal studies examining the development of tumors in immunodeficient mice (Kaplan et al., 1998; Shankaran et al., 2001; Smyth, Crowe, & Godfrey, 2001; Smyth et al., 2000), it was established that cytotoxic CD8 T-cells and NK cells controlled the incidence and severity of spontaneously occurring and chemically induced tumors. However, immune selective pressure also edited these tumors, enabling the expansion of tumor clones that had stopped expressing target antigens and making them less susceptible to immunological control. In addition, other immune elements, including regulatory T-cells (Treg) and several myeloid populations, were shown to suppress immunity, contributing to tumor outgrowth, angiogenesis, and metastasis (Coussens, Tinkle, Hanahan, & Werb, 2000; De Palma et al., 2005; Lin, Nguyen, Russell, & Pollard, 2001; Turk, Guevara-Patiño, Rizzuto, Engelhorn, & Houghton, 2004; Yang, DeBusk, et al., 2004). Nevertheless, early correlative studies of patients with many tumor types, including melanoma (Clark et al., 1989) and neurological tumors (Lauder & Aherne, 1972; Palma, Di Lorenzo, & Guidetti, 1978), demonstrated that the presence of intratumoral lymphocytes was associated with a positive prognosis and longer survival.

Different immune cell subsets have now been correlated with prevention of tumor establishment and outgrowth (Vesely, Kershaw, Schreiber, & Smyth, 2011) as well as a positive or negative prognosis in late-stage tumors (Fridman, Pagès, Sautès-Fridman, & Galon, 2012). In fact, the same cell types are often beneficial at both stages of tumor development. Cells that are present in the tumor mass and most often linked to a positive prognosis include cytotoxic lymphocytes (CD8 T-cells and NK cells) and CD4 T-cells with a Th1 (interferon-γ [IFNγ]-producing) phenotype. Cells in the tumor mass that represent myeloid lineages, including neutrophils, macrophages, and myeloid-derived suppressor cells, are most commonly associated with a negative prognosis. Other tumor-infiltrating cell types have not been consistently linked to a single prognostic outcome. In different studies, Th2 and Th17 cells, Treg, and NKT-cells have been linked to both positive and negative prognoses (Fridman et al., 2012). The reasons for these variable associations are unclear. For Treg, this could reflect the imprecision with which phenotypic markers (e.g., FoxP3) clearly identify true regulatory cells with suppressive function, as opposed to activated effector cells in humans (Tran, Ramsey, & Shevach, 2007; Wang, Ioan-Facsinay, van der Voort, Huizinga, & Toes, 2007). It has been proposed that Th17 cells might have different phenotypes or functions depending on the tumor type and therefore exert either pro- or antitumorigenic activity (Bailey et al., 2014; Wilke et al., 2011).

Recognizing that multiple subsets of immune cells are often present in tumors at the same time, their relative representations and function may be as important as their simple presence, as these create a balance between positive and negative influences. The ratio of CD8 T-cells to Treg or total CD4 T-cells has been shown to be prognostically important in ovarian, colorectal, and pancreatic cancer (Diederichsen, Hjelmborg, Christensen, Zeuthen, & Fenger, 2003; Ino et al., 2013; Preston et al., 2013; Sato et al., 2005). In addition, although high levels of CD8 T-cells in tumors have been linked to positive clinical outcomes more commonly than for any other cell type and in a number of different tumors, their functional status in the tumor is also relevant. For example, CD8 T-cells were only associated with longer survival of renal cell carcinoma patients if they were actively proliferating (Nakano et al., 2001). CD8 T-cells that expressed CD45RO, a marker of antigen experience, were associated with both enhanced expression of cytotoxicity genes and positive prognosis in colorectal cancer patients (Galon et al., 2006; Pagès et al., 2009). Gene signatures associated with cytotoxicity and IFNγ signaling as markers of effector CD8 T-cells have similarly been associated with a positive prognosis in many other tumor types (Galon, Angell, Bedognetti, & Marincola, 2013).

Interestingly, the precise localization of CD8 T-cells within the tumor also alters their prognostic significance. The density and location of CD8 T-cells in colorectal carcinomas, encompassed as an analysis termed the "Immunoscore," was shown to exceed traditional histopathological staging in prognostic power (Angell & Galon, 2013; Galon et al., 2006). CD8 T-cell presence in both the center of the tumor and the invasive margins was associated with a better outcome than the presence in only one location (Pagès et al., 2009). The presence of CD8 T-cells was associated with improved survival if they were localized to intraepithelial, but not stromal regions of ovarian carcinoma tumors (Sato et al., 2005). In metastatic melanoma, three distinct "immunotypes" have been defined based on the presence and intratumoral distribution of immune cells (Erdag et al., 2012). Immunotype A tumors were poorly or negligibly infiltrated by immune cells, and these patients had the poorest prognosis. Immunotype B tumors contained CD8 T-cells that remained perivascular. This phenotype was associated with an intermediate prognosis. Immunotype C tumors contained CD8 T-cells that extended well away from blood vessels throughout the tumor and were associated with the best overall prognosis. Therefore, even among patients with the same histological tumor type, there is a remarkable heterogeneity in overall CD8 T-cell representation and intratumoral distribution. Most importantly, this heterogeneity indicates that fundamental processes controlling T-cell infiltration into and migration within tumors vary.

2. CD8 T-CELL REPRESENTATION IN TUMORS AS A PREDICTIVE MARKER OF RESPONSIVENESS TO THERAPY

The emergence of clinically evident cancers reveals that despite the presence and activity of CD8 T-cells, tumors can escape their control (Vesely et al., 2011). Numerous strategies to harness and/or enhance the antitumor properties of CD8 T-cells have been developed, and in recent years, have led to encouraging successes. Melanoma has historically been the most studied tumor for immunotherapies, in part, because it is also the most responsive to a wide spectrum of such therapies. However, efficacy of certain treatments has also been shown in renal cell carcinoma, lung cancer, and bladder cancer. Regardless, only a fraction of patients with any of these cancers respond to immunotherapies. Efforts to identify the basis for responsiveness have suggested that a major determinant is the presence of effector CD8 T-cells in tumors prior to initiating therapy.

High-dose IL-2 has consistently been shown to elicit clinical responses, including complete responses, in a small fraction of patients (Rosenberg et al., 1994; Schwartzentruber et al., 2011). Gene expression profiling of pretreatment tumor biopsies has revealed that a pre-existing immune-related gene signature, indicating elevated representation of CD4 and CD8 T-cells and elevated expression of T-cell-derived cytokines and T-cell-attracting chemokines, is associated with clinical responses to IL-2 (Sullivan et al., 2009; Wang et al., 2002; Weiss et al., 2011). A similar association has also been observed with clinical responses to other immunotherapies, including therapeutic cancer vaccines (Gajewski, Louahed, & Brichard, 2010; Ulloa-Montoya et al., 2013), and treatment with the checkpoint blockade antibodies anti-CTLA-4 (Ji et al., 2012), and anti-PD-1/anti-PD-L1 (Herbst et al., 2014; Tumeh et al., 2014). The pretreatment presence of effector T-cells is also associated with enhanced responsiveness to some chemotherapy and radiotherapy treatments in colorectal cancer (Halama et al., 2011, 2009; Morris, Platell, & Iacopetta, 2008; Yasuda, Nirei, Sunami, Nagawa, & Kitayama, 2011), breast cancer (Denkert et al., 2010; Loi et al., 2013; West et al., 2011), head and neck cancer (Balermpas et al., 2014), and non-small cell lung cancer (Liu et al., 2012).

Given that the immunotherapies and traditional therapies outlined augment immunity and/or inhibit tumor growth through diverse and distinct mechanisms of action, the reason(s) that a pre-existing infiltrate of CD8 T-cells in the tumor is associated with clinical responses are not entirely clear. The connection is most easily explained for anti-PD-1/PD-L1 therapy and IL-2 therapies. IL-2 may act to expand the intratumoral effector T-cell population or rescue it from an anergic phenotype (Beverly, Kang, Lenardo, & Schwartz, 1992; Margolin, 2000). PD-1 expression on effector T-cells, and engagement with its ligand PD-L1, inhibits their secretion of effector cytokines, blunts their cytotoxic function, and promotes cell death, thereby protecting peripheral tissues from excessive immune-mediated damage (Keir, Butte, Freeman, & Sharpe, 2008). In tumors, the ligands PD-L1 and PD-L2 can be expressed on tumor and stromal cells and likewise restrict immune attack and drive T-cell apoptosis (Blank et al., 2004; Dong et al., 2002). In keeping with this, patients whose tumors or stroma express PD-L1 are more likely to respond to anti-PD-1 (Topalian et al., 2012; Tumeh et al., 2014). The pre-existing accumulation of effector CD8 T-cells in the tumor therefore represents the immediate target of anti-PD-1 therapy.

Anti-CTLA-4 is proposed to act primarily in the lymph node (LN) to enhance T-cell priming rather than locally in the tumor (Pardoll, 2012). This is supported by the emergence of a broader TCR repertoire among tumor-infiltrating lymphocytes upon treatment, likely reflecting expansion of lower affinity T-cells due to a lowered threshold of activation with CTLA-4 blockade (Cha et al., 2014; Kvistborg et al., 2014). In mouse models, anti-CTLA-4 can also deplete Treg (Bulliard et al., 2013; Simpson et al., 2013). Although this mechanism has not been demonstrated in humans, responsiveness to anti-CTLA-4 has been associated with the pre-existing level of intratumoral FoxP3^{+} cells (Hamid et al., 2011). IL-2, in addition to local effects in the tumor, could also support a more robust proliferative response in the LN. Therapeutic vaccination likewise aims to enhance the response to specific tumor antigens that occurs in tumor-draining LN. Finally, chemotherapies or radiotherapies may promote the immunogenic death of tumor cells acting as a natural vaccination to promote T-cell priming against antigens from the killed cells (Casares et al., 2005; Formenti & Demaria, 2013; Lugade et al., 2005; Zitvogel, Kepp, & Kroemer, 2011). Radiotherapy is also associated with abscopal effects, whereby local irradiation leads to regression of distant metastases. This phenomenon is poorly understood, but requires effector CD8 T-cells, indicating it is immune-mediated (Demaria et al., 2005, 2004; Postow et al., 2012).

Thus, for a variety of therapies, the presence and distribution of effector CD8 T-cells in the tumor microenvironment prior to therapy predicts a positive response. This is true even for interventions that do not seem to be directly targeting the CD8 T-cells already in the tumor. In all of these instances, we suggest that the prognostic significance of pre-existing CD8 T-cells in the tumor reflects a microenvironment, and a tumor-associated vasculature, that is permissive to CD8 T-cell accumulation. As a consequence, new CD8 effectors generated in local secondary lymphoid tissue by any of these treatments may more readily enter the tumor and control it.

The adoptive transfer of *ex vivo*-expanded lymphocytes has also shown clinical efficacy in a substantial percentage of treated patients with melanoma (Restifo, Dudley, & Rosenberg, 2012). The pre-existing presence of CD8 T-cells in the tumor is naturally a prerequisite for treatment, as that is the source of the cells that are harvested, expanded, and reinfused. New adoptive transfer therapies using T-cells derived from the blood rather than the tumor, which are genetically engineered to recognize tumor antigens, have recently been shown to have some antitumor activity in solid tumors (Beatty et al., 2014). It would be expected that the presence of endogenous T-cells in the responding patients' tumors is required, but this remains to be investigated.

3. DETERMINANTS OF CD8 T-CELL REPRESENTATION IN TUMORS AND OTHER TISSUES

The overall representation of T-cells in tissues, including tumors, is determined by the balance of several fundamental processes: cells entering tissues from the blood vasculature, cells leaving through draining lymphatics, and cells proliferating and dying *in situ*. To accumulate in a tumor at a peripheral site, however, typically effector T-cells are first activated by specific antigen in the draining LN (see Fig. 1). Tumors that are poorly infiltrated by effector T-cells may be poorly immunogenic due to a paucity of antigens. Consistent with this, we have observed that murine B16 melanoma tumors transfected to express ovalbumin as a strong neoantigen are infiltrated by larger numbers of effector CD8 T-cells than the parental B16 line, which is poorly antigenic (Peske et al., 2015). Similar results have been reported for other implantable murine tumors (Yu et al., 2005). Responses to anti-CTLA-4 or anti-PD-1/PD-L1, which are associated with a pre-existing CD8 T-cell infiltrate, have also been associated with mutational burden (Champiat, Ferté, Lebel-Binay, Eggermont, & Soria, 2014;

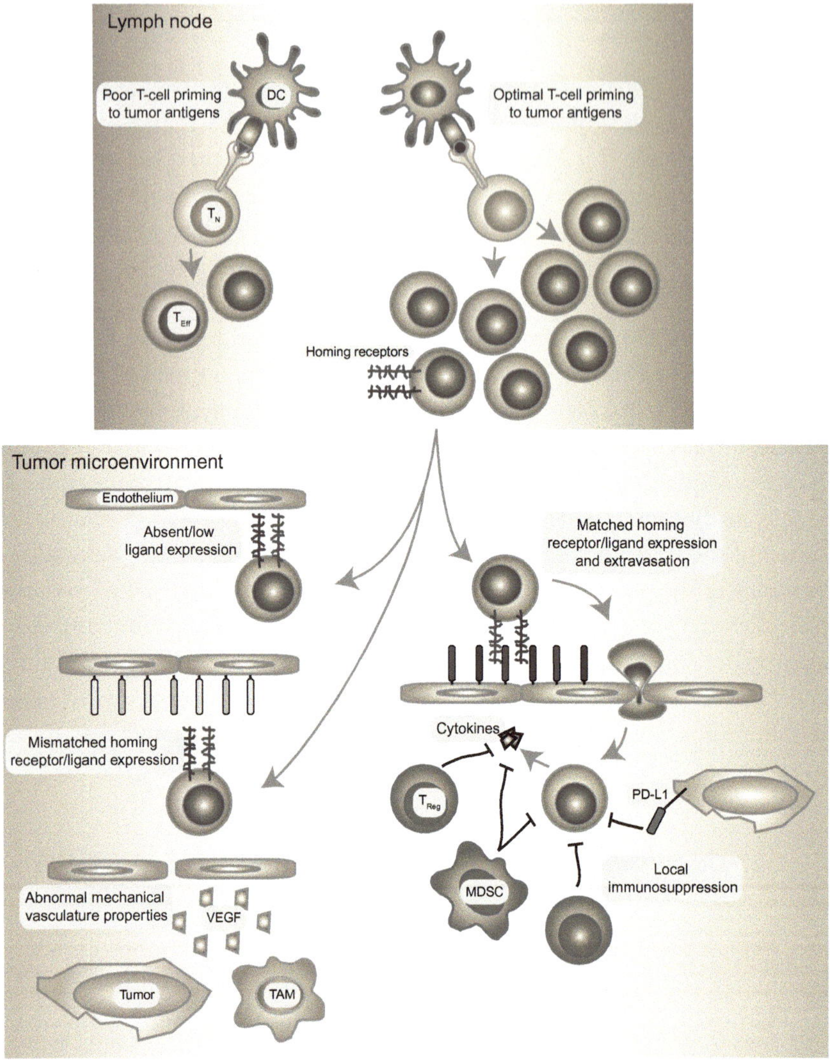

Figure 1 Factors controlling CD8 T-cell presence in tumors. The infiltration of CD8 T-cells into tumors is controlled by many factors. Initial naïve T-cell (T_N) priming to tumor antigens may be limited by poor tumor antigenicity or poor dendritic cell (DC) trafficking/maturation. If a large population of effector CD8 T-cells (T_{Eff}) is generated by spontaneous priming to tumor antigens, vaccination, or adoptive transfer, additional barriers may prevent the infiltration of these cells into the tumor. The tumor vasculature can express low levels of cognate ligands for the homing receptors expressed on the CD8 T-cell surface, or express ligands for homing receptors not expressed by the T-cells. High levels of VEGF produced by tumor and stromal cells such as tumor-associated macrophages (TAM) promote dysregulated angiogenesis, generating vasculature with abnormal mechanical properties that poorly supports CD8 T-cell infiltration. Activated T-cells that overcome these barriers and extravasate into the tumor can be suppressed by the tumor and other stromal populations, including regulatory T-cells (Treg) and myeloid-derived suppressor cells (MDSC). This limits their expression of inflammatory cytokines and inhibits further induction of ligand expression on the tumor vasculature. (See the color plate.)

Snyder et al., 2014), providing a link between T-cell representation and tumor antigenicity.

Poor representation of T-cells in tumors might also result from interference with dendritic cell (DC) maturation or trafficking. For example, type I IFN signaling is required to generate DCs capable of inducing antigen-specific antitumor CD8 T-cell responses in B16 tumor-bearing mice (Fuertes et al., 2011). Type I IFN is induced by tumor DNA that acts through the STING cytosolic DNA-sensing pathway in DC (Deng et al., 2014; Woo et al., 2014). Thus, defects in STING or type I IFN signaling might restrict DC activation and subsequent T-cell priming. Murine melanoma cells that failed to express chemokines that recruited cross-presenting DCs generated a poor T-cell response to an otherwise immunogenic tumor (Spranger, Bao, & Gajewski, 2014). High STAT-3 signaling, another common pathway activated in melanoma and other tumors, can also inhibit DC maturation thus limiting CD8 T-cell activation (Wang et al., 2004). In pancreatic tumors, the Kras driver mutation has been shown to prevent accumulation of T-cells by inducing the expression of GM-CSF, which promotes the infiltration of immunosuppressive myeloid-derived suppressor cells (Gabrilovich, Ostrand-Rosenberg, & Bronte, 2012; Pylayeva-Gupta, Lee, Hajdu, Miller, & Bar-Sagi, 2012; Vonderheide & Bayne, 2013).

In addition to the importance of these factors, there is also ample evidence to suggest that the tumor vasculature limits the representation of CD8 T-cells in tumors. Subcutaneous (SC) and intravenous (IV) routes of vaccination with bone marrow-derived DCs presenting tumor antigen both induce robust CD8 T-cell responses, but these differentially infiltrate and control tumors growing in SC sites or lungs (Mullins et al., 2003). The importance of vaccination route in enabling effective control of tumors growing in different anatomical locations has been confirmed with other vaccine modalities as well (Chang, Tai, Roffler, & Hwang, 2004; Hangalapura et al., 2011; Sandoval et al., 2013). This was shown to be related to the ability of vaccine-induced T-cells to enter tumors. Many other studies have also shown that even when circulating antigen-specific T-cells are present in blood, their accumulation in the tumor can be minimal (Lurquin et al., 2005; Marincola, Wang, Herlyn, Seliger, & Ferrone, 2003; Mullins et al., 2003; Thurner et al., 1999; Weiss et al., 2012). In this regard, limited infiltration of T-cells into tumors prevented rejection after Treg depletion in a B16 melanoma model (Quezada et al., 2008). Similarly, an exceedingly small number of adoptively transferred tumor-specific effector T-cells get into tumors, in both human and mouse studies

(Bernhard et al., 2008; Economou et al., 1996; Fisher et al., 1989; Ganss & Hanahan, 1998; Garbi, Arnold, Gordon, Hämmerling, & Ganss, 2004; Griffith et al., 1989; Kershaw et al., 2006; Pockaj et al., 1994). Finally, adoptively transferred T-cells controlled SC tumors but not gastric tumors in one murine study (Bourquin et al., 2010), suggesting that they can also differentially enter tumors based on their anatomical location. Detailed understanding of the homing characteristics of effector T-cells and tumor vasculature may explain why, even with robust effector T-cells in circulation, entry into tumors is limited.

3.1 Trafficking of Effector T-Cells into Tissues

Trafficking of leukocytes, including T-cells, from blood into lymphoid and peripheral tissues involves sequential interactions between homing receptors on leukocytes and corresponding ligands on vascular endothelial cells (Sackstein, 2005). An initial transient adhesion, in which leukocytes engage and roll slowly on the vascular surface, is followed by chemokine-mediated activation of the high-affinity conformation of integrins, leading to firm adhesion and transmigration into the underlying tissue (Butcher, 1991; Ley, Laudanna, Cybulsky, & Nourshargh, 2007). Effector differentiation in the LN upregulates expression of new homing receptors that enable CD8 T-cell entry into peripheral tissues where the corresponding vascular ligands are expressed (Mora & von Andrian, 2006).

The specific homing receptors upregulated on effector CD8 T-cells depend on the location of the priming LN and in turn on the properties of DCs and LN stromal cells that vary depending on the local environment (Campbell, Debes, Johnston, Wilson, & Butcher, 2003; Dudda et al., 2005; Hammerschmidt et al., 2008; Johansson-Lindbom et al., 2003; Masopust & Schenkel, 2013; Mora et al., 2003, 2005; Sigmundsdottir et al., 2007). For example, T-cells activated in gut-associated LN, or by DCs from gut-associated lymphoid tissues, upregulate the integrin α4β7 and the chemokine CCR9 (Campbell & Butcher, 2002; Mora et al., 2003). Conversely, T-cells activated in skin-associated LN, or by the corresponding DCs, express E-selectin ligand (ESL), P-selectin ligand (PSL), and the chemokine CCR10 (Dudda et al., 2005; Johansson-Lindbom et al., 2003; Mora et al., 2005; Sigmundsdottir et al., 2007).

Similar results are observed when T-cells are activated in different LN beds by exogenously administered DCs. Intraperitoneal (IP) immunization with bone marrow-derived DCs activates T-cells in the mesenteric and mediastinal LN that upregulates α4β7 integrin (Ferguson & Engelhard, 2010; Sheasley-O'Neill, Brinkman, Ferguson, Dispenza, & Engelhard, 2007). SC immunization activates T-cells in skin-draining LN, most of which upregulate ESL and PSL, while some express α4β1 integrin (Ferguson & Engelhard, 2010). IV immunization activates T-cells in the mediastinal LN and spleen that express α4β1 integrin without coexpression of either ESL or α4β7 integrin (Brinkman, Sheasley-O'Neill, Ferguson, & Engelhard, 2008; Ferguson & Engelhard, 2010; Sheasley-O'Neill et al., 2007). Finally, some homing receptors are upregulated on murine CD8 T-cells regardless of the site of activation. CXCR3, the receptor for CXCL9, 10, and 11 is upregulated on a substantial fraction of effector CD8 T-cells. A subset of these cells also expresses PSL, indicating that PSL expression is not restricted to cells primed in skin-draining LNs. This PSL^+ subset also coexpresses several other chemokine receptors (CCR3, 4, 5, and 6; Ferguson & Engelhard, 2010). Collectively, these results define three major populations of effector CD8 T-cells based on expression of molecules that initiate slow rolling and confer tissue specificity. By contrast, broad-based expression of chemokine receptors enables sensing of the presence of a variety of different inflammation-induced chemokines for the purposes of further immobilization and tissue entry.

Expression of the corresponding vascular ligands also varies depending on the anatomical location and inflammatory state of the underlying tissues. In some cases, this provides a basis for tissue-selective T-cell trafficking. E- and P-selectin on skin vasculature facilitate slow-rolling interactions with ESL^+ and PSL^+ effector T-cells (Austrup et al., 1997; Berg et al., 1991; Borges et al., 1997; Fuhlbrigge, Kieffer, Armerding, & Kupper, 1997; Fuhlbrigge, King, Dimitroff, Kupper, & Sackstein, 2002). E-selectin is homeostatically expressed at low levels only on skin vasculature (Brinkman, Rouhani, Srinivasan, & Engelhard, 2013; Chong, Murphy, Kupper, & Fuhlbrigge, 2004; Kupper & Fuhlbrigge, 2004). Transcription and translation leading to E-selectin expression within 4–6 h is enhanced by numerous inflammatory stimuli, including IL-1, tumor necrosis factor-alpha (TNFα), IFNγ, lipopolysaccharide (LPS), thrombin, and radiation (Hallahan, Clark, Kuchibhotla, Gewertz, & Collins, 1995; Kaplanski et al., 1997; Matsumoto et al., 2005, 2007; Yao et al., 1999; Zarbock, Ley, McEver, & Hidalgo, 2011). TNFα, IL-1, LPS, thrombin, histamine, and radiation also upregulate P-selectin within minutes as it is released from preformed stores in Weibel–Palade bodies on endothelial cells and alpha granules of platelets (Hariri et al., 2008; Yao et al., 1999). Inflammation induces transient expression of E- and P-selectin in a broad range of tissues (Barthel, Gavino, Descheny, & Dimitroff, 2007). Chemokines have also been implicated in selective T-cell trafficking to the skin. CCL27 and CCL17 are both homeostatically displayed on cutaneous venules and are upregulated by inflammatory stimuli (Homey et al., 2002; Kupper & Fuhlbrigge, 2004). CCL17 binds CCR4 on skin-homing CD4 T-cells to mediate integrin activation and induce extravasation (Andrew et al., 2001; Campbell et al., 1999), while CCL27 binds to CCR10 and promotes movement into the epidermis (Homey et al., 2002; Morales et al., 1999; Sigmundsdottir et al., 2007).

MAdCAM-1, a major ligand for α4β7 integrin, and CCL25, the ligand for CCR9, are selectively expressed on the vasculature of gut-associated tissues (e.g., intestinal lamina propria; Hammerschmidt et al., 2008; Rott, Briskin, Andrew, Berg, & Butcher, 1996). CCL25 is constitutively expressed at high levels on gut-associated vasculature and is not enhanced by inflammatory stimuli (Ericsson, Kotarsky, Svensson, Sigvardsson, & Agace, 2006), while MadCAM-1 is expressed constitutively at low levels and enhanced by TNFα and IL-1 (Ando et al., 2005). Low-affinity α4β7/MadCAM-1 interactions have been shown to initiate slow rolling of leukocytes (Chen, Salas, & Springer, 2003). Subsequent engagement of CCR9 with CCL25 induces the high-affinity forms of α4β7 integrin or LFA-1 which can mediate firm adhesion to gut vasculature (Berlin et al., 1995, 1993; Chen et al., 2003; De Château, Chen, Salas, & Springer, 2001; Salas, Shimaoka, Chen, Carman, & Springer, 2002).

Other vascular ligands are expressed more ubiquitously among different tissues, and therefore promote T-cell trafficking into a broader range of inflammatory sites. The integrin ligand VCAM-1 is constitutively expressed at low levels on vasculature of many tissues and is induced to much higher levels by TNFα, IFNγ, IL-1, LPS, thrombin, and radiation (Cook-Mills, Marchese, & Abdala-Valencia, 2011; Ferguson & Engelhard, 2010; Hubbard & Rothlein, 2000; Kaplanski et al., 1998; Lawrence & Springer, 1991; Mollà et al., 2003; Wang, Michie, Xu, & Suzuki, 2007). α4β1/VCAM-1 interactions contribute to T-cell trafficking into brain, lung, and interestingly, also the skin and gut (Baron, Madri, Ruddle, Hashim, & Janeway, 1993; Calzascia et al., 2005; Kenyon et al., 2009; Rott et al., 1996). In addition, α4β1/VCAM-1 interactions can support both slow rolling and firm adhesion of effector T-cells without chemokine-mediated activation, but possibly in cooperation with LFA-1 (Alon et al., 1995). Expression of certain chemokines is also induced during inflammation in multiple different tissues. CXCL9, 10, and 11, all ligands for CXCR3, are induced by IFNγ (Coursey, Bohat, Barbosa, Pflugfelder, & de Paiva, 2014; Tensen et al., 1999). CCL3, 4, and 5, all ligands for CCR5, are broadly induced by viruses and bacterial endotoxin (Sherry et al., 1988; Tsai et al., 2013) and promote T-cell infiltration into inflamed tissues (Abdi et al., 2002; Gregg, Nichols, Chen, Lu, & Engelhard, 2010; Hancock et al., 2000).

3.2 Trafficking of Effector T-Cells into Tumors

The homing receptor/ligand interactions required for T-cell entry into tumors are not as well characterized as for entry into peripheral tissues, and several important and related questions need to be considered. First, what homing receptor ligands are expressed on tumor vasculature? Does ligand expression vary based on anatomical site and/or tumor type? Are ligands expressed at sufficient levels to enable T-cell entry? Is tumor vascular ligand expression characteristic of the local peripheral tissue, or the tumor itself, and is it regulated positively or negatively by elements of the innate and adaptive immune systems? In many cases, the answers to these questions are only starting to be addressed.

Although tumors are sites at which significant T-cell-mediated death and inflammation may be occurring, the expression of many homing receptor ligands on tumor vasculature is low. E-selectin is often not expressed on the vasculature of squamous cell carcinomas of the skin or metastatic melanomas, despite being present on adjacent tissue vasculature (Clark et al., 2008; Weishaupt, Munoz, Buzney, Kupper, & Fuhlbrigge, 2007). MadCAM-1 is expressed at low levels on gastric adenocarcinoma vasculature relative to normal mucosal tissue (Enarsson et al., 2006). VCAM-1 and ICAM-1 expressions are also low on vasculature of melanoma, colorectal cancer, colorectal hepatic metastasis, and glioblastoma (Blank, Brown, Kacha, Markiewicz, & Gajewski, 2005; Dirkx et al., 2003; Weishaupt et al., 2007; Yoong, McNab, Hübscher, & Adams, 1998, ABW and VHE unpublished). Chemokines commonly associated with T-cell trafficking, including the CCR5 ligands CCL3, CCL4, and CCL5, or the CXCR3 ligands CXCL9, CXCL10, and CXCL11, are low in poorly infiltrated melanomas and colorectal carcinomas (Coppola et al., 2011; Harlin et al., 2009; Messina et al., 2012). Vascular endothelial growth factor (VEGF), endothelin B receptor, and CD73 are three factors that have been implicated in limiting ligand expression on vasculature, in part, through blocking inflammation-induced ligand upregulation (Buckanovich et al., 2008; Dirkx et al., 2003; Wang et al., 2011).

In some cases, expression of vascular ligands has also been shown to vary with the location of tumor growth or the tumor type. E-selectin was more often expressed at higher levels in Merkel cell carcinomas in the skin than in melanoma (Afanasiev et al., 2013; Weishaupt et al., 2007). In an assessment of several different implantable tumors growing subcutaneously, only a subset of tumors, including B16 melanoma, expressed vascular E-selectin (Seguin, Nicolazzi, Mignet, Scherman, & Chabot, 2012). We have found that the vasculature of B16 melanoma and Lewis Lung carcinoma tumors grown SC expresses E-selectin and relatively high levels of VCAM-1, while that of tumors grown IP expresses low levels of VCAM-1 and is negative for E-selectin (ABW and VHE unpublished). Conversely, MAdCAM-1 is expressed on a significantly higher fraction of the vasculature in IP B16 tumors compared to SC tumor vasculature. This indicates that homing receptor ligand expression on tumor vasculature resembles, and is presumably derived from, that of adjacent normal tissue. There is a paucity of information concerning expression of E-selectin, VCAM-1, and MAdCAM-1 among human tumor types and locations. Whether chemokines such as CCL27 and CCL25, which are normally expressed in skin and gut, are differentially expressed in tumors growing in different anatomic locations remain unknown.

Several studies have evaluated which homing receptor ligands enable infiltration of effector CD8 T-cells into tumors, either directly or as a correlation. VCAM-1 expression correlates with T-cell representation in pancreatic islet cell carcinoma and melanoma (Garbi et al., 2004; Lohr et al., 2011; Quezada et al., 2008), while ICAM-1 expression correlates with T-cell entry into melanoma, pancreatic islet carcinoma, and glioblastoma (Blank et al., 2005; Buckanovich et al., 2008; Fisher et al., 2011; Garbi et al., 2004; Lohr et al., 2011; Quezada et al., 2008). CD8 T-cell infiltration into SC B16 melanomas was also significantly reduced in ICAM-1$^{-/-}$ mice even following an inflammatory systemic hyperthermia therapy (Fisher et al., 2011). We have found that antibody blockade of $\alpha4\beta1$/VCAM-1 and LFA-1/ICAM-1 interactions significantly reduce the number of adoptively transferred $\alpha4\beta1^{+}$ effector CD8 T-cells that enter SC or IP B16 tumors (ABW and VHE unpublished). These molecular pairs are not redundant, suggesting that $\alpha4\beta1$/VCAM-1 acts to initiate slow rolling while LFA-1/ICAM-1 mediates arrest. Infiltration of adoptively transferred CXCR3$^{-/-}$ effector CD8 T-cells into SC or IP B16 tumors is almost entirely eliminated, implying that this is the major chemokine axis enabling entry (ABW and VHE unpublished). CXCR3 has also been associated with CD8 T-cell entry in other tumor models (Harlin et al., 2009; Kunz et al.,

1999; Mullins et al., 2004), and with increased survival in melanoma patients (Mullins et al., 2004). This also identifies an important role for the CXCR3 ligands CXCL9, 10, and 11. The direct role of VCAM-1, ICAM-1, and ligands for CXCR3 or other chemokine receptors in mediating T-cell entry into additional murine and human tumors still needs to be thoroughly examined.

E-selectin has also been implicated in CD8 T-cell entry into tumors. Low expression in melanomas was associated with an absence of ESL^+ CD8 T-cells (Clark et al., 2008). Higher vascular E-selectin expression among Merkel cell carcinomas in different patients was associated with larger numbers of CD8 T-cells, although it is unclear if the infiltrating T-cells were ESL^+ (Afanasiev et al., 2013). Fucosyltransferase IV and VII knockout CD8 T-cells cannot generate the carbohydrate structure to form functional ESL (Goelz et al., 1990, 1994; Knibbs et al., 1996; Maly et al., 1996) and their entry into SC B16-cOVA tumors is reduced compared to wild-type cells (Stark, Gurnani, Sad, & Krishnan, 2012). However, whether wild-type CD8 T-cell entry was dependent on either ESL or PSL (which is also fucosyltransferase dependent) or both was not determined. We have shown that adoptively transferred ESL^+ effector CD8 T-cells enter SC B16 tumors with $E\text{-selectin}^+$ vasculature more efficiently than IP tumors with $E\text{-selectin}^{neg}$ vasculature (ABW and VHE unpublished). Entry of ESL^+ effector CD8 T-cells into SC tumors growing in $E\text{-selectin}^{-/-}$ mice was also reduced compared to entry into SC tumors in wild-type mice, while blockade of P-selectin/PSL interactions with a recombinant P-selectin fusion protein had no effect (ABW and VHE unpublished). Thus, ESL/E-selectin interactions enable effector CD8 T-cell entry into skin-associated tumors where E-selectin is expressed on the vasculature.

Given the low level of MAdCAM-1 expression on SC tumor vasculature, it is not surprising that blocking antibodies to its receptor, α4β7, had no impact on T-cell entry into SC melanomas (Fisher et al., 2011). In human colorectal carcinoma patients, high MAdCAM-1 gene expression in tumor lysates correlates with the presence of CD8 T-cells (Mlecnik et al., 2010), but direct evidence that it mediates CD8 T-cell entry is lacking. The role of MAdCAM-1 in enabling T-cell infiltration into tumors deserves further scrutiny, especially in cancers of mucosal tissues or tumors that metastasize to mucosal sites.

Although selectin, integrin, and chemokine expression on tumor vasculature is generally low, it can still respond to inflammatory signals analogous to normal vasculature. For example, treating human squamous cell carcinomas with either the TLR7 agonist, imiquimod, or TNFα induced expression of E-selectin on the vasculature and significantly increased the number of ESL$^+$ CD8$^+$ T-cells in the tumor (Clark et al., 2008). Likewise, inflammation induced by systemic hyperthermia significantly increased the number of CD8 T-cells rolling on tumor vasculature, and this could be blocked by a cocktail of E- and P-selectin antibodies (Fisher et al., 2011). Additionally, treatment of pancreatic islet carcinomas with CpG upregulated VCAM-1 and ICAM-1 on tumor vasculature and significantly increased T-cell infiltration, likely due to enhanced homing ligand expression (Garbi et al., 2004). These data highlight that upregulation of homing receptor ligand expression on tumor-associated vasculature is an important maneuver to be developed in conjunction with other therapies that depend on immune infiltrates for their effectiveness.

3.3 Positive Feedback Loops in Vascular Ligand Expression

It is interesting that some of the proinflammatory cytokines that increase homing receptor ligand expression are also released by effector CD8 T-cells. This raises the possibility that early-stage effector CD8 T-cell entry into tumors could initiate a positive feedback loop in which their secretion of cytokines further upregulates homing receptor ligand expression, enhancing the entry of additional effector CD8 T-cells (see Fig. 2A). Indeed, exogenous antigen-specific T-cells that enter EL-4 thymoma increase accumulation of host T-cells as well (Boissonnas, Fetler, Zeelenberg, Hugues, & Amigorena, 2007). This increased accumulation was dependent on IFNγ released by the transferred cells, and associated with increased expression of several chemokines that are chemotactic for effector T-cells (Hollenbaugh & Dutton, 2006). We have found that B16-cOVA tumors grown in Rag1$^{-/-}$ mice, which lack B- and T-cells, express significantly lower levels of VCAM-1 and MAdCAM-1 (ABW and VHE unpublished). The adaptive immune effector activities that upregulate homing receptor ligand expression in these tumors remain to be elucidated. Importantly, the efficacy of PD-1 blockade in enhancing tumor control has been associated with induction of this positive feedback loop: enhanced IFNγ secretion by intratumoral CD8 T-cells in anti-PD-1-treated mice increased expression of chemokines, including CXCL10, and resulted in greater T-cell entry and tumor control (Peng et al., 2012).

3.4 Mechanical Properties of Vasculature

In normal angiogenesis, VEGF-activated endothelial cells detach from their neighbors and sprout in the direction of proangiogenic factors, including

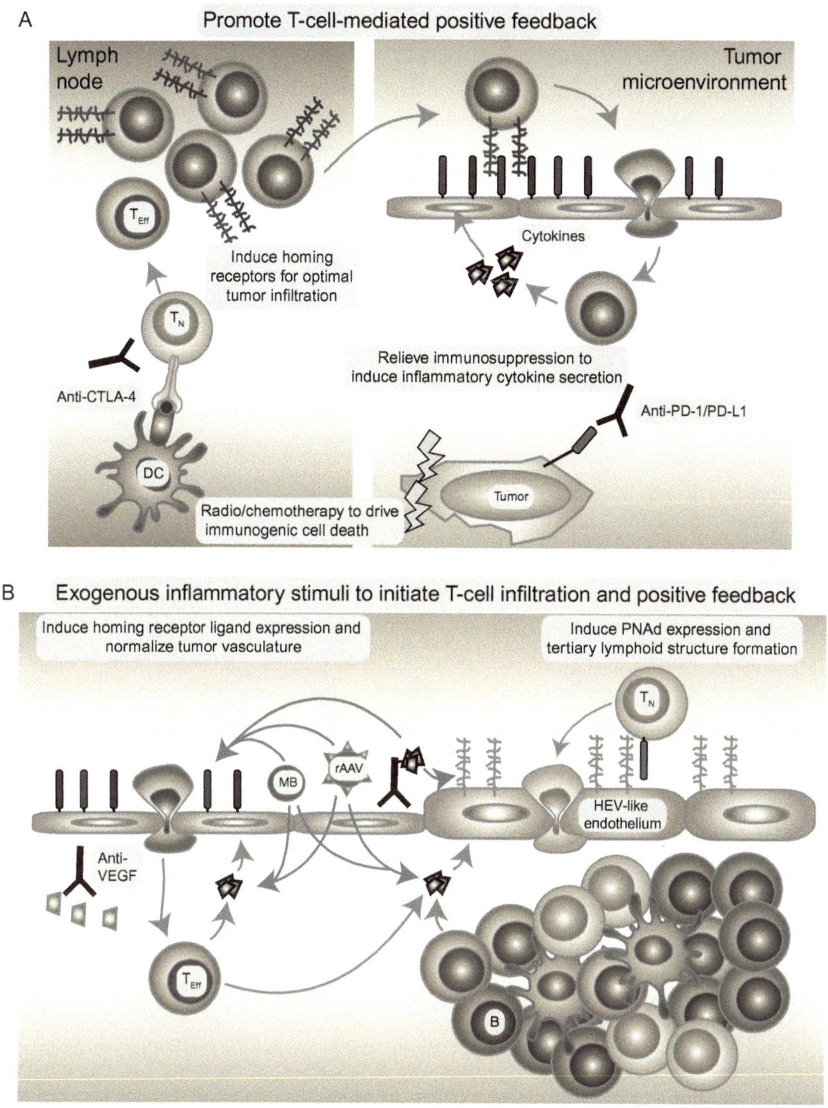

Figure 2 Strategies to promote CD8 T-cell infiltration into tumors. Several strategies could be pursued alone or in rational combinations to enhance infiltration of CD8 T-cells into tumors. To promote T-cell-mediated induction of homing receptor ligand expression (A), immunogenic cell death and treatment with anti-CTLA-4 can enhance the priming of naïve T-cells (T_N) to tumor antigens. Effector cells (T_{Eff}) expressing distinct patterns of homing receptors required to infiltrate certain tumor locations can be induced by distinct vaccination routes or generated for adoptive transfer by *in vitro* manipulation. Relieving local immunosuppression in the tumor microenvironment will enable activated T-cells infiltrating the tumor to secrete higher levels of inflammatory

(Continued)

VEGF itself (Weis & Cheresh, 2011). Proliferation results in the formation of tubes that recruit pericytes to provide stability. In a final resolution stage, the endothelial cells remodel and prune to form a functional vasculature. The enhanced availability of proangiogenic factors in tumors results in vessels that are disorganized, tortuous, leaky, and lack pericyte coverage. This abnormal architecture results in hypoxia in the tumor microenvironment and high intratumoral pressure. Loss of the gene encoding *Regulator of G-protein Signaling 5* resulted in normalization of this tumor vasculature and, intriguingly, also enhanced T-cell representation within tumors (Hamzah et al., 2008). This study concluded that this was due to a reduction in intratumoral pressure, which enabled more robust T-cell entry (Hamzah et al., 2008). This makes sense if fluid flow were a direct determinant of migration, but T-cells crawl on extracellular matrix to move within tissue. Instead, the decreased space between endothelial cells in normalized vasculature may create a more continuous vascular surface to support T-cell rolling as a prelude to entry. The effect of normalizing the tumor vasculature on vascular ligand expression was also not addressed. MadCAM-1 expression, for example, has been shown to be dependent on proximity of endothelial cells to one another (Ogawa et al., 2005), a property that could be altered by normalizing vasculature. While high-dose antiangiogenic therapy destroys vasculature and inhibits entry, low-dose antiangiogenic therapy may promote entry and enhance immunological tumor control alone or in combination with other strategies (Huang et al., 2012; Shrimali et al., 2010).

4. TUMORS DEVELOP HEV-LIKE VASCULATURE

Classically, naïve CD8 T-cells are thought to primarily recirculate through the blood and secondary lymphoid organs to scan antigen-presenting

Figure 2—Cont'd cytokines that further upregulate vascular ligands for T-cell homing receptors, generating a positive feedback loop. Expression of homing receptor ligands and T-cell infiltration can also be induced by exogenous inflammatory stimuli (B) including tumor-targeted delivery of inflammatory cytokines or cytokine genes via antibody–cytokine conjugates, microbubbles (MB), or engineered adeno-associated viruses (rAAV); systemic hyperthermia; or endothelin B receptor blockade. Anti-VEGF treatments can normalize tumor vasculature to support T-cell infiltration. Finally, tumor-targeted inflammatory stimuli that induce PNAd expression and tertiary lymphoid structure (TLS) formation can promote naïve T-cell infiltration into tumors and the local generation of an antitumor immune response. (See the color plate.)

cells for their cognate antigen (Von Andrian & Mackay, 2000). This tissue selectivity is based upon interactions of L-selectin and CCR7 with peripheral node addressin (PNAd) and CCL19/CCL21, respectively, which are normally selectively expressed on the specialized high endothelial venules (HEV) found in LN but not the vessels of peripheral tissues (Girard, Moussion, & Förster, 2012; Rosen, 2004). However, numerous recent studies have reported that PNAd and/or CCL21 are expressed in a variety of human tumors, including melanoma, breast, lung, ovarian, colorectal, and testicular cancers (Cipponi et al., 2012; Coppola et al., 2011; De Chaisemartin et al., 2011; Martinet et al., 2011, 2012; Messina et al., 2012; Sakai, Hoshino, Kitazawa, & Kobayashi, 2014). Several of these studies also showed that $PNAd^+$ HEV-like vasculature is associated with a positive prognosis (Avram et al., 2013; Martinet et al., 2011, 2012). These results suggest that inducing the development of HEV-like vasculature presents an alternative therapeutic path for enhancing intratumoral T-cell representation by enabling naïve T-cell entry into tumors, where they may become antitumor effectors.

4.1 Control of HEV in Lymph Nodes and Tertiary Lymphoid Structures

In the absence of an inflammatory insult, HEV that express PNAd and CCL21 are found exclusively in secondary lymphoid organs, including LN and MALT (e.g., PP, NALT), but not the spleen (Girard et al., 2012). In addition to their selective expression of ligands for naïve T-cell homing receptors, the endothelial cells of HEV can be distinguished from the flat endothelial cells found in other tissues by their plump, cuboidal morphology. This unique morphology also contributes to the trafficking function of HEV, enabling them to store incoming lymphocytes in "pockets" until there is room in the LN parenchyma to accommodate the entering cells (Mionnet et al., 2011).

HEV emerge in the developing LN during embryogenesis, but they do not develop their characteristic adhesion molecule expression pattern until after birth (Mebius, Streeter, Michie, Butcher, & Weissman, 1996). Still, development of HEV is presumed to depend on the same signals required for LN organogenesis as a whole. This process is dominated by signaling of the heterotrimeric form of lymphotoxin (LTα1β2) on lymphoid tissue-inducer cells through the lymphotoxin-β receptor (LTβR) on stromal organizer cells to induce chemokine secretion (Van de Pavert & Mebius, 2010). Mice deficient in LTα, LTβ, or LTβR lack most or all LN (Alimzhanov et al., 1997; De Togni et al., 1994; Fütterer et al., 1998; Koni et al., 1997). In the adult LN, the homeostatic maintenance of HEV morphology, expression of PNAd, and subsequent lymphocyte trafficking depend on LTα1β2 signals delivered by DCs directly to LTβR-expressing endothelial cells (Browning et al., 2005; Moussion & Girard, 2011), and are independent of B- and T-cells (Moussion & Girard, 2011). However, PNAd can be expressed on both the luminal and abluminal surfaces of HEVs (Rosen, 2004; Streeter, Rouse, & Butcher, 1988). LTβR signaling primarily controls luminal expression of PNAd on LN HEV (Browning et al., 2005). Furthermore, homeostatic expression of chemokine CCL21 is independent of LTβR (Browning et al., 2005; Liao & Ruddle, 2006). Thus, some, but not all specialized HEV characteristics depend on LTβR signaling.

When peripheral tissues are chronically inflamed, as in many autoimmune conditions, HEV-like blood vessels that express PNAd and/or CCL21 can develop (Rosen, 2004). This phenomenon has been reported in numerous human diseases and mouse models, including rheumatoid arthritis, Sjögren's syndrome, thyroiditis, atherosclerosis, allograft rejection, and bacterial or viral infection (Aloisi & Pujol-Borrell, 2006). In some of these conditions, $PNAd^+$ blood vessels have the unique cuboidal morphology of LN-resident HEV, while in others, the $PNAd^+$ vessels are composed of typical flat endothelial cells (Rosen, 2004). An additional feature of these inflamed tissues is the development of organized lymphocytic infiltrates around $PNAd^+$ blood vessels that are referred to as ectopic/tertiary lymphoid structures (TLS) or tertiary lymphoid organs (Aloisi & Pujol-Borrell, 2006; Drayton, Liao, Mounzer, & Ruddle, 2006). One set of criteria for defining a bona fide TLS has recently been proposed (Dieu-Nosjean, Goc, Giraldo, Sautès-Fridman, & Fridman, 2014). TLS are defined to consist of large infiltrates of B-cells and T-cells that are segregated into distinct zones, recapitulating the organization found in LN. They also contain follicular DCs and germinal centers where B-cells undergo class switching, and mature DCs capable of presenting antigen to and activating infiltrating T-cells. Not every report of TLS development has shown the structure contains all of these properties, but in general most have at least shown the accumulation of B-cells and T-cells in conjunction with antigen-presenting cells and stromal cells. The control of HEV-like vessels and TLS development in many models is similar to the mechanisms previously described for the LN. For example, in lung models of TLS that develop in response to flu or bacterial infections, DC are responsible for maintaining HEVs through LTβR signaling (GeurtsvanKessel et al., 2009;

Halle et al., 2009). Blockade of LTβR also prevents development of TLS and HEVs in many other models (Gatumu et al., 2009; Gräbner et al., 2009; Motallebzadeh et al., 2012; Rangel-Moreno et al., 2011).

4.2 Control of the Development of HEV-Like Vessels in Tumors

Although many studies have reported the existence of HEV-like vessels expressing PNAd and/or CCL21 in tumors, few have examined the cellular and molecular mechanisms leading to their spontaneous development. In human studies, the density of DCs expressing LTβ or markers of maturity has been correlated with the density of HEV-like vasculature (Martinet et al., 2013), consistent with the hypothesis that their development in tumors mirrors the pathways defined in LN. Data from several murine models, however, have implicated other cellular and molecular pathways. Recent work in our laboratory using ovalbumin-expressing B16 melanoma showed that development of HEV-like vasculature occurred in tumors growing in multiple anatomic locations in wild-type mice (Peske et al., 2015). Mechanistically, HEV-like vasculature was not induced by DC expression of LTβR, but instead required the secretion of homotrimeric $LT\alpha_3$ and IFNγ by activated effector CD8 T-cells and/or NK cells in the tumor microenvironment. These cytokines signaled through TNF receptors and the IFNγ receptor expressed on endothelial cells to induce PNAd and CCL21 expression. $PNAd^+$ blood vessels were also correlated with the presence of activated effector lymphocytes in a genetic model of melanoma driven by melanocyte-restricted $BRAF^{V600E}$ mutation and PTEN loss (Peske et al., 2015). A different study using methyl cholanthrene-induced fibrosarcomas found that the primary tumors that developed in wild-type mice did not contain HEV-like vasculature (Hindley et al., 2012). But when Treg were depleted, a fraction (~50%) of the tumors were well infiltrated with activated lymphocytes and contained blood vessels expressing PNAd and MAdCAM-1 (another HEV-associated molecule found on HEV in mesenteric LN and Peyer's patches, but not inguinal LN).

While these studies at first glance seem to point to disparate tumor-specific mechanisms leading to development of HEV-like vasculature, the results can be unified by positing that ongoing NK and/or T-cell-driven cytokine expression in the tumor microenvironment is necessary to establish and maintain HEV. Thus, in strongly antigenic tumors, effector lymphocytes receiving robust activation signals would secrete the required cytokines for HEV induction even in the presence of Treg. In less antigenic tumors, immunosuppression by Treg may dominate, necessitating their depletion to enable HEV induction by sufficiently activated effector lymphocytes. While DCs play a critical role in priming the effector T-cell response, their direct involvement in inducing HEV-like vasculature was not revealed in either murine model. The dependence of HEV-like vasculature in tumors on activated lymphocytes differs from the mechanisms defined in LN and non-tumor TLS. One possibility is that within the highly angiogenic tumor environment, endothelial cell control of HEV-like properties is altered. Indeed, differential responsiveness of $PNAd^+$ and $PNAd^-$ endothelial cells to VEGF has been documented for LN HEV (Chyou et al., 2008; Webster et al., 2006). Although endothelial cell morphology has not been carefully determined in all studies, control of PNAd expressed on flat venules in tumors (Peske et al., 2015) might differ from control on the morphologically distinct cuboidal HEV in LN.

4.3 Association of Tumor HEV with TLS

As highlighted above, $PNAd^+$ HEV-like vessels that emerge in inflamed tissues are often associated with organized TLS. Some studies have now determined if intratumoral HEV are similarly associated with organized lymphoid tissue. Not all have used the framework proposed by Dieu-Nosjean for identifying a TLS, or the organization described incompletely meets those standards. In addition, not all studies that stained for the presence of HEV also investigated if TLS were present. Including the studies that have identified HEV-like blood vessels associated with infiltrates of B- and T-cells even if they did not demonstrate fully segregated zones as in LN, HEV-associated TLS have been identified in numerous human tumors and animal models, including melanoma, lung, colorectal, and breast cancer (Goc, Fridman, Sautès-Fridman, & Dieu-Nosjean, 2013).

Importantly, HEV-like vessels also clearly develop in the absence of TLS. Primary human melanomas do contain HEV-like vessels expressing PNAd and CCL21 (Avram et al., 2013; Cipponi et al., 2012; Martinet et al., 2012). However, TLS are either entirely absent or present in only a small fraction of primary tumors (Cipponi et al., 2012; Ladányi et al., 2014). In contrast, metastases were more likely to contain TLS in association with HEV (Cipponi et al., 2012). The tissue of origin also plays a role in determining TLS presence in the metastasis. Lung metastases from primary colorectal cancers had a higher density of TLS than metastases from primary renal cell carcinomas (Remark et al., 2013). Interestingly, in our studies with ovalbumin-expressing B16 melanoma, HEV-like blood vessels develop in tumors growing at both IP and SC locations. However, associated TLS-like structures composed of an intermingled B- and T-cell infiltrate were only present in IP tumors (Peske et al., 2015). The absence of TLS in SC tumors was also observed using a B16 line transfected to express high levels of CCL21 (Shields, Kourtis, Tomei, Roberts, & Swartz, 2010). Thus, there are additional signals required to drive the maturation of an organized TLS along with those necessary for induction of PNAd on the vasculature.

One possibility is that certain sites receive the $LT\alpha_3$-mediated signals that induce PNAd expression, but poorly induce expression of chemokines such as CCL21 and CXCL13 if they fail to receive adequate IFNγ or LTβR signals. Certain anatomic locations of metastasis may also intrinsically be more or less able to support the development of TLS. For example, CXCL13 expression, which likely enables B-cell organization in the TLS (Henry & Kendall, 2010), is induced by retinoic acid signaling (Van de Pavert et al., 2009). Mucosal-associated sites where cells express high levels of retinoic acid-synthesizing enzymes may be more permissive to TLS neogenesis. In addition, transgenic overexpression of CCL21 induces TLS formation in the thyroid and pancreas (Luther et al., 2002; Marinkovic et al., 2006), but not the skin (Chen et al., 2002). Still, the skin does not have an absolute restriction on TLS development as cutaneous melanoma metastases (Cipponi et al., 2012) or SC tumors transfected to directly express LTα (Kim et al., 2004) can develop TLS. The skin might actively suppress TLS development via inhibitory factors or lack permissive signals present in mucosal sites, but this requires further investigation.

4.4 Tumor-Associated HEV-Like Vessels Support Enhanced Antitumor Immunity

While many human and murine tumors contain HEV, because their development is a consequence of a robust immune response, one possibility is that their linkage with a positive prognosis simply reflects the confounding variable of the presence of effector T-cells. However, it is now clear that intratumoral HEV also directly support an enhanced immune response. HEV-like vessels are the gateways for recruiting naïve T-cells into tumors (Peske et al., 2015). Once they have reached the tumor, naïve T-cells undergo priming and differentiation *in situ*, if they are specific for tumor antigens (Thompson, Enriquez, Fu, & Engelhard, 2010), leading to the significant restraint of tumor outgrowth (Peske et al., 2015). In some murine models where naïve T-cells are directed to the tumor in large numbers, tumors can even be completely eradicated (Yu et al., 2004). In contrast, another study demonstrated that a B16 cell line that directly secreted CCL21 developed HEV-like vessels as a component of a tolerogenic stromal environment enriched in Treg that inhibited antitumor immunity (Shields et al., 2010). While several other studies of the effects of either endogenous or exogenous CCL21 in the tumor microenvironment are consistent with the hypothesis that it is a beneficial factor promoting antitumor immunity (Kirk, Hartigan-O'Connor, Nickoloff, et al., 2001; Messina et al., 2012; Novak, Igoucheva, Cho, & Alexeev, 2007; Sharma et al., 2000; Turnquist et al., 2007; Yang, Hillinger, et al., 2004), these contrasting results suggest that the precise context in which the HEV-like blood vessels develop can be critical for determining their effect on antitumor immunity.

Furthermore, while TLS often form in relation to HEV-like vessels, it is not clear if they positively or negatively influence the development of local antitumor immunity. Histological- or gene expression-based evidence for the presence of TLS in human tumors is associated with a positive prognosis for several tumor types (Coppola et al., 2011; Dieu-Nosjean et al., 2008; Messina et al., 2012). This prognostic association may again be confounded by the fact that TLS form downstream of HEV induction as a consequence of an ongoing immune response. In a murine melanoma model where TLS-like structures (whether they included germinal centers and follicular DCs was not examined) were induced in the tumor in the absence of LN, priming of naïve T-cells still led to tumor eradication, suggesting the TLS was an effective locus for generating the antitumor immune response (Schrama et al., 2001, 2008). However, in B16-cOVA tumors, TLS-like structures develop only in IP tumors (Peske et al., 2015), but both IP and SC sites support the effective *in situ* priming and differentiation of tumor-specific naïve T-cells (Thompson et al., 2010). Furthermore, naïve T-cells primed in SC tumors in the absence of TLS still exert antitumor immune activity, delaying tumor outgrowth, and prolonging survival (Peske et al., 2015). Thus, the TLS does not appear to be absolutely required for intratumoral priming of naïve T-cells.

TLS may instead affect the antitumor immune response in more subtle ways. For example, chemokine expression in the TLS may simply help promote effective T-cell trafficking into the tumor. However, it is also possible that high levels of chemokines in TLS might retain T-cells in the structure around the vasculature, thereby restricting T-cell contact with the bulk of the tumor. Whether "Immunotype B" melanoma patients (Erdag et al., 2012), who have primarily perivascular lymphocytes and an intermediate prognosis, encompass the patients with intratumoral TLS is an interesting question. Another possibility is that the TLS primarily alters the function of intratumoral B-cells, which often dominate the structure. Intratumoral B-cells have been associated with either beneficial (DiLillo, Yanaba, & Tedder, 2010; Germain et al., 2014; Nielsen et al., 2012) or negative (Barbera-Guillem et al., 2000; DeNardo, Andreu, & Coussens, 2010) effects in different models. This could be related to whether or not the B-cells were present in the context of a TLS, which was not examined in all of these studies. Finally, the presence of TLS might improve the responsiveness to immunotherapies such as anti-CTLA-4/anti-PD-1 treatment, or vaccinations that are delivered directly to the tumor site. The overall contribution of the TLS to positive or negative effects on antitumor immunity therefore remains to be fully investigated, and will require more precise understanding of the factors driving their development.

5. ALTERING THE TUMOR VASCULATURE TO SUPPORT ENHANCED ENTRY OF NAÏVE AND EFFECTOR T-CELLS

5.1 Rationale for Modifying Tumor-Associated Vasculature

As we have reviewed, characteristics of the tumor vasculature determine whether or not tumors are permissive to the entry of both effector and naïve CD8 T-cells. Because the presence of CD8 T-cells in tumors is such a strong prognostic factor and predictor of responsiveness to immunotherapies, strategies that can alter the tumor vasculature to support the enhanced entry of T-cells hold the potential to extend the effectiveness of these immunotherapies to a much broader cross section of patients for whom they would otherwise be ineffective.

If a tumor contains only small numbers of CD8 T-cells, however, can altering just the properties of the vasculature actually have a meaningful effect? This is likely to depend on the precise nature of the tumor. For example, if the tumor has antigens that can be recognized by CD8 T-cells, but remains poorly infiltrated due to defects at the level of innate cell activation, or driver mutations that promote limited lymphocytic infiltration, then exogenous manipulations to initiate inflammation in the tumor or directly upregulate ligands for homing receptors would likely have a positive effect. Indeed in pancreatic cancer patients and murine models, vaccination and chemotherapy initiated accumulation of T-cells in the previously T-cell poor tumor (Lutz et al., 2014; Winograd et al., 2015). As effector T-cells reach the tumor in response to these interventions, they would secrete proinflammatory cytokines and initiate the positive feedback loop to support recruitment of additional effector CD8 T-cells into the tumor by maintaining an inflamed tumor vasculature. A similar effect would be expected in response to interventions designed to induce HEV-like blood vessels and promote naïve T-cell entry. Indeed, several studies have shown that maneuvers to induce intratumoral naïve T-cell priming, such as targeting of LTα to the tumor, or intratumoral vaccination with CCL21-secreting peptide-pulsed DCs, are effective, even in the absence of LN (Kirk, Hartigan-O'Connor, & Mule, 2001; Kirk, Hartigan-O'Connor, Nickoloff, et al., 2001; Schrama et al., 2008). Once naïve T-cells become activated, they would also be expected to contribute to the positive feedback loop, supporting the continual influx of T-cells through inflamed blood vessels.

There are still theoretical advantages to targeting the tumor to primarily enhance either naïve or effector T-cell entry. For example, the induction of HEV-like blood vessels appears to require LTα-TNFR signaling regardless of the site of tumor growth. Therefore, inducing vessels expressing PNAd and CCL21 at different anatomic locations may be easier than attempting to induce the different molecules involved in effector cell trafficking that may have a known tissue-selective preference for one site or another, such as E-selectin and MAdCAM-1. On the other hand, altering the vasculature to support entry of effector T-cells may work synergistically with current vaccination or adoptive transfer therapies by enhancing the very small fraction of transferred cells that enter the tumor.

5.2 Strategies for Modifying Tumor-Associated Vasculature

The simplest method for altering tumor-associated vasculature to support enhanced entry of CD8 T-cells would be through systemic administration of inflammatory stimuli, such as TNFα, LTα, LIGHT, and IFNγ, or agonistic antibodies targeting their receptors to induce upregulation of ligands for naïve and effector T-cell homing receptors. Unfortunately, this strategy is limited by the toxicity of these agents when given systemically. Therefore, an alternative strategy would be the concentrated delivery of inflammatory cytokines or other stimuli directly to the tumor site. While these strategies are still early in development, methods such as tumor endothelium-targeted microbubbles (Hernot & Klibanov, 2008) or engineered adeno-associated viruses that localize to specific tumor targets (Konkalmatt et al., 2013) are potential options (see Fig. 2). These methods could deliver a tumor vasculature-modifying drug or cytokine directly, shRNA sequences to knockdown inhibitory molecules, or even protein-coding nucleic acid sequences. These could potentially be the endothelial-expressed ligands themselves (e.g., E-selectin, VCAM-1, CXCL10), or an upstream cytokine known to induce their expression (e.g., TNFα, IFNγ, LTα).

Direct modulation of the tumor vasculature is not the only possibility; however, one interesting intervention involves a temporary induction of mild hyperthermia, which is associated with the expression of IL-6 to enhance ICAM-1 expression on tumor vasculature (Fisher et al., 2011). Inhibiting VEGF (Shrimali et al., 2010) or the endothelin B receptor that indirectly decreases expression of homing receptor ligands is another potential strategy (Buckanovich et al., 2008). Tissue engineering approaches to implant scaffolds to support development of TLS at the tumor site may also be feasible (Irvine, Stachowiak, & Hori, 2008). Furthermore, the matching of vaccination routes or *in vitro* treatments of adoptively transferred cells should be optimized to induce T-cell populations that express appropriate homing receptors to bind to the ligands expressed on tumor vasculature, which may vary with location of growth.

Interventions to enhance T-cell trafficking are not proposed to entirely supplant, but rather work in concert with current therapeutic strategies. For example, they may be combined with local radiotherapy or chemotherapy to enhance tumor antigenicity, or applied in combination with vaccination or adoptive transfer to increase the efficiency of CD8 T-cell entry into tumors. Rational combinations of immunotherapies are already showing increased efficacy in murine models and human patients (Victor et al., 2015). Modifying the tumor vasculature and microenvironment to support the entry of naïve and activated T-cells has the potential to further broaden the cohort of patients that will respond to current immunotherapies.

REFERENCES

Abdi, R., Smith, R. N., Makhlouf, L., Najafian, N., Luster, A. D., Auchincloss, H., et al. (2002). The role of CC chemokine receptor 5 (CCR5) in islet allograft rejection. *Diabetes*, *51*, 2489–2495.

Afanasiev, O. K., Nagase, K., Simonson, W., Vandeven, N., Blom, A., Koelle, D. M., et al. (2013). Vascular E-selectin expression correlates with CD8 lymphocyte infiltration and improved outcome in Merkel cell carcinoma. *The Journal of Investigative Dermatology*, *133*, 2065–2073. http://dx.doi.org/10.1038/jid.2013.36.

Alimzhanov, M. B., Kuprash, D. V., Kosco-Vilbois, M. H., Luz, A., Turetskaya, R. L., Tarakhovsky, A., et al. (1997). Abnormal development of secondary lymphoid tissues in lymphotoxin β-deficient mice. *Proceedings of the National Academy of Sciences of the United States of America*, *94*, 9302–9307.

Aloisi, F., & Pujol-Borrell, R. (2006). Lymphoid neogenesis in chronic inflammatory diseases. *Nature Reviews. Immunology*, *6*, 205–217.

Alon, R., Kassner, P. D., Carr, M. W., Finger, E. B., Hemler, M. E., & Springer, T. A. (1995). The integrin VLA-4 supports tethering and rolling in flow on VCAM-1. *The Journal of Cell Biology*, *128*, 1243–1253.

Ando, T., Jordan, P., Wang, Y., Itoh, M., Joh, T., Sasaki, M., et al. (2005). MAdCAM-1 expression and regulation in murine colonic endothelial cells in vitro. *Inflammatory Bowel Diseases*, *11*, 258–264.

Andrew, D. P., Ruffing, N., Kim, C. H., Miao, W., Heath, H., Li, Y., et al. (2001). C-C chemokine receptor 4 expression defines a major subset of circulating nonintestinal memory T cells of both Th1 and Th2 potential. *Journal of Immunology*, *166*, 103–111.

Angell, H., & Galon, J. (2013). From the immune contexture to the immunoscore: The role of prognostic and predictive immune markers in cancer. *Current Opinion in Immunology*, *25*, 261–267. http://dx.doi.org/10.1016/j.coi.2013.03.004.

Austrup, F., Vestweber, D., Borges, E., Lohning, M., Brauer, R., Herz, U., et al. (1997). P- and E-selectin mediate recruitment of T-helper-1 but not T-helper-2 cells into inflammed tissues. *Nature*, *385*, 81–83.

Avram, G., Sánchez-Sendra, B., Martín, J. M., Terrádez, L., Ramos, D., & Monteagudo, C. (2013). The density and type of MECA-79-positive high endothelial venules correlate with lymphocytic infiltration and tumour regression in primary cutaneous melanoma. *Histopathology*, *63*, 852–861. http://dx.doi.org/10.1111/his.12235.

Bailey, S. R., Nelson, M. H., Himes, R. A., Li, Z., Mehrotra, S., & Paulos, C. M. (2014). Th17 cells in cancer: The ultimate identity crisis. *Frontiers in Immunology*, *5*, 276. http://dx.doi.org/10.3389/fimmu.2014.00276.

Balermpas, P., Michel, Y., Wagenblast, J., Seitz, O., Weiss, C., Rödel, F., et al. (2014). Tumour-infiltrating lymphocytes predict response to definitive chemoradiotherapy in head and neck cancer. *British Journal of Cancer*, *110*, 501–509. http://dx.doi.org/10.1038/bjc.2013.640.

Barbera-Guillem, E., Nelson, M. B., Barr, B., Nyhus, J. K., May, K. F., Feng, L., et al. (2000). B lymphocyte pathology in human colorectal cancer. Experimental and clinical therapeutic effects of partial B cell depletion. *Cancer Immunology, Immunotherapy*, *48*, 541–549.

Baron, J. L., Madri, J. A., Ruddle, N. H., Hashim, G., & Janeway, C. A. (1993). Surface expression of alpha 4 integrin by CD4 T cells is required for their entry into brain parenchyma. *The Journal of Experimental Medicine*, *177*, 57–68.

Barthel, S. R., Gavino, J. D., Descheny, L., & Dimitroff, C. J. (2007). Targeting selectins and selectin ligands in inflammation and cancer. *Expert Opinion on Therapeutic Targets*, *11*, 1473–1491. http://dx.doi.org/10.1517/14728222.11.11.1473.

Beatty, G. L., Haas, A. R., Maus, M. V., Torigian, D. A., Soulen, M. C., Plesa, G., et al. (2014). Mesothelin-specific chimeric antigen receptor mRNA-engineered T cells induce antitumor activity in solid malignancies. *Cancer Immunology Research*, *2*, 112–120. http://dx.doi.org/10.1158/2326-6066.CIR-13-0170.

Berg, E. L., Yoshino, T., Rott, L. S., Robinson, M. K., Warnock, R. A., Kishimoto, T. K., et al. (1991). The cutaneous lymphocyte antigen is a skin lymphocyte homing receptor for the vascular lectin endothelial cell-leukocyte adhesion molecule 1. *The Journal of Experimental Medicine*, *174*, 1461–1466.

Berlin, C., Bargatze, R. F., Campbell, J. J., von Andrian, U. H., Szabo, M. C., Hasslen, S. R., et al. (1995). Alpha 4 integrins mediate lymphocyte attachment and rolling under physiologic flow. *Cell*, *80*, 413–422.

Berlin, C., Berg, E. L., Briskin, M. J., Andrew, D. P., Kilshaw, P. J., Holzmann, B., et al. (1993). Alpha 4 beta 7 integrin mediates lymphocyte binding to the mucosal vascular addressin MAdCAM-1. *Cell*, *74*, 185–195.

Bernhard, H., Neudorfer, J., Gebhard, K., Conrad, H., Hermann, C., Nährig, J., et al. (2008). Adoptive transfer of autologous, HER2-specific, cytotoxic T lymphocytes for the treatment of HER2-overexpressing breast cancer. *Cancer Immunology, Immunotherapy*, *57*, 271–280. http://dx.doi.org/10.1007/s00262-007-0355-7.

Beverly, B., Kang, S. M., Lenardo, M. J., & Schwartz, R. H. (1992). Reversal of in vitro T cell clonal anergy by IL-2 stimulation. *International Immunology*, *4*, 661–671.

Blank, C., Brown, I., Kacha, A. K., Markiewicz, M. A., & Gajewski, T. F. (2005). ICAM-1 contributes to but is not essential for tumor antigen cross-priming and CD8+ T cell-mediated tumor rejection in vivo. *Journal of Immunology*, *174*, 3416–3420.

Blank, C., Brown, I., Peterson, A. C., Spiotto, M., Iwai, Y., Honjo, T., et al. (2004). PD-L1/B7H-1 inhibits the effector phase of tumor rejection by T cell receptor (TCR) transgenic CD8+ T cells. *Cancer Research*, *64*, 1140–1145.

Boissonnas, A., Fetler, L., Zeelenberg, I. S., Hugues, S., & Amigorena, S. (2007). In vivo imaging of cytotoxic T cell infiltration and elimination of a solid tumor. *The Journal of Experimental Medicine*, *204*, 345–356. http://dx.doi.org/10.1084/jem.20061890.

Borges, E., Tietz, W., Steegmaier, M., Moll, T., Hallmann, R., Hamann, A., et al. (1997). P-selectin glycoprotein ligand-1 (PSGL-1) on T helper 1 but not on T helper 2 cells binds to P-selectin and supports migration into inflamed skin. *The Journal of Experimental Medicine*, *185*, 573–578.

Bourquin, C., von der Borch, P., Zoglmeier, C., Anz, D., Sandholzer, N., Suhartha, N., et al. (2010). Efficient eradication of subcutaneous but not of autochthonous gastric tumors by adoptive T cell transfer in an SV40 T antigen mouse model. *Journal of Immunology*, *185*, 2580–2588. http://dx.doi.org/10.4049/jimmunol.0903231.

Brinkman, C. C., Rouhani, S. J., Srinivasan, N., & Engelhard, V. H. (2013). Peripheral tissue homing receptors enable T cell entry into lymph nodes and affect the anatomical distribution of memory cells. *Journal of Immunology*, *191*, 2412–2425. http://dx.doi.org/10.4049/jimmunol.1300651.

Brinkman, C. C., Sheasley-O'Neill, S. L., Ferguson, A. R., & Engelhard, V. H. (2008). Activated CD8 T cells redistribute to antigen-free lymph nodes and exhibit effector and memory characteristics. *Journal of Immunology*, *181*, 1814–1824.

Browning, J. L., Allaire, N., Ngam-Ek, A., Notidis, E., Hunt, J., Perrin, S., et al. (2005). Lymphotoxin-beta receptor signaling is required for the homeostatic control of HEV differentiation and function. *Immunity*, *23*, 539–550. http://dx.doi.org/10.1016/j.immuni.2005.10.002.

Buckanovich, R. J., Facciabene, A., Kim, S., Benencia, F., Sasaroli, D., Balint, K., et al. (2008). Endothelin B receptor mediates the endothelial barrier to T cell homing to tumors and disables immune therapy. *Nature Medicine*, *14*, 28–36. http://dx.doi.org/10.1038/nm1699.

Bulliard, Y., Jolicoeur, R., Windman, M., Rue, S. M., Ettenberg, S., Knee, D. A., et al. (2013). Activating Fc γ receptors contribute to the antitumor activities of immunoregulatory receptor-targeting antibodies. *The Journal of Experimental Medicine*, *210*, 1685–1693. http://dx.doi.org/10.1084/jem.20130573.

Butcher, E. C. (1991). Leukocyte-endothelial cell recognition: Three (or more) steps to specificity and diversity. *Cell*, *67*, 1033–1036. http://dx.doi.org/10.1016/0092-8674(91)90279-8.

Calzascia, T., Masson, F., Di Berardino-Besson, W., Contassot, E., Wilmotte, R., urrand-Lions, M., et al. (2005). Homing phenotypes of tumor-specific CD8 T cells are predetermined at the tumor site by crosspresenting APCs. *Immunity*, *22*, 175–184.

Campbell, D. J., & Butcher, E. C. (2002). Rapid acquisition of tissue-specific homing phenotypes by CD4(+) T cells activated in cutaneous or mucosal lymphoid tissues. *The Journal of Experimental Medicine*, *195*, 135–141.

Campbell, D. J., Debes, G. F., Johnston, B., Wilson, E., & Butcher, E. C. (2003). Targeting T cell responses by selective chemokine receptor expression. *Seminars in Immunology*, *15*, 277–286. http://dx.doi.org/10.1016/j.smim.2003.08.005, S1044532303000642 [pii].

Campbell, J. J., Haraldsen, G., Pan, J., Rottman, J., Qin, S., Ponath, P., et al. (1999). The chemokine receptor CCR4 in vascular recognition by cutaneous but not intestinal memory T cells. *Nature*, *400*, 776–780.

Casares, N., Pequignot, M. O., Tesniere, A., Ghiringhelli, F., Roux, S., Chaput, N., et al. (2005). Caspase-dependent immunogenicity of doxorubicin-induced tumor cell death. *The Journal of Experimental Medicine*, *202*, 1691–1701. http://dx.doi.org/10.1084/jem.20050915.

Cha, E., Klinger, M., Hou, Y., Cummings, C., Ribas, A., Faham, M., et al. (2014). Improved survival with T cell clonotype stability after anti-CTLA-4 treatment in cancer patients. *Science Translational Medicine*, *6*, 238ra70. http://dx.doi.org/10.1126/scitranslmed.3008211.

Champiat, S., Ferté, C., Lebel-Binay, S., Eggermont, A., & Soria, J. C. (2014). Exomics and immunogenics: Bridging mutational load and immune checkpoints efficacy. *OncoImmunology*, *3*, e27817. http://dx.doi.org/10.4161/onci.27817.

Chang, C.-J., Tai, K.-F., Roffler, S., & Hwang, L.-H. (2004). The immunization site of cytokine-secreting tumor cell vaccines influences the trafficking of tumor-specific T lymphocytes and antitumor efficacy against regional tumors. *Journal of Immunology*, *173*, 6025–6032. http://dx.doi.org/10.4049/jimmunol.173.10.6025.

Chen, J., Salas, A., & Springer, T. A. (2003). Bistable regulation of integrin adhesiveness by a bipolar metal ion cluster. *Nature Structural & Molecular Biology*, *10*, 995–1001. http://dx.doi.org/10.1038/nsb1011.

Chen, S. C., Vassileva, G., Kinsley, D., Holzmann, S., Manfra, D., Wiekowski, M. T., et al. (2002). Ectopic expression of the murine chemokines CCL21a and CCL21b induces the formation of lymph node-like structures in pancreas, but not skin, of transgenic mice. *Journal of Immunology*, *168*, 1001–1008.

Chong, B. F., Murphy, J. E., Kupper, T. S., & Fuhlbrigge, R. C. (2004). E-selectin, thymus- and activation-regulated chemokine/CCL17, and intercellular adhesion molecule-1 are constitutively coexpressed in dermal microvessels: A foundation for a cutaneous immunosurveillance system. *Journal of Immunology*, *172*, 1575–1581.

Chyou, S., Ekland, E. H., Carpenter, A. C., Tzeng, T.-C. J., Tian, S., Michaud, M., et al. (2008). Fibroblast-type reticular stromal cells regulate the lymph node vasculature. *Journal of Immunology*, *181*, 3887–3896.

Cipponi, A., Mercier, M., Seremet, T., Baurain, J.-F., Théate, I., van den Oord, J., et al. (2012). Neogenesis of lymphoid structures and antibody responses occur in human melanoma metastases. *Cancer Research*, *72*, 3997–4007. http://dx.doi.org/10.1158/0008-5472.CAN-12-1377.

Clark, W. H., Jr., Elder, D. E., Guerry, D., 4th, Braitman, L. E., Trock, B. J., Schultz, D., et al. (1989). Model predicting survival in stage I melanoma based on tumor progression. *Journal of the National Cancer Institute*, *81*, 1893–1904.

Clark, R. A., Huang, S. J., Murphy, G. F., Mollet, I. G., Hijnen, D., Muthukuru, M., et al. (2008). Human squamous cell carcinomas evade the immune response by down-regulation of vascular E-selectin and recruitment of regulatory T cells. *The Journal of Experimental Medicine*, *205*, 2221–2234. http://dx.doi.org/10.1084/jem.20071190.

Coley, W. (1893). The treatment of malignant tumors by repeated inoculations of erysipelas. With a report of ten original cases. *The American Journal of the Medical Sciences*, *105*, 487–511.

Cook-Mills, J. M., Marchese, M. E., & Abdala-Valencia, H. (2011). Vascular cell adhesion molecule-1 expression and signaling during disease: Regulation by reactive oxygen species and antioxidants. *Antioxidants & Redox Signaling, 15*, 1607–1638. http://dx.doi.org/10.1089/ars.2010.3522.

Coppola, D., Nebozhyn, M., Khalil, F., Dai, H., Yeatman, T., Loboda, A., et al. (2011). Unique ectopic lymph node-like structures present in human primary colorectal carcinoma are identified by immune gene array profiling. *The American Journal of Pathology, 179*, 37–45. http://dx.doi.org/10.1016/j.ajpath.2011.03.007.

Coursey, T. G., Bohat, R., Barbosa, F. L., Pflugfelder, S. C., & de Paiva, C. S. (2014). Desiccating stress-induced chemokine expression in the epithelium is dependent on upregulation of NKG2D/RAE-1 and release of IFN-γ in experimental dry eye. *Journal of Immunology, 193*, 5264–5272. http://dx.doi.org/10.4049/jimmunol.1400016.

Coussens, L. M., Tinkle, C. L., Hanahan, D., & Werb, Z. (2000). MMP-9 supplied by bone marrow-derived cells contributes to skin carcinogenesis. *Cell, 103*, 481–490. http://dx.doi.org/10.1016/S0092-8674(00)00139-2.

De Chaisemartin, L., Goc, J., Damotte, D., Validire, P., Magdeleinat, P., Alifano, M., et al. (2011). Characterization of chemokines and adhesion molecules associated with T cell presence in tertiary lymphoid structures in human lung cancer. *Cancer Research, 71*, 6391–6399. http://dx.doi.org/10.1158/0008-5472.CAN-11-0952.

De Château, M., Chen, S., Salas, A., & Springer, T. A. (2001). Kinetic and mechanical basis of rolling through an integrin and novel Ca^{2+}-dependent rolling and Mg^{2+}-dependent firm adhesion modalities for the α4β7–MAdCAM-1 interaction. *Biochemistry, 40*, 13972–13979. http://dx.doi.org/10.1021/bi011582f.

De Palma, M., Venneri, M. A., Galli, R., Sergi, L. S., Politi, L. S., Sampaolesi, M., et al. (2005). Tie2 identifies a hematopoietic lineage of proangiogenic monocytes required for tumor vessel formation and a mesenchymal population of pericyte progenitors. *Cancer Cell, 8*, 211–226. http://dx.doi.org/10.1016/j.ccr.2005.08.002.

De Togni, P., Goellner, J., Ruddle, N. H., Streeter, P. R., Fick, A., Mariathasan, S., et al. (1994). Abnormal development of peripheral lymphoid organs in mice deficient in lymphotoxin. *Science, 264*, 703–707.

Demaria, S., Kawashima, N., Yang, A. M., Devitt, M. L., Babb, J. S., Allison, J. P., et al. (2005). Immune-mediated inhibition of metastases after treatment with local radiation and CTLA-4 blockade in a mouse model of breast cancer. *Clinical Cancer Research, 11*, 728–734.

Demaria, S., Ng, B., Devitt, M. L., Babb, J. S., Kawashima, N., Liebes, L., et al. (2004). Ionizing radiation inhibition of distant untreated tumors (abscopal effect) is immune mediated. *International Journal of Radiation Oncology, Biology, Physics, 58*, 862–870. http://dx.doi.org/10.1016/j.ijrobp.2003.09.012.

DeNardo, D. G., Andreu, P., & Coussens, L. M. (2010). Interactions between lymphocytes and myeloid cells regulate pro- versus anti-tumor immunity. *Cancer Metastasis Reviews, 29*, 309–316. http://dx.doi.org/10.1007/s10555-010-9223-6.

Deng, L., Liang, H., Xu, M., Yang, X., Burnette, B., Arina, A., et al. (2014). STING-dependent cytosolic DNA sensing promotes radiation-induced type i interferon-dependent antitumor immunity in immunogenic tumors. *Immunity, 41*, 843–852. http://dx.doi.org/10.1016/j.immuni.2014.10.019.

Denkert, C., Loibl, S., Noske, A., Roller, M., Müller, B. M., Komor, M., et al. (2010). Tumor-associated lymphocytes as an independent predictor of response to neoadjuvant chemotherapy in breast cancer. *Journal of Clinical Oncology, 28*, 105–113. http://dx.doi.org/10.1200/JCO.2009.23.7370.

Diederichsen, A. C. P., Hjelmborg,, J. v B., Christensen, P. B., Zeuthen, J., & Fenger, C. (2003). Prognostic value of the CD4+/CD8+ ratio of tumour infiltrating lymphocytes in colorectal cancer and HLA-DR expression on tumour cells. *Cancer Immunology, Immunotherapy*, *52*, 423–428. http://dx.doi.org/10.1007/s00262-003-0388-5.

Dieu-Nosjean, M.-C., Antoine, M., Danel, C., Heudes, D., Wislez, M., Poulot, V., et al. (2008). Long-term survival for patients with non-small-cell lung cancer with intratumoral lymphoid structures. *Journal of Clinical Oncology*, *26*, 4410–4417. http://dx.doi.org/10.1200/JCO.2007.15.0284.

Dieu-Nosjean, M.-C., Goc, J., Giraldo, N. A., Sautès-Fridman, C., & Fridman, W. H. (2014). Tertiary lymphoid structures in cancer and beyond. *Trends in Immunology*, *35*, 571–580. http://dx.doi.org/10.1016/j.it.2014.09.006.

DiLillo, D. J., Yanaba, K., & Tedder, T. F. (2010). B cells are required for optimal CD4+ and CD8+ T cell tumor immunity: Therapeutic B cell depletion enhances B16 melanoma growth in mice. *Journal of Immunology*, *184*, 4006–4016. http://dx.doi.org/10.4049/jimmunol.0903009.

Dirkx, A. E. M., oude Egbrink, M. G., Kuijpers, M. J., van der Niet, S. T., Heijnen, V. V., Bouma-ter Steege, J. C., et al. (2003). Tumor angiogenesis modulates leukocyte-vessel wall interactions in vivo by reducing endothelial adhesion molecule expression. *Cancer Research*, *63*, 2322–2329.

Dong, H., Strome, S. E., Salomao, D. R., Tamura, H., Hirano, F., Flies, D. B., et al. (2002). Tumor-associated B7-H1 promotes T-cell apoptosis: A potential mechanism of immune evasion. *Nature Medicine*, *8*, 793–800.

Drayton, D. L., Liao, S., Mounzer, R. H., & Ruddle, N. H. (2006). Lymphoid organ development: From ontogeny to neogenesis. *Nature Immunology*, *7*, 344–353.

Dudda, J. C., Lembo, A., Bachtanian, E., Huehn, J., Siewert, C., Hamann, A., et al. (2005). Dendritic cells govern induction and reprogramming of polarized tissue-selective homing receptor patterns of T cells: Important roles for soluble factors and tissue microenvironments. *European Journal of Immunology*, *35*, 1056–1065.

Economou, J. S., Belldegrun, A. S., Glaspy, J., Toloza, E. M., Figlin, R., Hobbs, J., et al. (1996). In vivo trafficking of adoptively transferred interleukin-2 expanded tumor-infiltrating lymphocytes and peripheral blood lymphocytes. Results of a double gene marking trial. *The Journal of Clinical Investigation*, *97*, 515–521. http://dx.doi.org/10.1172/JCI118443.

Enarsson, K., Johnsson, E., Lindholm, C., Lundgren, A., Pan-Hammarström, Q., Strömberg, E., et al. (2006). Differential mechanisms for T lymphocyte recruitment in normal and neoplastic human gastric mucosa. *Clinical Immunology*, *118*, 24–34. http://dx.doi.org/10.1016/j.clim.2005.08.001.

Erdag, G., Schaefer, J. T., Smolkin, M. E., Deacon, D. H., Shea, S. M., Dengel, L. T., et al. (2012). Immunotype and immunohistologic characteristics of tumor-infiltrating immune cells are associated with clinical outcome in metastatic melanoma. *Cancer Research*, *72*, 1070–1080. http://dx.doi.org/10.1158/0008-5472.CAN-11-3218.

Ericsson, A., Kotarsky, K., Svensson, M., Sigvardsson, M., & Agace, W. (2006). Functional characterization of the CCL25 promoter in small intestinal epithelial cells suggests a regulatory role for caudal-related homeobox (Cdx) transcription factors. *Journal of Immunology*, *176*, 3642–3651. http://dx.doi.org/10.4049/jimmunol.176.6.3642.

Ferguson, A. R., & Engelhard, V. H. (2010). CD8 T cells activated in distinct lymphoid organs differentially express adhesion proteins and coexpress multiple chemokine receptors. *Journal of Immunology*, *184*, 4079–4086. http://dx.doi.org/10.4049/jimmunol.0901903, jimmunol.0901903 [pii].

Fisher, D. T., Chen, Q., Skitzki, J. J., Muhitch, J. B., Zhou, L., Appenheimer, M. M., et al. (2011). IL-6 trans-signaling licenses mouse and human tumor microvascular gateways for trafficking of cytotoxic T cells. *The Journal of Clinical Investigation*, *121*, 3846–3859. http://dx.doi.org/10.1172/JCI44952.

Fisher, B., Packard, B. S., Read, E. J., Carrasquillo, J. A., Carter, C. S., Topalian, S. L., et al. (1989). Tumor localization of adoptively transferred indium-111 labeled tumor infiltrating lymphocytes in patients with metastatic melanoma. *Journal of Clinical Oncology, 7*, 250–261.

Formenti, S. C., & Demaria, S. (2013). Combining radiotherapy and cancer immunotherapy: A paradigm shift. *Journal of the National Cancer Institute, 105*, 256–265. http://dx.doi.org/10.1093/jnci/djs629.

Fridman, W. H., Pagès, F., Sautès-Fridman, C., & Galon, J. (2012). The immune contexture in human tumours: Impact on clinical outcome. *Nature Reviews. Cancer, 12*, 298–306. http://dx.doi.org/10.1038/nrc3245.

Fuertes, M. B., Kacha, A. K., Kline, J., Woo, S.-R., Kranz, D. M., Murphy, K. M., et al. (2011). Host type I IFN signals are required for antitumor CD8+ T cell responses through CD8{alpha}+ dendritic cells. *The Journal of Experimental Medicine, 208*, 2005–2016. http://dx.doi.org/10.1084/jem.20101159.

Fuhlbrigge, R. C., Kieffer, J. D., Armerding, D., & Kupper, T. S. (1997). Cutaneous lymphocyte antigen is a specialized form of PSGL-1 expressed on skin-homing T cells. *Nature, 389*, 978–981.

Fuhlbrigge, R. C., King, S. L., Dimitroff, C. J., Kupper, T. S., & Sackstein, R. (2002). Direct real-time observation of E- and P-selectin-mediated rolling on cutaneous lymphocyte-associated antigen immobilized on Western blots. *Journal of Immunology, 168*, 5645–5651.

Fütterer, A., Mink, K., Luz, A., Kosco-Vilbois, M. H., & Pfeffer, K. (1998). The lymphotoxin β receptor controls organogenesis and affinity maturation in peripheral lymphoid tissues. *Immunity, 9*, 59–70. http://dx.doi.org/10.1016/S1074-7613(00)80588-9.

Gabrilovich, D. I., Ostrand-Rosenberg, S., & Bronte, V. (2012). Coordinated regulation of myeloid cells by tumours. *Nature Reviews. Immunology, 12*, 253–268. http://dx.doi.org/10.1038/nri3175.

Gajewski, T. F., Louahed, J., & Brichard, V. G. (2010). Gene signature in melanoma associated with clinical activity. *Cancer Journal, 16*, 399–403. http://dx.doi.org/10.1097/PPO.0b013e3181eacbd8.

Galon, J., Angell, H. K., Bedognetti, D., & Marincola, F. M. (2013). The continuum of cancer immunosurveillance: Prognostic, predictive, and mechanistic signatures. *Immunity, 39*, 11–26. http://dx.doi.org/10.1016/j.immuni.2013.07.008.

Galon, J., Costes, A., Sanchez-Cabo, F., Kirilovsky, A., Mlecnik, B., Lagorce-Pagès, C., et al. (2006). Type, density, and location of immune cells within human colorectal tumors predict clinical outcome. *Science, 313*, 1960–1964. http://dx.doi.org/10.1126/science.1129139.

Ganss, R., & Hanahan, D. (1998). Tumor microenvironment can restrict the effectiveness of activated antitumor lymphocytes. *Cancer Research, 58*, 4673–4681.

Garbi, N., Arnold, B., Gordon, S., Hämmerling, G. J., & Ganss, R. (2004). CpG motifs as proinflammatory factors render autochthonous tumors permissive for infiltration and destruction. *Journal of Immunology, 172*, 5861–5869.

Gatumu, M. K., Skarstein, K., Papandile, A., Browning, J. L., Fava, R. A., & Bolstad, A. (2009). Blockade of lymphotoxin-beta receptor signaling reduces aspects of Sjögren syndrome in salivary glands of non-obese diabetic mice. *Arthritis Research & Therapy, 11*, R24. http://dx.doi.org/10.1186/ar2617.

Germain, C., Gnjatic, S., Tamzalit, F., Knockaert, S., Remark, R., Goc, J., et al. (2014). Presence of B cells in tertiary lymphoid structures is associated with a protective immunity in patients with lung cancer. *American Journal of Respiratory and Critical Care Medicine, 189*, 832–844. http://dx.doi.org/10.1164/rccm.201309-1611OC.

GeurtsvanKessel, C. H., Willart, M. A., Bergen, I. M., van Rijt, L. S., Muskens, F., Elewaut, D., et al. (2009). Dendritic cells are crucial for maintenance of tertiary lymphoid structures in the lung of influenza virus-infected mice. *The Journal of Experimental Medicine*, *206*, 2339–2349. http://dx.doi.org/10.1084/jem.20090410, jem.20090410 [pii].

Girard, J.-P., Moussion, C., & Förster, R. (2012). HEVs, lymphatics and homeostatic immune cell trafficking in lymph nodes. *Nature Reviews. Immunology*, *12*, 762–773. http://dx.doi.org/10.1038/nri3298.

Goc, J., Fridman, W.-H., Sautès-Fridman, C., & Dieu-Nosjean, M.-C. (2013). Characteristics of tertiary lymphoid structures in primary cancers. *OncoImmunology*, *2*, e26836. http://dx.doi.org/10.4161/onci.26836.

Goelz, S. E., Hession, C., Goff, D., Griffiths, B., Tizard, R., Newman, B., et al. (1990). ELFT: A gene that directs the expression of an ELAM-1 ligand. *Cell*, *63*, 1349–1356. http://dx.doi.org/10.1016/0092-8674(90)90430-M.

Goelz, S., Kumar, R., Potvin, B., Sundaram, S., Brickelmaier, M., & Stanley, P. (1994). Differential expression of an E-selectin ligand (SLex) by two Chinese hamster ovary cell lines transfected with the same alpha (1,3)-fucosyltransferase gene (ELFT). *The Journal of Biological Chemistry*, *269*, 1033–1040.

Gräbner, R., Lötzer, K., Döpping, S., Hildner, M., Radke, D., Beer, M., et al. (2009). Lymphotoxin β receptor signaling promotes tertiary lymphoid organogenesis in the aorta adventitia of aged ApoE$^{-/-}$ mice. *The Journal of Experimental Medicine*, *206*, 233–248. http://dx.doi.org/10.1084/jem.20080752.

Gregg, R. K., Nichols, L., Chen, Y., Lu, B., & Engelhard, V. H. (2010). Mechanisms of spatial and temporal development of autoimmune vitiligo in tyrosinase-specific TCR transgenic mice. *Journal of Immunology*, *184*, 1909–1917. http://dx.doi.org/10.4049/jimmunol.0902778, jimmunol.0902778 [pii].

Griffith, K. D., Read, E. J., Carrasquillo, J. A., Carter, C. S., Yang, J. C., Fisher, B., et al. (1989). In vivo distribution of adoptively transferred indium-111-labeled tumor infiltrating lymphocytes and peripheral blood lymphocytes in patients with metastatic melanoma. *Journal of the National Cancer Institute*, *81*, 1709–1717.

Halama, N., Michel, S., Kloor, M., Zoernig, I., Benner, A., Spille, A., et al. (2011). Localization and density of immune cells in the invasive margin of human colorectal cancer liver metastases are prognostic for response to chemotherapy. *Cancer Research*, *71*, 5670–5677. http://dx.doi.org/10.1158/0008-5472.CAN-11-0268.

Halama, N., Michel, S., Kloor, M., Zoernig, I., Pommerencke, T., von Knebel Doeberitz, M., et al. (2009). The localization and density of immune cells in primary tumors of human metastatic colorectal cancer shows an association with response to chemotherapy. *Cancer Immunity*, *9*, 1.

Hallahan, D., Clark, E. T., Kuchibhotla, J., Gewertz, B. L., & Collins, T. (1995). E-selectin gene induction by ionizing radiation is independent of cytokine induction. *Biochemical and Biophysical Research Communications*, *217*, 784–795. http://dx.doi.org/10.1006/bbrc.1995.2841.

Halle, S., Dujardin, H. C., Bakocevic, N., Fleige, H., Danzer, H., Willenzon, S., et al. (2009). Induced bronchus-associated lymphoid tissue serves as a general priming site for T cells and is maintained by dendritic cells. *The Journal of Experimental Medicine*, *206*, 2593–2601. http://dx.doi.org/10.1084/jem.20091472, jem.20091472 [pii].

Hamid, O., Schmidt, H., Nissan, A., Ridolfi, L., Aamdal, S., Hansson, J., et al. (2011). A prospective phase II trial exploring the association between tumor microenvironment biomarkers and clinical activity of ipilimumab in advanced melanoma. *Journal of Translational Medicine*, *9*, 204. http://dx.doi.org/10.1186/1479-5876-9-204.

Hammerschmidt, S. I., Ahrendt, M., Bode, U., Wahl, B., Kremmer, E., Förster, R., et al. (2008). Stromal mesenteric lymph node cells are essential for the generation of gut-homing T cells in vivo. *The Journal of Experimental Medicine*, *205*, 2483–2490. http://dx.doi.org/10.1084/jem.20080039.

Hamzah, J., Jugold, M., Kiessling, F., Rigby, P., Manzur, M., Marti, H. H., et al. (2008). Vascular normalization in Rgs5-deficient tumours promotes immune destruction. *Nature*, *453*, 410–414.

Hancock, W. W., Lu, B., Gao, W., Csizmadia, V., Faia, K., King, J. A., et al. (2000). Requirement of the chemokine receptor CXCR3 for acute allograft rejection. *The Journal of Experimental Medicine*, *192*, 1515–1520.

Hangalapura, B. N., Oosterhoff, D., Gupta, T., de Groot, J., Wijnands, P. G. J. T. B., van Beusechem, V. W., et al. (2011). Delivery route, MyD88 signaling and cross-priming events determine the anti-tumor efficacy of an adenovirus based melanoma vaccine. *Vaccine*, *29*, 2313–2321. http://dx.doi.org/10.1016/j.vaccine.2011.01.022.

Hariri, G., Zhang, Y., Fu, A., Han, Z., Brechbiel, M., Tantawy, M. N., et al. (2008). Radiation-guided P-selectin antibody targeted to lung cancer. *Annals of Biomedical Engineering*, *36*, 821–830. http://dx.doi.org/10.1007/s10439-008-9444-9.

Harlin, H., Meng, Y., Peterson, A. C., Zha, Y., Tretiakova, M., Slingluff, C., et al. (2009). Chemokine expression in melanoma metastases associated with CD8+ T-cell recruitment. *Cancer Research*, *69*, 3077–3085. http://dx.doi.org/10.1158/0008-5472.CAN-08-2281.

Henry, R. A., & Kendall, P. L. (2010). CXCL13 blockade disrupts B lymphocyte organization in tertiary lymphoid structures without altering B cell receptor bias or preventing diabetes in nonobese diabetic mice. *Journal of Immunology*, *185*, 1460–1465. http://dx.doi.org/10.4049/jimmunol.0903710.

Herbst, R. S., Soria, J.-C., Kowanetz, M., Fine, G. D., Hamid, O., Gordon, M. S., et al. (2014). Predictive correlates of response to the anti-PD-L1 antibody MPDL3280A in cancer patients. *Nature*, *515*, 563–567. http://dx.doi.org/10.1038/nature14011.

Hernot, S., & Klibanov, A. L. (2008). Microbubbles in ultrasound-triggered drug and gene delivery. *Advanced Drug Delivery Reviews*, *60*, 1153–1166. http://dx.doi.org/10.1016/j.addr.2008.03.005.

Hindley, J. P., Jones, E., Smart, K., Bridgeman, H., Lauder, S. N., Ondondo, B., et al. (2012). T-cell trafficking facilitated by high endothelial venules is required for tumor control after regulatory T-cell depletion. *Cancer Research*, *72*, 5473–5482. http://dx.doi.org/10.1158/0008-5472.CAN-12-1912.

Hollenbaugh, J. A., & Dutton, R. W. (2006). IFN-γ regulates donor CD8 T cell expansion, migration, and leads to apoptosis of cells of a solid tumor. *Journal of Immunology*, *177*, 3004–3011. http://dx.doi.org/10.4049/jimmunol.177.5.3004.

Homey, B., Alenius, H., Muller, A., Soto, H., Bowman, E. P., Yuan, W., et al. (2002). CCL27-CCR10 interactions regulate T cell-mediated skin inflammation. *Nature Medicine*, *8*, 157–165.

Huang, Y., Yuan, J., Righi, E., Kamoun, W. S., Ancukiewicz, M., Nezivar, J., et al. (2012). Vascular normalizing doses of antiangiogenic treatment reprogram the immunosuppressive tumor microenvironment and enhance immunotherapy. *Proceedings of the National Academy of Sciences of the United States of America*, *109*, 17561–17566. http://dx.doi.org/10.1073/pnas.1215397109.

Hubbard, A. K., & Rothlein, R. (2000). Intercellular adhesion molecule-1 (ICAM-1) expression and cell signaling cascades. *Free Radical Biology & Medicine*, *28*, 1379–1386.

Ino, Y., Yamazaki-Itoh, R., Shimada, K., Iwasaki, M., Kosuge, T., Kanai, Y., et al. (2013). Immune cell infiltration as an indicator of the immune microenvironment of pancreatic cancer. *British Journal of Cancer*, *108*, 914–923. http://dx.doi.org/10.1038/bjc.2013.32.

Irvine, D. J., Stachowiak, A. N., & Hori, Y. (2008). Lymphoid tissue engineering: Invoking lymphoid tissue neogenesis in immunotherapy and models of immunity. *Seminars in Immunology*, *20*, 137–146. http://dx.doi.org/10.1016/j.smim.2007.10.010.

Ji, R.-R., Chasalow, S. D., Wang, L., Hamid, O., Schmidt, H., Cogswell, J., et al. (2012). An immune-active tumor microenvironment favors clinical response to ipilimumab. *Cancer*

Immunology, Immunotherapy, 61, 1019–1031. http://dx.doi.org/10.1007/s00262-011-1172-6.
Johansson-Lindbom, B., Svensson, M., Wurbel, M. A., Malissen, B., Marquez, G., & Agace, W. (2003). Selective generation of gut tropic T cells in gut-associated lymphoid tissue (GALT): Requirement for GALT dendritic cells and adjuvant. *The Journal of Experimental Medicine, 198*, 963–969.
Kaplan, D. H., Shankaran, V., Dighe, A. S., Stockert, E., Aguet, M., Old, L. J., et al. (1998). Demonstration of an interferon gamma-dependent tumor surveillance system in immunocompetent mice. *Proceedings of the National Academy of Sciences of the United States of America, 95*, 7556–7561.
Kaplanski, G., Fabrigoule, M., Boulay, V., Dinarello, C. A., Bongrand, P., Kaplanski, S., et al. (1997). Thrombin induces endothelial type II activation in vitro: IL-1 and TNF-alpha-independent IL-8 secretion and E-selectin expression. *Journal of Immunology, 158*, 5435–5441.
Kaplanski, G., Marin, V., Fabrigoule, M., Boulay, V., Benoliel, A.-M., Bongrand, P., et al. (1998). Thrombin-activated human endothelial cells support monocyte adhesion in vitro following expression of intercellular adhesion molecule-1 (ICAM-1; CD54) and vascular cell adhesion molecule-1 (VCAM-1; CD106). *Blood, 92*, 1259–1267.
Keir, M. E., Butte, M. J., Freeman, G. J., & Sharpe, A. H. (2008). PD-1 and its ligands in tolerance and immunity. *Annual Review of Immunology, 26*, 677–704.
Kenyon, N. J., Liu, R., O'Roark, E. M., Huang, W., Peng, L., & Lam, K. S. (2009). An alpha4beta1 integrin antagonist decreases airway inflammation in ovalbumin-exposed mice. *European Journal of Pharmacology, 603*, 138–146. http://dx.doi.org/10.1016/j.ejphar.2008.11.063, S0014-2999(08)01216-8 [pii].
Kershaw, M. H., Westwood, J. A., Parker, L. L., Wang, G., Eshhar, Z., Mavroukakis, S. A., et al. (2006). A phase I study on adoptive immunotherapy using gene-modified T cells for ovarian cancer. *Clinical Cancer Research, 12*, 6106–6115. http://dx.doi.org/10.1158/1078-0432.CCR-06-1183.
Kim, H.-J., Kammertoens, T., Janke, M., Schmetzer, O., Qin, Z., Berek, C., et al. (2004). Establishment of early lymphoid organ infrastructure in transplanted tumors mediated by local production of lymphotoxin α and in the combined absence of functional B and T cells. *Journal of Immunology, 172*, 4037–4047.
Kirk, C. J., Hartigan-O'Connor, D., & Mule, J. J. (2001). The dynamics of the T-cell antitumor response: Chemokine-secreting dendritic cells can prime tumor-reactive T cells extranodally. *Cancer Research, 61*, 8794–8802.
Kirk, C. J., Hartigan-O'Connor, D., Nickoloff, B. J., Chamberlain, J. S., Giedlin, M., Aukerman, L., et al. (2001). T cell-dependent antitumor immunity mediated by secondary lymphoid tissue chemokine augmentation of dendritic cell-based immunotherapy. *Cancer Research, 61*, 2062–2070.
Knibbs, R. N., Craig, R. A., Natsuka, S., Chang, A., Cameron, M., Lowe, J. B., et al. (1996). The fucosyltransferase FucT-VII regulates E-selectin ligand synthesis in human T cells. *The Journal of Cell Biology, 133*, 911–920. http://dx.doi.org/10.1083/jcb.133.4.911.
Koni, P. A., Sacca, R., Lawton, P., Browning, J. L., Ruddle, N. H., & Flavell, R. A. (1997). Distinct roles in lymphoid organogenesis for lymphotoxins alpha and beta revealed in lymphotoxin beta-deficient mice. *Immunity, 6*, 491–500.
Konkalmatt, P. R., Deng, D., Thomas, S., Wu, M. T., Logsdon, C. D., French, B. A., et al. (2013). Plectin-1 targeted AAV vector for the molecular imaging of pancreatic cancer. *Frontiers in Oncology, 3*, 84. http://dx.doi.org/10.3389/fonc.2013.00084.
Kunz, M., Toksoy, A., Goebeler, M., Engelhardt, E., Bröcker, E., & Gillitzer, R. (1999). Strong expression of the lymphoattractant C-X-C chemokine Mig is associated with heavy infiltration of T cells in human malignant melanoma. *The Journal of Pathology, 189*, 552–558.

Kupper, T. S., & Fuhlbrigge, R. C. (2004). Immune surveillance in the skin: Mechanisms and clinical consequences. *Nature Reviews. Immunology*, *4*, 211–222.

Kvistborg, P., Philips, D., Kelderman, S., Hageman, L., Ottensmeier, C., Joseph-Pietras, D., et al. (2014). Anti-CTLA-4 therapy broadens the melanoma-reactive CD8+ T cell response. *Science Translational Medicine*, *6*, 254ra128. http://dx.doi.org/10.1126/scitranslmed.3008918.

Ladányi, A., Sebestyén, T., Mohos, A., Liszkay, G., Somlai, B., Tóth, E., et al. (2014). Ectopic lymphoid structures in primary cutaneous melanoma. *Pathology Oncology Research*, *20*, 981–985. http://dx.doi.org/10.1007/s12253-014-9784-8.

Lauder, I., & Aherne, W. (1972). The significance of lymphocytic infiltration in neuroblastoma. *British Journal of Cancer*, *26*, 321–330.

Lawrence, M. B., & Springer, T. A. (1991). Leukocytes roll on a selectin at physiologic flow rates: Distinction from and prerequisite for adhesion through integrins. *Cell*, *65*, 859–873.

Ley, K., Laudanna, C., Cybulsky, M. I., & Nourshargh, S. (2007). Getting to the site of inflammation: The leukocyte adhesion cascade updated. *Nature Reviews. Immunology*, *7*, 678–689.

Liao, S., & Ruddle, N. H. (2006). Synchrony of high endothelial venules and lymphatic vessels revealed by immunization. *Journal of Immunology*, *177*, 3369–3379.

Lin, E. Y., Nguyen, A. V., Russell, R. G., & Pollard, J. W. (2001). Colony-stimulating factor 1 promotes progression of mammary tumors to malignancy. *The Journal of Experimental Medicine*, *193*, 727–740. http://dx.doi.org/10.1084/jem.193.6.727.

Liu, H., Zhang, T., Ye, J., Li, H., Huang, J., Li, X., et al. (2012). Tumor-infiltrating lymphocytes predict response to chemotherapy in patients with advance non-small cell lung cancer. *Cancer Immunology, Immunotherapy*, *61*, 1849–1856. http://dx.doi.org/10.1007/s00262-012-1231-7.

Lohr, J., Ratliff, T., Huppertz, A., Ge, Y., Dictus, C., Ahmadi, R., et al. (2011). Effector T-cell infiltration positively impacts survival of glioblastoma patients and is impaired by tumor-derived TGF-β. *Clinical Cancer Research*, *17*, 4296–4308. http://dx.doi.org/10.1158/1078-0432.CCR-10-2557.

Loi, S., Sirtaine, N., Piette, F., Salgado, R., Viale, G., Eenoo, F. V., et al. (2013). Prognostic and predictive value of tumor-infiltrating lymphocytes in a phase III randomized adjuvant breast cancer trial in node-positive breast cancer comparing the addition of docetaxel to doxorubicin with doxorubicin-based chemotherapy. *Journal of Clinical Oncology*, *31*, 860–867. http://dx.doi.org/10.1200/JCO.2011.41.0902.

Lugade, A. A., Moran, J. P., Gerber, S. A., Rose, R. C., Frelinger, J. G., & Lord, E. M. (2005). Local radiation therapy of B16 melanoma tumors increases the generation of tumor antigen-specific effector cells that traffic to the tumor. *Journal of Immunology*, *174*, 7516–7523.

Lurquin, C., Lethé, B., Plaen, E. D., Corbière, V., Théate, I., van Baren, N., et al. (2005). Contrasting frequencies of antitumor and anti-vaccine T cells in metastases of a melanoma patient vaccinated with a MAGE tumor antigen. *The Journal of Experimental Medicine*, *201*, 249–257. http://dx.doi.org/10.1084/jem.20041378.

Luther, S. A., Bidgol, A., Hargreaves, D. C., Schmidt, A., Xu, Y., Paniyadi, J., et al. (2002). Differing activities of homeostatic chemokines CCL19, CCL21, and CXCL12 in lymphocyte and dendritic cell recruitment and lymphoid neogenesis. *Journal of Immunology*, *169*, 424–433.

Lutz, E. R., Wu, A. A., Bigelow, E., Sharma, R., Mo, G., Soares, K., et al. (2014). Immunotherapy converts nonimmunogenic pancreatic tumors into immunogenic foci of immune regulation. *Cancer Immunology Research*, *2*, 616–631. http://dx.doi.org/10.1158/2326-6066.CIR-14-0027.

Maly, P., Thall, A., Petryniak, B., Rogers, C. E., Smith, P. L., Marks, R. M., et al. (1996). The alpha(1, 3)fucosyltransferase Fuc-TVII controls leukocyte trafficking through an essential role in L-, E-, and P-selectin ligand biosynthesis. *Cell*, *86*(4), 643–653.

Margolin, K. A. (2000). Interleukin-2 in the treatment of renal cancer. *Seminars in Oncology*, *27*, 194–203.

Marincola, F. M., Wang, E., Herlyn, M., Seliger, B., & Ferrone, S. (2003). Tumors as elusive targets of T-cell-based active immunotherapy. *Trends in Immunology*, *24*, 334–341. http://dx.doi.org/10.1016/S1471-4906(03)00116-9.

Marinkovic, T., Garin, A., Yokota, Y., Fu, Y. X., Ruddle, N. H., Furtado, G. C., et al. (2006). Interaction of mature CD3+ CD4+ T cells with dendritic cells triggers the development of tertiary lymphoid structures in the thyroid. *The Journal of Clinical Investigation*, *116*, 2622–2632.

Martinet, L., Filleron, T., Guellec, S. L., Rochaix, P., Garrido, I., & Girard, J.-P. (2013). High endothelial venule blood vessels for tumor-infiltrating lymphocytes are associated with lymphotoxin β-producing dendritic cells in human breast cancer. *Journal of Immunology*, *191*, 2001–2008. http://dx.doi.org/10.4049/jimmunol.1300872.

Martinet, L., Garrido, I., Filleron, T., Le Guellec, S., Bellard, E., Fournie, J.-J., et al. (2011). Human solid tumors contain high endothelial venules: Association with T- and B-lymphocyte infiltration and favorable prognosis in breast cancer. *Cancer Research*, *71*, 5678–5687. http://dx.doi.org/10.1158/0008-5472.CAN-11-0431.

Martinet, L., Le Guellec, S., Filleron, T., Lamant, L., Meyer, N., Rochaix, P., et al. (2012). High endothelial venules (HEVs) in human melanoma lesions: Major gateways for tumor-infiltrating lymphocytes. *OncoImmunology*, *1*, 829–839. http://dx.doi.org/10.4161/onci.20492.

Masopust, D., & Schenkel, J. M. (2013). The integration of T cell migration, differentiation and function. *Nature Reviews. Immunology*, *13*, 309–320. http://dx.doi.org/10.1038/nri3442.

Matsumoto, M., Atarashi, K., Umemoto, E., Furukawa, Y., Shigeta, A., Miyasaka, M., et al. (2005). CD43 functions as a ligand for E-selectin on activated T cells. *Journal of Immunology*, *175*, 8042–8050.

Matsumoto, M., Shigeta, A., Furukawa, Y., Tanaka, T., Miyasaka, M., & Hirata, T. (2007). CD43 collaborates with P-selectin glycoprotein ligand-1 to mediate E-selectin-dependent T cell migration into inflamed skin. *Journal of Immunology*, *178*, 2499–2506, 178/4/2499 [pii].

Mebius, R. E., Streeter, P. R., Michie, S., Butcher, E. C., & Weissman, I. L. (1996). A developmental switch in lymphocyte homing receptor and endothelial vascular addressin expression regulates lymphocyte homing and permits CD4+ CD3- cells to colonize lymph nodes. *Proceedings of the National Academy of Sciences of the United States of America*, *93*, 11019–11024.

Messina, J. L., Fenstermacher, D. A., Eschrich, S., Qu, X., Berglund, A. E., Lloyd, M. C., et al. (2012). 12-Chemokine gene signature identifies lymph node-like structures in melanoma: Potential for patient selection for immunotherapy? *Scientific Reports*, *2*, 765. http://dx.doi.org/10.1038/srep00765.

Mionnet, C., Sanos, S. L., Mondor, I., Jorquera, A., Laugier, J.-P., Germain, R. N., et al. (2011). High endothelial venules as traffic control points maintaining lymphocyte population homeostasis in lymph nodes. *Blood*, *118*, 6115–6122. http://dx.doi.org/10.1182/blood-2011-07-367409.

Mlecnik, B., Tosolini, M., Charoentong, P., Kirilovsky, A., Bindea, G., Berger, A., et al. (2010). Biomolecular network reconstruction identifies T-cell homing factors associated with survival in colorectal cancer. *Gastroenterology*, *138*, 1429–1440. http://dx.doi.org/10.1053/j.gastro.2009.10.057.

Mollà, M., Gironella, M., Miquel, R., Tovar, V., Engel, P., Biete, A., et al. (2003). Relative roles of ICAM-1 and VCAM-1 in the pathogenesis of experimental radiation-induced intestinal inflammation. *International Journal of Radiation Oncology, Biology, Physics*, *57*, 264–273. http://dx.doi.org/10.1016/S0360-3016(03)00523-6.

Mora, J. R., Bono, M. R., Manjunath, N., Weninger, W., Cavanagh, L. L., Rosemblatt, M., et al. (2003). Selective imprinting of gut-homing T cells by Peyer's patch dendritic cells. *Nature, 424*, 88–93.

Mora, J. R., Cheng, G., Picarella, D., Briskin, M., Buchanan, N., & von Andrian, U. H. (2005). Reciprocal and dynamic control of CD8 T cell homing by dendritic cells from skin- and gut-associated lymphoid tissues. *The Journal of Experimental Medicine, 201*, 303–316.

Mora, J. R., & von Andrian, U. H. (2006). T-cell homing specificity and plasticity: New concepts and future challenges. *Trends in Immunology, 27*, 235–243.

Morales, J., Homey, B., Vicari, A. P., Hudak, S., Oldham, E., Hedrick, J., et al. (1999). CTACK, a skin-associated chemokine that preferentially attracts skin-homing memory T cells. *Proceedings of the National Academy of Sciences of the United States of America, 96*, 14470–14475.

Morris, M., Platell, C., & Iacopetta, B. (2008). Tumor-infiltrating lymphocytes and perforation in colon cancer predict positive response to 5-fluorouracil chemotherapy. *Clinical Cancer Research, 14*, 1413–1417. http://dx.doi.org/10.1158/1078-0432.CCR-07-1994.

Motallebzadeh, R., Rehakova, S., Conlon, T. M., Win, T. S., Callaghan, C. J., Goddard, M., et al. (2012). Blocking lymphotoxin signaling abrogates the development of ectopic lymphoid tissue within cardiac allografts and inhibits effector antibody responses. *The FASEB Journal, 26*, 51–62. http://dx.doi.org/10.1096/fj.11-186973.

Moussion, C., & Girard, J.-P. (2011). Dendritic cells control lymphocyte entry to lymph nodes through high endothelial venules. *Nature, 479*, 542–546. http://dx.doi.org/10.1038/nature10540.

Mullins, D. W., Sheasley, S. L., Ream, R. M., Bullock, T. N., Fu, Y. X., & Engelhard, V. H. (2003). Route of immunization with peptide-pulsed dendritic cells controls the distribution of memory and effector T cells in lymphoid tissues and determines the pattern of regional tumor control. *The Journal of Experimental Medicine, 198*, 1023–1034.

Mullins, I. M., Slingluff, C. L., Lee, J. K., Garbee, C. F., Shu, J., Anderson, S. G., et al. (2004). CXC chemokine receptor 3 expression by activated CD8+ T cells is associated with survival in melanoma patients with stage III disease. *Cancer Research, 64*, 7697–7701.

Nakano, O., Sato, M., Naito, Y., Suzuki, K., Orikasa, S., Aizawa, M., et al. (2001). Proliferative activity of intratumoral CD8+ T-lymphocytes as a prognostic factor in human renal cell carcinoma clinicopathologic demonstration of antitumor immunity. *Cancer Research, 61*, 5132–5136.

Nielsen, J. S., Sahota, R. A., Milne, K., Kost, S. E., Nesslinger, N. J., Watson, P. H., et al. (2012). CD20+ tumor-infiltrating lymphocytes have an atypical CD27- memory phenotype and together with CD8+ T cells promote favorable prognosis in ovarian cancer. *Clinical Cancer Research, 18*, 3281–3292. http://dx.doi.org/10.1158/1078-0432.CCR-12-0234.

Novak, L., Igoucheva, O., Cho, S., & Alexeev, V. (2007). Characterization of the CCL21-mediated melanoma-specific immune responses and in situ melanoma eradication. *Molecular Cancer Therapeutics, 6*, 1755–1764. http://dx.doi.org/10.1158/1535-7163.MCT-06-0709.

Ogawa, H., Binion, D. G., Heidemann, J., Theriot, M., Fisher, P. J., Johnson, N. A., et al. (2005). Mechanisms of MAdCAM-1 gene expression in human intestinal microvascular endothelial cells. *American Journal of Physiology. Cell Physiology, 288*, C272–C281. http://dx.doi.org/10.1152/ajpcell.00406.2003.

Pagès, F., Kirilovsky, A., Mlecnik, B., Asslaber, M., Tosolini, M., Bindea, G., et al. (2009). In situ cytotoxic and memory T cells predict outcome in patients with early-stage colorectal cancer. *Journal of Clinical Oncology, 27*, 5944–5951. http://dx.doi.org/10.1200/JCO.2008.19.6147.

Palma, L., Di Lorenzo, N., & Guidetti, B. (1978). Lymphocytic infiltrates in primary glioblastomas and recidivous gliomas. Incidence, fate, and relevance to prognosis in 228 operated cases. *Journal of Neurosurgery*, *49*, 854–861.

Pardoll, D. M. (2012). The blockade of immune checkpoints in cancer immunotherapy. *Nature Reviews. Cancer*, *12*, 252–264. http://dx.doi.org/10.1038/nrc3239.

Peng, W., Liu, C., Xu, C., Lou, Y., Chen, J., Yang, Y., et al. (2012). PD-1 blockade enhances T-cell migration to tumors by elevating IFN-γ inducible chemokines. *Cancer Research*, *72*, 5209–5218. http://dx.doi.org/10.1158/0008-5472.CAN-12-1187.

Peske, J. D., Thompson, E. D., Gemta, L., Baylis, R. A., Fu, Y.-X., & Engelhard, V. H. (2015). Effector lymphocyte-induced lymph node-like vasculature enables naïve T-cell entry into tumors and enhanced anti-tumor immunity. *Nature Communications*, *6*, 7114. http://dx.doi.org/10.1038/ncomms8114.

Pockaj, B. A., Sherry, R. M., Wei, J. P., Yannelli, J. R., Carter, C. S., Leitman, S. F., et al. (1994). Localization of 111indium-labeled tumor infiltrating lymphocytes to tumor in patients receiving adoptive immunotherapy. Augmentation with cyclophosphamide and correlation with response. *Cancer*, *73*, 1731–1737.

Postow, M. A., Callahan, M. K., Barker, C. A., Yamada, Y., Yuan, J., Kitano, S., et al. (2012). Immunologic correlates of the abscopal effect in a patient with melanoma. *The New England Journal of Medicine*, *366*, 925–931. http://dx.doi.org/10.1056/NEJMoa1112824.

Preston, C. C., Maurer, M. J., Oberg, A. L., Visscher, D. W., Kalli, K. R., Hartmann, L. C., et al. (2013). The ratios of CD8+ T cells to CD4+CD25+ FOXP3+ and FOXP3- T cells correlate with poor clinical outcome in human serous ovarian cancer. *PLoS One*, *8*, e80063. http://dx.doi.org/10.1371/journal.pone.0080063.

Pylayeva-Gupta, Y., Lee, K. E., Hajdu, C. H., Miller, G., & Bar-Sagi, D. (2012). Oncogenic Kras-induced GM-CSF production promotes the development of pancreatic neoplasia. *Cancer Cell*, *21*, 836–847. http://dx.doi.org/10.1016/j.ccr.2012.04.024.

Quezada, S. A., Peggs, K. S., Simpson, T. R., Shen, Y., Littman, D. R., & Allison, J. P. (2008). Limited tumor infiltration by activated T effector cells restricts the therapeutic activity of regulatory T cell depletion against established melanoma. *The Journal of Experimental Medicine*, *205*, 2125–2138. http://dx.doi.org/10.1084/jem.20080099.

Rangel-Moreno, J., Carragher, D. M., de la Luz Garcia-Hernandez, M., Hwang, J. Y., Kusser, K., Hartson, L., et al. (2011). The development of inducible bronchus-associated lymphoid tissue depends on IL-17. *Nature Immunology*, *12*, 639–646. http://dx.doi.org/10.1038/ni.2053.

Remark, R., Alifano, M., Cremer, I., Lupo, A., Dieu-Nosjean, M.-C., Riquet, M., et al. (2013). Characteristics and clinical impacts of the immune environments in colorectal and renal cell carcinoma lung metastases: Influence of tumor origin. *Clinical Cancer Research*, *19*, 4079–4091. http://dx.doi.org/10.1158/1078-0432.CCR-12-3847.

Restifo, N. P., Dudley, M. E., & Rosenberg, S. A. (2012). Adoptive immunotherapy for cancer: Harnessing the T cell response. *Nature Reviews. Immunology*, *12*, 269–281. http://dx.doi.org/10.1038/nri3191.

Rosen, S. D. (2004). Ligands for L-selectin: Homing, inflammation, and beyond. *Annual Review of Immunology*, *22*, 129–156.

Rosenberg, S. A., Yang, J. C., Topalian, S. L., Schwartzentruber, D. J., Weber, J. S., Parkinson, D. R., et al. (1994). Treatment of 283 consecutive patients with metastatic melanoma or renal cell cancer using high-dose bolus interleukin 2 [see comments]. *Journal of the American Medical Association*, *271*, 907–913.

Rott, L. S., Briskin, M. J., Andrew, D. P., Berg, E. L., & Butcher, E. C. (1996). A fundamental subdivision of circulating lymphocytes defined by adhesion to mucosal addressin cell adhesion molecule-1. Comparison with vascular cell adhesion molecule-1 and correlation with beta 7 integrins and memory differentiation. *Journal of Immunology, 156*, 3727–3736.

Sackstein, R. (2005). The lymphocyte homing receptors: Gatekeepers of the multistep paradigm. *Current Opinion in Hematology, 12*, 444–450.

Sakai, Y., Hoshino, H., Kitazawa, R., & Kobayashi, M. (2014). High endothelial venule-like vessels and lymphocyte recruitment in testicular seminoma. *Andrology, 2*, 282–289. http://dx.doi.org/10.1111/j.2047-2927.2014.00192.x.

Salas, A., Shimaoka, M., Chen, S., Carman, C. V., & Springer, T. (2002). Transition from rolling to firm adhesion is regulated by the conformation of the I domain of the integrin lymphocyte function-associated antigen-1. *The Journal of Biological Chemistry, 277*, 50255–50262. http://dx.doi.org/10.1074/jbc.M209822200.

Sandoval, F., Terme, M., Nizard, M., Badoual, C., Bureau, M.-F., Freyburger, L., et al. (2013). Mucosal imprinting of vaccine-induced CD8+ T cells is crucial to inhibit the growth of mucosal tumors. *Science Translational Medicine, 5*, 172ra20. http://dx.doi.org/10.1126/scitranslmed.3004888.

Sato, E., Olson, S. H., Ahn, J., Bundy, B., Nishikawa, H., Qian, F., et al. (2005). Intraepithelial CD8+ tumor-infiltrating lymphocytes and a high CD8+/regulatory T cell ratio are associated with favorable prognosis in ovarian cancer. *Proceedings of the National Academy of Sciences of the United States of America, 102*, 18538–18543. http://dx.doi.org/10.1073/pnas.0509182102, 0509182102 [pii].

Schrama, D., thor Straten,, P., Fischer, W. H., McLellan, A. D., Bröcker, E.-B., Reisfeld, R. A., et al. (2001). Targeting of lymphotoxin-α to the tumor elicits an efficient immune response associated with induction of peripheral lymphoid-like tissue. *Immunity, 14*, 111–121. http://dx.doi.org/10.1016/S1074-7613(01)00094-2.

Schrama, D., Voigt, H., Eggert, A. O., Xiang, R., Zhou, H., Schumacher, T. N. M., et al. (2008). Immunological tumor destruction in a murine melanoma model by targeted LTalpha independent of secondary lymphoid tissue. *Cancer Immunology, Immunotherapy, 57*, 85–95. http://dx.doi.org/10.1007/s00262-007-0352-x.

Schwartzentruber, D. J., Lawson, D. H., Richards, J. M., Conry, R. M., Miller, D. M., Treisman, J., et al. (2011). gp100 Peptide vaccine and interleukin-2 in patients with advanced melanoma. *The New England Journal of Medicine, 364*, 2119–2127. http://dx.doi.org/10.1056/NEJMoa1012863.

Seguin, J., Nicolazzi, C., Mignet, N., Scherman, D., & Chabot, G. (2012). Vascular density and endothelial cell expression of integrin alpha v beta 3 and E-selectin in murine tumours. *Tumour Biology, 33*, 1709–1717. http://dx.doi.org/10.1007/s13277-012-0428-x.

Shankaran, V., Ikeda, H., Bruce, A. T., White, J. M., Swanson, P. E., Old, L. J., et al. (2001). IFNgamma and lymphocytes prevent primary tumour development and shape tumour immunogenicity. *Nature, 410*, 1107–1111.

Sharma, S., Stolina, M., Luo, J., Strieter, R. M., Burdick, M., Zhu, L. X., et al. (2000). Secondary lymphoid tissue chemokine mediates T cell-dependent antitumor responses in vivo. *Journal of Immunology, 164*, 4558–4563.

Sheasley-O'Neill, S. L., Brinkman, C. C., Ferguson, A. R., Dispenza, M. C., & Engelhard, V. H. (2007). Dendritic cell immunization route determines integrin expression and lymphoid and nonlymphoid tissue distribution of CD8 T cells. *Journal of Immunology, 178*, 1512–1522.

Sherry, B., Tekamp-Olson, P., Gallegos, C., Bauer, D., Davatelis, G., Wolpe, S. D., et al. (1988). Resolution of the two components of macrophage inflammatory protein 1, and cloning and characterization of one of those components, macrophage inflammatory protein 1 beta. *The Journal of Experimental Medicine, 168*, 2251–2259. http://dx.doi.org/10.1084/jem.168.6.2251.

Shields, J. D., Kourtis, I. C., Tomei, A. A., Roberts, J. M., & Swartz, M. A. (2010). Induction of lymphoidlike stroma and immune escape by tumors that express the chemokine CCL21. *Science, 328*, 749–752. http://dx.doi.org/10.1126/science.1185837.

Shrimali, R. K., Yu, Z., Theoret, M. R., Chinnasamy, D., Restifo, N. P., & Rosenberg, S. A. (2010). Antiangiogenic agents can increase lymphocyte infiltration into tumor and enhance the effectiveness of adoptive immunotherapy of cancer. *Cancer Research, 70*, 6171–6180. http://dx.doi.org/10.1158/0008-5472.CAN-10-0153.

Sigmundsdottir, H., Pan, J., Debes, G. F., Alt, C., Habtezion, A., Soler, D., et al. (2007). DCs metabolize sunlight-induced vitamin D3 to "program" T cell attraction to the epidermal chemokine CCL27. *Nature Immunology, 8*, 285–293. http://dx.doi.org/10.1038/ni1433, ni1433 [pii].

Simpson, T. R., Li, F., Montalvo-Ortiz, W., Sepulveda, M. A., Bergerhoff, K., Arce, F., et al. (2013). Fc-dependent depletion of tumor-infiltrating regulatory T cells co-defines the efficacy of anti-CTLA-4 therapy against melanoma. *The Journal of Experimental Medicine, 210*, 1695–1710. http://dx.doi.org/10.1084/jem.20130579.

Smyth, M. J., Crowe, N. Y., & Godfrey, D. I. (2001). NK cells and NKT cells collaborate in host protection from methylcholanthrene-induced fibrosarcoma. *International Immunology, 13*, 459–463.

Smyth, M. J., Thia, K. Y., Street, S. E., MacGregor, D., Godfrey, D. I., & Trapani, J. A. (2000). Perforin-mediated cytotoxicity is critical for surveillance of spontaneous lymphoma. *The Journal of Experimental Medicine, 192*, 755–760.

Snyder, A., Makarov, V., Merghoub, T., Yuan, J., Zaretsky, J. M., Desrichard, A., et al. (2014). Genetic basis for clinical response to CTLA-4 blockade in melanoma. *The New England Journal of Medicine, 371*, 2189–2199. http://dx.doi.org/10.1056/NEJMoa1406498.

Spranger, S., Bao, R., & Gajewski, T. (2014). Melanoma-intrinsic β-catenin signaling prevents T cell infiltration and anti-tumor immunity. *Journal for Immunotherapy of Cancer, 2*, O15. http://dx.doi.org/10.1186/2051-1426-2-S3-O15.

Stark, F. C., Gurnani, K., Sad, S., & Krishnan, L. (2012). Lack of functional selectin ligand interactions compromises long term tumor protection by CD8+ T cells. *PLoS One, 7*, e32211. http://dx.doi.org/10.1371/journal.pone.0032211.

Streeter, P. R., Rouse, B. T., & Butcher, E. C. (1988). Immunohistologic and functional characterization of a vascular addressin involved in lymphocyte homing into peripheral lymph nodes. *The Journal of Cell Biology, 107*, 1853–1862.

Sullivan, R. J., Hoshida, Y., Brunet, J., Tahan, S., Aldridge, J., Kwabi, C., et al. (2009). A single center experience with high-dose (HD) IL-2 treatment for patients with advanced melanoma and pilot investigation of a novel gene expression signature as a predictor of response. *Journal of Clinical Oncology, 27*, 15s.

Tensen, C. P., Flier, J., van der Raaj-Helmer, E. M., Sampat-Sardjoepersad, S., Van Der Schors, R. C., Leurs, R., et al. (1999). Human IP-9: A keratinocyte-derived high affinity CXC-chemokine ligand for the IP-10/Mig receptor (CXCR3). *The Journal of Investigative Dermatology, 112*, 716–722.

Thompson, E. D., Enriquez, H. L., Fu, Y.-X., & Engelhard, V. H. (2010). Tumor masses support naive T cell infiltration, activation, and differentiation into effectors. *The Journal of Experimental Medicine, 207*, 1791–1804. http://dx.doi.org/10.1084/jem.20092454.

Thurner, B., Haendle, I., Roder, C., Dieckmann, D., Keikavoussi, P., Jonuleit, H., et al. (1999). Vaccination with MAGE-3A1 peptide-pulsed mature, monocyte-derived dendritic cells expands specific cytotoxic T cells and induces regression of some metastases in advanced stage IV melanoma. *The Journal of Experimental Medicine, 190*, 1669–1678.

Topalian, S. L., Hodi, F. S., Brahmer, J. R., Gettinger, S. N., Smith, D. C., McDermott, D. F., et al. (2012). Safety, activity, and immune correlates of anti-PD-1 antibody in cancer. *The New England Journal of Medicine, 366*, 2443–2454. http://dx.doi.org/10.1056/NEJMoa1200690.

Tran, D. Q., Ramsey, H., & Shevach, E. M. (2007). Induction of FOXP3 expression in naive human CD4+FOXP3 T cells by T-cell receptor stimulation is transforming growth factor-beta dependent but does not confer a regulatory phenotype. *Blood, 110*, 2983–2990. http://dx.doi.org/10.1182/blood-2007-06-094656.

Tsai, S.-C., Lin, S.-J., Lin, C.-J., Chou, Y.-C., Lin, J.-H., Yeh, T.-H., et al. (2013). Autocrine CCL3 and CCL4 induced by the oncoprotein LMP1 promote Epstein-Barr virus-triggered B cell proliferation. *Journal of Virology, 87*, 9041–9052. http://dx.doi.org/10.1128/JVI.00541-13.

Tumeh, P. C., Harview, C. L., Yearley, J. H., Shintaku, I. P., Taylor, E. J. M., Robert, L., et al. (2014). PD-1 blockade induces responses by inhibiting adaptive immune resistance. *Nature, 515*, 568–571. http://dx.doi.org/10.1038/nature13954.

Turk, M. J., Guevara-Patiño, J. A., Rizzuto, G. A., Engelhorn, M. E., & Houghton, A. N. (2004). Concomitant tumor immunity to a poorly immunogenic melanoma is prevented by regulatory T cells. *The Journal of Experimental Medicine, 200*, 771–782. http://dx.doi.org/10.1084/jem.20041130.

Turnquist, H. R., Lin, X., Ashour, A. E., Hollingsworth, M. A., Singh, R. K., Talmadge, J. E., et al. (2007). CCL21 induces extensive intratumoral immune cell infiltration and specific anti-tumor cellular immunity. *International Journal of Oncology, 30*, 631–639.

Ulloa-Montoya, F., Louahed, J., Dizier, B., Gruselle, O., Spiessens, B., Lehmann, F. F., et al. (2013). Predictive gene signature in MAGE-A3 antigen-specific cancer immunotherapy. *Journal of Clinical Oncology, 31*, 2388–2395. http://dx.doi.org/10.1200/JCO.2012.44.3762.

Van de Pavert, S. A., & Mebius, R. E. (2010). New insights into the development of lymphoid tissues. *Nature Reviews. Immunology, 10*, 664–674.

Van de Pavert, S. A., Olivier, B. J., Goverse, G., Vondenhoff, M. F., Greuter, M., Beke, P., et al. (2009). Chemokine CXCL13 is essential for lymph node initiation and is induced by retinoic acid and neuronal stimulation. *Nature Immunology, 10*, 1193–1199. http://dx.doi.org/10.1038/ni.1789.

Vesely, M., Kershaw, M., Schreiber, R., & Smyth, M. (2011). Natural innate and adaptive immunity to cancer. *Annual Review of Immunology, 29*, 235–271.

Victor, C. T.-S., Rech, A. J., Maity, A., Rengan, R., Pauken, K. E., Stelekati, E., et al. (2015). Radiation and dual checkpoint blockade activate non-redundant immune mechanisms in cancer. *Nature, 520*, 373–377. http://dx.doi.org/10.1038/nature14292, Advance online publication.

Von Andrian, U. H., & Mackay, C. R. (2000). T-cell function and migration. Two sides of the same coin. *The New England Journal of Medicine, 343*, 1020–1034.

Vonderheide, R. H., & Bayne, L. J. (2013). Inflammatory networks and immune surveillance of pancreatic carcinoma. *Current Opinion in Immunology, 25*, 200–205. http://dx.doi.org/10.1016/j.coi.2013.01.006.

Wang, L., Fan, J., Thompson, L. F., Zhang, Y., Shin, T., Curiel, T. J., et al. (2011). CD73 has distinct roles in nonhematopoietic and hematopoietic cells to promote tumor growth in mice. *The Journal of Clinical Investigation, 121*, 2371–2382. http://dx.doi.org/10.1172/JCI45559.

Wang, J., Ioan-Facsinay, A., van der Voort, E. I. H., Huizinga, T. W. J., & Toes, R. E. M. (2007). Transient expression of FOXP3 in human activated nonregulatory CD4+ T cells. *European Journal of Immunology, 37*, 129–138. http://dx.doi.org/10.1002/eji.200636435.

Wang, X., Michie, S. A., Xu, B., & Suzuki, Y. (2007). Importance of IFN-gamma-mediated expression of endothelial VCAM-1 on recruitment of CD8+ T cells into the brain

during chronic infection with Toxoplasma gondii. *Journal of Interferon & Cytokine Research, 27*, 329–338. http://dx.doi.org/10.1089/jir.2006.0154.
Wang, E., Miller, L. D., Ohnmacht, G. A., Mocellin, S., Perez-Diez, A., Petersen, D., et al. (2002). Prospective molecular profiling of melanoma metastases suggests classifiers of immune responsiveness. *Cancer Research, 62*, 3581–3586.
Wang, T., Niu, G., Kortylewski, M., Burdelya, L., Shain, K., Zhang, S., et al. (2004). Regulation of the innate and adaptive immune responses by Stat-3 signaling in tumor cells. *Nature Medicine, 10*, 48–54.
Webster, B., Ekland, E. H., Agle, L. M., Chyou, S., Ruggieri, R., & Lu, T. T. (2006). Regulation of lymph node vascular growth by dendritic cells. *The Journal of Experimental Medicine, 203*, 1903–1913. http://dx.doi.org/10.1084/jem.20052272.
Weis, S. M., & Cheresh, D. A. (2011). Tumor angiogenesis: Molecular pathways and therapeutic targets. *Nature Medicine, 17*, 1359–1370. http://dx.doi.org/10.1038/nm.2537.
Weishaupt, C., Munoz, K. N., Buzney, E., Kupper, T. S., & Fuhlbrigge, R. C. (2007). T-cell distribution and adhesion receptor expression in metastatic melanoma. *Clinical Cancer Research, 13*, 2549–2556. http://dx.doi.org/10.1158/1078-0432.CCR-06-2450.
Weiss, G. R., Grosh, W. W., Chianese-Bullock, K. A., Zhao, Y., Liu, H., Slingluff, C. L., et al. (2011). Molecular insights on the peripheral and intratumoral effects of systemic high-dose rIL-2 (aldesleukin) administration for the treatment of metastatic melanoma. *Clinical Cancer Research, 17*, 7440–7450. http://dx.doi.org/10.1158/1078-0432.CCR-11-1650.
Weiss, V. L., Lee, T. H., Song, H., Kouo, T. S., Black, C. M., Sgouros, G., et al. (2012). Trafficking of high avidity HER-2/neu-specific T cells into HER-2/neu-expressing tumors after depletion of effector/memory-like regulatory T cells. *PLoS One, 7*, e31962. http://dx.doi.org/10.1371/journal.pone.0031962.
West, N. R., Milne, K., Truong, P. T., Macpherson, N., Nelson, B. H., & Watson, P. H. (2011). Tumor-infiltrating lymphocytes predict response to anthracycline-based chemotherapy in estrogen receptor-negative breast cancer. *Breast Cancer Research, 13*, R126. http://dx.doi.org/10.1186/bcr3072.
Wiemann, B., & Starnes, C. O. (1994). Coley's toxins, tumor necrosis factor and cancer research: A historical perspective. *Pharmacology & Therapeutics, 64*, 529–564.
Wilke, C. M., Kryczek, I., Wei, S., Zhao, E., Wu, K., Wang, G., et al. (2011). Th17 cells in cancer: Help or hindrance? *Carcinogenesis, 32*, 643–649. http://dx.doi.org/10.1093/carcin/bgr019.
Winograd, R., Byrne, K. T., Evans, R. A., Odorizzi, P. M., Meyer, A. R. L., Bajor, D. L., et al. (2015). Induction of T-cell immunity overcomes complete resistance to PD-1 and CTLA-4 blockade and improves survival in pancreatic carcinoma. *Cancer Immunology Research, 3*, 399–411. http://dx.doi.org/10.1158/2326-6066.CIR-14-0215.
Woo, S.-R., Fuertes, M. B., Corrales, L., Spranger, S., Furdyna, M. J., Leung, M. Y. K., et al. (2014). STING-dependent cytosolic DNA sensing mediates innate immune recognition of immunogenic tumors. *Immunity, 41*, 830–842. http://dx.doi.org/10.1016/j.immuni.2014.10.017.
Yang, L., DeBusk, L. M., Fukuda, K., Fingleton, B., Green-Jarvis, B., Shyr, Y., et al. (2004). Expansion of myeloid immune suppressor Gr+CD11b+ cells in tumor-bearing host directly promotes tumor angiogenesis. *Cancer Cell, 6*, 409–421. http://dx.doi.org/10.1016/j.ccr.2004.08.031.
Yang, S.-C., Hillinger, S., Riedl, K., Zhang, L., Zhu, L., Huang, M., et al. (2004). Intratumoral administration of dendritic cells overexpressing CCL21 generates systemic antitumor responses and confers tumor immunity. *Clinical Cancer Research, 10*, 2891–2901. http://dx.doi.org/10.1158/1078-0432.CCR-03-0380.

Yao, L., Setiadi, H., Xia, L., Laszik, Z., Taylor, F. B., & McEver, R. P. (1999). Divergent inducible expression of P-selectin and E-selectin in mice and primates. *Blood*, *94*, 3820–3828.

Yasuda, K., Nirei, T., Sunami, E., Nagawa, H., & Kitayama, J. (2011). Density of CD4(+) and CD8(+) T lymphocytes in biopsy samples can be a predictor of pathological response to chemoradiotherapy (CRT) for rectal cancer. *Radiation Oncology*, *6*, 1–6. http://dx.doi.org/10.1186/1748-717X-6-49.

Yoong, K. F., McNab, G., Hübscher, S. G., & Adams, D. H. (1998). Vascular adhesion protein-1 and ICAM-1 support the adhesion of tumor-infiltrating lymphocytes to tumor endothelium in human hepatocellular carcinoma. *Journal of Immunology*, *160*, 3978–3988.

Yu, P., Lee, Y., Liu, W., Chin, R. K., Wang, J., Wang, Y., et al. (2004). Priming of naive T cells inside tumors leads to eradication of established tumors. *Nature Immunology*, *5*, 141–149.

Yu, P., Lee, Y., Liu, W., Krausz, T., Chong, A., Schreiber, H., et al. (2005). Intratumor depletion of CD4+ cells unmasks tumor immunogenicity leading to the rejection of late-stage tumors. *The Journal of Experimental Medicine*, *201*, 779–791. http://dx.doi.org/10.1084/jem.20041684.

Zarbock, A., Ley, K., McEver, R. P., & Hidalgo, A. (2011). Leukocyte ligands for endothelial selectins: Specialized glycoconjugates that mediate rolling and signaling under flow. *Blood*, *118*, 6743–6751. http://dx.doi.org/10.1182/blood-2011-07-343566.

Zitvogel, L., Kepp, O., & Kroemer, G. (2011). Immune parameters affecting the efficacy of chemotherapeutic regimens. *Nature Reviews. Clinical Oncology*, *8*, 151–160. http://dx.doi.org/10.1038/nrclinonc.2010.223.

CHAPTER NINE

Scavenger Receptors: Emerging Roles in Cancer Biology and Immunology

Xiaofei Yu*,†,‡, Chunqing Guo*,†,‡, Paul B. Fisher*,†,‡, John R. Subjeck§,1, Xiang-Yang Wang*,†,‡,1

*Department of Human and Molecular Genetics, Richmond, Virginia, USA
†VCU Institute of Molecular Medicine, Richmond, Virginia, USA
‡VCU Massey Cancer Center, Virginia Commonwealth University School of Medicine, Richmond, Virginia, USA
§Department of Cellular Stress Biology, Roswell Park Cancer Institute, Buffalo, New York, USA
[1]Corresponding authors: e-mail address: john.subjeck@roswellpark.org; xywang@vcu.edu

Contents

Abstract

Scavenger receptors constitute a large family of evolutionally conserved protein molecules that are structurally and functionally diverse. Although scavenger receptors were originally identified based on their capacity to scavenge modified lipoproteins, these molecules have been shown to recognize and bind to a broad spectrum of ligands, including modified and unmodified host-derived molecules or microbial components. As a major subset of innate pattern recognition receptors, scavenger receptors are

Advances in Cancer Research, Volume 128
ISSN 0065-230X
http://dx.doi.org/10.1016/bs.acr.2015.04.004

mainly expressed on myeloid cells and function in a wide range of biological processes, such as endocytosis, adhesion, lipid transport, antigen presentation, and pathogen clearance. In addition to playing a crucial role in maintenance of host homeostasis, scavenger receptors have been implicated in the pathogenesis of a number of diseases, e.g., atherosclerosis, neurodegeneration, or metabolic disorders. Emerging evidence has begun to reveal these receptor molecules as important regulators of tumor behavior and host immune responses to cancer. This review summarizes our current understanding on the newly identified, distinct functions of scavenger receptors in cancer biology and immunology. The potential of scavenger receptors as diagnostic biomarkers and novel targets for therapeutic interventions to treat malignancies is also highlighted.

1. INTRODUCTION

In late 1970s, Michael Brown and Joseph Goldstein initially identified scavenger receptors in macrophages and described their activity in the uptake of modified low-density lipoprotein (LDL), i.e., acetylated LDL (acLDL) (Goldstein, Ho, Basu, & Brown, 1979). Monty Krieger's group first cloned the scavenger receptors, i.e., prototype class A scavenger receptors, in 1990 (Kodama et al., 1990). With additional scavenger receptor family members identified, scavenger receptors are currently categorized into 10 classes (A–J) based on their sequence similarity or shared structural features. However, there is no or little sequence homology between different classes of scavenger receptors (Krieger, 1997; Whelan, Meehan, Golding, McConkey, & Bowdish, 2012). There are currently no known mammalian class C scavenger receptors, and the class C scavenger receptors have only been described in *Drosophila melanogaster* (Krieger, 1997). To address the inconsistencies and confusion of multiple names of scavenger receptors being used in the literature, a unified nomenclature system was recently proposed to describe the different classes of mammalian scavenger receptors (Prabhudas et al., 2014). It is now appreciated that these structurally heterogeneous scavenger receptors recognize a broad spectrum of ligands, including microbial pathogens or pathogen-derived molecular patterns (PAMPs), e.g., lipopolysaccharide (LPS) and lipoteichoic acid (LTA), as well as host-derived self-molecules or damage-associated molecular patterns, e.g., stress/heat shock proteins (HSPs), lipoproteins (Canton, Neculai, & Grinstein, 2013; Greaves & Gordon, 2009; Krieger et al., 1993; Pluddemann, Neyen, & Gordon, 2007). Based on their broad ligand-binding specificities during interaction with conserved microbial structures or endogenous self-molecules, scavenger receptors are considered to be an important subclass of the pattern recognition receptors (PRRs) in innate immunity (Gordon, 2002; Krieger, 1997). Scavenger receptors were recently defined as "cell surface receptors that typically bind multiple ligands and promote the removal of non-self or altered-self targets" (Prabhudas et al., 2014). These receptors often function by mechanisms that include adhesion, endocytosis, phagocytosis, transport, and signaling that ultimately lead to the elimination of degraded or harmful substances (Prabhudas et al., 2014).

Due to their property initially identified in the uptake of modified LDL, e.g., acLDL and oxidized LDL (oxLDL), by macrophages, the proatherogenic role of the scavenger receptors in atherosclerosis has been studied extensively (Kzhyshkowska, Neyen, & Gordon, 2012). However, their precise contribution to this disease remains unclear. Given their ability to recognize such a large repertoire of ligands, it is anticipated that scavenger receptors are critically involved in the maintenance of host homeostasis as well as in the pathogenesis of multiple diseases, e.g., type 2 diabetes mellitus (Kennedy & Kashyap, 2011), Alzheimer's disease (El Khoury et al., 2003; Wilkinson & El Khoury, 2012). The functional versatility of scavenger receptors in various diseases were recently discussed in several reviews by us or other researchers (Armengol et al., 2013; Canton et al., 2013; Kelley, Ozment, Li, Schweitzer, & Williams, 2014; Yu, Zuo, Subjeck, & Wang, 2012). Over the last few years, there is emerging evidence indicating that scavenger receptors act as an important regulator of tumor progression and host immune response to cancer (Neyen et al., 2013; Wang, Facciponte, Chen, Subjeck, & Repasky, 2007; Yi et al., 2011). Certain scavenger receptors have been exploited as diagnostic or prognostic markers in cancer of various types. In this review, we highlight recent insights into these previously under-appreciated functions of the mammalian scavenger receptors in cancer biology and immunology. We will also discuss the feasibility of developing scavenger receptor-targeted therapeutic strategies for cancer treatment.

2. SCAVENGER RECEPTORS IN CANCER IMMUNOBIOLOGY

2.1 Class A Scavenger Receptor

2.1.1 Scavenger Receptor Class A

Scavenger receptor class A (SR-A), also called SCARA1/SR-A1, macrophage scavenger receptor 1 (MSR1) or CD204, was the first scavenger receptor cloned and represents the prototypic member of class A scavenger receptors (Kodama et al., 1990). A signature for all the class A scavenger receptors, including SR-A, is a distinct collagenous domain (Kodama et al., 1990; Rohrer, Freeman, Kodama, Penman, & Krieger, 1990). SR-A is a phagocytic PRR expressed primarily on tissue macrophages and dendritic cells (DCs). SR-A recognizes a diverse array of "self" and "nonself" ligands, including modified LDLs (acLDL, oxLDL), Gram-positive and Gram-negative bacteria, molecules of microbial origin or PAMPs (e.g., LPS, double strand RNA, unmethylated bacterial CpG DNA), hepatitis C virus, HSPs, proteoglycans, and β-amyloid (Pluddemann et al., 2007). The role of SR-A in atherosclerosis has been extensively studied because it was the first receptor identified for modified lipoproteins that are pertinent to the development of vascular disease (Kzhyshkowska et al., 2012; Suzuki et al., 1997). However, controversies still exist with regard to the precise contribution of SR-A to atherosclerosis (Kuchibhotla et al., 2008; Moore et al., 2005). SR-A is also involved in the maintenance of tissue homeostasis by clearance of modified self-components and apoptotic cells, host defense against invading microorganisms, and disease pathogenesis, such as neurodegeneration (Canton et al., 2013; El Khoury et al., 1996; Frenkel et al., 2013; Gordon, 2002; Kelley et al., 2014; Suzuki et al., 1997; Yu et al., 2012). However, accumulating evidence is now revealing important roles for SR-A in cancer.

Tumor-associated macrophages (TAMs) are a major stromal component in the tumor microenvironment (TME) (Lewis & Pollard, 2006). TAMs not only support survival and growth of tumors but also contribute to tumor metastasis, and immune evasion (Guo, Buranych, Sarkar, Fisher, & Wang, 2013; Lewis & Pollard, 2006; Qian & Pollard, 2010). Highly plastic macrophages mainly originate from circulating monocytes infiltrating peripheral tissues and acquire distinct characteristics as a result of environmental cues (Murdoch, Muthana, Coffelt, & Lewis, 2008). Macrophages can be generally categorized into two populations with distinct functional phenotypes: classically activated or M1 macrophages with proinflammatory and tumor-suppressive features, alternatively activated or M2 macrophages with anti-inflammatory, proangiogenic, immunosuppressive, and tumor-promoting activities. Macrophage polarization is increasingly recognized as an important pathogenic factor in inflammatory and neoplastic diseases (Labonte, Tosello-Trampont, & Hahn, 2014; Sica et al., 2008). It has been well documented that TAMs often show an M2-like phenotype and contribute to cancer cell proliferation, invasion and metastasis, tumor angiogenesis, matrix remodeling, and immune suppression (Guo, Buranych, et al., 2013). Immunohistochemistry studies in lung cancer (Ohtaki et al., 2010), liver cancer (Yeung et al., 2014), T cell leukemia/lymphoma (Saito et al., 2014), esophageal squamous cell carcinoma (Shigeoka et al., 2013), and pancreatic cancer (Yoshikawa et al., 2012) demonstrate that SR-A expression in tumor tissues is restricted to TAMs and that high level of SR-A is associated with a more aggressive cancer phenotype. Furthermore, an increased number of SR-A^+ TAMs has been shown to correlate with histological grade and poor prognosis in numerous cancers (Hirayama et al., 2012; Hou, Chao, Tung, Wang, & Shan, 2014; Kawamura, Komohara, Takaishi, Katabuchi, & Takeya, 2009; Kurahara et al., 2011; Sugimoto et al., 2014; Yoshikawa et al., 2012).

Although accumulating evidence points to a potential role of SR-A in TAM polarization toward an M2-like phenotype, the underlying mechanism remains elusive. Mer tyrosine kinase (MerTK), the major apoptotic cell receptor on macrophages, was recently shown to have a central role in M2 polarization of macrophages and favor an anti-inflammatory, immunosuppressive microenvironment (Graham, DeRyckere, Davies, & Earp, 2014; Zizzo, Hilliard, Monestier, & Cohen, 2012). Indeed, SR-A was reported to be required for the optimized function of MerTK during engulfment of apoptotic cells and subsequent resolution of inflammation (Todt, Hu, & Curtis, 2008). While the detailed interplay between SR-A and MerTK in ingesting of apoptotic cells is unclear, it is reasonable to believe that abundant apoptotic tumor cells in the TME together with elevated expression of SR-A and MerTK are critically involved in the programing of TAMs and immunosuppressive mechanisms in the TME.

Elevation of SR-A in TAMs implicates its potential involvement in their functions. However, studies of the functional regulation of TAMs by SR-A during tumor growth and progression are very limited. SR-A was recently reported to inhibit the production of tumoricidal molecules by TAMs, e.g., nitric oxide, interferon (IFN)-β, and IFN-γ, which caused outgrowth of EL4 lymphoma (Komohara et al., 2009). SR-A-mediated inhibition of IFN-β secretion seems to be consistent with a previous work showing that SR-A suppressed the TLR4-mediated interferon regulatory factor (IRF)-3/IFN-β pathway in endoplasmic reticulum (ER)-stressed macrophages (Seimon, Obstfeld, Moore, Golenbock, & Tabas, 2006). Using SR-A-deficient mice, Neyen et al. demonstrated that SR-A on TAMs was necessary for invasion and metastasis of ovarian and pancreatic tumors (Neyen et al., 2013). In this study, several potential SR-A ligands (e.g., Galectin-1, Fibronectin, Vimentin, and Matrilin-2) present in the supernatants of tumor cell-macrophage coculture were identified (Neyen et al., 2013). While the effect of SR-A engagement by these putative ligands on tumor progression was not examined, these molecules have been implicated in mesenchymal–epithelial transition (EMT) and are known to promote tumor cell invasiveness (Bacigalupo et al., 2014; Shankar et al., 2010; Thiery, 2002). However, tumor-suppressive activities of SR-A were also reported. SR-A can inhibit Lewis lung carcinoma in mice via modulating proangiogenic factors, e.g., vascular endothelial growth factor (VEGF) and matrix metalloproteinase-9 (MMP9) (Ben et al., 2012). SR-A in leukemia stem cell of chronic myeloid leukemia (CML) has been suggested as a tumor suppressor gene. In this study, SR-A deletion accelerated CML development and increased the self-renewal and differentiation capacity of leukemia stem cells through PI3K-AKT-GSK-3β and β-Catenin pathways (Chen et al., 2011). Although the discrepancies on SR-A action in these studies have not been addressed, SR-A appears to be of significance in the development of novel therapeutic strategies directed to target SR-A^+ TAMs for therapeutic benefits.

Single-nucleotide polymorphisms are a type of genetic variation associated with population diversity, genome evolution, and disease susceptibility. Epidemiology and pathological studies have established an intimate link between chronic inflammation and cancer development (McLean & El-Omar, 2009). The polymorphisms of multiple genes involved in regulation of inflammatory response have been associated with higher cancer risk (Caruso et al., 2009). *Sra* gene is located on chromosome 8p22, a genetic region that is associated with multiple tumor susceptibility phenotypes (Low et al., 2011). Genetic variations of *Sra* have been associated with the increased susceptibility of prostate cancer (Miller et al., 2003; Xu et al., 2002), although the conclusion was queried by other studies (Rennert et al., 2008; Seppala et al., 2003; Wang et al., 2003). Several common and rare missense polymorphisms variants in the *Sra* gene were also associated with a high risk of prostate cancer (Xu et al., 2002). Significant differences in the spectrum of mutations and sequence variants in the *Sra* gene have been found among various racial groups and populations (Hsing et al., 2007; Rennert et al., 2008; Sun, Turner, Xu, Gronberg, & Isaacs, 2007). A T+25C polymorphism located in the 5′ untranslated region of the *Sra* gene was recently suggested to increase lung cancer risk via down-regulating SR-A expression (Ben et al., 2012). While more work is clearly required to validate these findings, it is possible that screening of *Sra* polymorphisms may help identify populations at risk of cancer prior to disease onset.

The identification of SR-A as a negative regulator of antitumor immune response provides new insight into the functional diversity of this innate PRR (Wang et al., 2007). This finding was derived from our research in understanding the immunogenicity of HSPs or molecular chaperones as immunostimulatory adjuvants in cancer vaccination therapy (Murshid, Gong, & Calderwood, 2008; Srivastava, 2002; Wang, Facciponte, & Subjeck, 2006; Wang & Subjeck, 2013). A primary feature of chaperone molecules in cancer immunotherapy is their capacity to deliver polypeptide antigens efficiently to specialized antigen-presenting cells (APCs), such as DCs, and introduce these antigenic targets into the major histocompatibility complex (MHC) class I pathway for cross-presentation, resulting in priming $CD8^+$ cytotoxic T lymphocytes (CTLs). Given the superior antigen cross-presenting capacity of HSPs, there has been an intensive search for dedicated receptors or binding structures on APCs that specifically recognize HSPs. Surprisingly, SR-A, with a promiscuous binding feature, was found to bind a number of HSPs, including Hsp110, Grp94, and Grp170 (Berwin et al., 2003; Facciponte, Wang, & Subjeck, 2007). Although SR-A clearly participated in binding and uptake of these HSPs, the exact contribution of the SR-A to antitumor immunity generated by HSP-based vaccines was not addressed.

We first examined the impact of SR-A on vaccination-induced antitumor immune response using SR-A-deficient mice (Wang et al., 2007). We made a striking observation that, in contrast to our initial prediction that SR-A-deficiency should reduce HSP vaccine activity, lack of SR-A was found to profoundly enhance a protective antitumor immune response upon administration of HSP-based chaperone vaccines (Wang et al., 2007). Additionally, SR-A absence restored the immunogenicity of poorly immunogenic murine melanoma and lung tumor cells, as indicated by improved antitumor efficacy after immunization with irradiated tumor cells as cell-based vaccines. Although an early study reported that SR-A knockout animals showed no defect in clearance of apoptotic cells (Komohara et al., 2005; Platt, Suzuki, Kodama, & Gordon, 2000), it is evident that immune tolerance to dying tumor cells was broken in the absence of SR-A. Our finding indeed was supported by a study from the Karlsson group, which suggested that class A scavenger receptors function as regulators of immune tolerance to apoptotic cells (Wermeling et al., 2007). The SR-A absence enhanced antitumor immune response was dependent on a CTL response, because depletion of $CD8^+$ T cells or phagocytic cells (presumably APCs) abolished the antitumor activity of vaccines in $SRA^{-/-}$ mice. Furthermore, we demonstrated that $SRA^{-/-}$ mice similarly developed enhanced immune response upon vaccination with Freund's complete adjuvant or LPS, suggesting that SR-A dampens the immunostimulatory activities of adjuvants of both mammalian and non-mammalian origins and that in these contexts SR-A represents an immune suppressor of antigen/tumor-specific T cell responses (Qian et al., 2011; Wang et al., 2007).

Monophosphoryl lipid A (MPL) is a chemically modified low toxic LPS that targets TLR4 signaling and has been tested in multiple vaccine trials (Baldridge et al., 2004). We showed that SR-A attenuated antitumor CTL response elicited by ovalbumin (OVA)-MPL immunization (Yi et al., 2009). Furthermore, the lack of SR-A appeared to render DCs more responsive to LPS stimulation as indicated by elevation of costimulatory molecules and production of proinflammatory factors, e.g., tumor necrosis factor α (TNF-α). SR-A-altered immunogenicity of DCs in response to TLR4 activation correlates with a previously suggested role of SR-A in limiting DC maturation and activation (Becker, Cotena, Gordon, & Platt, 2006). Our subsequent studies revealed that SR-A downregulated the activation TLR4-NF-κB signaling pathway in DCs by directly interacting with the TNF receptor-associated factor 6 (TRAF6), resulting in inhibition of TRAF6 dimerization and ubiquitination (Yu et al., 2011). Intriguingly, the attenuation of NF-κB activity by SR-A appeared to be independent of its ligand-binding domain, suggesting that the signaling-regulatory feature of SR-A may be uncoupled from its endocytic functions. These results not only elucidate a novel mechanism by which SR-A restricts TLR4 activation and consequent inflammatory response but also provide molecular basis of SR-A-mediated suppression of functional activation of APCs in TLR4-targeting vaccination-induced CTL response. In addition to $CD8^+$ T cells, SR-A can also limit the activation of $CD4^+$ T cells by inhibiting the function of DCs treated with anti-CD40 antibodies and IFN-γ (Yi et al., 2012).

In light of the fact that the immunogenicity of dying tumor cells increases in $SR\text{-}A^{-/-}$ mice, we examined the regulatory effect of SR-A in cross-presentation of cell-associated antigen using OVA-expressing RM1 prostate tumor model. While SR-A deficiency does not significantly influence the phagocytic ability of DCs, $SR\text{-}A^{-/-}$ DCs displayed increased capacity in cross-presenting OVA antigen from dying RM1 cells and generated a much more potent antigen-specific T cell response compared with wild-type DCs, which resulted in improved tumor inhibition in both prophylactic and therapeutic settings (Guo, Yi, Yu, Hu, et al., 2012).

The immunosuppressive activity of SR-A in antitumor immunity was also supported by independent studies from other groups. Inhibition of SR-A by fucoidan, a sulfated polysaccharide from the Fucus species and other brown algae that is capable of blocking SR-A function (Tateno, Ogawa, Muramoto, Kamiya, & Saneyoshi, 2002), can enhance the cross-presentation of NY-ESO-1, a cancer-testis antigen, leading to an increased CTL activation against NY-ESO-1 positive cancers (Hu et al., 2010). Herber et al. demonstrated that, in tumor-bearing mice and in cancer patients, SR-A-mediated excessive lipid uptake and accumulation in DCs endowed them with tolerogenic properties, which caused a profound defect in DC function and impaired antitumor immunity (Herber et al., 2010). This study provides an additional insight into the dysfunctional APCs in tumor-bearing host and a new mechanism by which SR-A downregulates the immunogenicity of APCs.

APCs, particularly DCs and macrophages, are sentinels distributed throughout the body. These cells play a central role not only in maintaining immune tolerance to self-antigens but also direct effective immune responses to eliminate "danger," such as invading pathogens (Banchereau & Steinman, 1998). These findings also raise an intriguing question as to whether SR-A may be involved in tumor-induced immune tolerance during tumor growth and progression. DCs are known to capture antigen from live tumor cells via a "nibbling" process that is dependent on cell–cell contact, and this has been shown to be mediated by SR-A (Harshyne, Zimmer, Watkins, & Barratt-Boyes, 2003). SR-A was responsible for the acquisition and cross-presentation of tumor antigen gp100 from melanoma cells to T cells; however, this study did not address the potential significance of this SR-A activity *in vivo*. It is likely that SR-A-mediated transfer of live cell-associated antigen by DCs may lead to immune tolerance under a steady state or immune escape during tumor development. It is conceivable that the immunoregulatory effect of SR-A may depend on the context of their ligation and other receptors engaged simultaneously, as well as factors released from cells. Recently, we showed that SR-A is essential for maintenance of tissue homeostasis in a mouse model of immune-mediated liver injury (Zuo et al., 2013). Genetic SR-A ablation highly sensitized mice to concanavalin A (Con A)-induced hepatitis. Mechanistic studies revealed that SR-A on myeloid cells mobilized in response to tissue injury functions as a negative regulator limiting the activation of T cells that produce cytotoxic cytokine IFN-γ. This result is analogous to our finding of SR-A in suppressing the effector function of tumor-specific T cells in cancer immunotherapy. Together, our studies of SR-A in cancer- and immune-mediated tissue injury establish SR-A on myeloid cells, including DCs, as a key regulator involved in host immune homeostasis and tumor-induced immune tolerance (Fig. 1).

2.1.2 Macrophage Receptor with Collagenous Structure

Macrophage receptor with collagenous structure (MARCO also referred to as SR-A6) is considered a dominant receptor for unopsonized particles and bacteria in the lung (Elomaa et al., 1995; van der Laan et al., 1999), due to its restricted expression in distinct populations of macrophages in lung, spleen, and lymph node. Most studies have been centered on the role of MARCO in the host defense against respiratory tract infections and pneumoconiosis induced by crystalline silica or cigarette smoke (Thakur, Hamilton, & Holian, 2008; Thomsen, Nordestgaard, Kobzik, & Dahl, 2013). However, several lines of evidence recently implicated MARCO as a regulator of DC function and antitumor immunity. An early study reported that MARCO was involved in actin cytoskeleton rearrangements during the phenotypic and functional maturation of DCs (Granucci et al., 2003). It was shown that MARCO was highly elevated in DCs upon pulsing with mouse tumor lysate (Matsushita, Komine, Grolleau-Julius, Pilon-Thomas, & Mule, 2010). Intriguingly, treatment of tumor lysate-pulsed DCs with anti-MARCO antibodies promoted these cells to traffic to draining lymph nodes and facilitated the induction of tumor-reactive IFN-γ producing T cells for tumor inhibition (Matsushita et al., 2010). Komine et al. recently found that MARCO$^{-/-}$ DCs displayed increased motility in response to the chemokine CCL-21 *in vivo* and migrated more efficiently after injection into mice (Komine, Kuhn, Matsushita, Mule, & Pilon-Thomas, 2013). Immunization with tumor lysate-pulsed DCs derived from MARCO$^{-/-}$ mice, compared to WT counterparts, significantly enhanced T cell-mediated antitumor immune responses and prolonged the survival of B16 melanoma-bearing mice (Komine et al., 2013). These observations are generally in line with our results of SR-A function in DC-induced antitumor immunity. Since MARCO is also expressed on human monocyte-derived DCs (Matsushita et al., 2010), the strategies that target MARCO on these cells may improve the therapeutic efficacy DC-based anticancer vaccination.

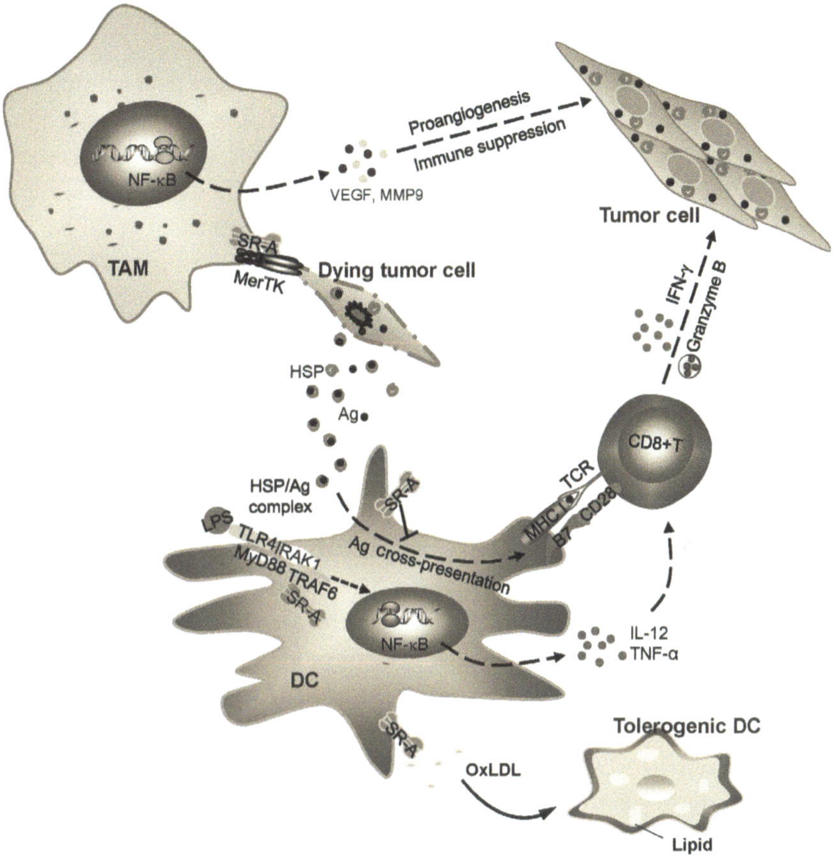

Figure 1 A schematic representation of tumor-promoting functions of scavenger receptor class A (SR-A). The increased expression of SR-A may interact with and engage Mer tyrosine kinase (MerTK) signaling during interaction with dying tumor cells in the tumor microenvironment (TME), which facilitates the polarization of tumor-associated macrophages (TAMs) toward an M2-like phenotype. Proangiogenic and immunosuppressive activity of TAMs contributes to tumor progression and invasion, metastasis. The SR-A also inhibits the antigen-cross-presenting functions and activation of on dendritic cells (DCs) in response to vaccines, such as antigen (Ag) carried by heat shock proteins (HSPs) or formulated with toll-like receptor (TLR) agonists (e.g., LPS). It is executed by SR-A interference of activation of TNF receptor-associated factor 6 (TRAF6) in DCs, which leads to downregulation of TLR4-NF-κB signaling and production of immunostimulatory cytokines (e.g., TNF-α, IL-12) that are crucial for expansion and tumoricidal activity of $CD8^+$ cytotoxic T lymphocytes (CTLs). Additionally, SR-A-mediated excessive lipid accumulation can skew DCs differentiation toward a tolerogenic phenotype in the TME, which suppresses the functions of effector T cells and promotes cancer escape from the immune attack. (See the color plate.)

2.1.3 Scavenger Receptor Class A, Member 3 and Member 5 (SCARA3 and SCARA5)

Unlike SR-A and MARCO that are primarily expressed in myeloid cells, two other class A scavenger receptor, SCARA3 (also referred to as cellular stress response 1 [CSR1], SR-A3) and SCARA5 (SR-A5), can be detected in a variety of tissues or cells (Whelan et al., 2012). The methylation of the *Scara3* gene promoter, and to a lesser extent downregulation of SCARA3 protein expression, has been associated with a high rate of prostate cancer metastasis. Forced overexpression of SCARA3 in prostate cancer cell lines (DU145 and PC3) resulted in inhibition of tumor growth and invasion, suggesting that SCARA3 may be a potent tumor suppressor gene in prostate cancer (Yu et al., 2006). However, analysis of clinical samples from 351 multiple myeloma (MM) patients showed an inverse correlation between the level of *Scara3* gene, disease progression and favorable clinical outcome (Brown et al., 2013). SCARA3 expression in MM can be upregulated by ionizing radiation (IR) or chemotherapeutic drugs, which is believed to protect cells from oxidative stress by scavenging IR- or drug-generated reactive oxygen species, and therefore contribute to the resistance of MM to cancer therapeutics (Brown et al., 2013). Genomic analyses suggested that SCARA3 overexpression in ovarian carcinoma and primary peritoneal carcinoma correlates with disease progression and recurrence (Bock, Nymoen, Brenne, Kaern, & Davidson, 2012; Han, Tokino, & Nakamura, 1998). While the discrepancies on SCARA3 association with cancer progression or therapeutic resistance is unclear, future studies should examine the protein levels of SCARA3 in patient samples using immunohistochemistry, since the studies involving ovarian cancer or MM only analyzed the mRNA levels of SCARA3.

SCARA5 is unable to endocytose-modified LDLs, but it can mediate the scavenging of serum ferritin from cell surface or iron delivery (Li et al., 2009). SCARA5 expression was frequently downregulated in various cancer cell lines and tumor samples (Yan et al., 2012). Promoter hypermethylation and allelic imbalance-induced SCARA5 suppression has been detected in patient specimens with hepatocellular carcinoma (HCC) (Huang, Zheng, et al., 2010). Forced SCARA5 overexpression in HCC cell line can reverse its malignant phenotype *in vitro* and suppress its tumorigenesis and metastasis through the focal adhesion kinase (FAK)–Src-p130Cas signaling pathway (Huang, Zheng, et al., 2010). Mechanistic studies demonstrated that DNA methyltransferase 1 is responsible for the *Scara5* promoter silence by physically associating with Snail1, a transcription factor that can directly bind to the E-box elements in *Scara5* promoter. Snail1-mediated *SCARA5* suppression in tumor cells is essential for EMT-induced cell migration, a crucial event in cancer metastasis (Liu et al., 2013; Son & Moon, 2010). Yan et al. further demonstrated that systemic delivery of SCARA5 by using the *Scara5*-cationic liposome complex markedly inhibited subcutaneous glioma tumors and spontaneous lung tumors in mice (Yan et al., 2012). Upregulation of SCARA5 also resulted in the inactivation of signal transducer and activator of transcription 3 (STAT3), as well as downregulation of STAT3-regulated genes that have been implicated in tumor progression and metastasis, including cyclinB1, cyclinD1, AKT, survivin, VEGF-A, and MMP9 (Yan et al., 2012). These studies provide a rationale for using SCARA5 as a therapeutic agent for potential cancer control.

2.2 Class B Scavenger Receptor

2.2.1 Thrombospondin Receptor CD36

CD36 (also referred to as SR-B2), initially identified as a receptor for thrombospondin (TSP), is the prototype class B scavenger receptor (Asch, Barnwell, Silverstein, & Nachman, 1987). As one of the most widely studied scavenger receptors, CD36 plays an important role in the recognition and endocytic uptake of oxidized phospholipids, modified LDL, apoptotic cells, or amyloid proteins (Stewart et al., 2010), and is involved in the regulation of many aspects of inflammatory processes in atherosclerosis and Alzheimer's disease (Endemann et al., 1993; Philips, Rubin, & Perrimon, 2005; Ren, Silverstein, Allen, & Savill, 1995; Sun et al., 2006). Since TSP-1/2, the ligands of CD36, are the potent endogenous inhibitors of angiogenesis, the role of CD36 in controlling tumor neovascularization has been studied (Hale et al., 2012). On endothelial cells, the interaction between CD36 and TSP-1/2 initiated sequential intracellular signaling cascades involving phosphorylation of nonreceptor tyrosine kinase Fyn, the mitogen-activated protein kinase (MAPK) p38 and c-Jun N-terminal kinase, which resulted in the activation of proapoptotic signals such as caspase 3 cleavage, induction of Fas/Fas ligand and TNF-α (Jimenez et al., 2000; Simantov, Febbraio, & Silverstein, 2005; Volpert et al., 2002). Genetic depletion of *Cd36* gene in mice enhanced the growth of syngeneic tumors, associated with increased tumoral vascularity (Hale et al., 2012). Given the importance of TSP-mediated suppression of tumor angiogenesis, a TSP-2 and IgG-Fc fusion protein (N-TSP2-Fc) was administrated to mice-bearing human breast tumor xenografts (MDA-MB-435, MDA-MB-231). N-TSP2-Fc significantly inhibited the growth and metastasis of breast tumors in a CD36-dependent manner (Koch et al., 2011).

Low-CD36 expression has been associated with higher metastasis grade or worse prognosis in colon cancer, breast cancer, and ovarian cancer (Rachidi, Qin, Sun, Zheng, & Li, 2013; Uray, Liang, & Hyder, 2004). It was shown that the highly aggressive breast tumor MDA-MB-231 expresses much less CD36 than the less aggressive MCF-7 and T47-D cells (Uray et al., 2004). This may be explained by the binding capacity of CD36 for collagen in extracellular matrix (ECM). Low expression of CD36 may reduce tumor cell adhesion to ECM, thus causing increased cell mobility and metastatic potential (Uray et al., 2004). Paradoxically, the expression level of CD36 in glioblastoma was found to negatively correlate with patient prognosis (Hale et al., 2014). Interestingly, CD36 appeared to be enriched on a subset of glioblastoma cancer stem cells (CSCs). CD36 reduction resulted in concomitant loss of self-renewal and tumor initiation capacity in these cells (Hale et al., 2014), suggesting that the selectively enhanced expression of scavenger receptors, such as CD36, may provide survival, and metabolic advantages in CSCs.

CD36 has been called "fatty acid translocase" due to its abundant presence in cell types involved in fatty acid metabolism, such as adipocytes, hepatocytes, cardiomyocytes, and intestinal enterocytes (Coburn et al., 2000; Drover et al., 2008; Zhou et al., 2008). CD36-mediated binding and transportation of long-chain fatty acids may facilitate intracellular lipid accumulation, a hallmark of aggressive cancer cells (Nieva et al., 2012). Surprisingly, a recent study showed that repressed CD36 expression in fibroblast from mammary tissue is responsible for pathologic changes in mammary gland hyperplasia and breast cancer, including impaired adipocyte differentiation, excessive ECM deposition, and is associated with increased risk of aggressive breast cancer in patients (DeFilippis et al., 2012). This finding underscores a crucial role of the pro-oncogenic tissue state via repression of CD36 in supporting tumorigenesis and suggests that strategies to modulate CD36 may help prevent the progression of breast cancer in women who are at high risk. While the mechanism underlying tumorigenesis promoted by the repression of CD36 is not completely understood, it is clear from steatohepatitis and obesity models that aberrant fatty acid levels can upregulate CD36 expression and affect the activity of CD36 in nonadipose cells, e.g., cardiomyocytes and vascular smooth muscle cells (Angin et al., 2012; Lau, Chu, & Weiss,

2004). Further studies are necessary to define whether dysregulated lipid metabolism may alter the expression of CD36 and its function during cancer development.

2.2.2 Scavenger Receptor Class B, Member 1 (SR-BI)

Scavenger Receptor Class B, Member 1 SR-BI (also known as SCARB1 or SR-B1) was the first identified receptor for high-density lipoprotein (HDL). SR-BI and CD36 share considerable sequence homology and mediate the transport of modified LDL, native HDL, and very low-density lipoprotein (VLDL). SR-BI is ubiquitously expressed in multiple tissues, but it is more densely expressed in organs involved in cholesterol metabolism, e.g., liver, adrenal, and gonad (Landschulz, Pathak, Rigotti, Krieger, & Hobbs, 1996; Nakagawa-Toyama et al., 2005). HDL is one of the major carriers for cholesterol, which is an important regulator of cancer development (Cruz, Mo, McConathy, Sabnis, & Lacko, 2013). Epidemiologic studies suggest that low levels of HDL cholesterol and HDL particles are risk markers of cancer development and prognosis (Kotani et al., 2013; Vilchez, Martinez-Ruiz, Sancho-Rodriguez, Martinez-Hernandez, & Noguera-Velasco, 2014). As the primary receptor responsible for the selective internalization of cholesteryl ester from HDL molecules, the role of SR-BI in cancer development recently received increasing attention.

Abundant expression of SR-BI, which participates in selective uptake of HDL-cholesteryl ester (HDL-CE), has been observed in human choriocarcinoma cells, malignant human epithelial cells, prostate cancer cells, breast cancer cells, and hepatoma cells (Graf, Roswell, & Smart, 2001; Mooberry, Nair, Paranjape, McConathy, & Lacko, 2010; Wadsack, Hirschmugl, et al., 2003; Wadsack, Hrzenjak, et al., 2003). In breast cancer, SR-BI protein levels were found to be significantly elevated in malignant tissues compared with surrounding histologically disease-free tissues (Cao et al., 2004). Overexpression of SR-BI protected breast cancer MCF-7 cells against TNF-α-induced apoptosis, whereas expression of the extracellular domain of SR-BI (amino acids 1–464) significantly inhibited the cell proliferation (Cao et al., 2004). This truncated SR-BI retained the HDL uptake capacity, but lacked the C-terminal intracellular region that is believed to regulate HDL signaling, indicating that SR-BI may be able to define the growth behavior of breast cancer cells in the presence of HDL. Another study revealed that SR-BI-mediated AKT signaling was required for sustained proliferation, mobility, and invasiveness of breast cancer cells in response to stimulation of HDL-CE (Danilo et al., 2013).

Cholesterol is the precursor of bioactive steroid hormones, such as androgen. Prostate cancer patients who have received androgen deprivation therapy commonly develop recurrence that is more aggressive and castration resistant. SR-BI expression was significantly elevated upon progression to castration-resistance in the LNCaP xenograft model, suggesting an essential role that SR-BI may play in regulation of cholesterol uptake during prostate cancer development and progression (Leon et al., 2010). Recently, small-interfering RNA (siRNA)-mediated downregulation of SR-BI was reported to effectively inhibit the production of prostate-specific antigen, and the viability of prostate cancer cells, implicating a possible therapeutic effect of SR-BI in the treatment of the castration-resistant disease (Twiddy, Cox, & Wasan, 2012).

2.3 Class D Scavenger Receptor

CD68, also known as macrosialin in mice, is the only known member of the class D scavenger receptors. CD68 is a glycosylated type I membrane protein that belongs to the lysosome-associated membrane protein family of molecules (Song, Lee, & Schindler, 2011). CD68 is predominantly expressed in late endosomes and lysosomes of macrophages, but is also found on the surface of DCs and osteoclasts (Jiang et al., 1998; Ramprasad et al., 1995). CD68 has been widely used as a pan-macrophage marker (Holness & Simmons, 1993). Increased macrophage ($CD68^+$) index is associated with high vascularity and nodal metastasis, as well as reduced overall survival in human breast cancer (Leek et al., 1996). In a large cohort study involving 1322 patients with breast cancer, higher numbers of $CD68^+$ macrophages predicted worse breast cancer-specific survival and a shorter disease-free interval (Mahmoud et al., 2012). A multicenter study also suggested that patients with lower $CD68^+$ TAMs level showed improved metastasis-free survival (Jezequel et al., 2012), which further supports the predictive value of $CD68^+$ TAMs in human breast cancer. Recently, multivariate analyses showed that the number of $CD68^+$ cells was also an independent and significant factor for poor prognosis in patients with myxoid liposarcoma (Nabeshima et al., 2015).

Angiogenesis is a critical event in tumor growth and metastasis. The high density of $CD68^+$ TAMs is accompanied with high stromal and serum levels of VEGF. There is an association between expressions of CD68 and Ras in the angiogenesis of breast cancer (Li et al., 2015). Upregulation of VEGF in macrophages by IR is believed to decrease the antitumor efficacy of radiotherapy (Meng et al., 2010), suggesting that the CD68$^+$ TAMs may also be an indicator for the outcome of cancer treatment, such as radiotherapy. Despite its wide use as a predictor for cancer prognosis, the functions of CD68 in TAMs, the major inflammatory component of the tumor stroma, are largely unknown.

2.4 Class E Scavenger Receptor

2.4.1 Lectin-Like Oxidized LDL Receptor 1

Lectin-like oxidized LDL receptor 1 (LOX-1), also called oxidized low-density lipoprotein receptor 1 (OLR1), is a major class E scavenger receptor for oxLDL, advanced glycation end products (AGEs), bacteria, and apoptotic cells (Huysamen & Brown, 2009; Oka et al., 1998; Sawamura et al., 1997; Shimaoka et al., 2001). LOX-1 is primarily expressed in endothelial cells, cardiomyocytes, smooth muscle cells, B cells, macrophages, DCs, and platelets (Delneste et al., 2002; Dunn et al., 2008; Huysamen & Brown, 2009; Jeannin et al., 2005; Joo et al., 2014; Nickel et al., 2009). LOX-1 has been implicated in multiple physiological and pathophysiological processes, e.g., lipid metabolism, cholesterol biosynthesis, and atherogenesis (Huysamen & Brown, 2009; Mehta et al., 2007). Recent studies identified LOX-1 as a possible link between obesity, dyslipidemia, and cancer (Hirsch et al., 2010; Khaidakov et al., 2011). Hirsch and colleagues conducted a study to identify the cancer cell-specific transcriptional signature by comparing the oncogene Src or telomerase/Ras transformed mammary epithelial cells (MCF10A) or primary fibroblasts with their parental nontransformed cells (Hirsch et al., 2010). This signature revealed several common genes related to metabolic disorders, inflammation and carcinogenesis, indicating the importance of lipid metabolism in cellular transformation. Interestingly, upregulation of LOX-1 in the transformed cells was shown to contribute to the cellular transformation and maintenance of the transformed state by stimulating inflammatory signaling (e.g., IL-6, IL-8, and IL-1β) and hypoxia-regulated pathways (VEGF, HIF-1α, carbonic anhydrase 9) in an NF-κB-dependent manner. LOX-1 knockdown or blockade in transformed cells impaired their anchorage-independent growth, cell migration as well as invasion. In addition to supporting tumor growth in mouse xenograft models, LOX-1 was shown to be highly expressed in the patient specimens with late stage metastatic breast cancer and prostate cancer. These results provide supporting evidence that the activation of LOX-1 pathway may be a major event in tumorigenesis.

This hypothesis was tested further by Khaidakov et al. using a LOX-1 deficient mouse model (Khaidakov et al., 2011). LOX-1 abrogation resulted in broad suppression of NF-κB-targeted genes that are related to cell proliferation, migration, apoptosis, angiogenesis, and immune defense. Deficiency of LOX-1 also caused profound inhibition of rate-limiting enzymes involved in lipogenesis. Overexpression of LOX1 activated an NF-κB-dependent anti-apoptosis pathway (BCL2, BCL2A1, and TNFAIP3) as well as lipogenesis in MCF10A normal mammary epithelial cells and HCC1143 breast cancer cells, suggesting that LOX-1 acts as an oncogene promoting tumorigenesis (Khaidakov et al., 2011). Supporting evidence also came from a study showing that upregulation of endothelial LOX-1 by TNF-α facilitated the adhesion and trans-endothelial migration of MDA-MB-231 breast cancer cells (Liang, Zhang, & Fu, 2007).

Several studies have documented the involvement of LOX-1 in host immune responses, especially T cell immunity (Delneste et al., 2002; Jeannin et al., 2005; Joo et al., 2014; Parlato et al., 2010). LOX-1 on DCs can capture PAMPs and collaborate with TLR2 to activate DCs for enhanced cellular responses (Jeannin et al., 2005). In addition, LOX-1 on mouse or human DCs functions as a receptor for Hsp60 (Xie et al., 2010) and Hsp70 (Delneste et al., 2002; Theriault, Adachi, & Calderwood, 2006). LOX-1 was shown to mediate the delivery of Hsp60-fused antigen into the MHC class I presentation pathway (Xie et al., 2010). Anti-LOX-1-neutralizing antibodies can inhibit Hsp70 binding to DCs, Hsp70-induced antigen cross-presentation, as well as subsequent antigen-specific $CD8^+$ T cell response for tumor inhibition (Delneste et al., 2002). Furthermore, human monocyte-derived DCs capture antigens for cross-presentation via LOX-1 and a LOX-1-dependent pathway is essential for IFN-α to render DCs fully competent for cross-priming $CD8^+$ effector T cells (Parlato et al., 2010). A recent study highlighted combined expression of LOX-1 on DCs and B cells in supporting humoral responses (Joo et al., 2014). While LOX-1 signaling on DCs promotes B cell differentiation via the production of the TNF superfamily ligands APRIL and BAFF, LOX-1 signaling on B cells upregulates C–C chemokine receptor type 7 (CCR7), promoting cellular migration toward lymphoid tissues. Together, these findings suggest that LOX-1 may be exploited for the rational design of novel cancer vaccines to augment both cellular and humoral immunity.

2.4.2 *β*-Glucan Receptor Dectin-1

β-Glucan, a naturally derived polysaccharide present in the cell walls of plants, bacteria, and fungi including mushrooms, has been shown to stimulate the function of innate immune cells, e.g., macrophages, DCs, granulocytes, natural killer (NK) cells, and augment adaptive immune responses that inhibit tumor growth and metastasis (Lee & Kim, 2014; Yoon, Koppula, & Lee, 2013). β-Glucan has been approved as an immunoadjuvant therapeutic for cancer treatment in some countries (Ina, Kataoka, & Ando, 2013; Wang, Bi, Zou, & Gu, 2012). A recent study has shown that β-Glucan exerts multiple antitumor effects in a Dectin-1-dependent manner (Aleem, 2013). Increased tumor growth and lung metastasis was observed in Dectin-$1^{-/-}$ mice with subcutaneous B16 melanomas as compared with WT mice (Chiba et al., 2014).

Dectin-1, a type II transmembrane protein with a C-type lectin-like carbohydrate recognition domain, is the major β-Glucan receptor on myeloid DCs, macrophages, monocytes, and B cells (Agrawal, Gupta, & Agrawal, 2010). Dectin-1 has been shown to induce NF-κB-targeted inflammatory cytokines in cooperation with TLR2/TLR6 upon β-Glucan stimulation (Moreira et al., 2011; Yadav & Schorey, 2006). Unlike other scavenger receptors that lack conserved signaling motif, Dectin-1 in DCs can directly trigger production of inflammatory cytokines (TNF-α, IL-6, IL-2, IL-23) through its cytoplasmic domain containing an immunoreceptor tyrosine-based activation motif (ITAM), phosphorylation of downstream kinase Syk, and adaptor protein caspase recruitment domain 9 (CARD9), thus inducing the Th17 and Th1 responses (Carter, Thompson, Reid, Wong, & Tough, 2006b; LeibundGut-Landmann et al., 2007; Strasser et al., 2012; Taylor et al., 2007). In addition to inducing the differentiation of naïve CD4 T cells into Th17 cells, Dectin-1 is able to directly trigger the secretion of IL-17 from TCRγδ T cells, which are essential for antifungal immunity (Martin, Hirota, Cua, Stockinger, & Veldhoen, 2009).

Dectin-1 engagement can also drive $CD8^+$ T cell responses. Curdlan, a selective β-Glucan agonist and a ligand for Dectin-1, is a potent adjuvant to prime the expansion and differentiation of CTL precursors *in vitro* and *in vivo* (Leibundgut-Landmann, Osorio, Brown, & Reis e Sousa, 2008). Antibody-mediated Dectin-1 ligation induces CTL, $CD4^+$ T cell, and antibody responses, which protected mice against melanoma challenge (Leibundgut-Landmann et al., 2008). A recent study showed that Dectin-1 contributes to NK cell-mediated tumor killing (Chiba et al.,

2014). Upon recognition of the *N*-Glycan structures that are highly expressed on tumor cells, Dectin-1-Syk pathway triggers nuclear translocation of IRF5 and induction of genes (e.g., *Fam26f*) that are known to enhance the tumoricidal activity of NK cells. Therefore, the ability of Dectin-1 to mobilize both innate and adaptive components of the host immune system makes it a promising target for cancer immunotherapy.

2.5 Class F Scavenger Receptor

Scavenger receptor expressed by endothelial cells-I (SREC-I), also named scavenger receptor class F, member 1 (SCARF1), was identified as an endothelial receptor for modified LDL (Adachi, Tsujimoto, Arai, & Inoue, 1997). A recent study showed that SREC-I, similar to CED-1, was involved in the clearance of apoptotic cells (Ramirez-Ortiz et al., 2013). SREC-I is also expressed in phagocytic cells (e.g., macrophages, DCs) and functions to bind immunostimulatory HSPs, including calreticulin (Berwin, Delneste, Lovingood, Post, & Pizzo, 2004), Hsp70 (Theriault et al., 2006), Hsp90 (Murshid, Gong, & Calderwood, 2010), Hsp110, and Grp170 (Facciponte et al., 2007). The early study showed that Hsp70 isolated from tumor-DC fusions (Hsp70.PC-F) were highly immunogenic and induced potent antitumor immunity (Enomoto et al., 2006). Although SREC-I is present at relatively low levels in murine bone marrow-derived DCs, its expression is elevated upon exposure to the Hsp70 vaccine (Gong et al., 2009). This study also demonstrated that SREC-I together with TLRs is required for T cell responses generated by Hsp70.PC-F vaccine, indicating a positive cross-talk between these two sets of PRRs (Gong et al., 2009). Indeed, a tightly orchestrated cooperation between signaling and endocytic PRRs involving SREC-I, SR-A, and TLR2 during the recognition of the hepatitis C virus by DCs was recently reported (Beauvillain et al., 2010).

Molecular studies revealed that SREC-I-mediated internalization of Hsp90–OVA peptide complexes through a Cdc42-regulated, dynamin-independent endocytic pathway. These Hsp90 complexes were transported from the GPI-anchored protein-enriched early endosomal compartment to recycling endosomes. Peptides that did not require additional processing were loaded directly onto MHC class I in endosomes, whereas extended peptides were targeted for cytosomal processing by aminopeptidases and proteases (Murshid et al., 2010). The requirement of cytosomal processing pathway for generating antigenic peptide epitopes from extended polypeptides carried by HSPs is consistent with our recent study of Grp170-enhanced cross-presentation of melanoma antigen gp100 (Wang, Chang, et al., 2013). We demonstrated that Grp170 efficiently facilitated the gp100 protein access to the ER. The interaction of gp100 with molecular components involved in ER-associated protein dislocation and/or degradation, strengthened by Grp170-based chaperoning, resulted in cytosolic translocation of tumor antigen for ubiquitination and proteasome-dependent processing (Wang, Chang, et al., 2013). However, whether SREC-I is involved in transporting or directing of internalized Grp170-gp100 complex to the ER, and required for resultant activation of tumor antigen-specific CTLs remains to be determined.

2.6 Class G Scavenger Receptor

Scavenger receptor for phosphatidylserine and oxidized lipoprotein (SR-PSOX), the single family member of class G scavenger receptor, not only binds phosphatidylserine and oxidized lipoprotein but also functions as a chemokine named CXC chemokine ligand (CXCL) 16, which can recruit NKT cells, T cells via interacting with the orphan G-protein coupled chemokine receptor CXCR6 (Geissmann et al., 2005; Kim et al., 2001; Matloubian, David, Engel, Ryan, & Cyster, 2000; Shimaoka et al., 2000). The transmembrane form of SR-PSOX/CXCL16 (TM-CXCL16) is mainly expressed on macrophages, DCs, monocytes, B cells, liver sinusoidal endothelial cells, and various types of tumor cells, where it acts as an adhesion molecule to promote the activation of antigen-specific, primary and secondary T cell responses (Heydtmann et al., 2005; Matsumura & Demaria, 2010; Matsumura et al., 2008). SR-PSOX/CXCL16 was shown to facilitate interaction between DCs and $CD8^+$ T cells, and to guide T cell movements in the splenic red pulp (Matloubian et al., 2000). Additionally, binding and scavenging of both Gram-negative and Gram-positive bacteria by the membrane-anchored form of CXL16 on macrophages or DCs are dependent on its chemokine domain, indicating an important role of TM-CXCL16 in the host defense involving both innate and adaptive responses (Shimaoka et al., 2003). There also exists a soluble form of SR-PSOX/CXCL16 (sCXCL16) with similar chemotactic activity, which is generated by constitutive or inducible cleavage through the activation of cell surface disintegrin-like metalloproteinases ADAM10 and ADAM17 (Abel et al., 2004; Pupovac, Foster, & Sluyter, 2013; Schramme, Abdel-Bakky, Kampfer-Kolb, Pfeilschifter, & Gutwein, 2008). Shedding of SR-PSOX/CXCL16 from cell surface can be triggered by the treatment with TNF-α, IL-1β, IFN-γ, phorbol 12-myristate 13-acetate (PMA), extracellular ATP, or radiation (Gutwein et al., 2009; Matsumura & Demaria, 2010; Pupovac et al., 2013).

SR-PSOX/CXCL16 and its binding partner CXCR6, as well as its processing enzyme ADAM10 and ADAM17, are overexpressed in many tumor cells, including prostate, breast, colorectal, gastric, liver, ovarian, pancreatic, cervical, lung cancer, glial tumors, and Ewing sarcoma (Gooden et al., 2014; Hattermann, Held-Feindt, Ludwig, & Mentlein, 2013; Huang, Zhang, Cui, Zhao, & Zheng, 2013; Na et al., 2014; Wente et al., 2008). Increasing evidence supports the involvement of sCXCL16 in tumor progression, e.g., promoting proliferation, migration, and invasiveness of CXCR6^{+} cancer cells (Lu et al., 2008; Schramme et al., 2008; Xing et al., 2012). The elevated level of sCXCL16 in serum has been considered an independent predictor for poor survival in ovarian cancer patients and those with colorectal cancer who have developed the recurrence of liver metastases (Gooden et al., 2014; Matsushita et al., 2012). Independent studies also support the association of SR-PSOX/CXCL16 with poor prognosis in various cancers. Analysis of 354 prostate cancer samples revealed that SR-PSOX/CXCL16 expression was significantly increased in patients with perineural invasion, lymph node and bone metastasis, large tumor burden, and high pathological disease stage (Ha et al., 2011). In 92 patient samples of epithelial ovarian cancer, expression of SR-PSOX/CXCL16 and CXCR6 was significantly related to lymph node metastasis and reduced median survival (Guo, Cui, Zhang, & Huang, 2011). Studies using 461 specimens from 12 different cancers indicated that the elevation of SR-PSOX/CXCL16 and CXCR6 on both tumor cells and adjacent T cells may facilitate the formation of proinflammatory TME via recruiting tumor-infiltrating leukocytes, which enhances tumor cell proliferation and invasiveness (Darash-Yahana et al., 2009). The involvement of sCXCL16 in promoting neutrophil infiltration, angiogenesis, and formation of tumor-promoting inflammatory environment has also been shown in HCC patients (Gao et al., 2012).

A feed-forward signaling loop between tumor cells and mesenchymal stem cells (MSCs), which can be triggered by the engagement of CXCL16-CXCR6, was recently proposed (Chaturvedi, Gilkes, Takano, & Semenza, 2014; Jung et al., 2013). Tumor cell-produced sCXCL16 recruits CXCR6^{+} MSCs to the tumor site. CXCL12 secreted from these recruited MSCs will in turn bind to its receptor CXCR4 on tumor cells, resulting in enhanced cancer invasiveness and metastasis (Chaturvedi et al., 2014; Jung et al., 2013). Another study showed that activation of CXCL16-CXCR6 axis enhanced prostate cancer progression and metastasis, which was associated with the upregulation of proangiogenic factor IL-8 and VEGF that depended on the CXCR6/AKT/mTOR signaling pathway (Wang, Lu, Koch, Zhang, & Taichman, 2008).

A different finding was made in studies that involved 104 patient samples of renal cell carcinoma (RCC) and 58 samples of colorectal carcinoma (CRC) (Gutwein et al., 2009; Hojo et al., 2007). In these two studies, TM-CXCL16 correlated inversely with tumor stage and a high level of tumoral TM-CXCL16 appeared to be a prognostic marker for long-term survival. Immunohistochemistry and flow cytometry analyses showed that SR-PSOX/CXCL16 was located predominantly in the membrane and cytosol of RCC cell lines (Gutwein et al., 2009). In line with these clinical data, overexpression of TM-CXCL16 in breast cancer MDA-MB-231 cells suppressed their invasiveness *in vitro* and tumorigenesis *in vivo* (Fang et al., 2014). IR can upregulate the expression of TM-CXCL16 and promote the shedding of sCXCL16, which results in improved therapeutic efficacy by recruiting $CD8^+CXCR6^+$ effector T cells (Matsumura & Demaria, 2010; Matsumura et al., 2008). These results clearly demonstrate the different functions of SR-PSOX/CXCL16 in various cancers or therapeutic settings. Understanding the context-dependent activities of SR-PSOX/CXCL16 is essential for developing therapeutics to block cancer progression and invasion.

2.7 Class H Scavenger Receptor

Stabilin-1, also referred to as Fasciclin, epidermal growth factor-like and lamin-type epidermal growth factor-like, and link domain-containing scavenger receptor-1 (FEEL-1), or common lymphatic endothelial and vascular endothelial receptor-1 (CLEVER-1), and stabilin-2/FEEL-2 are the current known class H scavenger receptor members (Adachi & Tsujimoto, 2002; Irjala et al., 2003; Politz et al., 2002). Stabilin-1 and stabilin-2, which bind several ligands, including oxLDL, acLDL, hyaluronan (HA), heparin, and matricellular protein such as secreted protein acidic and rich in cysteine (SPARC), play important roles in clearance of these "unwanted" self-substances (Qian et al., 2009; Rost & Sumanas, 2014; Workman & Sage, 2011). Stabilin-1 was also reported to bind Hsp70–peptide complexes and mediate its internalization (Theriault et al., 2006). However, its role in modulating Hsp70 vaccine-induced antitumor immune response is unknown. Stabilin-1 and stabilin-2 are constitutively present on tissue resident macrophages, lymphatic endothelial cells, and sinusoidal endothelial cells in bone marrow and liver (Qian et al., 2009; Shetty et al., 2011). However, their expression changes on vasculature at the sites of chronic inflammation or tumor, where they mediate the trafficking of lymphocytes, granulocytes, and monocytes to the inflamed tissues (David et al., 2012; Karikoski et al., 2009).

An early study suggested stabilin-1 as a multifunctional scavenger receptor that could link endocytic clearance, intracellular sorting, and transcytosis in macrophages (Kzhyshkowska & Krusell, 2009). SPARC, a nonstructural glycoprotein crucial for angiogenesis, wound healing, and tissue remodeling, plays a significant role in altering cancer cell activity and remodeling the TME (Nagaraju, Dontula, El-Rayes, & Lakka, 2014). Given that stabilin-1^+ macrophages can actively uptake and degrade circulating SPARC, it is conceivable that aberrant clearance of SPARC may contribute to tumor progression and metastasis (Nagaraju et al., 2014). Indeed, the expression of stabilin-1 in TAMs decreased during the progression of glioma and melanoma (David et al., 2012). Stabilin-1 on liver sinusoidal endothelial cells was shown to preferentially facilitate the recruitment of $CD4^+FoxP3^+$ regulatory T cells (Treg) to the liver tissue with HCC, which could disable the immune effector functions and facilitate tumor escape (Shetty et al., 2011).

The role of stabilin-1 in tumor growth was further validated using cell-specific stabilin-1 knockout mice (Karikoski et al., 2014). Elevation of stabilin-1 in tumor vasculature enhanced the binding of immunosuppressive leukocytes to the intratumoral blood vessels and promoted tumor cell trafficking via the lymphatics. Growth of primary tumors, not of metastases, was inhibited in mice that lacked stabilin-1 in macrophages or in vascular endothelium. The absence of functional stabilin-1 resulted in diminished tumor infiltration by immunosuppressive leukocytes and suppressed tumor progression, suggesting that stabilin-1 represents a novel target for overcoming immune evasion and blocking lymphatic spread of cancer (Karikoski et al., 2014).

HA, a major component of the ECM, is highly increased in tumor progression, which correlates with high tumor grade and poor prognosis (Karbownik & Nowak, 2013). The binding of HA to its receptor activates signaling pathways that stimulate cell proliferation, invasiveness, multidrug resistance, and EMT in many tumors (Workman & Sage, 2011). Antibody blockade or genetic ablation of stabilin-2, which disrupted HA–stabilin-2 interaction, led to elevated circulating HA levels and prevented tumor metastasis (Sironen et al., 2011), suggesting that functional inhibition of stabilin-2 may be a potential approach to suppressing tumor progression. In addition, stabilin-2 expression levels have been linked to the outcome of cancer patients. Tissue microarray analysis of 296 samples from patients with HCC showed that loss of stabilin-2 expression in peri-tumorous liver tissue correlated with increased survival (Geraud et al., 2013). Based on its differential expression in prostate cancer patients versus healthy controls, stabilin-2 has been identified as a potential early diagnostic biomarker for detecting indolent and advanced prostate cancer (Neuhaus et al., 2013).

2.8 Class I Scavenger Receptor

CD163 is the prototype class I scavenger receptor for haptoglobin–hemoglobin (Hp–Hb) complexes. CD163 is exclusively expressed on monocytes/macrophages or hematopoietic malignancies with monocytic/histiocytic differentiation (Nguyen et al., 2005). CD163 expression is tightly regulated by inflammatory responses, where anti-inflammatory signals (e.g., IL-10, glucocorticoid) induce CD163 expression, but proinflammatory signals (e.g., LPS, TNF-α, IFN-γ) suppress CD163 synthesis (Buechler et al., 2000). Studies of CD163 regulation in multiple tumor models indicate that the high level of CD163 is a feature of macrophages undergoing differentiation toward the "alternatively activated" M2 phenotype (Edin et al., 2012; Fujimura, Kambayashi, Furudate, Kakizaki, & Aiba, 2013; Gordon & Martinez, 2010; Komohara, Ohnishi, Kuratsu, & Takeya, 2008; Tiainen et al., 2014; van Dongen et al., 2010). CD163-involved macrophage polarization may be related to its function of scavenging Hp–Hb complexes. Release of Hb into plasma is a phenomenon occurred during physiologic or pathologic intravascular hemolysis, e.g., inflammation and hemorrhage in the tumor. Free form of Hb in the circulation forms complexes with plasma glycoprotein Hp, which results in the high-affinity interaction of CD163 with Hp–Hb complexes in a calcium-dependent manner (Madsen et al., 2004). The binding of the complexes to CD163$^+$ TAMs stimulates the induction of stress-responsive hemo oxygenase-1 (HO-1), a heme-detoxification enzyme that is also involved in macrophage polarization toward an M2 phenotype and important for production of anti-inflammatory cytokine IL-10 (Naito, Takagi, & Higashimura, 2014; Sierra-Filardi, Vega, Sanchez-Mateos, Corbi, & Puig-Kroger, 2010; Weis, Weigert, von Knethen, & Brune, 2009). Thus, the CD163–HO-1–IL-10 axis may be an important contributor to the formation of immunosuppressive TME.

CD68 and CD163 are often used to identify macrophages in tissue sections (Kong et al., 2013). Compared to CD68 that is commonly used as a pan-macrophage marker (Holness & Simmons, 1993), CD163 is regarded as a specific monocyte/macrophage marker for M2 macrophages (Ambarus et al., 2012; Lau et al., 2004; Qian & Pollard, 2010). The presence of $CD163^{+}$ macrophages was suggested to have a stronger association with less favorable clinicopathological features than $CD68^{+}$ macrophages (Medrek, Ponten, Jirstrom, & Leandersson, 2012). Numerous studies demonstrate that elevated CD163 expression correlates with advanced cancer stages, unfavorable prognosis, early distant recurrence, and reduced patient survival in various types of cancer, which include melanoma (Jensen et al., 2009), meningioma (Kanno et al., 2013), breast cancer (Mansfield, Heikkila, von Smitten, Vakkila, & Leidenius, 2012; Shabo, Stal, Olsson, Dore, & Svanvik, 2008; Tiainen et al., 2014), colorectal cancer (Edin et al., 2012; Shabo, Olsson, Elkarim, Sun, & Svanvik, 2014), oral squamous cell carcinoma (He, Bao, et al., 2014; Wang et al., 2014), ovarian carcinoma (Reinartz et al., 2014), HCC (Kong et al., 2013), angiosarcoma (Fujimura et al., 2013), glioma (Komohara et al., 2008), and gastrointestinal stromal tumors (van Dongen et al., 2010), and hematopoietic malignancies, such as T cell leukemia/lymphoma (Komohara et al., 2013), acute myeloid leukemia (Garcia, Gardner, & Reichard, 2008), and classical Hodgkin lymphoma (Klein et al., 2014; Koh, Park, Yoon, Suh, & Huh, 2014). A recent study showed that relapse of head and neck cancer after chemoradiotherapy also correlated with $CD163^{+}$ macrophages in primary tumor and $CD11b^{+}$ myeloid cells in recurrences (Balermpas et al., 2014).

Several studies reported that the tumor cell itself in breast cancer, rectal cancer, bladder cancer, and meningioma expresses CD163 and that the CD163 levels are associated with metastatic grade, early recurrence, and reduced patient survival (Kanno et al., 2013; Maniecki et al., 2012; Shabo, Olsson, Sun, & Svanvik, 2009; Shabo et al., 2008). It was found that IR-induced CD163 expression on tumor cells rendered these cells more resistant to radiotherapy (Shabo et al., 2008). Two mechanisms have been proposed to explain how tumor cells express macrophage surface markers such as CD163, which include the heterotypic cell fusion of cancer cells with TAMs or a generic molecular exchange between those cells via exosome-mediated transfer (Shabo & Svanvik, 2011). $CD163^{+}$ tumor cells are also suggested to constitute a subpopulation of cancer cells, which are associated with EMT and increased metastatic activity induced by TAMs. Upregulation of granulocyte colony-stimulating factor (G-CSF) is believed to be responsible for suppressed apoptosis and enhanced proliferation in $CD163^+$ tumor cells (Kanno et al., 2013).

CD163 was recently identified as a receptor for TNF-like weak inducer of apoptosis (TWEAK), a member of the TNF superfamily that is involved in proinflammatory responses, proangiogenesis, and tissue remodeling (Bover et al., 2007; Michaelson & Burkly, 2009; Moreno et al., 2009). In tumor cells, binding of TWEAK to its receptor FGF-inducible molecule 14 (Fn14) results in stimulation of tumor cell proliferation, migration and invasion, as well as NF-κB signaling and gene expression that promotes tumor growth, angiogenesis, and immune suppression (Cheng, Whitsett, Tran, & Winkles, 2014; Yin et al., 2014, 2013). On macrophages, TWEAK selectively binds to the scavenger receptor cysteine-rich domain of the CD163. CD163-mediated TWEAK scavenging by macrophages contributes to its degradation and sequestration in TME, which may prevent TWEAK from exerting its tumor-promoting functions, which suggests a potential antitumor benefit of TWEAK–CD163 interaction in macrophages (Bover et al., 2007).

CD163 not only exists as a membrane-bound form, but also is present as a soluble form (sCD163) in plasma and other tissue fluids. ADAM17 was shown to cleave CD163 ectodomain, thereby downregulating the surface expression of CD163 (Etzerodt, Maniecki, Moller, Moller, & Moestrup, 2010; Etzerodt et al., 2014). Intriguingly, sCD163 has the abilities to inhibit T cell proliferation (Hogger & Sorg, 2001) and to promote recognition and phagocytosis of *Staphylococcus aureus* (Kneidl et al., 2012). Circulating sCD163 level has been suggested to be a prognostic biomarker for cancer patients with poor outcome and may reflect increased activity of $CD163^+$ TAMs (Andersen, Abildgaard, Maniecki, Moller, & Andersen, 2014; Jones et al., 2013; No, Moon, Kim, & Kim, 2013; Sugaya et al., 2012). The role of sCD163 in cancer is poorly understood. It is possible that sCD163 may also be involved in TAM polarization by competing for binding to Hp–Hb complexes.

2.9 Class J Scavenger Receptor

Receptor for advanced glycation endproducts (RAGE), the only member of the class J SR group, also belongs to the immunoglobulin (IgG) superfamily. RAGE has a broad spectrum of ligands, including advanced glycation endproducts, prototype of high mobility group (HMGB) family proteins (e.g., HMGB1, amphoterin), glycosaminoglycan, amyloid A peptides, members of the S100/calgranulin protein family, collagen I and IV, β-amyloid, integrin Mac-1, and complement C3 (Yamagishi, Matsui, & Fukami, 2015). Among six isoforms of RAGE mRNA splicing variants identified so far (Hudson, Carter, et al., 2008), only two functionally relevant isoforms have been well studied. These include a full-transmembrane form, which can initiate signaling through its intracellular domain, and a truncated, endogenous secretory form of RAGE (esRAGE), which can function as a decoy receptor (Cheng et al., 2005). The ectodomain of RAGE can be proteolytically cleaved off by MMP9 and/or ADAM-10 to generate another soluble form of RAGE (sRAGE) with the similar decoy activity (Allmen, Koch, Fritz, & Legler, 2008; Raucci et al., 2008). Reduced or silenced esRAGE expression has been found in nonsmall cell lung carcinoma patients with significantly lower survival rate (Kobayashi et al., 2007). A meta-analysis of cancer patients, including breast, pancreatic, liver, lung, and colorectal cancers, showed that sRAGE level was inversely associated with the significant risk of cancer, indicating a protective role of circulating sRAGE in the development of cancer (He, Zhang, et al., 2014).

More than 30 gene polymorphisms in *RAGE* have been identified in multiple cancers, including renal caner, oral cancer, breast cancer, colorectal cancer, lung cancer, ovarian cancer, pancreatic cancer, nasopharyngeal carcinoma, and gastric cancer (Cheng et al., 2005; Chocholaty et al., 2014; Gu et al., 2008; Krechler et al., 2010; Pan et al., 2013; Qian, Sun, Zhang, Ke, & Zhu, 2014; Su, Chien, Lin, Chen, & Yang, 2015; Zhang et al., 2013; Zhou, Deng, Li, Yin, & Ye, 2014). A comprehensive meta-analysis suggested that the 82G/S polymorphism (3374 cancer cases vs. 3757 controls) in the *RAGE* promoter region is associated with a significantly increased risk of cancer, where −374T/A polymorphism (2936 cancer cases vs. 3,338 control) is associated with a reduced risk of cancer (Xia et al., 2015). Therefore, the polymorphisms of *RAGE* may be used as a potential marker for early screening or diagnosis of certain types of cancers.

Co-overexpression of RAGE and its ligands are commonly found in many types of cancer and are associated with cancer progression and poor outcome (Moser et al., 2014; Yamagishi et al., 2015; Zhao et al., 2014). Accumulating evidence suggests that the multiligand-RAGE axis plays crucial roles in tumorigenesis, e.g., enhancing tumor angiogenesis and hypoxia resistance, promoting tumor cell proliferation and invasion, orchestrating the immunosuppressive TME (Chen et al., 2014; Kang et al., 2014; Nasser et al., 2015). An array of signaling pathways have been linked with the tumor-promoting activities of RAGE, including the activation of

MAPKs, PI3K/Akt, NF-κB, Jak/STAT, Src kinase, and Rho GTPases Diaphanous-1 (Dukic-Stefanovic, Gasic-Milenkovic, Deuther-Conrad, & Munch, 2003; Hofmann et al., 1999; Hudson, Kalea, et al., 2008; Kim et al., 2008; Palumbo et al., 2009; Reddy et al., 2006; Toure et al., 2008). Both Erk1 and Erk2 have been identified as direct RAGE-binding partners (Ishihara, Tsutsumi, Kawane, Nakajima, & Kasaoka, 2003). HMGB1, S100A4, S100A7-mediated RAGE-Erk1/2 activation were shown to inhibit tumor cell autophagy and apoptosis, promote tumor cell proliferation, increase cell mobility and invasiveness (Dahlmann et al., 2014; Nasser et al., 2015; Yamagishi et al., 2015; Zhang, Wu, Zhang, Han, & Lin, 2015). HMGB1 interaction with RAGE were also reported to provoke the proliferation of lung cancer cells and inhibit their apoptosis by regulating Bax and Bcl-2 levels through PI3K/Akt signaling pathway (Xu et al., 2014). In oncogene *Kras* mutation-driven pancreatic cancer, hypoxia induced RAGE expression in an NF-κB-dependent but HIF-1α-independent manner. Consequently, overexpressed RAGE directly interacted with KRAS, further sustaining KRAS downstream signaling pathways (Raf-Mek-Erk and PI3K-Akt) and driving tumor progression (Kang et al., 2014).

In studies that evaluated the functional significance of RAGE in cancer development, it was shown that RAGE-deficient mice displayed reduced tumor growth, metastasis, and tumor vascularization, as well as decreased infiltration of M2 TAMs and tumor-associated inflammation (Medrek et al., 2012). In both mouse glioma and breast cancer models, systemic blockade of RAGE by administration of RAGE-neutralizing antibodies or soluble RAGE resulted in profound inhibition of tumor growth and metastasis (Chen et al., 2014; Nasser et al., 2015). However, an antitumor effect of RAGE was recently reported in embryonal rhabdomyosarcoma (ERMS) (Chiappalupi, Riuzzi, Fulle, Donato, & Sorci, 2014). RAGE is expressed in muscle tissue during embryonic development and can maintain myogenesis via a Cdc42-Rac1-MKK6-p38-dependent and myogenin-dependent repression of Pax7, a critical transcription factor for self-renewal and biogenesis of muscle satellite cells (Riuzzi, Sorci, Sagheddu, & Donato, 2012). Highly expressed Pax7 was found to promote the migration and invasiveness of ERMS cells and in turn cause reduction of RAGE. Overexpression of RAGE in human ERMS cells can downregulate Pax7 and reduce metastasis. Additional studies are needed to define the distinct effects of RAGE on cancers of different types, which should be considered during the design of RAGE-targeted antitumor therapeutics.

3. SCAVENGER RECEPTORS IN CANCER THERAPY

3.1 Scavenger Receptor-Based Delivery of Antineoplastic Drugs

To date, systemic delivery of anticancer therapeutics to targeted cancer cells and tissues remains a major challenge. Barriers to effective targeted drug delivery include systemic toxicity or side effects, poor solubility and biostability, and high entrapment and first-pass metabolism by the liver. Recently, a variety of biomimetic lipoprotein nanoparticles carrying therapeutic agents to target cancer cells that highly express certain scavenger receptors have been tested in preclinical applications. HDL consists of apolipoproteins A–I and lipophilic components (e.g., cholesteryl ester, cholesterol, and phospholipids). HDL-based nanoparticles (8–11 nm in diameter) are ideal drug carriers because their shielded hydrophobic core is suitable for accommodating lipophilic drugs. These nanoparticles may be selectively targeted to tumor cells based on the expression of their high-affinity receptor SR-BI (Ng, Lovell, & Zheng, 2011). HDL particles are completely biodegradable and do not trigger any immune response, since all components of HDL are considered self and already present in the human body. Due to their small size, these nanoparticles can easily escape the removal by the reticuloendothelial system. Importantly, the overexpression of the major HDL receptor SR-BI on cancer cells potentiates the binding and uptake of HDL-CE, a nutrient for rapid dividing tumor cells (Ng et al., 2011).

HDL can capture exogenous and endogenous circulating microRNA (miRNA) and deliver them to SR-BI$^+$ target cells to induce differential gene expression (Vickers, Palmisano, Shoucri, Shamburek, & Remaley, 2011). Therefore, recombinant HDL has been exploited to deliver siRNA that targets key molecules involved in cancer growth and metastasis. RNAi-HDL nanoparticles that directly deliver siRNA for VEGF or VEGFR2 to SR-BI-overexpressed tumor endothelial cells strongly inhibit neovascularization and tumor growth in mice established with orthotopic Lewis lung or MCF-7 breast cancer (Ding et al., 2014; Tripathy, Vinokour, McMahon, Volpert, & Thaxton, 2014). RNAi-HDL nanoparticle targeting signal transducer and activator transcription 3 (STAT3) or FAK resulted in the suppression of ovarian and colorectal cancers (Shahzad et al., 2011). Recombinant HDL nanoparticles have also been used to deliver chemotherapeutic drugs, e.g., paclitaxel or α-tocopheryl-succinate, to SR-BI$^+$ cancers (Hrzenjak et al., 2004; Mooberry et al.,

2010; Shin et al., 2012). It was recently reported that a highly biocompatible HDL-mimicking peptide-phospholipid scaffold nanocarrier not only can serve as a cargo to deliver therapeutic drugs to SR-BI^{+} nasopharyngeal carcinoma but also can exert direct antitumor efficacy *in vivo* (Zheng et al., 2013).

SR-A has also been suggested as a targeting molecule for nanoparticle-based drug delivery. SR-A can efficiently mediate opsonin-independent internalization of dextran-coated superparamagnetic iron oxide (SPIO) nanoparticles via its positively charged extracellular collagenous domain (Chao et al., 2013, 2012). SPIO-based delivery platform may be used for early detection of metastases in cancer patients or used as a carrier to deliver chemotherapeutics into tumors (Chiang, Tseng, Liao, & Chen, 2015; Jafari et al., 2015). SR-A was shown to specifically express on the immunosuppressive vascular leukocytes (VCLs) in mouse and human ovarian cancer. Administration of toxin-conjugated anti-SR-A antibodies to mice with peritoneal ovarian tumors resulted in selective depletion of these SR-A-expressing cell population and effectively reduced tumor burden and ascites accumulation (Bak, Walters, Takeya, Conejo-Garcia, & Berwin, 2007).

3.2 Scavenger Receptors and Immune Modulation Therapy

Given the immunosuppressive activity of SR-A in vaccination-generated antitumor response, manipulation of SR-A expression or blockade of SR-A function is expected to enhance the potency of cancer vaccines. Large stress/HSP, such as Hsp110 and Grp170, when complexed with tumor antigen (e.g., Gp100) have demonstrated superior antitumor efficacy primarily through enhancing antigen cross-presentation and activation of tumor-specific CTLs (Wang, Chang, et al., 2013; Wang et al., 2007; Wang & Subjeck, 2013; Wang et al., 2010). The promising preclinical results of this recombinant chaperone vaccine (i.e., Hsp110-gp100) have led to an ongoing Phase I melanoma clinical trial at Roswell Park Cancer Institute. Due to the presence of various HSP-binding receptors on APCs, including scavenger receptors, these HSP-based vaccines are believed to selectively target endogenous DCs. Hence, downregulation of SR-A in DCs may be used in conjunction with HSP vaccines for improved antitumor immunity (Qian et al., 2011). We recently evaluated the feasibility of reducing SR-A expression levels to enhance the potency of DC-based vaccine in preclinical cancer models (Yi et al., 2011; Yu & Wang, 2012). We demonstrated that lentivirus-mediated delivery of a short hairpin RNA (shRNA) for SR-A resulted in efficient downregulation of SR-A in DCs. SR-A-silenced DCs carrying tumor antigen gp100 were much more immunogenic than mock-modified DCs in provoking an antigen-specific $CD8^+$ CTL response. Tumor-specific CTLs elicited by SR-A-silenced DC-gp100 vaccine exhibited increased effector functions (e.g., cytokine production and tumoricidal activity), which markedly inhibited established melanoma and metastases (Yi et al., 2011). In the setting of combined radiotherapy and *in situ* DC vaccine therapy, we showed that intratumoral administration of unmodified DCs failed to synergize with radiotherapy (Guo, Yi, Yu, Zuo, et al., 2012). However, administration of SR-A-silenced DCs, when combined with local radiotherapy, profoundly suppressed mouse prostate cancers (e.g., RM1 and TRAMP-C2) and distant metastases, and prolonged the lifespan of tumor-bearing animals, which depended on $CD8^+$ cells and IFN-γ (Guo, Yi, Yu, Zuo, et al., 2012). Therefore, these studies provide preclinical evidence supporting the principle of silencing SR-A in DCs as a means to break tolerance against tumor-associated antigens.

In addition to the genetic approach for downregulating SR-A expression, small molecule inhibitors (SMIs) may also be exploited for potential therapeutic benefits. Sennoside B, a small molecule from screening of bioactive SMI libraries, was reported to effectively reduce SR-A-mediated antigen transfer and inhibit T cell proliferation *in vitro* and *in vivo* (Raycroft, Harvey, Bruck, & Mamula, 2012). However, the effect of this compound on vaccine-induced antitumor immunity has not been examined. An apolipoprotein A–I mimetic peptide, which can compete with a range of SR-A ligands, was shown to block SR-A-mediated adhesion (Navab, Anantharamaiah, Reddy, Van Lenten, & Fogelman, 2008) and inhibit tumor growth and metastasis in mice-bearing ovarian and pancreatic cancers (Neyen et al., 2013).

It has been well established that DCs function as the essential link between the innate and adaptive arms of the immune system (Todt et al., 2008). Various vaccination and immunotherapeutic strategies aim to target DCs because of their pivotal role in adaptive immunity (Guo, Manjili, et al., 2013). While our studies provide a rationale for selectively blocking immunosuppressive SR-A to improve DC-based cancer vaccines, other scavenger receptors on DCs provide an opportunity to target antigens preferentially to DCs for processing and presentation. Anti-Dectin-1/2 antibodies conjugated to OVA antigen induced significant expansion of T cells in the draining lymph nodes of mice and IFN-γ production by T cells (Carter, Thompson, Reid, Wong, & Tough, 2006a, 2006b). In addition, β1,3-d-glucan conjugated to OVA, which can be rapidly phagocytosed by DCs possibly via Dectin-1/2, provoked DC maturation and stimulated >100-fold more efficiently OVA-specific OT-I and OT-II T cells (Huang, Ostroff, Lee, Specht, & Levitz, 2010), suggesting that antigen targeted to Dectin-1/2 on DCs may facilitate efficient antigen capture and concurrently induce DC activation. Anti-LOX-1 antibodies have also been successfully to target antigens to DCs to induce antigen-specific CTL response (Li et al., 2012) and antitumor immunity (Delneste et al., 2002), indicating that scavenger receptor targeting of tumor antigens is a promising strategy for cancer immunotherapy.

4. CONCLUDING REMARKS

The large repertoire of ligands recognized by scavenger receptors defines their broad range of functions in many physiologic and pathologic conditions, e.g., lipid metabolism, tissue homeostasis, inflammation, atherosclerosis, and autoimmune disorders. Recently, these innate PRRs are emerging as important regulators of tumorigenesis, cancer invasion, and the antitumor immune response (Table 1). However, the extent and the mechanism of their involvement in cancer biology and immunology have not yet been fully appreciated because research focused on these scavenger receptors in these areas is in its infancy. The overexpression of certain SRs (e.g., SR-A, CD163) on TAMs and their use as cancer diagnostic or prognosis markers strongly suggest their potential involvement in the functional regulation of TAMs during tumor progression, including tumor cell proliferation and mobility, tumor angiogenesis, and immune suppression. However, the molecular underpinnings of the distinct actions of specific scavenger receptors in these processes are largely unknown. The recent discovery of the immunosuppressive activity of SR-A in vaccination-induced T cell activation and antitumor immune response was striking, given its established role in DC-mediated capture of immunostimulatory HSPs and associated tumor antigens. Our proof-of-principle studies demonstrated the feasibility of SR-A blockade to improve the antitumor efficacy of DC vaccines. In contrast, antigen targeting to certain scavenger receptors, such as LOX-1, may lead to enhanced T cell response and tumor eradication, further stressing the functional versatility and complexity of these scavenger receptors. More work is needed to determine the relative contribution of

Table 1 Diverse Functions of Scavenger Receptors in Cancer

Name	Family	Expression	Roles	References
SR-A	Class A	Myeloid cells and LSEC	Inhibition of NO, IFN-β and IFN-γ production by TAMs	Komohara et al. (2009) Neyen et al. (2013)
			Required for tumor cell invasion	Wang et al. (2007), Yi et al. (2009), Yi et al. (2011), Guo, Yi, Yu, Hu, et al. (2012), and Guo, Yi, Yu, Zuo, et al. (2012)
			Inhibits DC activation and antigen cross-presentation	
			Induction of tolerogenic DCs	Herber et al. (2010)
			Regulation of tumor angiogenesis	Ben et al. (2012)
			Suppression of leukemia stem cells	Chen et al. (2011)
MARCO	Class A	Myeloid cells	Modulation of DC-based cancer vaccine	Matsushita et al. (2010) and Komine et al. (2013)
SCARA3	Class A	Ubiquitous expression	Tumor suppressor gene in prostate cancer	Yu et al. (2006)
			Multiple myeloma therapeutic resistance	Brown et al. (2013)
SCARA5	Class A	Selected ECs	Inhibition of tumorigenesis and metastasis	Huang, Zheng, et al. (2010)
			Tumor suppressor gene	Liu et al. (2013) and Yan et al. (2012)
CD36	Class B	Phagocytic cells and ECs	Inhibition of tumor angiogenesis	Jimenez et al. (2000), Simantov et al. (2005), Volpert et al. (2002)
			Biomarkers	DeFilippis et al. (2012), Hale et al. (2014), Rachidi et al. (2013), and Uray et al. (2004)

SR-BI	Class B	Ubiquitous expression	Protection of tumor cells from apoptosis Mediates invasiveness of breast cancer Required for prostate cancer tumor development	Cao et al. (2004) Danilo et al. (2013) Leon et al. (2010) and Twiddy et al. (2012)
CD68	Class D	Macrophages, DCs, and osteoclast	Biomarkers	Jezequel et al. (2012), Leek et al. (1996), Mahmoud et al. (2012), and Nabeshima et al. (2015)
LOX-1	Class E	ECs, smooth muscle cells, macrophages, and neutrophils	Participation in cancer cell transformation Activation of NF-κB-dependent tumorigenic pathway Cross-presentation of HSP-associated antigen	Hirsch et al. (2010) Khaidakov et al. (2011) Delneste et al. (2002)
Dectin-1	Class E	Myeloid cells, B cells, and monocytes	Induction of CTLs Contributes to tumoricidal activity of NK cells	Leibundgut-Landmann et al. (2008) Chiba et al. (2014)
SREC-I	Class F	Myeloid cells and ECs	Cross-presentation of HSP-associated antigen	Gong et al. (2009)
SR-PSOX/CXCL16	Class G	Myeloid cells, B cells, monocytes, LSECs, and some tumor cells	sCXCL16 facilitates tumor progression TM-CXCL16 inhibits tumorigenesis Biomarkers	Chaturvedi et al. (2014), Jung et al. (2013), Lu et al. (2008), Shimaoka et al. (2003), Xing et al. (2012) and Wang et al. (2008) Fang et al. (2014) Gooden et al. (2014), Hattermann et al. (2013), Huang et al. (2013), Na et al. (2014), and Wente et al. (2008)

Continued

Table 1 Diverse Functions of Scavenger Receptors in Cancer—cont'd

Name	Family	Expression	Roles	References
Stabilin-1	Class H	Macrophage, lymphatic, and sinusoidal ECs	Scavenging circulating SPARC Recruitment of Tregs Cancer immune evasion and metastasis	Nagaraju et al. (2014) Shetty et al. (2011) Karikoski et al. (2014)
Stabilin-2	Class H	Macrophage, lymphatic, and sinusoidal ECs	Scavenging circulating HA Biomarkers	Sironen et al. (2011) Geraud et al. (2013) and Neuhaus et al. (2013)
CD163	Class I	Monocytes, macrophages, and some tumor cells	Promoting immunosuppressive TME Scavenging circulating TWEAK Biomarkers	Sierra-Filardi et al. (2010) Bover et al. (2007) Andersen et al. (2014), Edin et al. (2012), Fujimura et al. (2013), Garcia et al. (2008) and He, Bao, et al. (2014)
RAGE	Class J	Myeloid cells, neutrophils, and T and B lymphocytes	Promoting tumorigenesis Biomarkers	Chen et al. (2014), Kang et al. (2014), Nasser et al. (2015), Wang, Chang, et al. (2013), and Xu et al. (2014) Kang et al. (2014), Kobayashi et al. (2007), and He, Zhang, et al. (2014)

CTL, cytotoxic T lymphocyte; DC, dendritic cell; EC, endothelial cells; HA, hyaluronan; HSP, heat shock protein; IFN-β, interferon-β; LOX-1, lectin-like oxidized low-density lipoprotein (LDL) receptor-1; LSEC, liver sinusoidal endothelial cells; MARCO, macrophage receptor with collagenous structure; NK, natural killer; NO, nitric oxide; RAGE, receptor for advanced glycation endproducts; SR-A, scavenger receptor class A; SREC-I, scavenger receptor expressed by endothelial cell-I; SR-PSOX, scavenger receptor for phosphatidylserine and oxidized lipoprotein; SCARA3, scavenger receptor class A member 3; SPARC, secreted protein acidic and rich in cysteine; TAM, tumor-associated macrophages; TM-CXCL16, transmembrane form of CXC chemokine ligand 16; TME, tumor microenvironment, TWEAK, TNF-like weak inducer of apoptosis; Treg, regulatory T cell.

scavenger receptors to the functional activation of APCs and resultant antitumor immunity. Furthermore, additional studies are necessary to elucidate the molecular basis of how the ligand-specific interaction and various coreceptors may dictate or influence the outcome of engaging these scavenger receptors in homeostatic state and pathological settings. A better understating of the immunobiology of scavenger receptors will facilitate the development of rational approaches to target functionally distinct receptors for drug delivery, diagnostic imaging, antigen capture and processing, and antagonizing immune suppression, which are expected to lead to improved outcomes in cancer treatment.

ACKNOWLEDGMENTS

The present study was supported in part by National Institutes of Health (NIH) Grants CA175033, CA154708, CA099326, Department of Defense (DOD) W81XWH-11-1-0481, W81XWH-13-1-0162, the National Foundation for Cancer Research and NCI Cancer Center Support Grant to VCU Massey Cancer Center P30CA16059. X-Y.W. is the Harrison Endowed Scholar in Cancer Research in the VCU Massey Cancer Center. P.B.F. holds the Thelma Newmeyer Corman Chair in Cancer Research in the VCU Massey Cancer Center.

Competing Interests: None declared.

REFERENCES

Abel, S., Hundhausen, C., Mentlein, R., Schulte, A., Berkhout, T. A., Broadway, N., et al. (2004). The transmembrane CXC-chemokine ligand 16 is induced by IFN-gamma and TNF-alpha and shed by the activity of the disintegrin-like metalloproteinase ADAM10. *Journal of Immunology*, *172*, 6362–6372.

Adachi, H., & Tsujimoto, M. (2002). FEEL-1, a novel scavenger receptor with in vitro bacteria-binding and angiogenesis-modulating activities. *The Journal of Biological Chemistry*, *277*, 34264–34270.

Adachi, H., Tsujimoto, M., Arai, H., & Inoue, K. (1997). Expression cloning of a novel scavenger receptor from human endothelial cells. *The Journal of Biological Chemistry*, *272*, 31217–31220.

Agrawal, S., Gupta, S., & Agrawal, A. (2010). Human dendritic cells activated via dectin-1 are efficient at priming Th17, cytotoxic CD8 T and B cell responses. *PLoS One*, *5*, e13418.

Aleem, E. (2013). beta-Glucans and their applications in cancer therapy: Focus on human studies. *Anti-Cancer Agents in Medicinal Chemistry*, *13*, 709–719.

Allmen, E. U., Koch, M., Fritz, G., & Legler, D. F. (2008). V domain of RAGE interacts with AGEs on prostate carcinoma cells. *Prostate*, *68*, 748–758.

Ambarus, C. A., Krausz, S., van Eijk, M., Hamann, J., Radstake, T. R., Reedquist, K. A., et al. (2012). Systematic validation of specific phenotypic markers for in vitro polarized human macrophages. *Journal of Immunological Methods*, *375*, 196–206.

Andersen, M. N., Abildgaard, N., Maniecki, M. B., Moller, H. J., & Andersen, N. F. (2014). Monocyte/macrophage-derived soluble CD163: A novel biomarker in multiple myeloma. *European Journal of Haematology*, *93*, 41–47.

Angin, Y., Steinbusch, L. K., Simons, P. J., Greulich, S., Hoebers, N. T., Douma, K., et al. (2012). CD36 inhibition prevents lipid accumulation and contractile dysfunction in rat cardiomyocytes. *The Biochemical Journal*, *448*, 43–53.

Armengol, C., Bartoli, R., Sanjurjo, L., Serra, I., Amezaga, N., Sala, M., et al. (2013). Role of scavenger receptors in the pathophysiology of chronic liver diseases. *Critical Reviews in Immunology*, *33*, 57–96.

Asch, A. S., Barnwell, J., Silverstein, R. L., & Nachman, R. L. (1987). Isolation of the thrombospondin membrane receptor. *The Journal of Clinical Investigation*, *79*, 1054–1061.

Bacigalupo, M. L., Manzi, M., Espelt, M. V., Gentilini, L. D., Compagno, D., Laderach, D. J., et al. (2014). Galectin-1 triggers epithelial-mesenchymal transition in human hepatocellular carcinoma cells. *Journal of Cellular Physiology*, *230*, 1298–1309.

Bak, S. P., Walters, J. J., Takeya, M., Conejo-Garcia, J. R., & Berwin, B. L. (2007). Scavenger receptor-A-targeted leukocyte depletion inhibits peritoneal ovarian tumor progression. *Cancer Research*, *67*, 4783–4789.

Baldridge, J. R., McGowan, P., Evans, J. T., Cluff, C., Mossman, S., Johnson, D., et al. (2004). Taking a Toll on human disease: Toll-like receptor 4 agonists as vaccine adjuvants and monotherapeutic agents. *Expert Opinion on Biological Therapy*, *4*, 1129–1138.

Balermpas, P., Rodel, F., Liberz, R., Oppermann, J., Wagenblast, J., Ghanaati, S., et al. (2014). Head and neck cancer relapse after chemoradiotherapy correlates with CD163+ macrophages in primary tumour and CD11b+ myeloid cells in recurrences. *British Journal of Cancer*, *111*, 1509–1518.

Banchereau, J., & Steinman, R. M. (1998). Dendritic cells and the control of immunity. *Nature*, *392*, 245–252.

Beauvillain, C., Meloni, F., Sirard, J. C., Blanchard, S., Jarry, U., Scotet, M., et al. (2010). The scavenger receptors SRA-1 and SREC-I cooperate with TLR2 in the recognition of the hepatitis C virus non-structural protein 3 by dendritic cells. *Journal of Hepatology*, *52*, 644–651.

Becker, M., Cotena, A., Gordon, S., & Platt, N. (2006). Expression of the class A macrophage scavenger receptor on specific subpopulations of murine dendritic cells limits their endotoxin response. *European Journal of Immunology*, *36*, 950–960.

Ben, J., Jin, G., Zhang, Y., Ma, B., Bai, H., Chen, J., et al. (2012). Class A scavenger receptor deficiency exacerbates lung tumorigenesis by cultivating a procarcinogenic microenvironment in humans and mice. *American Journal of Respiratory and Critical Care Medicine*, *186*, 763–772.

Berwin, B., Delneste, Y., Lovingood, R. V., Post, S. R., & Pizzo, S. V. (2004). SREC-I, a type F scavenger receptor, is an endocytic receptor for calreticulin. *The Journal of Biological Chemistry*, *279*, 51250–51257.

Berwin, B., Hart, J. P., Rice, S., Gass, C., Pizzo, S. V., Post, S. R., et al. (2003). Scavenger receptor-A mediates gp96/GRP94 and calreticulin internalization by antigen-presenting cells. *The EMBO Journal*, *22*, 6127–6136.

Bock, A. J., Nymoen, D. A., Brenne, K., Kaern, J., & Davidson, B. (2012). SCARA3 mRNA is overexpressed in ovarian carcinoma compared with breast carcinoma effusions. *Human Pathology*, *43*, 669–674.

Bover, L. C., Cardo-Vila, M., Kuniyasu, A., Sun, J., Rangel, R., Takeya, M., et al. (2007). A previously unrecognized protein-protein interaction between TWEAK and CD163: Potential biological implications. *Journal of Immunology*, *178*, 8183–8194.

Brown, C. O., Schibler, J., Fitzgerald, M. P., Singh, N., Salem, K., Zhan, F., et al. (2013). Scavenger receptor class A member 3 (SCARA3) in disease progression and therapy resistance in multiple myeloma. *Leukemia Research*, *37*, 963–969.

Buechler, C., Ritter, M., Orso, E., Langmann, T., Klucken, J., & Schmitz, G. (2000). Regulation of scavenger receptor CD163 expression in human monocytes and macrophages by pro- and antiinflammatory stimuli. *Journal of Leukocyte Biology*, *67*, 97–103.

Canton, J., Neculai, D., & Grinstein, S. (2013). Scavenger receptors in homeostasis and immunity. *Nature Reviews. Immunology, 13*, 621–634.

Cao, W. M., Murao, K., Imachi, H., Yu, X., Abe, H., Yamauchi, A., et al. (2004). A mutant high-density lipoprotein receptor inhibits proliferation of human breast cancer cells. *Cancer Research, 64*, 1515–1521.

Carter, R. W., Thompson, C., Reid, D. M., Wong, S. Y., & Tough, D. F. (2006a). Induction of CD8+ T cell responses through targeting of antigen to Dectin-2. *Cellular Immunology, 239*, 87–91.

Carter, R. W., Thompson, C., Reid, D. M., Wong, S. Y., & Tough, D. F. (2006b). Preferential induction of CD4+ T cell responses through in vivo targeting of antigen to dendritic cell-associated C-type lectin-1. *Journal of Immunology, 177*, 2276–2284.

Caruso, C., Balistreri, C. R., Candore, G., Carruba, G., Colonna-Romano, G., Di Bona, D., et al. (2009). Polymorphisms of pro-inflammatory genes and prostate cancer risk: A pharmacogenomic approach. *Cancer Immunology, Immunotherapy, 58*, 1919–1933.

Chao, Y., Karmali, P. P., Mukthavaram, R., Kesari, S., Kouznetsova, V. L., Tsigelny, I. F., et al. (2013). Direct recognition of superparamagnetic nanocrystals by macrophage scavenger receptor SR-AI. *ACS Nano, 7*, 4289–4298.

Chao, Y., Makale, M., Karmali, P. P., Sharikov, Y., Tsigelny, I., Merkulov, S., et al. (2012). Recognition of dextran-superparamagnetic iron oxide nanoparticle conjugates (Feridex) via macrophage scavenger receptor charged domains. *Bioconjugate Chemistry, 23*, 1003–1009.

Chaturvedi, P., Gilkes, D. M., Takano, N., & Semenza, G. L. (2014). Hypoxia-inducible factor-dependent signaling between triple-negative breast cancer cells and mesenchymal stem cells promotes macrophage recruitment. *Proceedings of the National Academy of Sciences of the United States of America, 111*, E2120–E2129.

Chen, Y., Sullivan, C., Peng, C., Shan, Y., Hu, Y., Li, D., et al. (2011). A tumor suppressor function of the Msr1 gene in leukemia stem cells of chronic myeloid leukemia. *Blood, 118*, 390–400.

Chen, X., Zhang, L., Zhang, I. Y., Liang, J., Wang, H., Ouyang, M., et al. (2014). RAGE expression in tumor-associated macrophages promotes angiogenesis in glioma. *Cancer Research, 74*, 7285–7297.

Cheng, C., Tsuneyama, K., Kominami, R., Shinohara, H., Sakurai, S., Yonekura, H., et al. (2005). Expression profiling of endogenous secretory receptor for advanced glycation end products in human organs. *Modern Pathology, 18*, 1385–1396.

Cheng, E., Whitsett, T. G., Tran, N. L., & Winkles, J. A. (2014). The TWEAK receptor Fn14 is a Src-inducible protein and a positive regulator of Src-driven cell invasion. *Molecular Cancer Research, 13*, 575–583.

Chiang, C. S., Tseng, Y. H., Liao, B. J., & Chen, S. Y. (2015). Magnetically targeted nanocapsules for PAA-cisplatin-conjugated cores in PVA/SPIO shells via surfactant-free emulsion for reduced nephrotoxicity and enhanced lung cancer therapy. *Advanced Healthcare Materials, 4*, 1066–1075. http://dx.doi.org/10.1002/adhm.201400794.

Chiappalupi, S., Riuzzi, F., Fulle, S., Donato, R., & Sorci, G. (2014). Defective RAGE activity in embryonal rhabdomyosarcoma cells results in high PAX7 levels that sustain migration and invasiveness. *Carcinogenesis, 35*, 2382–2392.

Chiba, S., Ikushima, H., Ueki, H., Yanai, H., Kimura, Y., Hangai, S., et al. (2014). Recognition of tumor cells by Dectin-1 orchestrates innate immune cells for anti-tumor responses. *eLife, 3*, e04177.

Chocholaty, M., Jachymova, M., Schmidt, M., Havlova, K., Krepelova, A., Zima, T., et al. (2014). Polymorphisms of the receptor for advanced glycation end-products and glyoxalase I in patients with renal cancer. *Tumour Biology, 36*, 2121–2126.

Coburn, C. T., Knapp, F. F., Jr., Febbraio, M., Beets, A. L., Silverstein, R. L., & Abumrad, N. A. (2000). Defective uptake and utilization of long chain fatty acids in

muscle and adipose tissues of CD36 knockout mice. *The Journal of Biological Chemistry*, *275*, 32523–32529.
Cruz, P. M., Mo, H., McConathy, W. J., Sabnis, N., & Lacko, A. G. (2013). The role of cholesterol metabolism and cholesterol transport in carcinogenesis: A review of scientific findings, relevant to future cancer therapeutics. *Frontiers in Pharmacology*, *4*, 119.
Dahlmann, M., Okhrimenko, A., Marcinkowski, P., Osterland, M., Herrmann, P., Smith, J., et al. (2014). RAGE mediates S100A4-induced cell motility via MAPK/ERK and hypoxia signaling and is a prognostic biomarker for human colorectal cancer metastasis. *Oncotarget*, *5*, 3220–3233.
Danilo, C., Gutierrez-Pajares, J. L., Mainieri, M. A., Mercier, I., Lisanti, M. P., & Frank, P. G. (2013). Scavenger receptor class B type I regulates cellular cholesterol metabolism and cell signaling associated with breast cancer development. *Breast Cancer Research*, *15*, R87.
Darash-Yahana, M., Gillespie, J. W., Hewitt, S. M., Chen, Y. Y., Maeda, S., Stein, I., et al. (2009). The chemokine CXCL16 and its receptor, CXCR6, as markers and promoters of inflammation-associated cancers. *PLoS One*, *4*, e6695.
David, C., Nance, J. P., Hubbard, J., Hsu, M., Binder, D., & Wilson, E. H. (2012). Stabilin-1 expression in tumor associated macrophages. *Brain Research*, *1481*, 71–78.
DeFilippis, R. A., Chang, H., Dumont, N., Rabban, J. T., Chen, Y. Y., Fontenay, G. V., et al. (2012). CD36 repression activates a multicellular stromal program shared by high mammographic density and tumor tissues. *Cancer Discovery*, *2*, 826–839.
Delneste, Y., Magistrelli, G., Gauchat, J., Haeuw, J., Aubry, J., Nakamura, K., et al. (2002). Involvement of LOX-1 in dendritic cell-mediated antigen cross-presentation. *Immunity*, *17*, 353–362.
Ding, Y., Wang, Y., Zhou, J., Gu, X., Wang, W., Liu, C., et al. (2014). Direct cytosolic siRNA delivery by reconstituted high density lipoprotein for target-specific therapy of tumor angiogenesis. *Biomaterials*, *35*, 7214–7227.
Drover, V. A., Nguyen, D. V., Bastie, C. C., Darlington, Y. F., Abumrad, N. A., Pessin, J. E., et al. (2008). CD36 mediates both cellular uptake of very long chain fatty acids and their intestinal absorption in mice. *The Journal of Biological Chemistry*, *283*, 13108–13115.
Dukic-Stefanovic, S., Gasic-Milenkovic, J., Deuther-Conrad, W., & Munch, G. (2003). Signal transduction pathways in mouse microglia N-11 cells activated by advanced glycation endproducts (AGEs). *Journal of Neurochemistry*, *87*, 44–55.
Dunn, S., Vohra, R. S., Murphy, J. E., Homer-Vanniasinkam, S., Walker, J. H., & Ponnambalam, S. (2008). The lectin-like oxidized low-density-lipoprotein receptor: A pro-inflammatory factor in vascular disease. *The Biochemical Journal*, *409*, 349–355.
Edin, S., Wikberg, M. L., Dahlin, A. M., Rutegard, J., Oberg, A., Oldenborg, P. A., et al. (2012). The distribution of macrophages with a M1 or M2 phenotype in relation to prognosis and the molecular characteristics of colorectal cancer. *PLoS One*, *7*, e47045.
El Khoury, J., Hickman, S. E., Thomas, C. A., Cao, L., Silverstein, S. C., & Loike, J. D. (1996). Scavenger receptor-mediated adhesion of microglia to beta-amyloid fibrils. *Nature*, *382*, 716–719.
El Khoury, J. B., Moore, K. J., Means, T. K., Leung, J., Terada, K., Toft, M., et al. (2003). CD36 mediates the innate host response to beta-amyloid. *The Journal of Experimental Medicine*, *197*, 1657–1666.
Elomaa, O., Kangas, M., Sahlberg, C., Tuukkanen, J., Sormunen, R., Liakka, A., et al. (1995). Cloning of a novel bacteria-binding receptor structurally related to scavenger receptors and expressed in a subset of macrophages. *Cell*, *80*, 603–609.
Endemann, G., Stanton, L. W., Madden, K. S., Bryant, C. M., White, R. T., & Protter, A. A. (1993). CD36 is a receptor for oxidized low density lipoprotein. *The Journal of Biological Chemistry*, *268*, 11811–11816.

Enomoto, Y., Bharti, A., Khaleque, A. A., Song, B., Liu, C., Apostolopoulos, V., et al. (2006). Enhanced immunogenicity of heat shock protein 70 peptide complexes from dendritic cell-tumor fusion cells. *Journal of Immunology, 177*, 5946–5955.

Etzerodt, A., Maniecki, M. B., Moller, K., Moller, H. J., & Moestrup, S. K. (2010). Tumor necrosis factor alpha-converting enzyme (TACE/ADAM17) mediates ectodomain shedding of the scavenger receptor CD163. *Journal of Leukocyte Biology, 88*, 1201–1205.

Etzerodt, A., Rasmussen, M. R., Svendsen, P., Chalaris, A., Schwarz, J., Galea, I., et al. (2014). Structural basis for inflammation-driven shedding of CD163 ectodomain and tumor necrosis factor-alpha in macrophages. *The Journal of Biological Chemistry, 289*, 778–788.

Facciponte, J. G., Wang, X. Y., & Subjeck, J. R. (2007). Hsp110 and Grp170, members of the Hsp70 superfamily, bind to scavenger receptor-A and scavenger receptor expressed by endothelial cells-I. *European Journal of Immunology, 37*, 2268–2279.

Fang, Y., Henderson, F. C., Jr., Yi, Q., Lei, Q., Li, Y., & Chen, N. (2014). Chemokine CXCL16 expression suppresses migration and invasiveness and induces apoptosis in breast cancer cells. *Mediators of Inflammation, 2014*, 478641.

Frenkel, D., Wilkinson, K., Zhao, L., Hickman, S. E., Means, T. K., Puckett, L., et al. (2013). Scara1 deficiency impairs clearance of soluble amyloid-beta by mononuclear phagocytes and accelerates Alzheimer's-like disease progression. *Nature Communications, 4*, 2030.

Fujimura, T., Kambayashi, Y., Furudate, S., Kakizaki, A., & Aiba, S. (2013). Immunomodulatory effect of bisphosphonate Risedronate sodium on CD163+ arginase 1+ M2 macrophages: The development of a possible supportive therapy for angiosarcoma. *Clinical & Developmental Immunology, 2013*, 325412.

Gao, Q., Zhao, Y. J., Wang, X. Y., Qiu, S. J., Shi, Y. H., Sun, J., et al. (2012). CXCR6 upregulation contributes to a proinflammatory tumor microenvironment that drives metastasis and poor patient outcomes in hepatocellular carcinoma. *Cancer Research, 72*, 3546–3556.

Garcia, C., Gardner, D., & Reichard, K. K. (2008). CD163: A specific immunohistochemical marker for acute myeloid leukemia with monocytic differentiation. *Applied Immunohistochemistry & Molecular Morphology, 16*, 417–421.

Geissmann, F., Cameron, T. O., Sidobre, S., Manlongat, N., Kronenberg, M., Briskin, M. J., et al. (2005). Intravascular immune surveillance by CXCR6+ NKT cells patrolling liver sinusoids. *PLoS Biology, 3*, e113.

Geraud, C., Mogler, C., Runge, A., Evdokimov, K., Lu, S., Schledzewski, K., et al. (2013). Endothelial transdifferentiation in hepatocellular carcinoma: Loss of Stabilin-2 expression in peri-tumorous liver correlates with increased survival. *Liver International, 33*, 1428–1440.

Goldstein, J. L., Ho, Y. K., Basu, S. K., & Brown, M. S. (1979). Binding site on macrophages that mediates uptake and degradation of acetylated low density lipoprotein, producing massive cholesterol deposition. *Proceedings of the National Academy of Sciences of the United States of America, 76*, 333–337.

Gong, J., Zhu, B., Murshid, A., Adachi, H., Song, B., Lee, A., et al. (2009). T cell activation by heat shock protein 70 vaccine requires TLR signaling and scavenger receptor expressed by endothelial cells-1. *Journal of Immunology, 183*, 3092–3098.

Gooden, M. J., Wiersma, V. R., Boerma, A., Leffers, N., Boezen, H. M., ten Hoor, K. A., et al. (2014). Elevated serum CXCL16 is an independent predictor of poor survival in ovarian cancer and may reflect pro-metastatic ADAM protease activity. *British Journal of Cancer, 110*, 1535–1544.

Gordon, S. (2002). Pattern recognition receptors: Doubling up for the innate immune response. *Cell, 111*, 927–930.

Gordon, S., & Martinez, F. O. (2010). Alternative activation of macrophages: Mechanism and functions. *Immunity*, *32*, 593–604.

Graf, G. A., Roswell, K. L., & Smart, E. J. (2001). 17beta-Estradiol promotes the up-regulation of SR-BII in HepG2 cells and in rat livers. *Journal of Lipid Research*, *42*, 1444–1449.

Graham, D. K., DeRyckere, D., Davies, K. D., & Earp, H. S. (2014). The TAM family: Phosphatidylserine sensing receptor tyrosine kinases gone awry in cancer. *Nature Reviews. Cancer*, *14*, 769–785.

Granucci, F., Petralia, F., Urbano, M., Citterio, S., Di Tota, F., Santambrogio, L., et al. (2003). The scavenger receptor MARCO mediates cytoskeleton rearrangements in dendritic cells and microglia. *Blood*, *102*, 2940–2947.

Greaves, D. R., & Gordon, S. (2009). The macrophage scavenger receptor at 30 years of age: Current knowledge and future challenges. *Journal of Lipid Research*, *50*(Suppl.), S282–S286.

Gu, H., Yang, L., Sun, Q., Zhou, B., Tang, N., Cong, R., et al. (2008). Gly82Ser polymorphism of the receptor for advanced glycation end products is associated with an increased risk of gastric cancer in a Chinese population. *Clinical Cancer Research*, *14*, 3627–3632.

Guo, C., Buranych, A., Sarkar, D., Fisher, P. B., & Wang, X. Y. (2013). The role of tumor-associated macrophages in tumor vascularization. *Vascular Cell*, *5*, 20.

Guo, L., Cui, Z. M., Zhang, J., & Huang, Y. (2011). Chemokine axes CXCL12/CXCR4 and CXCL16/CXCR6 correlate with lymph node metastasis in epithelial ovarian carcinoma. *Chinese Journal of Cancer*, *30*, 336–343.

Guo, C., Manjili, M. H., Subjeck, J. R., Sarkar, D., Fisher, P. B., & Wang, X. Y. (2013). Therapeutic cancer vaccines: Past, present, and future. *Advances in Cancer Research*, *119*, 421–475.

Guo, C., Yi, H., Yu, X., Hu, F., Zuo, D., Subjeck, J. R., et al. (2012). Absence of scavenger receptor A promotes dendritic cell-mediated cross-presentation of cell-associated antigen and antitumor immune response. *Immunology and Cell Biology*, *90*, 101–108.

Guo, C., Yi, H., Yu, X., Zuo, D., Qian, J., Yang, G., et al. (2012). In situ vaccination with CD204 gene-silenced dendritic cell, not unmodified dendritic cell, enhances radiation therapy of prostate cancer. *Molecular Cancer Therapeutics*, *11*, 2331–2341.

Gutwein, P., Schramme, A., Sinke, N., Abdel-Bakky, M. S., Voss, B., Obermuller, N., et al. (2009). Tumoural CXCL16 expression is a novel prognostic marker of longer survival times in renal cell cancer patients. *European Journal of Cancer*, *45*, 478–489.

Ha, H. K., Lee, W., Park, H. J., Lee, S. D., Lee, J. Z., & Chung, M. K. (2011). Clinical significance of CXCL16/CXCR6 expression in patients with prostate cancer. *Molecular Medicine Reports*, *4*, 419–424.

Hale, J. S., Li, M., Sinyuk, M., Jahnen-Dechent, W., Lathia, J. D., & Silverstein, R. L. (2012). Context dependent role of the CD36–thrombospondin–histidine-rich glycoprotein axis in tumor angiogenesis and growth. *PLoS One*, *7*, e40033.

Hale, J. S., Otvos, B., Sinyuk, M., Alvarado, A. G., Hitomi, M., Stoltz, K., et al. (2014). Cancer stem cell-specific scavenger receptor 36 drives glioblastoma progression. *Stem Cells*, *32*, 1746–1758.

Han, H. J., Tokino, T., & Nakamura, Y. (1998). CSR, a scavenger receptor-like protein with a protective role against cellular damage caused by UV irradiation and oxidative stress. *Human Molecular Genetics*, *7*, 1039–1046.

Harshyne, L. A., Zimmer, M. I., Watkins, S. C., & Barratt-Boyes, S. M. (2003). A role for class A scavenger receptor in dendritic cell nibbling from live cells. *Journal of Immunology*, *170*, 2302–2309.

Hattermann, K., Held-Feindt, J., Ludwig, A., & Mentlein, R. (2013). The CXCL16-CXCR6 chemokine axis in glial tumors. *Journal of Neuroimmunology*, *260*, 47–54.

He, L., Bao, H., Xue, J., Zheng, L., Zhang, Q., Sun, L., et al. (2014). Circulating soluble advanced glycation end product is inversely associated with the significant risk of developing cancer: Evidence from a meta-analysis. *Tumour Biology*, *35*, 8749–8755.

He, K. F., Zhang, L., Huang, C. F., Ma, S. R., Wang, Y. F., Wang, W. M., et al. (2014). CD163 + tumor-associated macrophages correlated with poor prognosis and cancer stem cells in oral squamous cell carcinoma. *BioMed Research International*, *2014*, 838632.

Herber, D. L., Cao, W., Nefedova, Y., Novitskiy, S. V., Nagaraj, S., Tyurin, V. A., et al. (2010). Lipid accumulation and dendritic cell dysfunction in cancer. *Nature Medicine*, *16*, 880–886.

Heydtmann, M., Lalor, P. F., Eksteen, J. A., Hubscher, S. G., Briskin, M., & Adams, D. H. (2005). CXC chemokine ligand 16 promotes integrin-mediated adhesion of liver-infiltrating lymphocytes to cholangiocytes and hepatocytes within the inflamed human liver. *Journal of Immunology*, *174*, 1055–1062.

Hirayama, S., Ishii, G., Nagai, K., Ono, S., Kojima, M., Yamauchi, C., et al. (2012). Prognostic impact of CD204-positive macrophages in lung squamous cell carcinoma: Possible contribution of Cd204-positive macrophages to the tumor-promoting microenvironment. *Journal of Thoracic Oncology*, *7*, 1790–1797.

Hirsch, H. A., Iliopoulos, D., Joshi, A., Zhang, Y., Jaeger, S. A., Bulyk, M., et al. (2010). A transcriptional signature and common gene networks link cancer with lipid metabolism and diverse human diseases. *Cancer Cell*, *17*, 348–361.

Hofmann, M. A., Drury, S., Fu, C., Qu, W., Taguchi, A., Lu, Y., et al. (1999). RAGE mediates a novel proinflammatory axis: A central cell surface receptor for S100/calgranulin polypeptides. *Cell*, *97*, 889–901.

Hogger, P., & Sorg, C. (2001). Soluble CD163 inhibits phorbol ester-induced lymphocyte proliferation. *Biochemical and Biophysical Research Communications*, *288*, 841–843.

Hojo, S., Koizumi, K., Tsuneyama, K., Arita, Y., Cui, Z., Shinohara, K., et al. (2007). High-level expression of chemokine CXCL16 by tumor cells correlates with a good prognosis and increased tumor-infiltrating lymphocytes in colorectal cancer. *Cancer Research*, *67*, 4725–4731.

Holness, C. L., & Simmons, D. L. (1993). Molecular cloning of CD68, a human macrophage marker related to lysosomal glycoproteins. *Blood*, *81*, 1607–1613.

Hou, Y. C., Chao, Y. J., Tung, H. L., Wang, H. C., & Shan, Y. S. (2014). Coexpression of CD44-positive/CD133-positive cancer stem cells and CD204-positive tumor-associated macrophages is a predictor of survival in pancreatic ductal adenocarcinoma. *Cancer*, *120*, 2766–2777.

Hrzenjak, A., Reicher, H., Wintersperger, A., Steinecker-Frohnwieser, B., Sedlmayr, P., Schmidt, H., et al. (2004). Inhibition of lung carcinoma cell growth by high density lipoprotein-associated alpha-tocopheryl-succinate. *Cellular and Molecular Life Sciences*, *61*, 1520–1531.

Hsing, A. W., Sakoda, L. C., Chen, J., Chokkalingam, A. P., Sesterhenn, I., Gao, Y. T., et al. (2007). MSR1 variants and the risks of prostate cancer and benign prostatic hyperplasia: A population-based study in China. *Carcinogenesis*, *28*, 2530–2536.

Hu, Y., Cheng, S. C., Chan, K. T., Ke, Y., Xue, B., Sin, F. W., et al. (2010). Fucoidin enhances dendritic cell-mediated T-cell cytotoxicity against NY-ESO-1 expressing human cancer cells. *Biochemical and Biophysical Research Communications*, *392*, 329–334.

Huang, H., Ostroff, G. R., Lee, C. K., Specht, C. A., & Levitz, S. M. (2010). Robust stimulation of humoral and cellular immune responses following vaccination with antigen-loaded beta-glucan particles. *mBio*, *1*, e00164-10.

Huang, Y., Zhang, J., Cui, Z. M., Zhao, J., & Zheng, Y. (2013). Expression of the CXCL12/CXCR4 and CXCL16/CXCR6 axes in cervical intraepithelial neoplasia and cervical cancer. *Chinese Journal of Cancer*, *32*, 289–296.

Huang, J., Zheng, D. L., Qin, F. S., Cheng, N., Chen, H., Wan, B. B., et al. (2010). Genetic and epigenetic silencing of SCARA5 may contribute to human hepatocellular carcinoma by activating FAK signaling. *The Journal of Clinical Investigation, 120*, 223–241.

Hudson, B. I., Carter, A. M., Harja, E., Kalea, A. Z., Arriero, M., Yang, H., et al. (2008). Identification, classification, and expression of RAGE gene splice variants. *FASEB Journal, 22*, 1572–1580.

Hudson, B. I., Kalea, A. Z., Del Mar Arriero, M., Harja, E., Boulanger, E., D'Agati, V., et al. (2008). Interaction of the RAGE cytoplasmic domain with diaphanous-1 is required for ligand-stimulated cellular migration through activation of Rac1 and Cdc42. *The Journal of Biological Chemistry, 283*, 34457–34468.

Huysamen, C., & Brown, G. D. (2009). The fungal pattern recognition receptor, Dectin-1, and the associated cluster of C-type lectin-like receptors. *FEMS Microbiology Letters, 290*, 121–128.

Ina, K., Kataoka, T., & Ando, T. (2013). The use of lentinan for treating gastric cancer. *Anti-Cancer Agents in Medicinal Chemistry, 13*, 681–688.

Irjala, H., Elima, K., Johansson, E. L., Merinen, M., Kontula, K., Alanen, K., et al. (2003). The same endothelial receptor controls lymphocyte traffic both in vascular and lymphatic vessels. *European Journal of Immunology, 33*, 815–824.

Ishihara, K., Tsutsumi, K., Kawane, S., Nakajima, M., & Kasaoka, T. (2003). The receptor for advanced glycation end-products (RAGE) directly binds to ERK by a D-domain-like docking site. *FEBS Letters, 550*, 107–113.

Jafari, A., Salouti, M., Shayesteh, S. F., Heidari, Z., Rajabi, A. B., Boustani, K., et al. (2015). Synthesis and characterization of Bombesin-superparamagnetic iron oxide nanoparticles as a targeted contrast agent for imaging of breast cancer using MRI. *Nanotechnology, 26*, 075101.

Jeannin, P., Bottazzi, B., Sironi, M., Doni, A., Rusnati, M., Presta, M., et al. (2005). Complexity and complementarity of outer membrane protein A recognition by cellular and humoral innate immunity receptors. *Immunity, 22*, 551–560.

Jensen, T. O., Schmidt, H., Moller, H. J., Hoyer, M., Maniecki, M. B., Sjoegren, P., et al. (2009). Macrophage markers in serum and tumor have prognostic impact in American Joint Committee on Cancer stage I/II melanoma. *Journal of Clinical Oncology, 27*, 3330–3337.

Jezequel, P., Campion, L., Spyratos, F., Loussouarn, D., Campone, M., Guerin-Charbonnel, C., et al. (2012). Validation of tumor-associated macrophage ferritin light chain as a prognostic biomarker in node-negative breast cancer tumors: A multicentric 2004 national PHRC study. *International Journal of Cancer, 131*, 426–437.

Jiang, Z., Shih, D. M., Xia, Y. R., Lusis, A. J., de Beer, F. C., de Villiers, W. J., et al. (1998). Structure, organization, and chromosomal mapping of the gene encoding macrosialin, a macrophage-restricted protein. *Genomics, 50*, 199–205.

Jimenez, B., Volpert, O. V., Crawford, S. E., Febbraio, M., Silverstein, R. L., & Bouck, N. (2000). Signals leading to apoptosis-dependent inhibition of neovascularization by thrombospondin-1. *Nature Medicine, 6*, 41–48.

Jones, K., Vari, F., Keane, C., Crooks, P., Nourse, J. P., Seymour, L. A., et al. (2013). Serum CD163 and TARC as disease response biomarkers in classical Hodgkin lymphoma. *Clinical Cancer Research, 19*, 731–742.

Joo, H., Li, D., Dullaers, M., Kim, T. W., Duluc, D., Upchurch, K., et al. (2014). C-type lectin-like receptor LOX-1 promotes dendritic cell-mediated class-switched B cell responses. *Immunity, 41*, 592–604.

Jung, Y., Kim, J. K., Shiozawa, Y., Wang, J., Mishra, A., Joseph, J., et al. (2013). Recruitment of mesenchymal stem cells into prostate tumours promotes metastasis. *Nature Communications, 4*, 1795.

Kang, R., Hou, W., Zhang, Q., Chen, R., Lee, Y. J., Bartlett, D. L., et al. (2014). RAGE is essential for oncogenic KRAS-mediated hypoxic signaling in pancreatic cancer. *Cell Death & Disease*, *5*, e1480.

Kanno, H., Nishihara, H., Wang, L., Yuzawa, S., Kobayashi, H., Tsuda, M., et al. (2013). Expression of CD163 prevents apoptosis through the production of granulocyte colony-stimulating factor in meningioma. *Neuro-Oncology*, *15*, 853–864.

Karbownik, M. S., & Nowak, J. Z. (2013). Hyaluronan: Towards novel anti-cancer therapeutics. *Pharmacological Reports*, *65*, 1056–1074.

Karikoski, M., Irjala, H., Maksimow, M., Miiluniemi, M., Granfors, K., Hernesniemi, S., et al. (2009). Clever-1/Stabilin-1 regulates lymphocyte migration within lymphatics and leukocyte entrance to sites of inflammation. *European Journal of Immunology*, *39*, 3477–3487.

Karikoski, M., Marttila-Ichihara, F., Elima, K., Rantakari, P., Hollmen, M., Kelkka, T., et al. (2014). Clever-1/stabilin-1 controls cancer growth and metastasis. *Clinical Cancer Research*, *20*, 6452–6464.

Kawamura, K., Komohara, Y., Takaishi, K., Katabuchi, H., & Takeya, M. (2009). Detection of M2 macrophages and colony-stimulating factor 1 expression in serous and mucinous ovarian epithelial tumors. *Pathology International*, *59*, 300–305.

Kelley, J. L., Ozment, T. R., Li, C., Schweitzer, J. B., & Williams, D. L. (2014). Scavenger receptor-A (CD204): A two-edged sword in health and disease. *Critical Reviews in Immunology*, *34*, 241–261.

Kennedy, D. J., & Kashyap, S. R. (2011). Pathogenic role of scavenger receptor CD36 in the metabolic syndrome and diabetes. *Metabolic Syndrome and Related Disorders*, *9*, 239–245.

Khaidakov, M., Mitra, S., Kang, B. Y., Wang, X., Kadlubar, S., Novelli, G., et al. (2011). Oxidized LDL receptor 1 (OLR1) as a possible link between obesity, dyslipidemia and cancer. *PLoS One*, *6*, e20277.

Kim, C. H., Kunkel, E. J., Boisvert, J., Johnston, B., Campbell, J. J., Genovese, M. C., et al. (2001). Bonzo/CXCR6 expression defines type 1-polarized T-cell subsets with extralymphoid tissue homing potential. *The Journal of Clinical Investigation*, *107*, 595–601.

Kim, J. Y., Park, H. K., Yoon, J. S., Kim, S. J., Kim, E. S., Ahn, K. S., et al. (2008). Advanced glycation end product (AGE)-induced proliferation of HEL cells via receptor for AGE-related signal pathways. *International Journal of Oncology*, *33*, 493–501.

Klein, J. L., Nguyen, T. T., Bien-Willner, G. A., Chen, L., Foyil, K. V., Bartlett, N. L., et al. (2014). CD163 immunohistochemistry is superior to CD68 in predicting outcome in classical Hodgkin lymphoma. *American Journal of Clinical Pathology*, *141*, 381–387.

Kneidl, J., Loffler, B., Erat, M. C., Kalinka, J., Peters, G., Roth, J., et al. (2012). Soluble CD163 promotes recognition, phagocytosis and killing of Staphylococcus aureus via binding of specific fibronectin peptides. *Cellular Microbiology*, *14*, 914–936.

Kobayashi, S., Kubo, H., Suzuki, T., Ishizawa, K., Yamada, M., He, M., et al. (2007). Endogenous secretory receptor for advanced glycation end products in non-small cell lung carcinoma. *American Journal of Respiratory and Critical Care Medicine*, *175*, 184–189.

Koch, M., Hussein, F., Woeste, A., Grundker, C., Frontzek, K., Emons, G., et al. (2011). CD36-mediated activation of endothelial cell apoptosis by an N-terminal recombinant fragment of thrombospondin-2 inhibits breast cancer growth and metastasis in vivo. *Breast Cancer Research and Treatment*, *128*, 337–346.

Kodama, T., Freeman, M., Rohrer, L., Zabrecky, J., Matsudaira, P., & Krieger, M. (1990). Type I macrophage scavenger receptor contains alpha-helical and collagen-like coiled coils. *Nature*, *343*, 531–535.

Koh, Y. W., Park, C. S., Yoon, D. H., Suh, C., & Huh, J. (2014). CD163 expression was associated with angiogenesis and shortened survival in patients with uniformly treated classical Hodgkin lymphoma. *PLoS One*, *9*, e87066.

Komine, H., Kuhn, L., Matsushita, N., Mule, J. J., & Pilon-Thomas, S. (2013). Examination of MARCO activity on dendritic cell phenotype and function using a gene knockout mouse. *PLoS One*, *8*, e67795.

Komohara, Y., Niino, D., Saito, Y., Ohnishi, K., Horlad, H., Ohshima, K., et al. (2013). Clinical significance of CD163(+) tumor-associated macrophages in patients with adult T-cell leukemia/lymphoma. *Cancer Science*, *104*, 945–951.

Komohara, Y., Ohnishi, K., Kuratsu, J., & Takeya, M. (2008). Possible involvement of the M2 anti-inflammatory macrophage phenotype in growth of human gliomas. *The Journal of Pathology*, *216*, 15–24.

Komohara, Y., Takemura, K., Lei, X. F., Sakashita, N., Harada, M., Suzuki, H., et al. (2009). Delayed growth of EL4 lymphoma in SR-A-deficient mice is due to upregulation of nitric oxide and interferon-gamma production by tumor-associated macrophages. *Cancer Science*, *100*, 2160–2166.

Komohara, Y., Terasaki, Y., Kaikita, K., Suzuki, H., Kodama, T., & Takeya, M. (2005). Clearance of apoptotic cells is not impaired in mouse embryos deficient in class A scavenger receptor types I and II (CD204). *Developmental Dynamics*, *232*, 67–74.

Kong, L. Q., Zhu, X. D., Xu, H. X., Zhang, J. B., Lu, L., Wang, W. Q., et al. (2013). The clinical significance of the CD163+ and CD68+ macrophages in patients with hepatocellular carcinoma. *PLoS One*, *8*, e59771.

Kotani, K., Sekine, Y., Ishikawa, S., Ikpot, I. Z., Suzuki, K., & Remaley, A. T. (2013). High-density lipoprotein and prostate cancer: An overview. *Journal of Epidemiology/Japan Epidemiological Association*, *23*, 313–319.

Krechler, T., Jachymova, M., Mestek, O., Zak, A., Zima, T., & Kalousova, M. (2010). Soluble receptor for advanced glycation end-products (sRAGE) and polymorphisms of RAGE and glyoxalase I genes in patients with pancreas cancer. *Clinical Biochemistry*, *43*, 882–886.

Krieger, M. (1997). The other side of scavenger receptors: Pattern recognition for host defense. *Current Opinion in Lipidology*, *8*, 275–280.

Krieger, M., Acton, S., Ashkenas, J., Pearson, A., Penman, M., & Resnick, D. (1993). Molecular flypaper, host defense, and atherosclerosis. Structure, binding properties, and functions of macrophage scavenger receptors. *The Journal of Biological Chemistry*, *268*, 4569–4572.

Kuchibhotla, S., Vanegas, D., Kennedy, D. J., Guy, E., Nimako, G., Morton, R. E., et al. (2008). Absence of CD36 protects against atherosclerosis in ApoE knock-out mice with no additional protection provided by absence of scavenger receptor A I/II. *Cardiovascular Research*, *78*, 185–196.

Kurahara, H., Shinchi, H., Mataki, Y., Maemura, K., Noma, H., Kubo, F., et al. (2011). Significance of M2-polarized tumor-associated macrophage in pancreatic cancer. *The Journal of Surgical Research*, *167*, e211–e219.

Kzhyshkowska, J., & Krusell, L. (2009). Cross-talk between endocytic clearance and secretion in macrophages. *Immunobiology*, *214*, 576–593.

Kzhyshkowska, J., Neyen, C., & Gordon, S. (2012). Role of macrophage scavenger receptors in atherosclerosis. *Immunobiology*, *217*, 492–502.

Labonte, A. C., Tosello-Trampont, A. C., & Hahn, Y. S. (2014). The role of macrophage polarization in infectious and inflammatory diseases. *Molecules and Cells*, *37*, 275–285.

Landschulz, K. T., Pathak, R. K., Rigotti, A., Krieger, M., & Hobbs, H. H. (1996). Regulation of scavenger receptor, class B, type I, a high density lipoprotein receptor, in liver and steroidogenic tissues of the rat. *The Journal of Clinical Investigation*, *98*, 984–995.

Lau, S. K., Chu, P. G., & Weiss, L. M. (2004). CD163: A specific marker of macrophages in paraffin-embedded tissue samples. *American Journal of Clinical Pathology*, *122*, 794–801.

Lee, D. H., & Kim, H. W. (2014). Innate immunity induced by fungal beta-glucans via dectin-1 signaling pathway. *International Journal of Medicinal Mushrooms*, *16*, 1–16.

Leek, R. D., Lewis, C. E., Whitehouse, R., Greenall, M., Clarke, J., & Harris, A. L. (1996). Association of macrophage infiltration with angiogenesis and prognosis in invasive breast carcinoma. *Cancer Research, 56*, 4625–4629.

LeibundGut-Landmann, S., Gross, O., Robinson, M. J., Osorio, F., Slack, E. C., Tsoni, S. V., et al. (2007). Syk- and CARD9-dependent coupling of innate immunity to the induction of T helper cells that produce interleukin 17. *Nature Immunology, 8*, 630–638.

Leibundgut-Landmann, S., Osorio, F., Brown, G. D., & Reis e Sousa, C. (2008). Stimulation of dendritic cells via the dectin-1/Syk pathway allows priming of cytotoxic T-cell responses. *Blood, 112*, 4971–4980.

Leon, C. G., Locke, J. A., Adomat, H. H., Etinger, S. L., Twiddy, A. L., Neumann, R. D., et al. (2010). Alterations in cholesterol regulation contribute to the production of intratumoral androgens during progression to castration-resistant prostate cancer in a mouse xenograft model. *Prostate, 70*, 390–400.

Lewis, C. E., & Pollard, J. W. (2006). Distinct role of macrophages in different tumor microenvironments. *Cancer Research, 66*, 605–612.

Li, W., Liang, R. R., Zhou, C., Wu, M. Y., Lian, L., Yuan, G. F., et al. (2015). The association between expressions of Ras and CD68 in the angiogenesis of breast cancers. *Cancer Cell International, 15*, 17.

Li, J. Y., Paragas, N., Ned, R. M., Qiu, A., Viltard, M., Leete, T., et al. (2009). Scara5 is a ferritin receptor mediating non-transferrin iron delivery. *Developmental Cell, 16*, 35–46.

Li, D., Romain, G., Flamar, A. L., Duluc, D., Dullaers, M., Li, X. H., et al. (2012). Targeting self- and foreign antigens to dendritic cells via DC-ASGPR generates IL-10-producing suppressive CD4+ T cells. *The Journal of Experimental Medicine, 209*, 109–121.

Liang, M., Zhang, P., & Fu, J. (2007). Up-regulation of LOX-1 expression by TNF-alpha promotes trans-endothelial migration of MDA-MB-231 breast cancer cells. *Cancer Letters, 258*, 31–37.

Liu, J., Hu, G., Chen, D., Gong, A. Y., Soori, G. S., Dobleman, T. J., et al. (2013). Suppression of SCARA5 by Snail1 is essential for EMT-associated cell migration of A549 cells. *Oncogenesis, 2*, e73.

Low, J. S., Tao, Q., Ng, K. M., Goh, H. K., Shu, X. S., Woo, W. L., et al. (2011). A novel isoform of the 8p22 tumor suppressor gene DLC1 suppresses tumor growth and is frequently silenced in multiple common tumors. *Oncogene, 30*, 1923–1935.

Lu, Y., Wang, J., Xu, Y., Koch, A. E., Cai, Z., Chen, X., et al. (2008). CXCL16 functions as a novel chemotactic factor for prostate cancer cells in vitro. *Molecular Cancer Research, 6*, 546–554.

Madsen, M., Moller, H. J., Nielsen, M. J., Jacobsen, C., Graversen, J. H., van den Berg, T., et al. (2004). Molecular characterization of the haptoglobin.hemoglobin receptor CD163. Ligand binding properties of the scavenger receptor cysteine-rich domain region. *The Journal of Biological Chemistry, 279*, 51561–51567.

Mahmoud, S. M., Lee, A. H., Paish, E. C., Macmillan, R. D., Ellis, I. O., & Green, A. R. (2012). Tumour-infiltrating macrophages and clinical outcome in breast cancer. *Journal of Clinical Pathology, 65*, 159–163.

Maniecki, M. B., Etzerodt, A., Ulhoi, B. P., Steiniche, T., Borre, M., Dyrskjot, L., et al. (2012). Tumor-promoting macrophages induce the expression of the macrophage-specific receptor CD163 in malignant cells. *International Journal of Cancer, 131*, 2320–2331.

Mansfield, A. S., Heikkila, P., von Smitten, K., Vakkila, J., & Leidenius, M. (2012). The presence of sinusoidal CD163(+) macrophages in lymph nodes is associated with favorable nodal status in patients with breast cancer. *Virchows Archiv, 461*, 639–646.

Martin, B., Hirota, K., Cua, D. J., Stockinger, B., & Veldhoen, M. (2009). Interleukin-17-producing gammadelta T cells selectively expand in response to pathogen products and environmental signals. *Immunity, 31*, 321–330.

Matloubian, M., David, A., Engel, S., Ryan, J. E., & Cyster, J. G. (2000). A transmembrane CXC chemokine is a ligand for HIV-coreceptor Bonzo. *Nature Immunology, 1*, 298–304.
Matsumura, S., & Demaria, S. (2010). Up-regulation of the pro-inflammatory chemokine CXCL16 is a common response of tumor cells to ionizing radiation. *Radiation Research, 173*, 418–425.
Matsumura, S., Wang, B., Kawashima, N., Braunstein, S., Badura, M., Cameron, T. O., et al. (2008). Radiation-induced CXCL16 release by breast cancer cells attracts effector T cells. *Journal of Immunology, 181*, 3099–3107.
Matsushita, N., Komine, H., Grolleau-Julius, A., Pilon-Thomas, S., & Mule, J. J. (2010). Targeting MARCO can lead to enhanced dendritic cell motility and anti-melanoma activity. *Cancer Immunology, Immunotherapy, 59*, 875–884.
Matsushita, K., Toiyama, Y., Tanaka, K., Saigusa, S., Hiro, J., Uchida, K., et al. (2012). Soluble CXCL16 in preoperative serum is a novel prognostic marker and predicts recurrence of liver metastases in colorectal cancer patients. *Annals of Surgical Oncology, 19*(Suppl 3), S518–S527.
McLean, M. H., & El-Omar, E. M. (2009). Genetic aspects of inflammation. *Current Opinion in Pharmacology, 9*, 370–374.
Medrek, C., Ponten, F., Jirstrom, K., & Leandersson, K. (2012). The presence of tumor associated macrophages in tumor stroma as a prognostic marker for breast cancer patients. *BMC Cancer, 12*, 306.
Mehta, J. L., Sanada, N., Hu, C. P., Chen, J., Dandapat, A., Sugawara, F., et al. (2007). Deletion of LOX-1 reduces atherogenesis in LDLR knockout mice fed high cholesterol diet. *Circulation Research, 100*, 1634–1642.
Meng, Y., Beckett, M. A., Liang, H., Mauceri, H. J., van Rooijen, N., Cohen, K. S., et al. (2010). Blockade of tumor necrosis factor alpha signaling in tumor-associated macrophages as a radiosensitizing strategy. *Cancer Research, 70*, 1534–1543.
Michaelson, J. S., & Burkly, L. C. (2009). Therapeutic targeting of TWEAK/Fnl4 in cancer: Exploiting the intrinsic tumor cell killing capacity of the pathway. *Results and Problems in Cell Differentiation, 49*, 145–160.
Miller, D. C., Zheng, S. L., Dunn, R. L., Sarma, A. V., Montie, J. E., Lange, E. M., et al. (2003). Germ-line mutations of the macrophage scavenger receptor 1 gene: Association with prostate cancer risk in African-American men. *Cancer Research, 63*, 3486–3489.
Mooberry, L. K., Nair, M., Paranjape, S., McConathy, W. J., & Lacko, A. G. (2010). Receptor mediated uptake of paclitaxel from a synthetic high density lipoprotein nanocarrier. *Journal of Drug Targeting, 18*, 53–58.
Moore, K. J., Kunjathoor, V. V., Koehn, S. L., Manning, J. J., Tseng, A. A., Silver, J. M., et al. (2005). Loss of receptor-mediated lipid uptake via scavenger receptor A or CD36 pathways does not ameliorate atherosclerosis in hyperlipidemic mice. *The Journal of Clinical Investigation, 115*, 2192–2201.
Moreira, A. P., Cavassani, K. A., Ismailoglu, U. B., Hullinger, R., Dunleavy, M. P., Knight, D. A., et al. (2011). The protective role of TLR6 in a mouse model of asthma is mediated by IL-23 and IL-17A. *The Journal of Clinical Investigation, 121*, 4420–4432.
Moreno, J. A., Munoz-Garcia, B., Martin-Ventura, J. L., Madrigal-Matute, J., Orbe, J., Paramo, J. A., et al. (2009). The CD163-expressing macrophages recognize and internalize TWEAK: Potential consequences in atherosclerosis. *Atherosclerosis, 207*, 103–110.
Moser, B., Janik, S., Schiefer, A. I., Mullauer, L., Bekos, C., Scharrer, A., et al. (2014). Expression of RAGE and HMGB1 in thymic epithelial tumors, thymic hyperplasia and regular thymic morphology. *PLoS One, 9*, e94118.
Murdoch, C., Muthana, M., Coffelt, S. B., & Lewis, C. E. (2008). The role of myeloid cells in the promotion of tumour angiogenesis. *Nature Reviews. Cancer, 8*, 618–631.
Murshid, A., Gong, J., & Calderwood, S. K. (2008). Heat-shock proteins in cancer vaccines: Agents of antigen cross-presentation. *Expert Review of Vaccines, 7*, 1019–1030.

Murshid, A., Gong, J., & Calderwood, S. K. (2010). Heat shock protein 90 mediates efficient antigen cross presentation through the scavenger receptor expressed by endothelial cells-I. *Journal of Immunology, 185*, 2903–2917.

Na, K. Y., Kim, H. S., Jung, W. W., Sung, J. Y., Kalil, R. K., Kim, Y. W., et al. (2014). CXCL16 and CXCR6 in Ewing sarcoma family tumor. *Human Pathology, 45*, 753–760.

Nabeshima, A., Matsumoto, Y., Fukushi, J., Iura, K., Matsunobu, T., Endo, M., et al. (2015). Tumour-associated macrophages correlate with poor prognosis in myxoid liposarcoma and promote cell motility and invasion via the HB-EGF-EGFR-PI3K/Akt pathways. *British Journal of Cancer, 112*, 547–555.

Nagaraju, G. P., Dontula, R., El-Rayes, B. F., & Lakka, S. S. (2014). Molecular mechanisms underlying the divergent roles of SPARC in human carcinogenesis. *Carcinogenesis, 35*, 967–973.

Naito, Y., Takagi, T., & Higashimura, Y. (2014). Heme oxygenase-1 and anti-inflammatory M2 macrophages. *Archives of Biochemistry and Biophysics, 564*, 83–88.

Nakagawa-Toyama, Y., Hirano, K., Tsujii, K., Nishida, M., Miyagawa, J., Sakai, N., et al. (2005). Human scavenger receptor class B type I is expressed with cell-specific fashion in both initial and terminal site of reverse cholesterol transport. *Atherosclerosis, 183*, 75–83.

Nasser, M. W., Wani, N., Ahirwar, D. K., Powell, C. A., Ravi, J., Elbaz, M. M., et al. (2015). RAGE mediates S100A7-induced breast cancer growth and metastasis by modulating the tumor microenvironment. *Cancer Research, 75*, 974–985.

Navab, M., Anantharamaiah, G. M., Reddy, S. T., Van Lenten, B. J., & Fogelman, A. M. (2008). Apo A-1 mimetic peptides as atheroprotective agents in murine models. *Current Drug Targets, 9*, 204–209.

Neuhaus, J., Schiffer, E., von Wilcke, P., Bauer, H. W., Leung, H., Siwy, J., et al. (2013). Seminal plasma as a source of prostate cancer peptide biomarker candidates for detection of indolent and advanced disease. *PLoS One, 8*, e67514.

Neyen, C., Pluddemann, A., Mukhopadhyay, S., Maniati, E., Bossard, M., Gordon, S., et al. (2013). Macrophage scavenger receptor a promotes tumor progression in murine models of ovarian and pancreatic cancer. *Journal of Immunology, 190*, 3798–3805.

Ng, K. K., Lovell, J. F., & Zheng, G. (2011). Lipoprotein-inspired nanoparticles for cancer theranostics. *Accounts of Chemical Research, 44*, 1105–1113.

Nguyen, T. T., Schwartz, E. J., West, R. B., Warnke, R. A., Arber, D. A., & Natkunam, Y. (2005). Expression of CD163 (hemoglobin scavenger receptor) in normal tissues, lymphomas, carcinomas, and sarcomas is largely restricted to the monocyte/macrophage lineage. *The American Journal of Surgical Pathology, 29*, 617–624.

Nickel, T., Schmauss, D., Hanssen, H., Sicic, Z., Krebs, B., Jankl, S., et al. (2009). oxLDL uptake by dendritic cells induces upregulation of scavenger-receptors, maturation and differentiation. *Atherosclerosis, 205*, 442–450.

Nieva, C., Marro, M., Santana-Codina, N., Rao, S., Petrov, D., & Sierra, A. (2012). The lipid phenotype of breast cancer cells characterized by Raman microspectroscopy: Towards a stratification of malignancy. *PLoS One, 7*, e46456.

No, J. H., Moon, J. M., Kim, K., & Kim, Y. B. (2013). Prognostic significance of serum soluble CD163 level in patients with epithelial ovarian cancer. *Gynecologic and Obstetric Investigation, 75*, 263–267.

Ohtaki, Y., Ishii, G., Nagai, K., Ashimine, S., Kuwata, T., Hishida, T., et al. (2010). Stromal macrophage expressing CD204 is associated with tumor aggressiveness in lung adenocarcinoma. *Journal of Thoracic Oncology, 5*, 1507–1515.

Oka, K., Sawamura, T., Kikuta, K., Itokawa, S., Kume, N., Kita, T., et al. (1998). Lectin-like oxidized low-density lipoprotein receptor 1 mediates phagocytosis of aged/apoptotic cells in endothelial cells. *Proceedings of the National Academy of Sciences of the United States of America, 95*, 9535–9540.

Palumbo, R., De Marchis, F., Pusterla, T., Conti, A., Alessio, M., & Bianchi, M. E. (2009). Src family kinases are necessary for cell migration induced by extracellular HMGB1. *Journal of Leukocyte Biology, 86*, 617–623.

Pan, H., Niu, W., He, L., Wang, B., Cao, J., Zhao, F., et al. (2013). Contributory role of five common polymorphisms of RAGE and APE1 genes in lung cancer among Han Chinese. *PLoS One, 8*, e69018.

Parlato, S., Romagnoli, G., Spadaro, F., Canini, I., Sirabella, P., Borghi, P., et al. (2010). LOX-1 as a natural IFN-alpha-mediated signal for apoptotic cell uptake and antigen presentation in dendritic cells. *Blood, 115*, 1554–1563.

Philips, J. A., Rubin, E. J., & Perrimon, N. (2005). Drosophila RNAi screen reveals CD36 family member required for mycobacterial infection. *Science, 309*, 1251–1253.

Platt, N., Suzuki, H., Kodama, T., & Gordon, S. (2000). Apoptotic thymocyte clearance in scavenger receptor class A-deficient mice is apparently normal. *Journal of Immunology, 164*, 4861–4867.

Pluddemann, A., Neyen, C., & Gordon, S. (2007). Macrophage scavenger receptors and host-derived ligands. *Methods, 43*, 207–217.

Politz, O., Gratchev, A., McCourt, P. A., Schledzewski, K., Guillot, P., Johansson, S., et al. (2002). Stabilin-1 and −2 constitute a novel family of fasciclin-like hyaluronan receptor homologues. *The Biochemical Journal, 362*, 155–164.

Prabhudas, M., Bowdish, D., Drickamer, K., Febbraio, M., Herz, J., Kobzik, L., et al. (2014). Standardizing scavenger receptor nomenclature. *Journal of Immunology, 192*, 1997–2006.

Pupovac, A., Foster, C. M., & Sluyter, R. (2013). Human P2X7 receptor activation induces the rapid shedding of CXCL16. *Biochemical and Biophysical Research Communications, 432*, 626–631.

Qian, H., Johansson, S., McCourt, P., Smedsrod, B., Ekblom, M., & Johansson, S. (2009). Stabilins are expressed in bone marrow sinusoidal endothelial cells and mediate scavenging and cell adhesive functions. *Biochemical and Biophysical Research Communications, 390*, 883–886.

Qian, B. Z., & Pollard, J. W. (2010). Macrophage diversity enhances tumor progression and metastasis. *Cell, 141*, 39–51.

Qian, F., Sun, B. L., Zhang, W. Y., Ke, J., & Zhu, J. (2014). Gly82Ser polymorphism of the receptor for advanced glycation end-product (RAGE) potential high risk in patients with colorectal cancer. *Tumour Biology, 35*, 3171–3175.

Qian, J., Yi, H., Guo, C., Yu, X., Zuo, D., Chen, X., et al. (2011). CD204 suppresses large heat shock protein-facilitated priming of tumor antigen gp100-specific T cells and chaperone vaccine activity against mouse melanoma. *Journal of Immunology, 187*, 2905–2914.

Rachidi, S. M., Qin, T., Sun, S., Zheng, W. J., & Li, Z. (2013). Molecular profiling of multiple human cancers defines an inflammatory cancer-associated molecular pattern and uncovers KPNA2 as a uniform poor prognostic cancer marker. *PLoS One, 8*, e57911.

Ramirez-Ortiz, Z. G., Pendergraft, W. F., 3rd, Prasad, A., Byrne, M. H., Iram, T., Blanchette, C. J., et al. (2013). The scavenger receptor SCARF1 mediates the clearance of apoptotic cells and prevents autoimmunity. *Nature Immunology, 14*, 917–926.

Ramprasad, M. P., Fischer, W., Witztum, J. L., Sambrano, G. R., Quehenberger, O., & Steinberg, D. (1995). The 94- to 97-kDa mouse macrophage membrane protein that recognizes oxidized low density lipoprotein and phosphatidylserine-rich liposomes is identical to macrosialin, the mouse homologue of human CD68. *Proceedings of the National Academy of Sciences of the United States of America, 92*, 9580–9584.

Raucci, A., Cugusi, S., Antonelli, A., Barabino, S. M., Monti, L., Bierhaus, A., et al. (2008). A soluble form of the receptor for advanced glycation endproducts (RAGE) is produced by proteolytic cleavage of the membrane-bound form by the sheddase a disintegrin and metalloprotease 10 (ADAM10). *FASEB Journal, 22*, 3716–3727.

Raycroft, M. T., Harvey, B. P., Bruck, M. J., & Mamula, M. J. (2012). Inhibition of antigen trafficking through scavenger receptor A. *The Journal of Biological Chemistry*, *287*, 5310–5316.

Reddy, M. A., Li, S. L., Sahar, S., Kim, Y. S., Xu, Z. G., Lanting, L., et al. (2006). Key role of Src kinase in S100B-induced activation of the receptor for advanced glycation end products in vascular smooth muscle cells. *The Journal of Biological Chemistry*, *281*, 13685–13693.

Reinartz, S., Schumann, T., Finkernagel, F., Wortmann, A., Jansen, J. M., Meissner, W., et al. (2014). Mixed-polarization phenotype of ascites-associated macrophages in human ovarian carcinoma: Correlation of CD163 expression, cytokine levels and early relapse. *International Journal of Cancer*, *134*, 32–42.

Ren, Y., Silverstein, R. L., Allen, J., & Savill, J. (1995). CD36 gene transfer confers capacity for phagocytosis of cells undergoing apoptosis. *The Journal of Experimental Medicine*, *181*, 1857–1862.

Rennert, H., Zeigler-Johnson, C., Mittal, R. D., Tan, Y. C., Sadowl, C. M., Edwards, J., et al. (2008). Analysis of the RNASEL/HPC1, and macrophage scavenger receptor 1 in Asian-Indian advanced prostate cancer. *Urology*, *72*, 456–460.

Riuzzi, F., Sorci, G., Sagheddu, R., & Donato, R. (2012). HMGB1-RAGE regulates muscle satellite cell homeostasis through p38-MAPK- and myogenin-dependent repression of Pax7 transcription. *Journal of Cell Science*, *125*, 1440–1454.

Rohrer, L., Freeman, M., Kodama, T., Penman, M., & Krieger, M. (1990). Coiled-coil fibrous domains mediate ligand binding by macrophage scavenger receptor type II. *Nature*, *343*, 570–572.

Rost, M. S., & Sumanas, S. (2014). Hyaluronic acid receptor Stabilin-2 regulates Erk phosphorylation and arterial–venous differentiation in zebrafish. *PLoS One*, *9*, e88614.

Saito, Y., Komohara, Y., Niino, D., Horlad, H., Ohnishi, K., Takeya, H., et al. (2014). Role of CD204-positive tumor-associated macrophages in adult T-cell leukemia/lymphoma. *Journal of Clinical and Experimental Hematopathology*, *54*, 59–65.

Sawamura, T., Kume, N., Aoyama, T., Moriwaki, H., Hoshikawa, H., Aiba, Y., et al. (1997). An endothelial receptor for oxidized low-density lipoprotein. *Nature*, *386*, 73–77.

Schramme, A., Abdel-Bakky, M. S., Kampfer-Kolb, N., Pfeilschifter, J., & Gutwein, P. (2008). The role of CXCL16 and its processing metalloproteinases ADAM10 and ADAM17 in the proliferation and migration of human mesangial cells. *Biochemical and Biophysical Research Communications*, *370*, 311–316.

Seimon, T. A., Obstfeld, A., Moore, K. J., Golenbock, D. T., & Tabas, I. (2006). Combinatorial pattern recognition receptor signaling alters the balance of life and death in macrophages. *Proceedings of the National Academy of Sciences of the United States of America*, *103*, 19794–19799.

Seppala, E. H., Ikonen, T., Autio, V., Rokman, A., Mononen, N., Matikainen, M. P., et al. (2003). Germ-line alterations in MSR1 gene and prostate cancer risk. *Clinical Cancer Research*, *9*, 5252–5256.

Shabo, I., Olsson, H., Elkarim, R., Sun, X. F., & Svanvik, J. (2014). Macrophage infiltration in tumor stroma is related to tumor cell expression of CD163 in colorectal cancer. *Cancer Microenvironment*, 7, 61–69.

Shabo, I., Olsson, H., Sun, X. F., & Svanvik, J. (2009). Expression of the macrophage antigen CD163 in rectal cancer cells is associated with early local recurrence and reduced survival time. *International Journal of Cancer*, *125*, 1826–1831.

Shabo, I., Stal, O., Olsson, H., Dore, S., & Svanvik, J. (2008). Breast cancer expression of CD163, a macrophage scavenger receptor, is related to early distant recurrence and reduced patient survival. *International Journal of Cancer*, *123*, 780–786.

Shabo, I., & Svanvik, J. (2011). Expression of macrophage antigens by tumor cells. *Advances in Experimental Medicine and Biology, 714*, 141–150.
Shahzad, M. M., Mangala, L. S., Han, H. D., Lu, C., Bottsford-Miller, J., Nishimura, M., et al. (2011). Targeted delivery of small interfering RNA using reconstituted high-density lipoprotein nanoparticles. *Neoplasia, 13*, 309–319.
Shankar, J., Messenberg, A., Chan, J., Underhill, T. M., Foster, L. J., & Nabi, I. R. (2010). Pseudopodial actin dynamics control epithelial-mesenchymal transition in metastatic cancer cells. *Cancer Research, 70*, 3780–3790.
Shetty, S., Weston, C. J., Oo, Y. H., Westerlund, N., Stamataki, Z., Youster, J., et al. (2011). Common lymphatic endothelial and vascular endothelial receptor-1 mediates the transmigration of regulatory T cells across human hepatic sinusoidal endothelium. *Journal of Immunology, 186*, 4147–4155.
Shigeoka, M., Urakawa, N., Nakamura, T., Nishio, M., Watajima, T., Kuroda, D., et al. (2013). Tumor associated macrophage expressing CD204 is associated with tumor aggressiveness of esophageal squamous cell carcinoma. *Cancer Science, 104*, 1112–1119.
Shimaoka, T., Kume, N., Minami, M., Hayashida, K., Kataoka, H., Kita, T., et al. (2000). Molecular cloning of a novel scavenger receptor for oxidized low density lipoprotein, SR-PSOX, on macrophages. *The Journal of Biological Chemistry, 275*, 40663–40666.
Shimaoka, T., Kume, N., Minami, M., Hayashida, K., Sawamura, T., Kita, T., et al. (2001). LOX-1 supports adhesion of Gram-positive and Gram-negative bacteria. *Journal of Immunology, 166*, 5108–5114.
Shimaoka, T., Nakayama, T., Kume, N., Takahashi, S., Yamaguchi, J., Minami, M., et al. (2003). Cutting edge: SR-PSOX/CXC chemokine ligand 16 mediates bacterial phagocytosis by APCs through its chemokine domain. *Journal of Immunology, 171*, 1647–1651.
Shin, J. Y., Yang, Y., Heo, P., Lee, J. C., Kong, B., Cho, J. Y., et al. (2012). pH-responsive high-density lipoprotein-like nanoparticles to release paclitaxel at acidic pH in cancer chemotherapy. *International Journal of Nanomedicine, 7*, 2805–2816.
Sica, A., Larghi, P., Mancino, A., Rubino, L., Porta, C., Totaro, M. G., et al. (2008). Macrophage polarization in tumour progression. *Seminars in Cancer Biology, 18*, 349–355.
Sierra-Filardi, E., Vega, M. A., Sanchez-Mateos, P., Corbi, A. L., & Puig-Kroger, A. (2010). Heme oxygenase-1 expression in M-CSF-polarized M2 macrophages contributes to LPS-induced IL-10 release. *Immunobiology, 215*, 788–795.
Simantov, R., Febbraio, M., & Silverstein, R. L. (2005). The antiangiogenic effect of thrombospondin-2 is mediated by CD36 and modulated by histidine-rich glycoprotein. *Matrix Biology, 24*, 27–34.
Sironen, R. K., Tammi, M., Tammi, R., Auvinen, P. K., Anttila, M., & Kosma, V. M. (2011). Hyaluronan in human malignancies. *Experimental Cell Research, 317*, 383–391.
Son, H., & Moon, A. (2010). Epithelial-mesenchymal transition and cell invasion. *Toxicological Research, 26*, 245–252.
Song, L., Lee, C., & Schindler, C. (2011). Deletion of the murine scavenger receptor CD68. *Journal of Lipid Research, 52*, 1542–1550.
Srivastava, P. (2002). Interaction of heat shock proteins with peptides and antigen presenting cells: Chaperoning of the innate and adaptive immune responses. *Annual Review of Immunology, 20*, 395–425.
Stewart, C. R., Stuart, L. M., Wilkinson, K., van Gils, J. M., Deng, J., Halle, A., et al. (2010). CD36 ligands promote sterile inflammation through assembly of a Toll-like receptor 4 and 6 heterodimer. *Nature Immunology, 11*, 155–161.
Strasser, D., Neumann, K., Bergmann, H., Marakalala, M. J., Guler, R., Rojowska, A., et al. (2012). Syk kinase-coupled C-type lectin receptors engage protein kinase C-sigma to elicit Card9 adaptor-mediated innate immunity. *Immunity, 36*, 32–42.
Su, S., Chien, M., Lin, C., Chen, M., & Yang, S. (2015). RAGE gene polymorphism and environmental factor in the risk of oral cancer. *Journal of Dental Research, 94*, 403–411.

Sugaya, M., Miyagaki, T., Ohmatsu, H., Suga, H., Kai, H., Kamata, M., et al. (2012). Association of the numbers of CD163(+) cells in lesional skin and serum levels of soluble CD163 with disease progression of cutaneous T cell lymphoma. *Journal of Dermatological Science*, *68*, 45–51.

Sugimoto, M., Mitsunaga, S., Yoshikawa, K., Kato, Y., Gotohda, N., Takahashi, S., et al. (2014). Prognostic impact of M2 macrophages at neural invasion in patients with invasive ductal carcinoma of the pancreas. *European Journal of Cancer*, *50*, 1900–1908.

Sun, M., Finnemann, S. C., Febbraio, M., Shan, L., Annangudi, S. P., Podrez, E. A., et al. (2006). Light-induced oxidation of photoreceptor outer segment phospholipids generates ligands for CD36-mediated phagocytosis by retinal pigment epithelium: A potential mechanism for modulating outer segment phagocytosis under oxidant stress conditions. *The Journal of Biological Chemistry*, *281*, 4222–4230.

Sun, J., Turner, A., Xu, J., Gronberg, H., & Isaacs, W. (2007). Genetic variability in inflammation pathways and prostate cancer risk. *Urologic Oncology*, *25*, 250–259.

Suzuki, H., Kurihara, Y., Takeya, M., Kamada, N., Kataoka, M., Jishage, K., et al. (1997). A role for macrophage scavenger receptors in atherosclerosis and susceptibility to infection. *Nature*, *386*, 292–296.

Tateno, H., Ogawa, T., Muramoto, K., Kamiya, H., & Saneyoshi, M. (2002). Rhamnose-binding lectins from steelhead trout (Oncorhynchus mykiss) eggs recognize bacterial lipopolysaccharides and lipoteichoic acid. *Bioscience, Biotechnology, and Biochemistry*, *66*, 604–612.

Taylor, P. R., Tsoni, S. V., Willment, J. A., Dennehy, K. M., Rosas, M., Findon, H., et al. (2007). Dectin-1 is required for beta-glucan recognition and control of fungal infection. *Nature Immunology*, *8*, 31–38.

Thakur, S. A., Hamilton, R. F., Jr., & Holian, A. (2008). Role of scavenger receptor a family in lung inflammation from exposure to environmental particles. *Journal of Immunotoxicology*, *5*, 151–157.

Theriault, J. R., Adachi, H., & Calderwood, S. K. (2006). Role of scavenger receptors in the binding and internalization of heat shock protein 70. *Journal of Immunology*, *177*, 8604–8611.

Thiery, J. P. (2002). Epithelial-mesenchymal transitions in tumour progression. *Nature Reviews. Cancer*, *2*, 442–454.

Thomsen, M., Nordestgaard, B. G., Kobzik, L., & Dahl, M. (2013). Genetic variation in the scavenger receptor MARCO and its association with chronic obstructive pulmonary disease and lung infection in 10,604 individuals. *Respiration; International Review of Thoracic Diseases*, *85*, 144–153.

Tiainen, S., Tumelius, R., Rilla, K., Hamalainen, K., Tammi, M., Tammi, R., et al. (2014). High numbers of macrophages, especially M2-like (CD163-positive), correlate with hyaluronan accumulation and poor outcome in breast cancer. *Histopathology*, *66*, 873–883.

Todt, J. C., Hu, B., & Curtis, J. L. (2008). The scavenger receptor SR-A I/II (CD204) signals via the receptor tyrosine kinase Mertk during apoptotic cell uptake by murine macrophages. *Journal of Leukocyte Biology*, *84*, 510–518.

Toure, F., Zahm, J. M., Garnotel, R., Lambert, E., Bonnet, N., Schmidt, A. M., et al. (2008). Receptor for advanced glycation end-products (RAGE) modulates neutrophil adhesion and migration on glycoxidated extracellular matrix. *The Biochemical Journal*, *416*, 255–261.

Tripathy, S., Vinokour, E., McMahon, K. M., Volpert, O. V., & Thaxton, C. S. (2014). High density lipoprotein nanoparticles deliver RNAi to endothelial cells to inhibit angiogenesis. *Particle and Particle Systems Characterization*, *31*, 1141–1150.

Twiddy, A. L., Cox, M. E., & Wasan, K. M. (2012). Knockdown of scavenger receptor class B type I reduces prostate specific antigen secretion and viability of prostate cancer cells. *Prostate*, *72*, 955–965.

Uray, I. P., Liang, Y., & Hyder, S. M. (2004). Estradiol down-regulates CD36 expression in human breast cancer cells. *Cancer Letters*, *207*, 101–107.
van der Laan, L. J., Dopp, E. A., Haworth, R., Pikkarainen, T., Kangas, M., Elomaa, O., et al. (1999). Regulation and functional involvement of macrophage scavenger receptor MARCO in clearance of bacteria in vivo. *Journal of Immunology*, *162*, 939–947.
van Dongen, M., Savage, N. D., Jordanova, E. S., Briaire-de Bruijn, I. H., Walburg, K. V., Ottenhoff, T. H., et al. (2010). Anti-inflammatory M2 type macrophages characterize metastasized and tyrosine kinase inhibitor-treated gastrointestinal stromal tumors. *International Journal of Cancer*, *127*, 899–909.
Vickers, K. C., Palmisano, B. T., Shoucri, B. M., Shamburek, R. D., & Remaley, A. T. (2011). MicroRNAs are transported in plasma and delivered to recipient cells by high-density lipoproteins. *Nature Cell Biology*, *13*, 423–433.
Vilchez, J. A., Martinez-Ruiz, A., Sancho-Rodriguez, N., Martinez-Hernandez, P., & Noguera-Velasco, J. A. (2014). The real role of prediagnostic high-density lipoprotein cholesterol and the cancer risk: A concise review. *European Journal of Clinical Investigation*, *44*, 103–114.
Volpert, O. V., Zaichuk, T., Zhou, W., Reiher, F., Ferguson, T. A., Stuart, P. M., et al. (2002). Inducer-stimulated Fas targets activated endothelium for destruction by anti-angiogenic thrombospondin-1 and pigment epithelium-derived factor. *Nature Medicine*, *8*, 349–357.
Wadsack, C., Hirschmugl, B., Hammer, A., Levak-Frank, S., Kozarsky, K. F., Sattler, W., et al. (2003). Scavenger receptor class B, type I on non-malignant and malignant human epithelial cells mediates cholesteryl ester-uptake from high density lipoproteins. *The International Journal of Biochemistry & Cell Biology*, *35*, 441–454.
Wadsack, C., Hrzenjak, A., Hammer, A., Hirschmugl, B., Levak-Frank, S., Desoye, G., et al. (2003). Trophoblast-like human choriocarcinoma cells serve as a suitable in vitro model for selective cholesteryl ester uptake from high density lipoproteins. *European Journal of Biochemistry/FEBS*, *270*, 451–462.
Wang, J. L., Bi, Z., Zou, J. W., & Gu, X. M. (2012). Combination therapy with lentinan improves outcomes in patients with esophageal carcinoma. *Molecular Medicine Reports*, *5*, 745–748.
Wang, L., Chang, E. W., Wong, S. C., Ong, S. M., Chong, D. Q., & Ling, K. L. (2013). Increased myeloid-derived suppressor cells in gastric cancer correlate with cancer stage and plasma S100A8/A9 proinflammatory proteins. *Journal of Immunology*, *190*, 794–804.
Wang, X. Y., Facciponte, J., Chen, X., Subjeck, J. R., & Repasky, E. A. (2007). Scavenger receptor-A negatively regulates antitumor immunity. *Cancer Research*, *67*, 4996–5002.
Wang, X. Y., Facciponte, J. G., & Subjeck, J. R. (2006). Molecular chaperones and cancer immunotherapy. *Handbook of Experimental Pharmacology*, *172*, 305–329.
Wang, J., Lu, Y., Koch, A. E., Zhang, J., & Taichman, R. S. (2008). CXCR6 induces prostate cancer progression by the AKT/mammalian target of rapamycin signaling pathway. *Cancer Research*, *68*, 10367–10376.
Wang, L., McDonnell, S. K., Cunningham, J. M., Hebbring, S., Jacobsen, S. J., Cerhan, J. R., et al. (2003). No association of germline alteration of MSR1 with prostate cancer risk. *Nature Genetics*, *35*, 128–129.
Wang, X. Y., & Subjeck, J. R. (2013). High molecular weight stress proteins: Identification, cloning and utilisation in cancer immunotherapy. *International Journal of Hyperthermia*, *29*, 364–375.
Wang, X. Y., Sun, X., Chen, X., Facciponte, J., Repasky, E. A., Kane, J., et al. (2010). Superior antitumor response induced by large stress protein chaperoned protein antigen compared with peptide antigen. *Journal of Immunology*, *184*, 6309–6319.
Wang, S., Sun, M., Gu, C., Wang, X., Chen, D., Zhao, E., et al. (2014). Expression of CD163, interleukin-10, and interferon-gamma in oral squamous cell carcinoma: Mutual relationships and prognostic implications. *European Journal of Oral Sciences*, *122*, 202–209.

Weis, N., Weigert, A., von Knethen, A., & Brune, B. (2009). Heme oxygenase-1 contributes to an alternative macrophage activation profile induced by apoptotic cell supernatants. *Molecular Biology of the Cell, 20*, 1280–1288.

Wente, M. N., Gaida, M. M., Mayer, C., Michalski, C. W., Haag, N., Giese, T., et al. (2008). Expression and potential function of the CXC chemokine CXCL16 in pancreatic ductal adenocarcinoma. *International Journal of Oncology, 33*, 297–308.

Wermeling, F., Chen, Y., Pikkarainen, T., Scheynius, A., Winqvist, O., Izui, S., et al. (2007). Class A scavenger receptors regulate tolerance against apoptotic cells, and autoantibodies against these receptors are predictive of systemic lupus. *The Journal of Experimental Medicine, 204*, 2259–2265.

Whelan, F. J., Meehan, C. J., Golding, G. B., McConkey, B. J., & Bowdish, D. M. (2012). The evolution of the class A scavenger receptors. *BMC Evolutionary Biology, 12*, 227.

Wilkinson, K., & El Khoury, J. (2012). Microglial scavenger receptors and their roles in the pathogenesis of Alzheimer's disease. *International Journal of Alzheimer's Disease, 2012*, 489456.

Workman, G., & Sage, E. H. (2011). Identification of a sequence in the matricellular protein SPARC that interacts with the scavenger receptor stabilin-1. *Journal of Cellular Biochemistry, 112*, 1003–1008.

Xia, W., Xu, Y., Mao, Q., Dong, G., Shi, R., Wang, J., et al. (2015). Association of RAGE polymorphisms and cancer risk: A meta-analysis of 27 studies. *Medical Oncology, 32*, 442.

Xie, J., Zhu, H., Guo, L., Ruan, Y., Wang, L., Sun, L., et al. (2010). Lectin-like oxidized low-density lipoprotein receptor-1 delivers heat shock protein 60-fused antigen into the MHC class I presentation pathway. *Journal of Immunology, 185*, 2306–2313.

Xing, Y. N., Xu, X. Y., Nie, X. C., Yang, X., Yu, M., Xu, H. M., et al. (2012). Role and clinicopathologic significance of CXC chemokine ligand 16 and chemokine (C-X-C motif) receptor 6 expression in gastric carcinomas. *Human Pathology, 43*, 2299–2307.

Xu, J., Zheng, S. L., Komiya, A., Mychaleckyj, J. C., Isaacs, S. D., Hu, J. J., et al. (2002). Germline mutations and sequence variants of the macrophage scavenger receptor 1 gene are associated with prostate cancer risk. *Nature Genetics, 32*, 321–325.

Xu, X., Zhu, H., Wang, T., Sun, Y., Ni, P., Liu, Y., et al. (2014). Exogenous high-mobility group box 1 inhibits apoptosis and promotes the proliferation of lewis cells via RAGE/TLR4-dependent signal pathways. *Scandinavian Journal of Immunology, 79*, 386–394.

Yadav, M., & Schorey, J. S. (2006). The beta-glucan receptor dectin-1 functions together with TLR2 to mediate macrophage activation by mycobacteria. *Blood, 108*, 3168–3175.

Yamagishi, S., Matsui, T., & Fukami, K. (2015). Role of receptor for advanced glycation end products (RAGE) and its ligands in cancer risk. *Rejuvenation Research, 18*, 48–56.

Yan, N., Zhang, S., Yang, Y., Cheng, L., Li, C., Dai, L., et al. (2012). Therapeutic upregulation of Class A scavenger receptor member 5 inhibits tumor growth and metastasis. *Cancer Science, 103*, 1631–1639.

Yeung, O. W., Lo, C., Ling, C., Qi, X., Geng, W., Li, C., et al. (2014). Alternatively activated (M2) macrophages promote tumour growth and invasiveness in hepatocellular carcinoma. *Journal of Hepatology, 62*, 607–616.

Yi, H., Guo, C., Yu, X., Gao, P., Qian, J., Zuo, D., et al. (2011a). Targeting the immunoregulator SRA/CD204 potentiates specific dendritic cell vaccine-induced T-cell response and antitumor immunity. *Cancer Research, 71*, 6611–6620.

Yi, H., Yu, X., Gao, P., Wang, Y., Baek, S. H., Chen, X., et al. (2009). Pattern recognition scavenger receptor SRA/CD204 down-regulates Toll-like receptor 4 signaling-dependent CD8 T-cell activation. *Blood, 113*, 5819–5828.

Yi, H., Zuo, D., Yu, X., Hu, F., Manjili, M. H., Chen, Z., et al. (2012). Suppression of antigen-specific CD4+ T cell activation by SRA/CD204 through reducing the immunostimulatory capability of antigen-presenting cell. *Journal of Molecular Medicine (Berlin, Germany), 90*, 413–426.

Yin, J., Liu, Y. N., Tillman, H., Barrett, B., Hewitt, S., Ylaya, K., et al. (2014). AR-regulated TWEAK-FN14 pathway promotes prostate cancer bone metastasis. *Cancer Research*, *74*, 4306–4317.

Yin, X., Luistro, L., Zhong, H., Smith, M., Nevins, T., Schostack, K., et al. (2013). RG7212 anti-TWEAK mAb inhibits tumor growth through inhibition of tumor cell proliferation and survival signaling and by enhancing the host antitumor immune response. *Clinical Cancer Research*, *19*, 5686–5698.

Yoon, T. J., Koppula, S., & Lee, K. H. (2013). The effects of beta-glucans on cancer metastasis. *Anti-Cancer Agents in Medicinal Chemistry*, *13*, 699–708.

Yoshikawa, K., Mitsunaga, S., Kinoshita, T., Konishi, M., Takahashi, S., Gotohda, N., et al. (2012). Impact of tumor-associated macrophages on invasive ductal carcinoma of the pancreas head. *Cancer Science*, *103*, 2012–2020.

Yu, G., Tseng, G. C., Yu, Y. P., Gavel, T., Nelson, J., Wells, A., et al. (2006). CSR1 suppresses tumor growth and metastasis of prostate cancer. *The American Journal of Pathology*, *168*, 597–607.

Yu, X., & Wang, X. Y. (2012). Antagonizing the innate pattern recognition receptor CD204 to improve dendritic cell-targeted cancer immunotherapy. *Oncoimmunology*, *1*, 770–772.

Yu, X., Yi, H., Guo, C., Zuo, D., Wang, Y., Kim, H. L., et al. (2011). Pattern precognition scavenger receptor CD204 attenuates toll-like receptor 4-induced NF-{kappa}B activation by directly inhibiting ubiquitination of tumor necrosis factor (TNF) receptor-associated factor 6. *The Journal of Biological Chemistry*, *286*, 18795–18806.

Yu, X., Zuo, D., Subjeck, J. R., & Wang, X.-Y. (2012). Scavenger receptor A (SRA/CD204): A multifaceted regulator of inflammatory response and immunity. In Masoud H. Manjili (Ed.), *Cytokines: Mechanisms, functions and abnormalities* (pp. 173–196). New York: NOVA Science.

Zhang, S., Hou, X., Zi, S., Wang, Y., Chen, L., & Kong, B. (2013). Polymorphisms of receptor for advanced glycation end products and risk of epithelial ovarian cancer in Chinese patients. *Cellular Physiology and Biochemistry*, *31*, 525–531.

Zhang, Q. Y., Wu, L. Q., Zhang, T., Han, Y. F., & Lin, X. (2015). Autophagy-mediated HMGB1 release promotes gastric cancer cell survival via RAGE activation of extracellular signal-regulated kinases 1/2. *Oncology Reports*, *33*, 1630–1638.

Zhao, C. B., Bao, J. M., Lu, Y. J., Zhao, T., Zhou, X. H., Zheng, D. Y., et al. (2014). Co-expression of RAGE and HMGB1 is associated with cancer progression and poor patient outcome of prostate cancer. *American Journal of Cancer Research*, *4*, 369–377.

Zheng, Y., Liu, Y., Jin, H., Pan, S., Qian, Y., Huang, C., et al. (2013). Scavenger receptor B1 is a potential biomarker of human nasopharyngeal carcinoma and its growth is inhibited by HDL-mimetic nanoparticles. *Theranostics*, *3*, 477–486.

Zhou, D. N., Deng, Y. F., Li, R. H., Yin, P., & Ye, C. S. (2014). Concurrent alterations of RAGE, RECK, and MMP9 protein expression are relevant to Epstein-Barr virus infection, metastasis, and survival in nasopharyngeal carcinoma. *International Journal of Clinical and Experimental Pathology*, 7, 3245–3254.

Zhou, J., Febbraio, M., Wada, T., Zhai, Y., Kuruba, R., He, J., et al. (2008). Hepatic fatty acid transporter Cd36 is a common target of LXR, PXR, and PPARgamma in promoting steatosis. *Gastroenterology*, *134*, 556–567.

Zizzo, G., Hilliard, B. A., Monestier, M., & Cohen, P. L. (2012). Efficient clearance of early apoptotic cells by human macrophages requires M2c polarization and MerTK induction. *Journal of Immunology*, *189*, 3508–3520.

Zuo, D., Yu, X., Guo, C., Wang, H., Qian, J., Yi, H., et al. (2013). Scavenger receptor a restrains T-cell activation and protects against concanavalin A-induced hepatic injury. *Hepatology*, *57*, 228–238.

INDEX

Note: Page numbers followed by "*f*" indicate figures and "*t*" indicate tables.

D

P

R

S

T

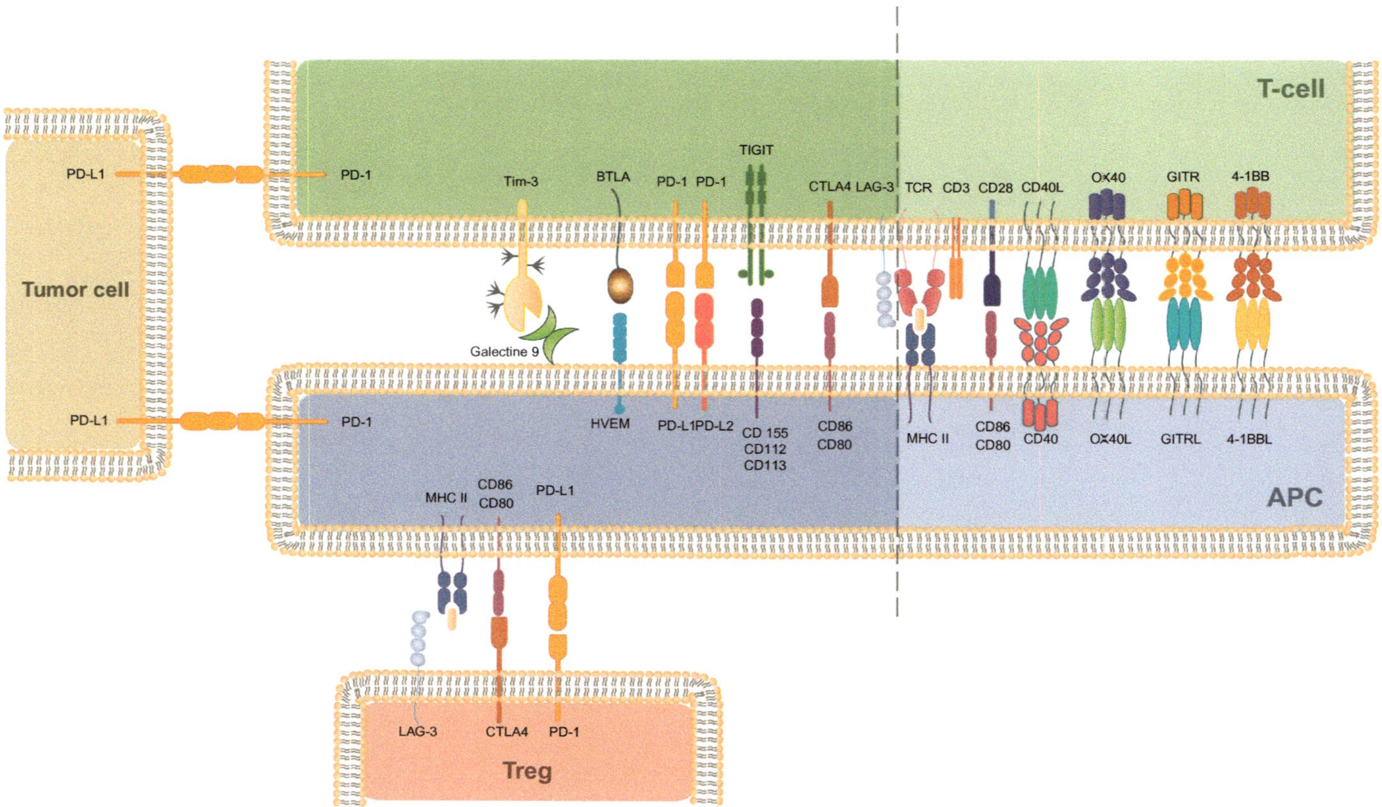

Figure 1, Danny N. Khalil *et al.* (See Page 6 of this volume.)

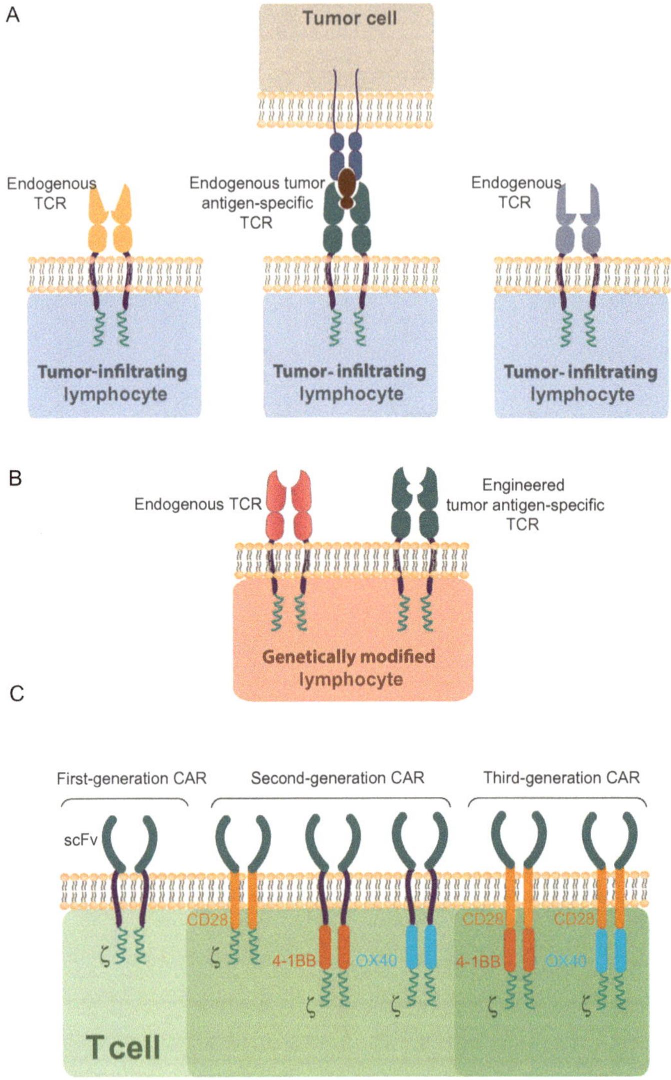

Figure 2, Danny N. Khalil *et al.* (See Page 27 of this volume.)

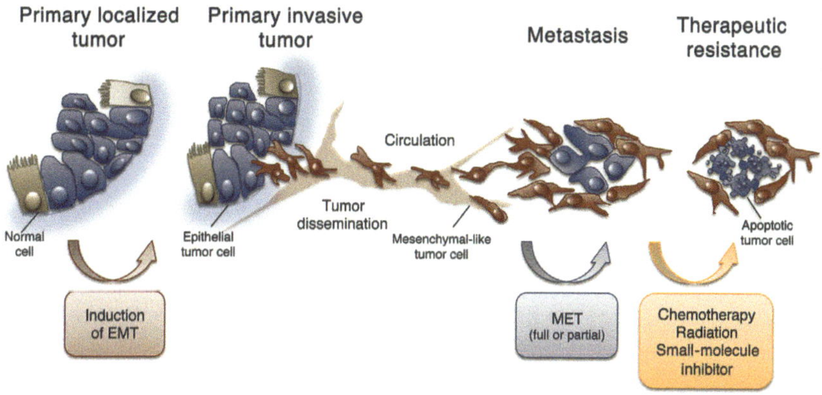

Figure 1, Claudia Palena and Duane H. Hamilton (See Page 72 of this volume.)

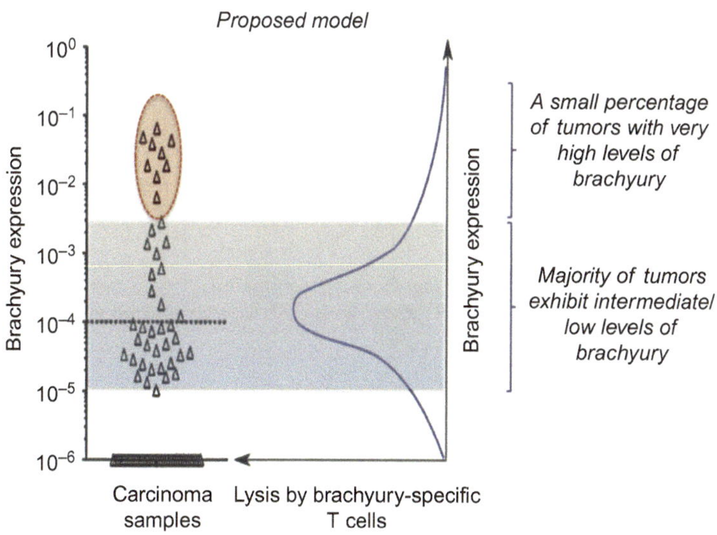

Figure 2, Claudia Palena and Duane H. Hamilton (See Page 84 of this volume.)

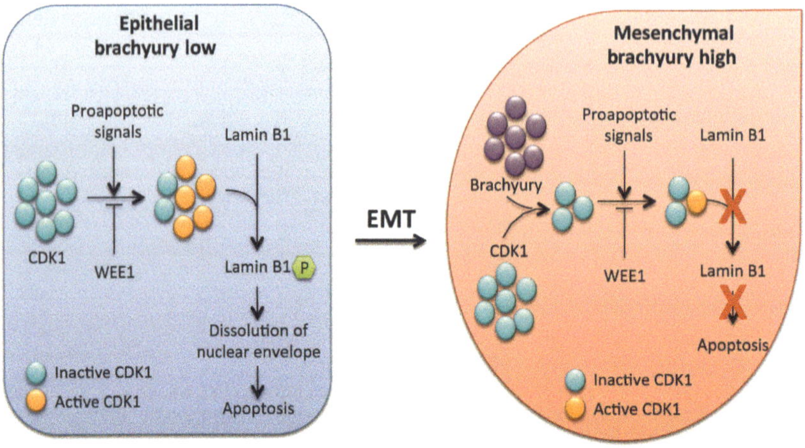

Figure 3, Claudia Palena and Duane H. Hamilton (See Page 85 of this volume.)

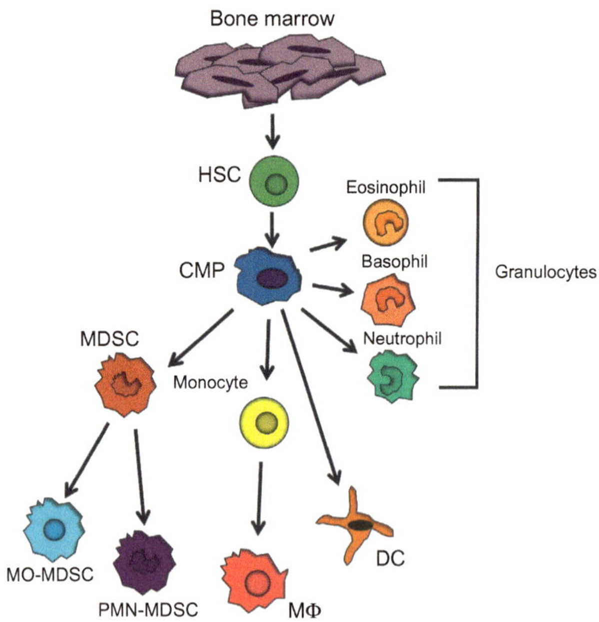

Figure 1, Katherine H. Parker *et al.* (See Page 98 of this volume.)

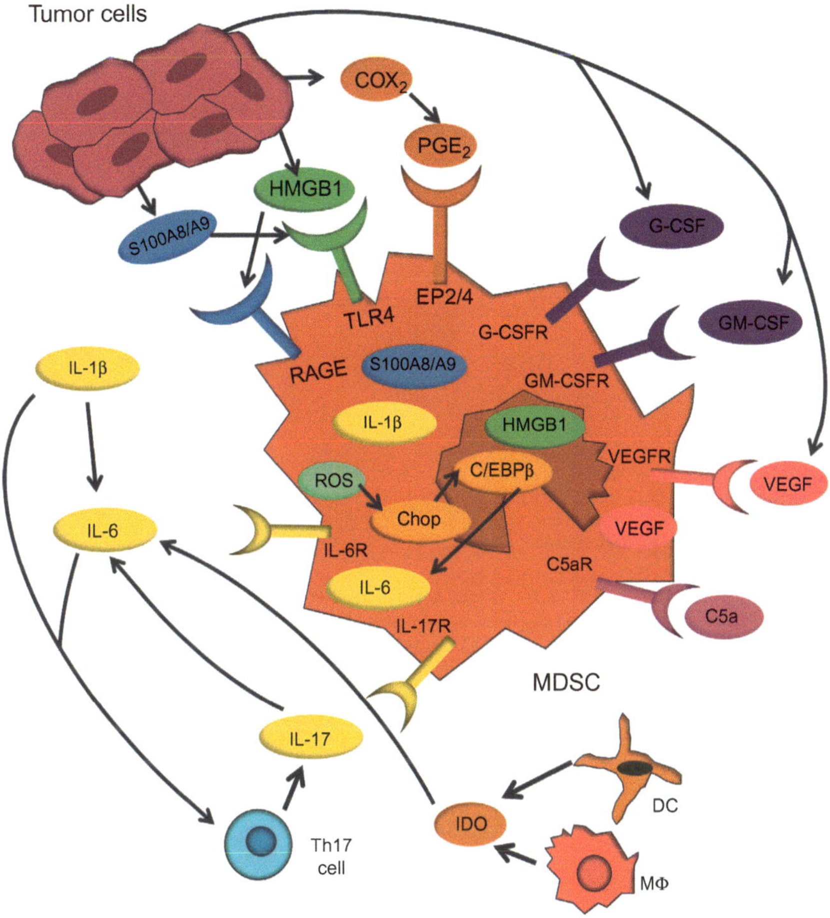

Figure 2, Katherine H. Parker *et al.* (See Page 102 of this volume.)

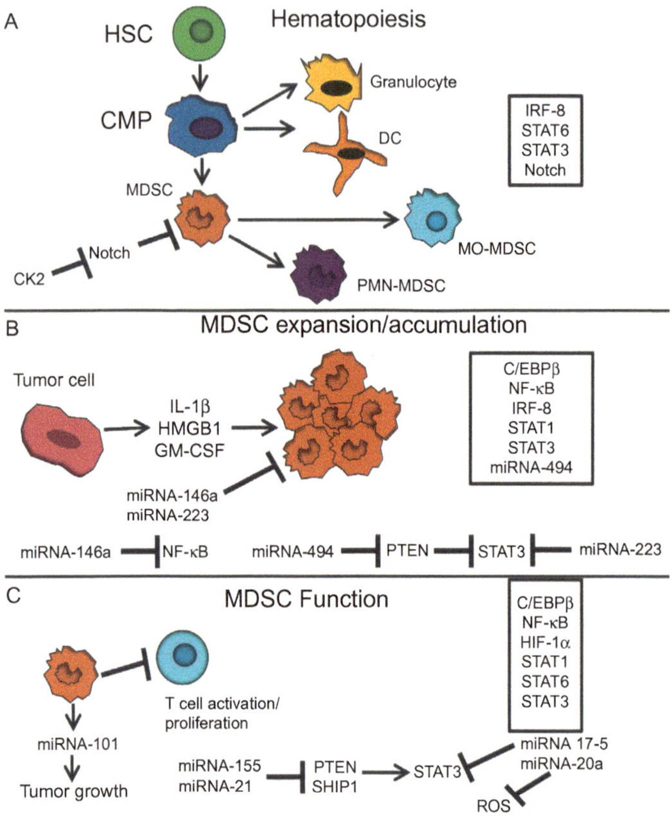

Figure 3, Katherine H. Parker *et al.* (See Page 108 of this volume.)

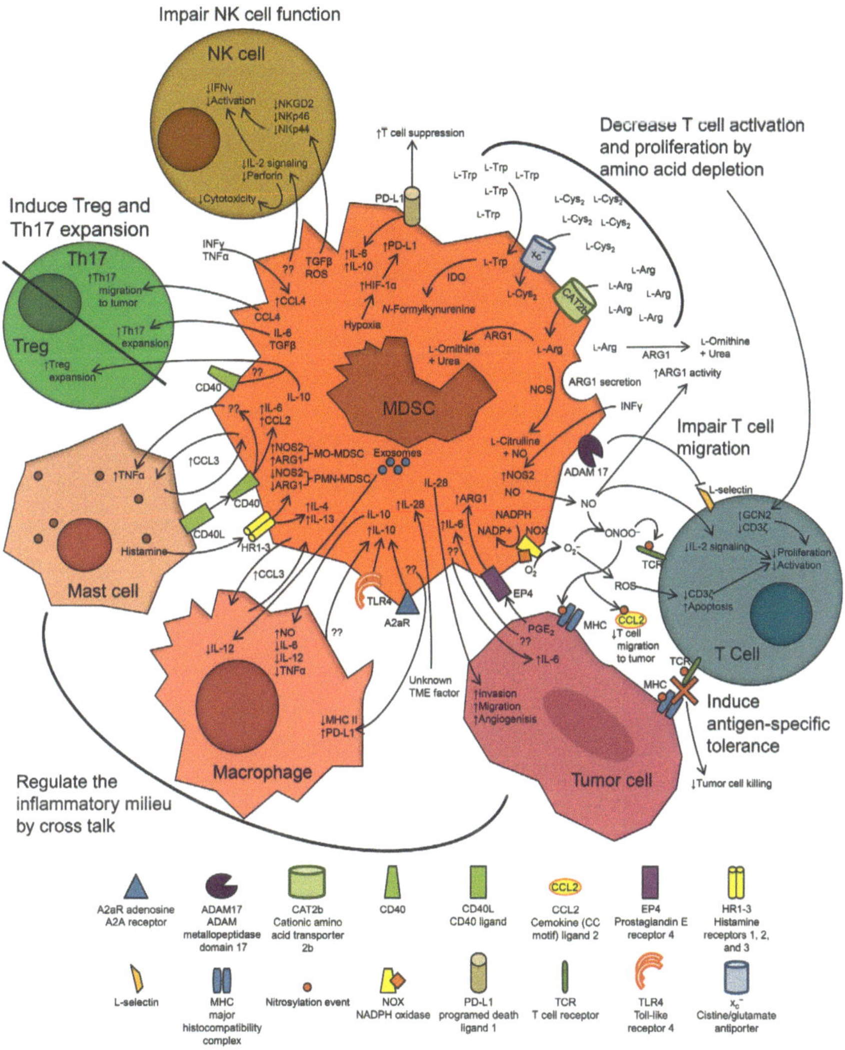

Figure 4, Katherine H. Parker *et al.* (See Page 113 of this volume.)

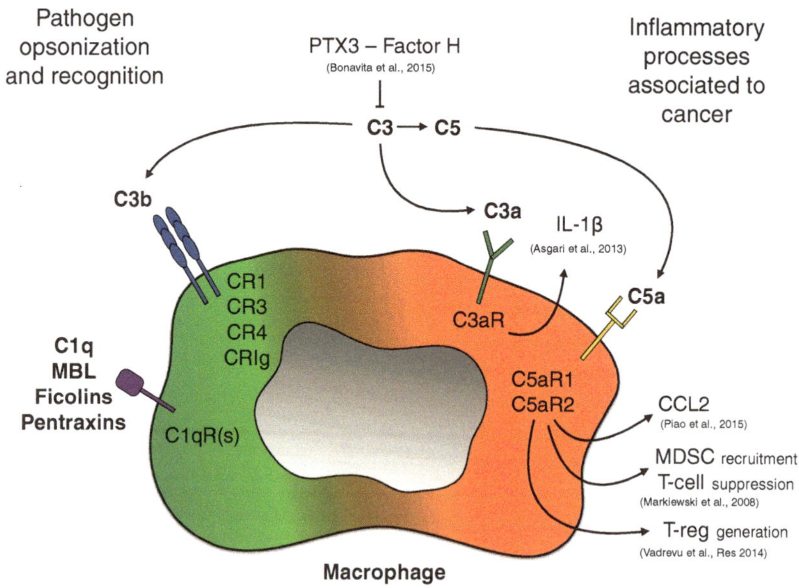

Figure 1, Eduardo Bonavita *et al.* (See Page 149 of this volume.)

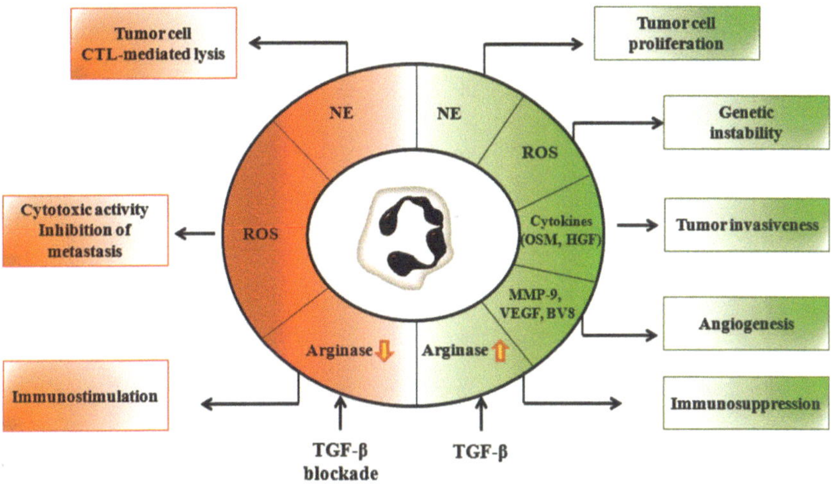

Figure 2, Eduardo Bonavita *et al.* (See Page 154 of this volume.)

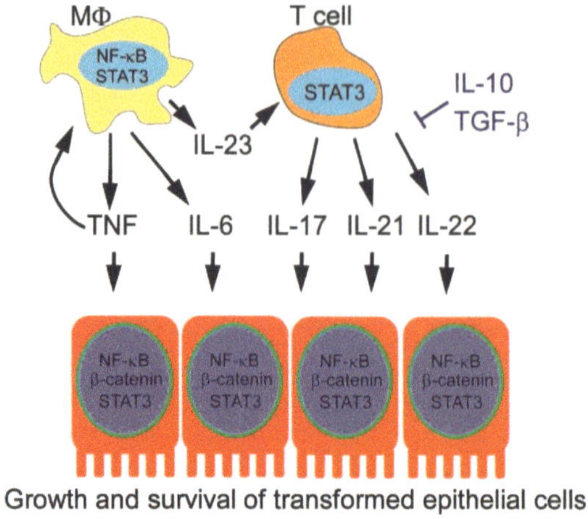

Figure 1, Kepeng Wang and Michael Karin (See Page 175 of this volume.)

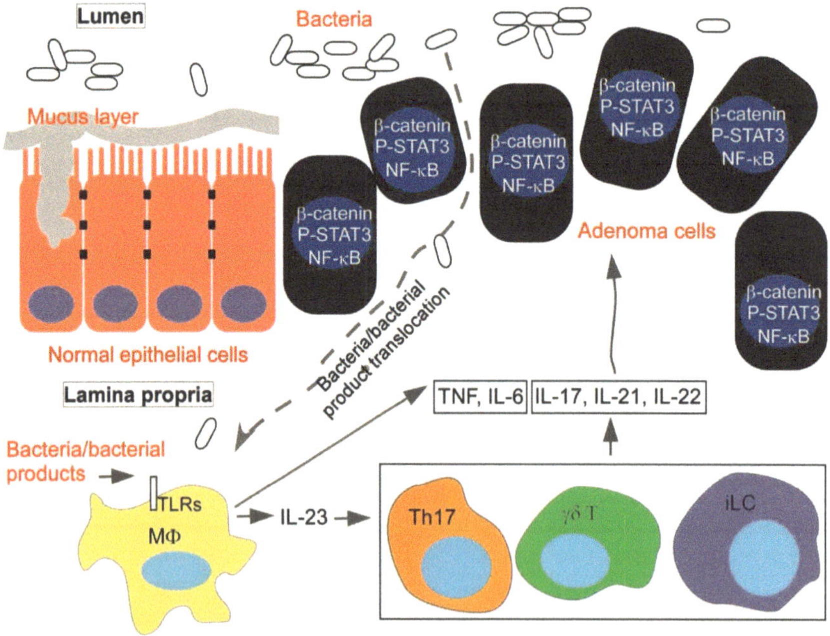

Figure 2, Kepeng Wang and Michael Karin (See Page 187 of this volume.)

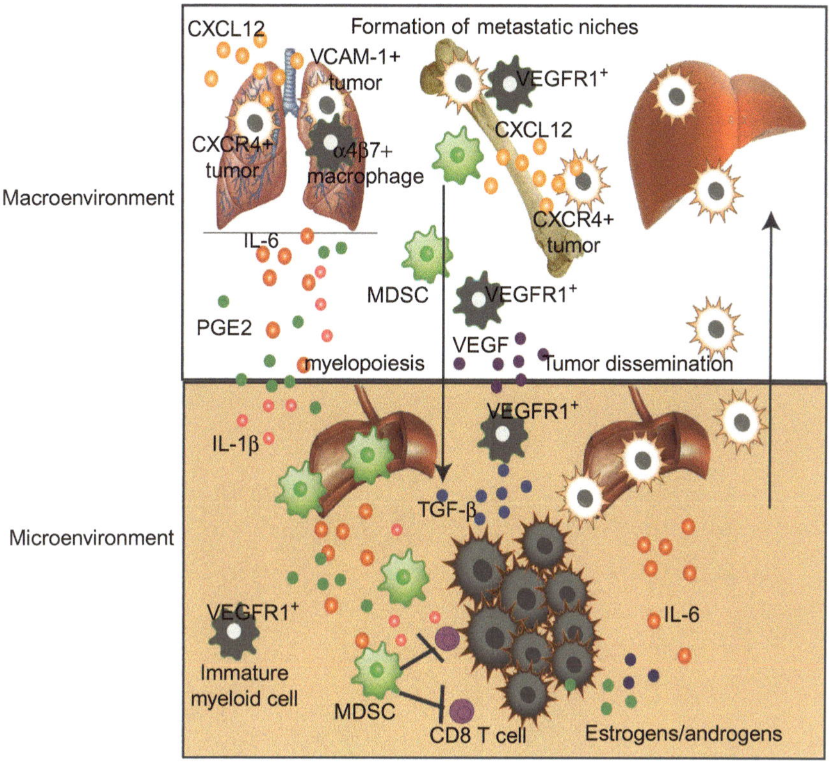

Figure 1, Melanie R. Rutkowski *et al.* (See Page 243 of this volume.)

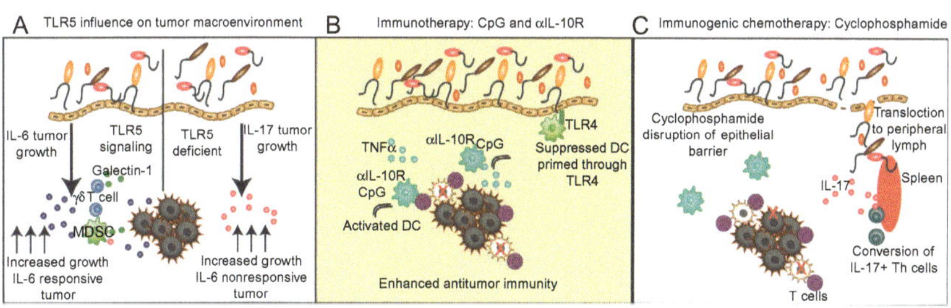

Figure 2, Melanie R. Rutkowski *et al.* (See Page 250 of this volume.)

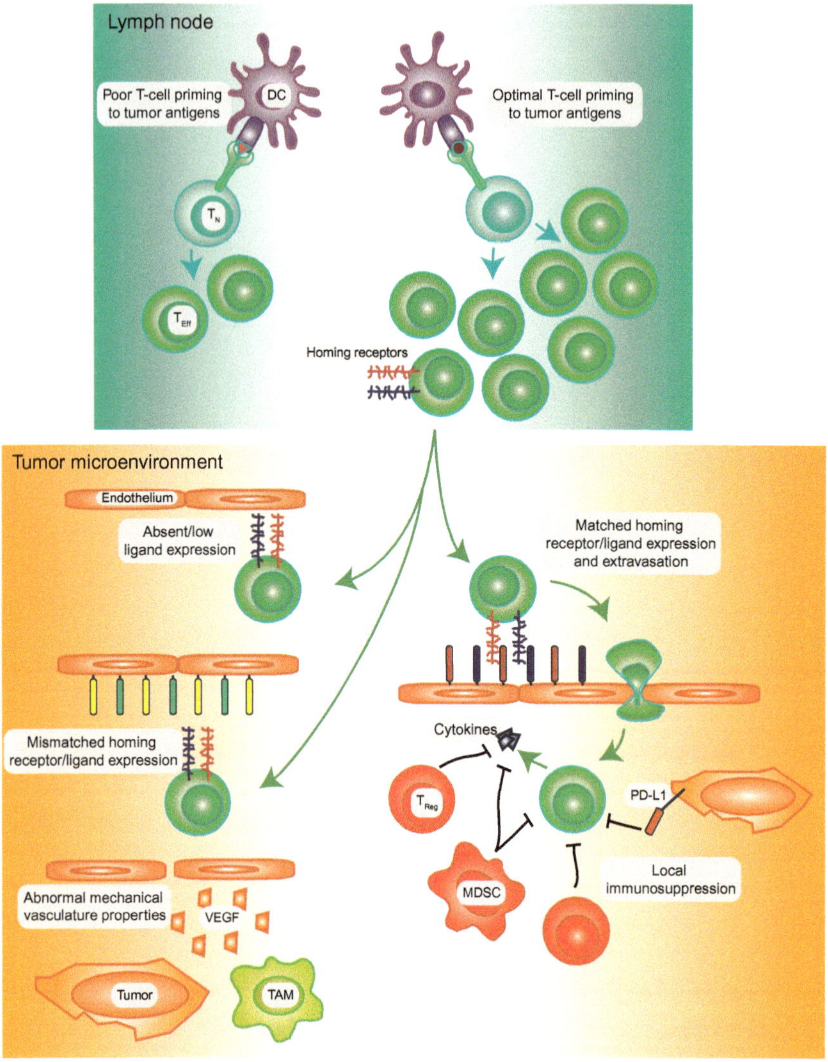

Figure 1, J. David Peske *et al.* (See Page 270 of this volume.)

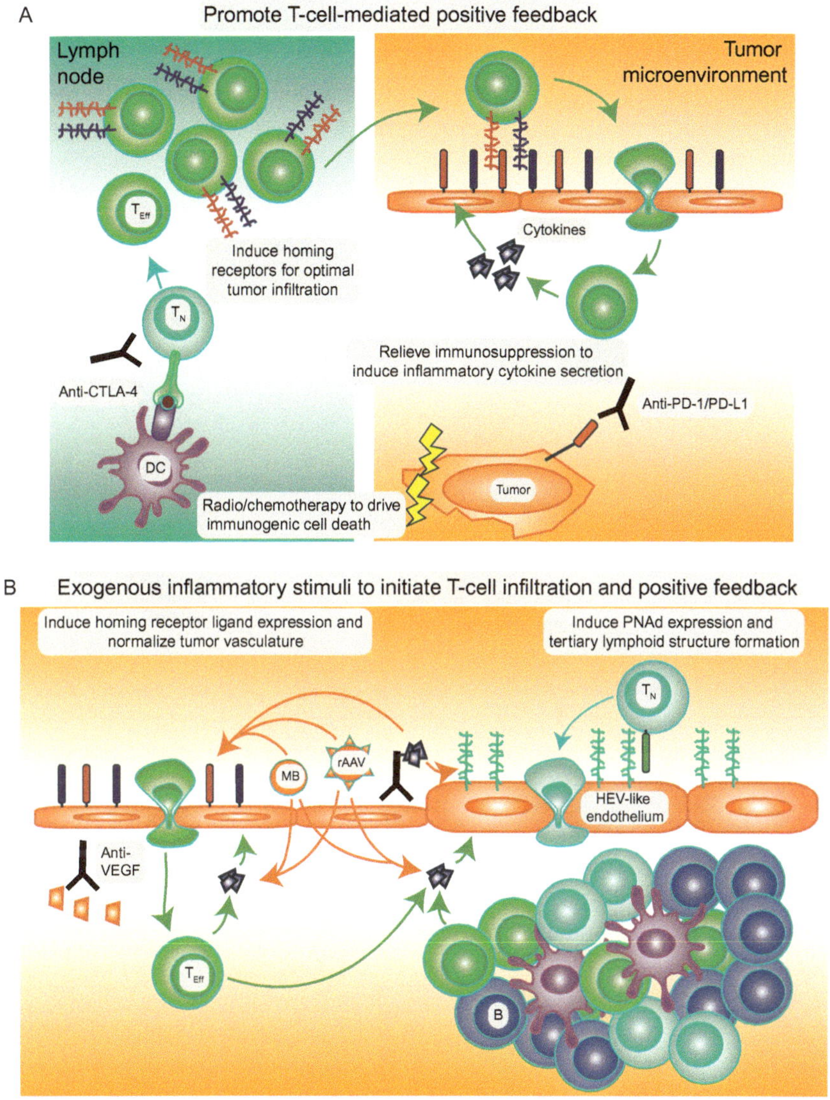

Figure 2, J. David Peske *et al.* (See Page 279 of this volume.)

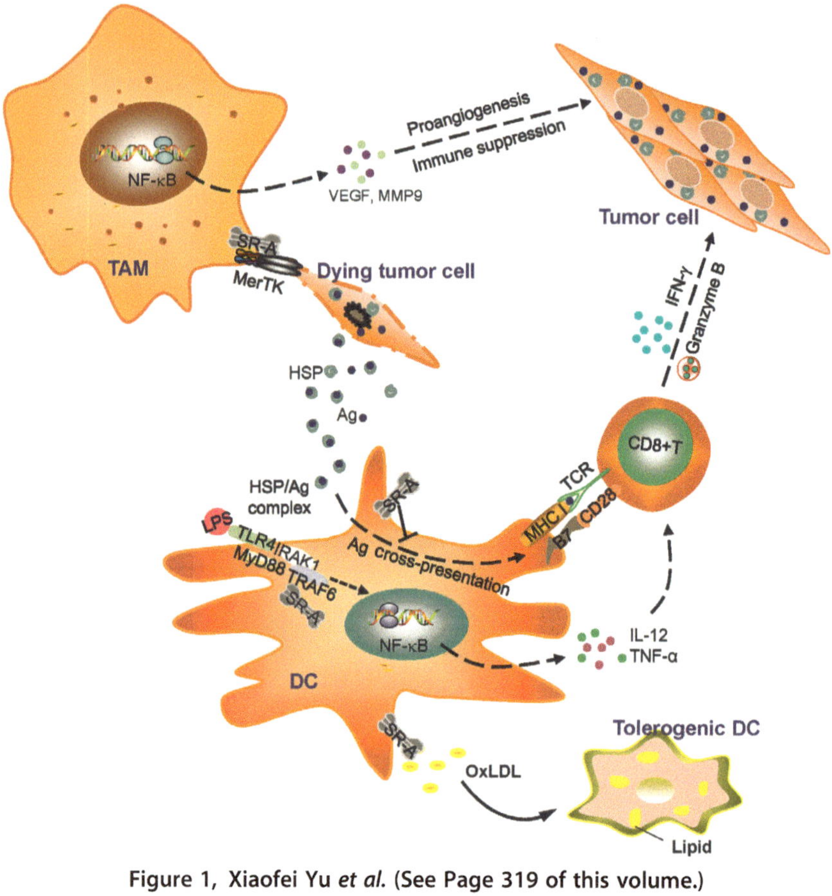

Figure 1, Xiaofei Yu *et al.* (See Page 319 of this volume.)

FSC
www.fsc.org
MIX
Papier | Fördert gute Waldnutzung
FSC® C083411

Kolibri 360 GmbH
Ferdinand-Jühlke-Straße 7
99095 Erfurt, Deutschland
produktsicherheit@kolibri360.de